Lippincott's Illustrated Reviews: Microbiology

Third Edition

Lippincott's Illustrated Reviews: Microbiology

Third Edition

Cynthia Nau Cornelissen, Ph.D.
Department of Microbiology and Immunology
School of Medicine
Virginia Commonwealth University
Richmond, Virginia

Bruce D. Fisher, M.D.
Department of Medicine
Jersey Shore University Medical Center
Neptune, New Jersey
Department of Medicine
University of Medicine and Dentistry of New Jersey–
Robert Wood Johnson Medical School
Piscataway, New Jersey

Richard A. Harvey, Ph.D.
Department of Biochemistry
University of Medicine and Dentistry of New Jersey–
Robert Wood Johnson Medical School
Piscataway, New Jersey

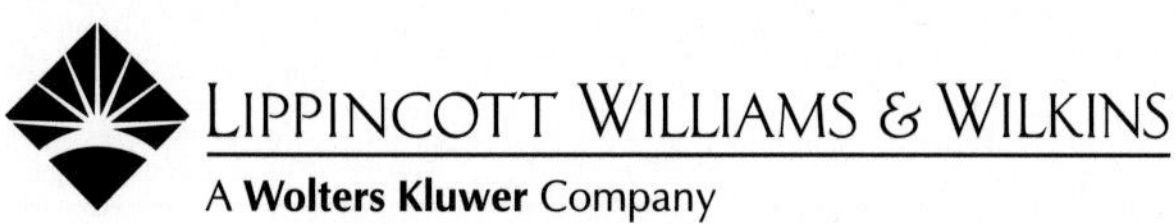

A **Wolters Kluwer** Company
Philadelphia • Baltimore • New York • London
Buenos Aires • Hong Kong • Sydney • Tokyo

Acknowledgments

Cynthia Nau Cornelissen is grateful to her husband, Christopher and to her children, Jeremy and Emily, for their support and encouragement during this endeavor.

Bruce D. Fisher is grateful to his wife Doris, for constant support and encouragement; to Elliot Frank, MD, FACP, Chair of the Department of Medicine at Jersey Shore University Medical Center, esteemed colleague and consummate clinician-educator; and to Donald Armstrong, MD, MACP, for mentorship, guidance, and inspiration for over 35 years.

Richard Harvey is grateful to the many friends and colleagues who generously contributed their time and effort to help us make this book as accurate and useful as possible.

Without talented artists, an Illustrated Review would be impossible, and we have been particularly fortunate in working with Michael Cooper throughout this project. His artistic sense and computer graphics expertise have greatly added to our ability to bring microbiology "stories" alive for our readers. We are also highly appreciative of Dr. Hae Sook Kim and Linda Duckenfield, SM/MT (ASCP), for assistance in preparing photomicrographs.

The editors and production staff of Lippincott Williams & Wilkins were a constant source of encouragement and discipline. We particularly want to acknowledge the tremendously supportive and creative contributions of our editor, Susan Rhyner, whose imagination and positive attitude helped us bring this complex project to completion. The design, content, editing, and assembly of the book have been greatly enhanced through the efforts of Kelly Horvath.

Acquisitions Editor: Susan Rhyner
Product Manager: Angela Collins
Marketing Manager: Joy Fisher-Williams
Vendor Manager: Alicia Jackson
Cover Design: Holly McLaughlin
Development Editor: Kelly Horvath
Third Edition

351 West Camden Street
Baltimore, MD 21201

Two Commerce Square; 2001 Market Street
Philadelphia, PA 19103

Printed in China

9 8 7 6 5 4 3 2 1

Library of Congress Cataloging-in-Publication Data
Cornelissen, Cynthia Nau.
Microbiology / Cynthia Nau Cornelissen, Bruce D. Fisher, Richard A. Harvey. -- 3rd ed.
p. ; cm. -- (Lippincott's illustrated reviews)
Includes index.
Rev. ed. of: Microbiology / Richard A. Harvey, Pamela C. Champe, Bruce D. Fisher. c2007.
Summary: "Lippincott's Illustrated Reviews: Microbiology, Third Edition enables rapid review and assimilation of large amounts of complex information about medical microbiology. The book has the hallmark features for which Lippincott's Illustrated Reviews volumes are so popular: an outline format, 450 full-color illustrations, end-of-chapter summaries, review questions, plus an entire section of clinical case studies with full-color illustrations. NEW TO THIS EDITION: an online testbank of 100 review questions"--Provided by publisher.
ISBN 978-1-60831-733-2 (pbk.)
I. Fisher, Bruce D., M.D. II. Harvey, Richard A., Ph. D. III. Title. IV. Series: Lippincott's illustrated reviews.
[DNLM: 1. Microbiological Phenomena--Outlines. QW 18.2]
579--dc23

To purchase additional copies of this book, call our customer service department at **(800) 638-3030** or fax orders to **(301) 223-2320**. International customers should call **(301) 223-2300**.

Visit Lippincott Williams & Wilkins on the Internet: http://www.lww.com. Lippincott Williams & Wilkins customer service representatives are available from 8:30 am to 6:00 pm, EST.

RRS1207

Unique Clinical Features

Summaries of bacteria and their diseases

Summary of common diseases

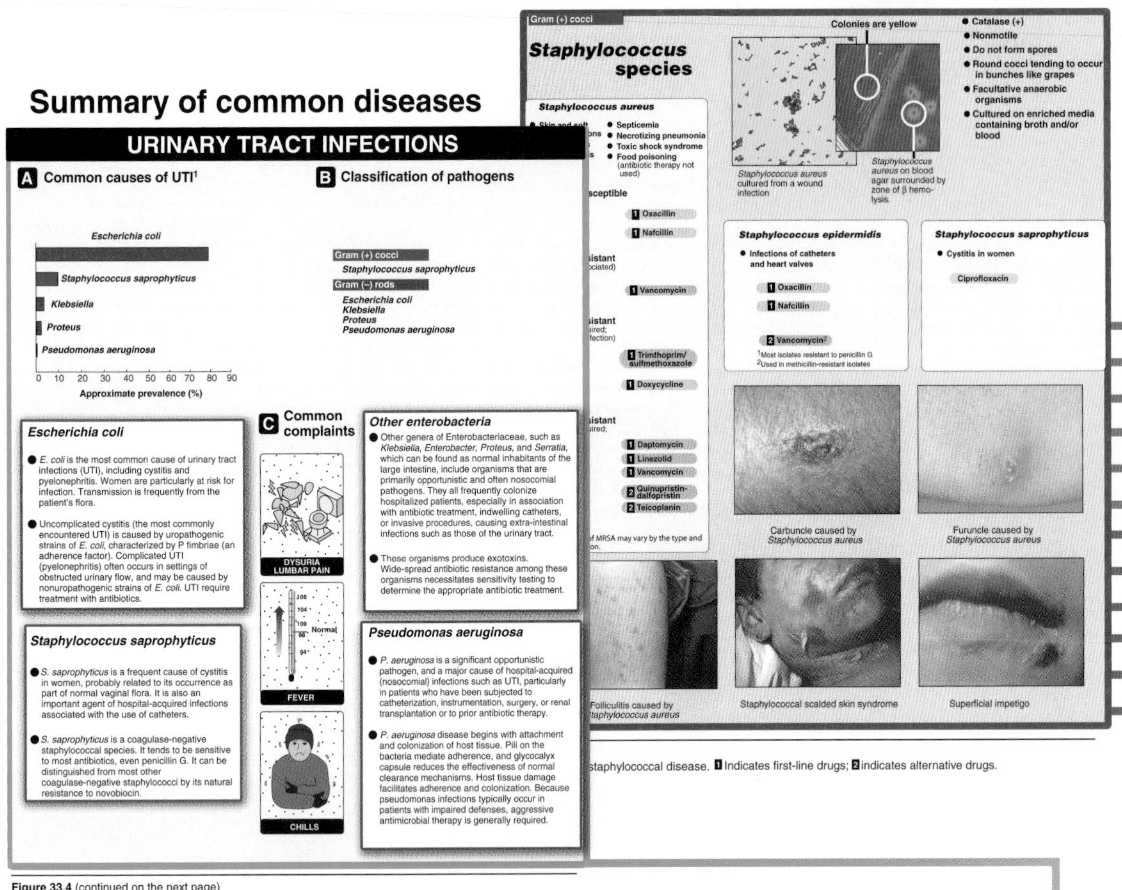

Gram (+) cocci
Staphylococcus species
Colonies are yellow
Catalase (+)
Nonmotile
Do not form spores
Round cocci tending to occur in bunches like grapes
Facultative anaerobic organisms
Cultured on enriched media containing broth and/or blood
Staphylococcus aureus
Septicemia
Necrotizing pneumonia
Toxic shock syndrome
Food poisoning (antibiotic therapy not used)
Staphylococcus aureus cultured from a wound infection
Staphylococcus aureus on blood agar surrounded by zone of β hemolysis.
Oxacillin
Nafcillin
Vancomycin
Trimethoprim/ sulfmethoxazole
Doxycycline
Daptomycin
Linezolid
Vancomycin
Quinupristin-dalfopristin
Teicoplanin
Staphylococcus epidermidis
Infections of catheters and heart valves
Oxacillin
Nafcillin
Vancomycin
Most isolates resistant to penicillin G
Used in methicillin-resistant isolates
Staphylococcus saprophyticus
Cystitis in women
Ciprofloxacin
Carbuncle caused by Staphylococcus aureus
Furuncle caused by Staphylococcus aureus
Staphylococcal scalded skin syndrome
Superficial impetigo
staphylococcal disease. 1 Indicates first-line drugs; 2 indicates alternative drugs.
URINARY TRACT INFECTIONS
A Common causes of UTI
B Classification of pathogens
Escherichia coli
Staphylococcus saprophyticus
Klebsiella
Proteus
Pseudomonas aeruginosa
0 10 20 30 40 50 60 70 80 90
Approximate prevalence (%)
Gram (+) cocci
Staphylococcus saprophyticus
Gram (–) rods
Escherichia coli
Klebsiella
Proteus
Pseudomonas aeruginosa
Escherichia coli
E. coli is the most common cause of urinary tract infections (UTI), including cystitis and pyelonephritis. Women are particularly at risk for infection. Transmission is frequently from the patient's flora.
Uncomplicated cystitis (the most commonly encountered UTI) is caused by uropathogenic strains of E. coli, characterized by P fimbriae (an adherence factor). Complicated UTI (pyelonephritis) often occurs in settings of obstructed urinary flow, and may be caused by nonuropathogenic strains of E. coli. UTI require treatment with antibiotics.
C Common complaints
DYSURIA LUMBAR PAIN
Normal
FEVER
CHILLS
Other enterobacteria
Other genera of Enterobacteriaceae, such as Klebsiella, Enterobacter, Proteus, and Serratia, which can be found as normal inhabitants of the large intestine, include organisms that are primarily opportunistic and often nosocomial pathogens. They all frequently colonize hospitalized patients, especially in association with antibiotic treatment, indwelling catheters, or invasive procedures, causing extra-intestinal infections such as those of the urinary tract.
These organisms produce exotoxins. Wide-spread antibiotic resistance among these organisms necessitates sensitivity testing to determine the appropriate antibiotic treatment.
Staphylococcus saprophyticus
S. saprophyticus is a frequent cause of cystitis in women, probably related to its occurrence as part of normal vaginal flora. It is also an important agent of hospital-acquired infections associated with the use of catheters.
S. saprophyticus is a coagulase-negative staphylococcal species. It tends to be sensitive to most antibiotics, even penicillin G. It can be distinguished from most other coagulase-negative staphylococci by its natural resistance to novobiocin.
Pseudomonas aeruginosa
P. aeruginosa is a significant opportunistic pathogen, and a major cause of hospital-acquired (nosocomial) infections such as UTI, particularly in patients who have been subjected to catheterization, instrumentation, surgery, or renal transplantation or to prior antibiotic therapy.
P. aeruginosa disease begins with attachment and colonization of host tissue. Pili on the bacteria mediate adherence, and glycocalyx capsule reduces the effectiveness of normal clearance mechanisms. Host tissue damage facilitates adherence and colonization. Because pseudomonas infections typically occur in patients with impaired defenses, aggressive antimicrobial therapy is generally required.
Figure 33.4 (continued on the next page)
Disease summary of urinary tract infections. Uncomplicated cystitis.

Illustrated Case Studies

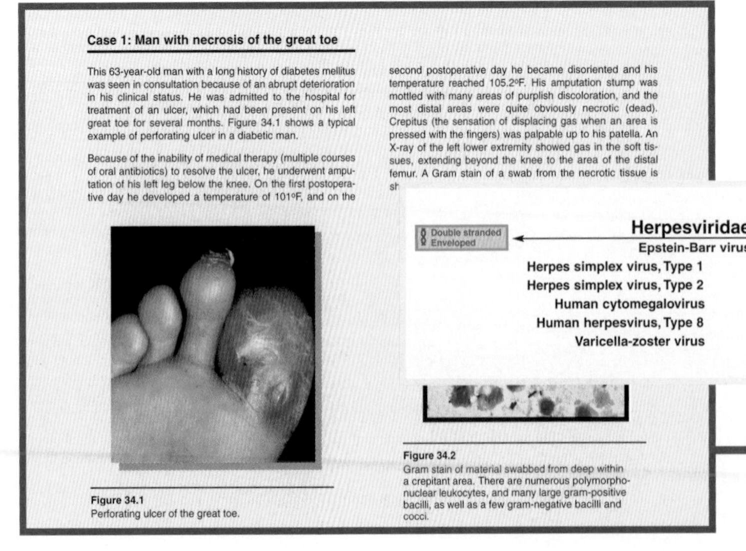

Quick Review

Double stranded
Enveloped

Herpesviridae

Epstein-Barr virus
Herpes simplex virus, Type 1
Herpes simplex virus, Type 2
Human cytomegalovirus
Human herpesvirus, Type 8
Varicella-zoster virus

Common characteristics

- Linear, double-stranded DNA genome
- Replicate in the nucleus
- Envelope contains antigenic, species-specific glycoproteins
- In the tegument between the envelope and capsid are a number of virus-coded enzymes and transcription factors essential for initiation of the infectious cycle
- All herpesviruses can enter a latent state following primary infection, to be reactivated at a later time

Contents

UNIT I:
The Microbial World

Introduction to Microbiology 1

I. OVERVIEW

Microorganisms can be found in every ecosystem and in close association with every type of multicellular organism. They populate the healthy human body by the billions as benign passengers (normal flora, see p. 7) and even as participants in bodily functions. For example, bacteria play a role in the degradation of intestinal contents. In this volume, we primarily consider the role of microorganisms (that is, bacteria, fungi, protozoa, helminths, and viruses) in the initiation and spread of human diseases. Those relatively few species of microorganisms that are harmful to humans, either by production of toxic compounds or by direct infection, are characterized as pathogens.

Most infectious disease is initiated by colonization (the establishment of proliferating microorganisms on the skin or mucous membranes) as shown in Figure 1.1. The major exceptions are diseases caused by introduction of organisms directly into the bloodstream or internal organs. Microbial colonization may result in: 1) elimination of the microorganism without affecting the host; 2) infection in which the organisms multiply and cause the host to react by making an immune or other type of response or 3) a transient or prolonged carrier state. Infectious disease occurs when the organism causes tissue damage and impairment of body function.

II. PROKARYOTIC PATHOGENS

All prokaryotic organisms are classified as bacteria, whereas eukaryotic organisms include fungi, protozoa, and helminths as well as humans. Prokaryotic organisms are divided into two major groups: the eubacteria, which include all bacteria of medical importance, and the archaebacteria, a collection of evolutionarily distinct organisms. Cells of prokaryotic and eukaryotic organisms differ in several significant structural features as illustrated in Figure 1.2.

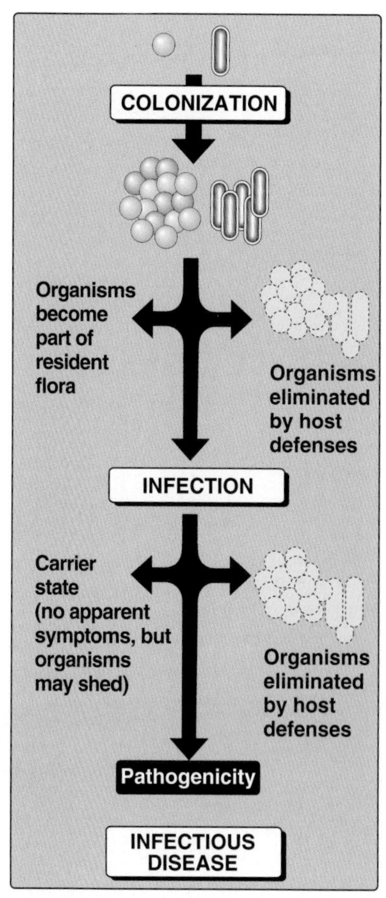

Figure 1.1
Some possible outcomes following exposure to microorganisms.

CHARACTERISTIC	PROKARYOTIC CELLS	EUKARYOTIC CELLS
Chromosome	Usually single, circular[1]	Multiple
Nucleus	No nuclear envelope or nucleoli	Membrane bound, nucleoli present
Membrane-bound organelles	Not present	Present (examples include mitochondria and endoplasmic reticulum)
Cell wall	Usually present, many contain peptidoglycan	Present in plant cells, no peptidoglycan
Plasma membrane	No carbohydrates, most lack sterols	Sterols and carbohydrates present
Ribosome	70S	80S (70S in organelles)
Average size	0.2–2 mm in diameter	10–100 mm in diameter

Figure 1.2
Comparison of prokaryotic and eukaryotic cells. [1]Some bacteria have more than one circular molecule as their genome. *Vibrios*, for example, have two circular chromosomes. *Borrellia* have linear chromosomes and a wide array of different sized plasmids.

A. Typical bacteria

Most bacteria have shapes that can be described as a rod, sphere, or corkscrew. Prokarytoic cells are smaller than eukaryotic cells (Figure 1.3). Nearly all bacteria, with the exception of the mycoplasma, have a rigid cell wall surrounding the cell membrane that determines the shape of the organism. The cell wall also determines whether the bacterium is classified as gram positive or gram negative (see p. 21). External to the cell wall may be flagella, pili, and/or a capsule. Bacterial cells divide by binary fission. However, many bacteria exchange genetic information carried on plasmids (small, specialized genetic elements capable of self-replication) including the information necessary for establishment of antibiotic resistance. Bacterial structure, metabolism, and genetics as well as the wide variety of human diseases caused by bacteria are described in detail in Unit II, beginning on p. 49.

B. Atypical bacteria

Atypical bacteria include groups of organisms such as *Mycoplasma*, *Chlamydia*, and *Rickettsia* that, although prokaryotic, lack significant characteristic structural components or metabolic capabilities that separate them from the larger group of typical bacteria.

III. FUNGI

Fungi are nonphotosynthetic, generally saprophytic, eukaryotic organisms. Some fungi are filamentous and are commonly called molds, whereas others (that is, the yeasts) are unicellular (see p. 203). Fungal reproduction may be asexual, sexual, or both, and all fungi produce spores. Pathogenic fungi can cause diseases, ranging from skin infections (superficial mycoses) to serious, systemic infections (deep mycoses).

IV. PROTOZOA

Protozoa are single-celled, nonphotosynthetic, eukaryotic organisms that come in various shapes and sizes. Many protozoa are free living, but others are among the most clinically important parasites of humans. Members of this group infect all major tissues and organs of the body. They can be intracellular parasites, or extracellular parasites in the blood, urogenital region, or intestine. Transmission is generally by ingestion of an infective stage of the parasite or by insect bite. Protozoa cause a variety of diseases that are discussed in Chapter 21, p. 217.

V. HELMINTHS

Helminths are groups of worms that live as parasites. They are multicellular, eukaryotic organisms with complex body organization. They are divided into three main groups: tapeworms (cestodes), flukes (trematodes), and roundworms (nematodes). Helminths are parasitic, receiving nutrients by ingesting or absorbing digestive contents or ingesting or absorbing body fluids or tissues. Almost any organ in the body can be parasitized.

VI. VIRUSES

Viruses are obligate intracellular parasites that do not have a cellular structure. Rather, a virus consists of molecule(s) of DNA (DNA virus) or RNA (RNA virus), but not both, surrounded by a protein coat. A virus may also have an envelope derived from the plasma membrane of the host cell from which the virus is released. Viruses contain the genetic information necessary for directing their own replication but require the host's cellular structures and enzymatic machinery to complete the process of their own reproduction. The fate of the host cell following viral infection ranges from rapid lysis and release of many progeny virions to gradual, prolonged release of viral particles.

VII. ORGANIZING THE MICROORGANISMS

The authors have adopted two color-coded graphic formats: 1) an expanded hierarchical organization and 2) lists of clinically important bacteria and viruses.

A. Hierarchical organization

A hierarchical organization resembles a family tree. These graphs in Figures 1.4 and 1.5 divide bacteria and viruses into groups based on the characteristics of the microorganisms.

B. Lists of important bacteria and viruses

The hierarchical organizations described above are informative and useful as a study aids. However, they, at times, may provide the reader with too much information in a cumbersome configuration. The authors have thus adopted a second, simpler color-coded list format to represent the clinically important groups of bacteria and viruses. For example, bacteria are organized into eight groups according to Gram staining, morphology, and biochemical or other characteristics. The ninth item of the list, labeled "Other," is used to represent any organism not included in one of the other eight categories (Figure 1.6). In a similar way, viral pathogens are organized into seven groups based on the nature of their genome, symmetry of organization, and the presence or absence of a lipid envelope (Figure 1.7).

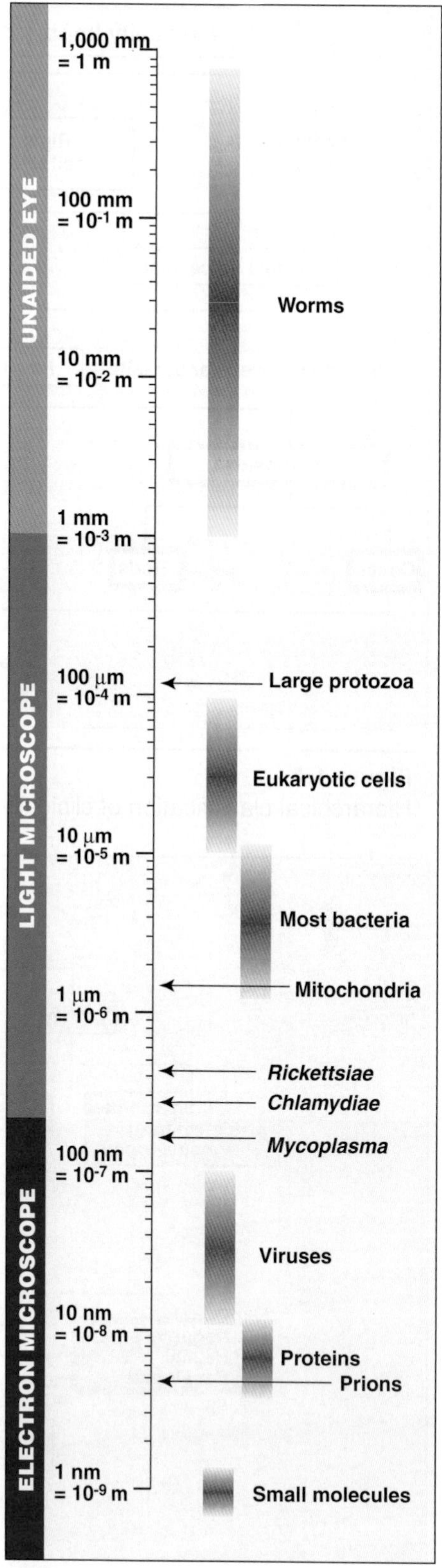

Figure 1.3
Relative size of organisms and molecules.

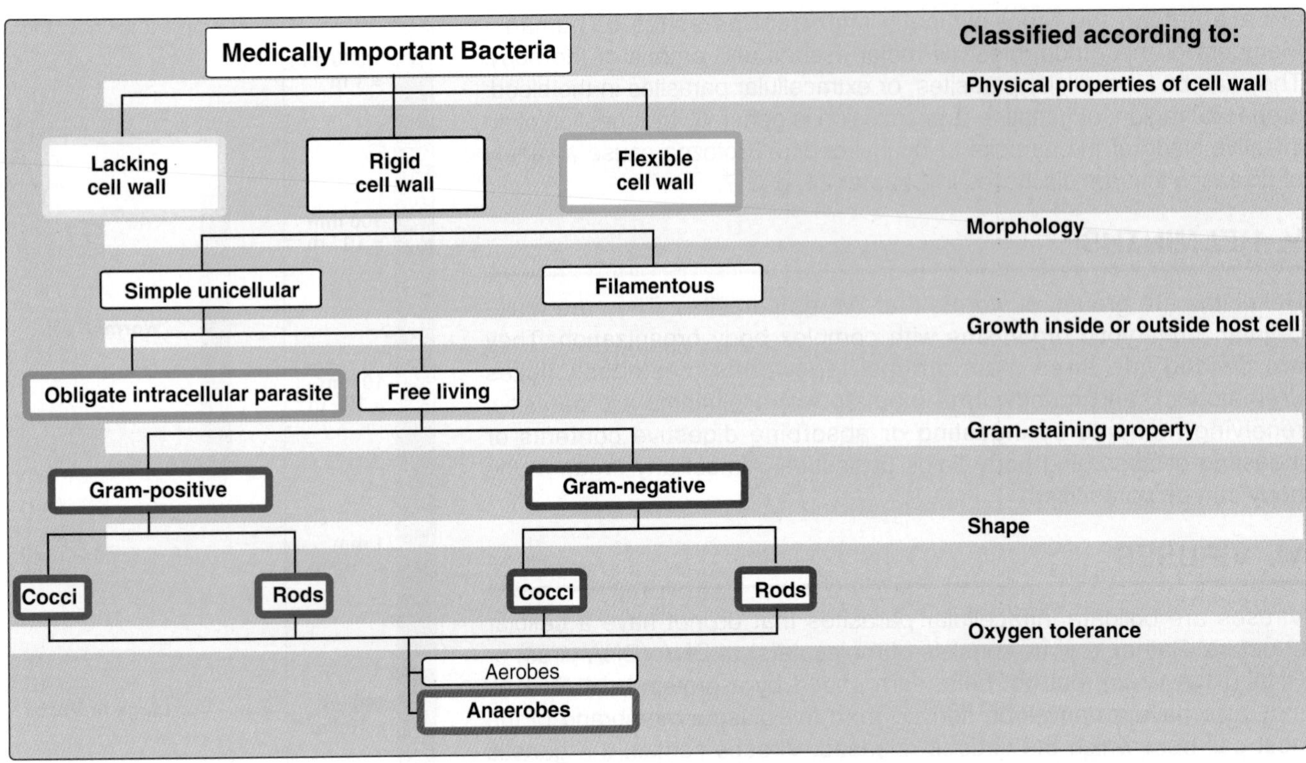

Figure 1.4
Hierarchical classification of clinically important bacteria according to six distinguishing characteristics.

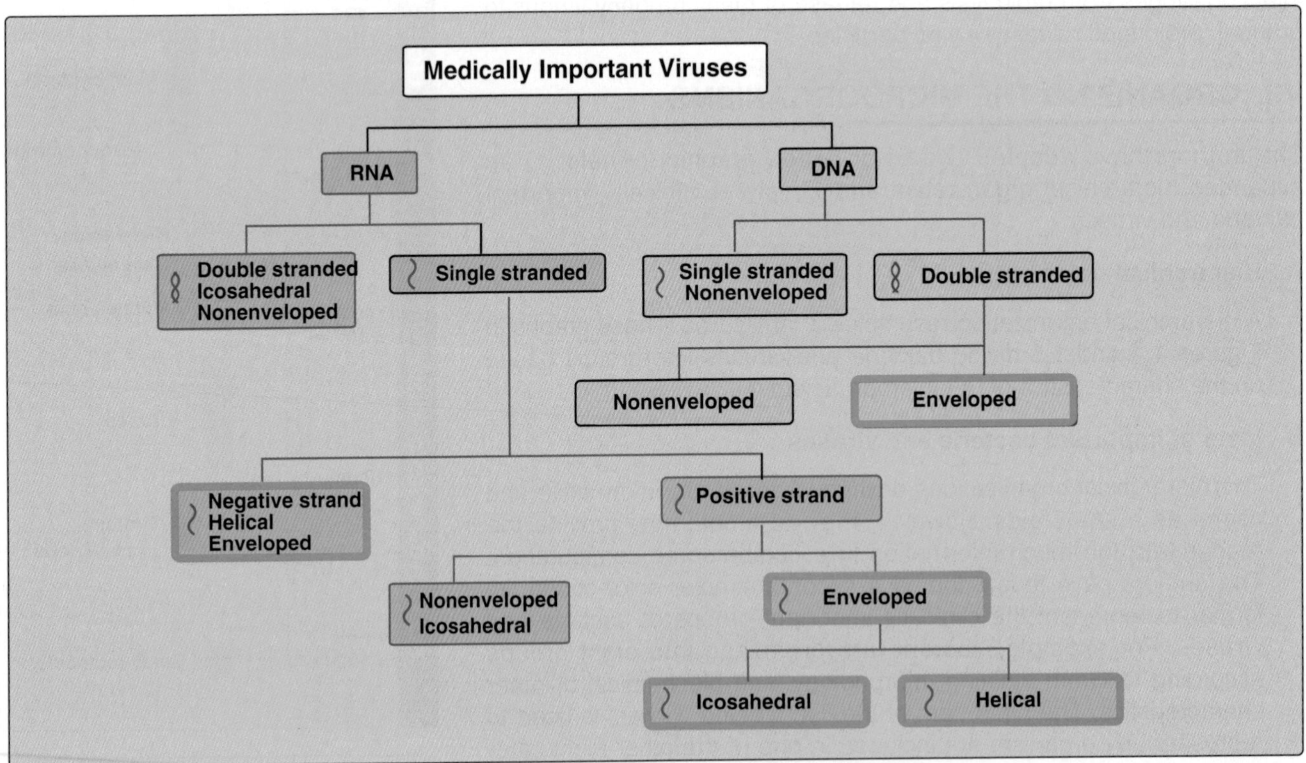

Figure 1.5
Classification of medically important virus families.

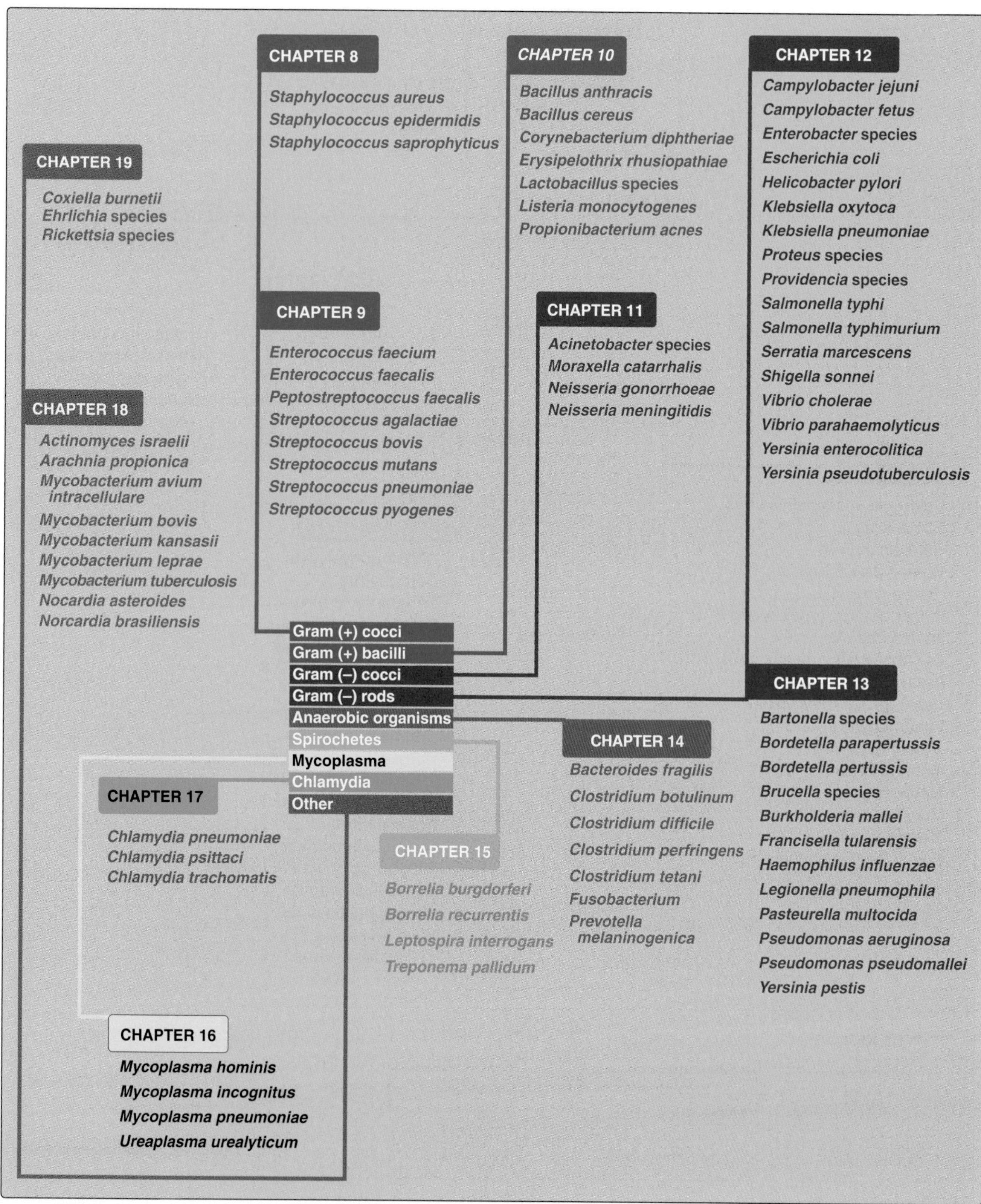

Figure 1.6
Medically important bacteria discussed in this book, organized into similar groups based on morphology, biochemistry, and/or staining properties.

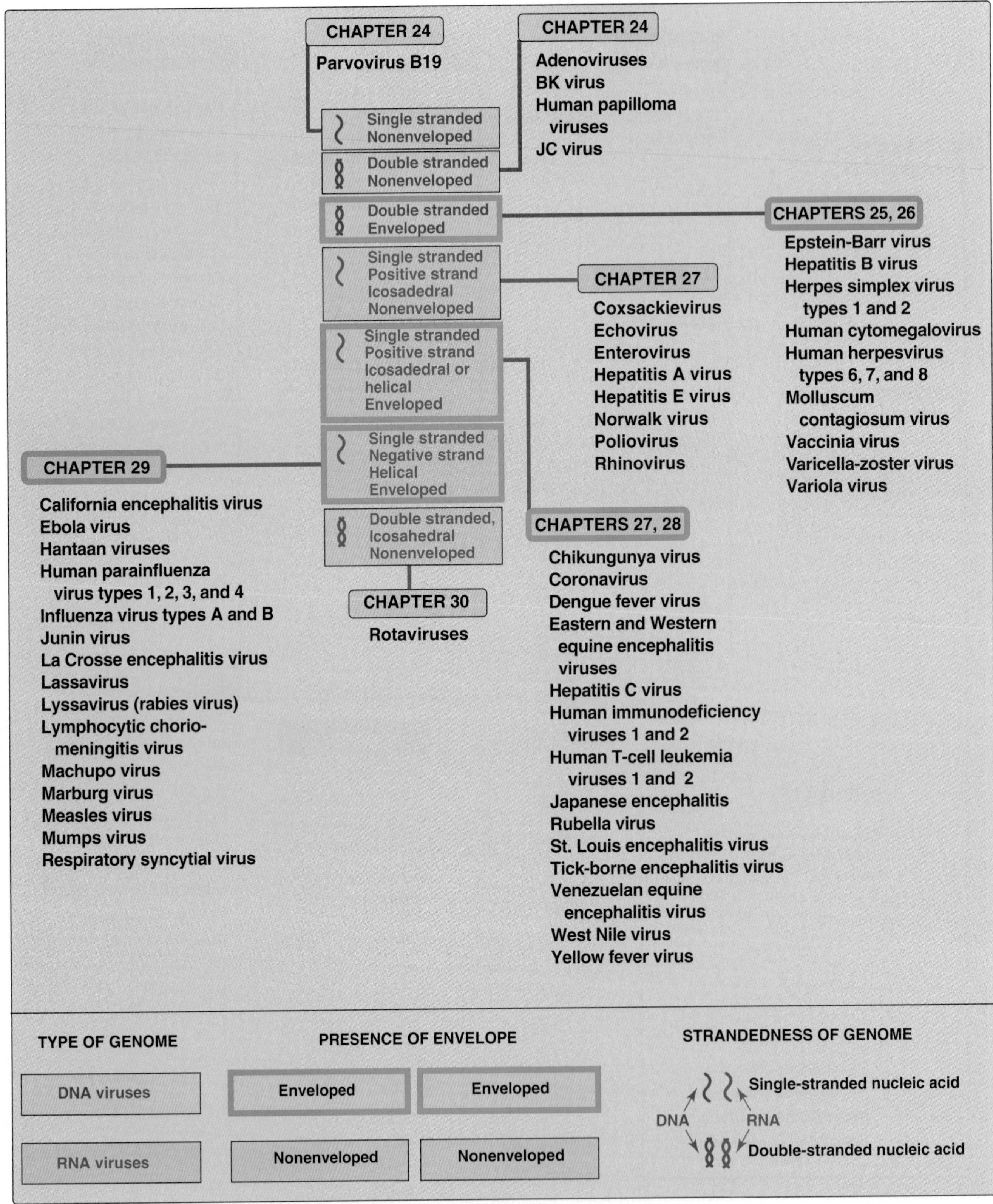
CHAPTER 24
Parvovirus B19
CHAPTER 24
Adenoviruses
BK virus
Human papilloma viruses
JC virus
Single stranded Nonenveloped
Double stranded Nonenveloped
Double stranded Enveloped
CHAPTERS 25, 26
Epstein-Barr virus
Hepatitis B virus
Herpes simplex virus types 1 and 2
Human cytomegalovirus
Human herpesvirus types 6, 7, and 8
Molluscum contagiosum virus
Vaccinia virus
Varicella-zoster virus
Variola virus
Single stranded Positive strand Icosadedral Nonenveloped
CHAPTER 27
Coxsackievirus
Echovirus
Enterovirus
Hepatitis A virus
Hepatitis E virus
Norwalk virus
Poliovirus
Rhinovirus
Single stranded Positive strand Icosadedral or helical Enveloped
CHAPTERS 27, 28
Chikungunya virus
Coronavirus
Dengue fever virus
Eastern and Western equine encephalitis viruses
Hepatitis C virus
Human immunodeficiency viruses 1 and 2
Human T-cell leukemia viruses 1 and 2
Japanese encephalitis
Rubella virus
St. Louis encephalitis virus
Tick-borne encephalitis virus
Venezuelan equine encephalitis virus
West Nile virus
Yellow fever virus
Single stranded Negative strand Helical Enveloped
CHAPTER 29
California encephalitis virus
Ebola virus
Hantaan viruses
Human parainfluenza virus types 1, 2, 3, and 4
Influenza virus types A and B
Junin virus
La Crosse encephalitis virus
Lassavirus
Lyssavirus (rabies virus)
Lymphocytic chorio-meningitis virus
Machupo virus
Marburg virus
Measles virus
Mumps virus
Respiratory syncytial virus
Double stranded, Icosahedral Nonenveloped
CHAPTER 30
Rotaviruses
TYPE OF GENOME
DNA viruses
RNA viruses
PRESENCE OF ENVELOPE
Enveloped
Enveloped
Nonenveloped
Nonenveloped
STRANDEDNESS OF GENOME
Single-stranded nucleic acid
DNA
RNA
Double-stranded nucleic acid

Figure 1.7
Medically important viruses discussed in this book, organized into similar groups based on the nature of the genome and the presence or absence of a lipid envelope.

Normal Flora

2

I. OVERVIEW

The human body is continuously inhabited by many different microorganisms (mostly bacteria, but also fungi and other microorganisms), which, under normal circumstances in a healthy individual, are harmless and may even be beneficial. These microorganisms are termed "normal flora." The normal flora are also termed commensals, which literally means "organisms that dine together." Except for occasional transient invaders, the internal organs and systems are sterile, including the spleen, pancreas, liver, bladder, central nervous system, and blood. A healthy newborn enters the world in essentially sterile condition, but, after birth, it rapidly acquires normal flora from food and the environment, including from other humans.

II. THE HUMAN MICROBIOME

The human microbiome is the total number and diversity of microbes found in and on the human body. In the past, the ability to cultivate organisms from tissues and clinical samples was the gold standard for identification of normal flora and bacterial pathogens. However, the recent application of culture-independent molecular detection methods based on DNA sequencing (see p. 28) indicates that the human body contains a far greater bacterial diversity than previously recognized. Unlike classic microbiologic culture methods, molecular detection requires neither prior knowledge of an organism nor the ability to culture it. Thus, molecular methods are capable of detecting fastidious and nonculturable species. Even using advanced molecular techniques, it is difficult to define the human microbiome because microbial species present vary from individual to individual as a result of physiologic differences, diet, age, and geographic habitat. Despite these limitations, it is useful to be aware of the dominant types and distribution of resident flora, because such knowledge provides an understanding of the possible infections that result from injury to a particular body site.

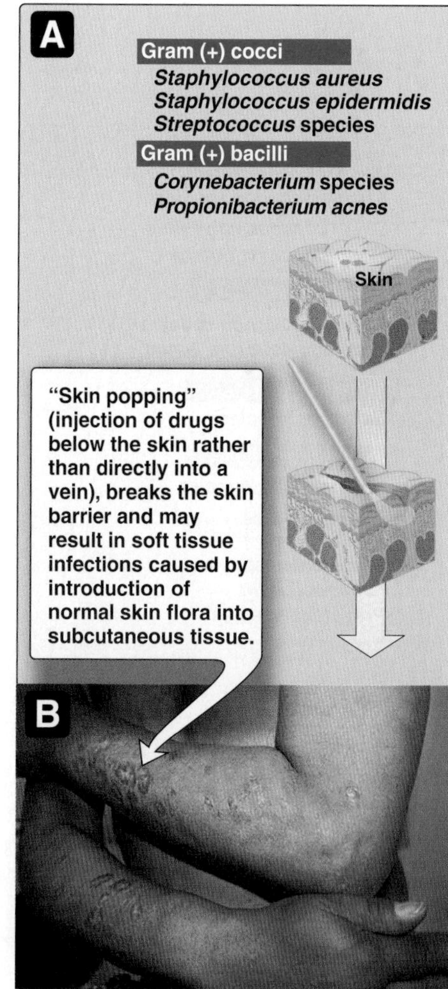

Figure 2.1
A. Examples of bacteria that inhabit the skin. B. Arm of individual who injects drugs by "skin popping."

Gram (+) cocci

Staphylococcus aureus
Staphylococcus epidermidis
Streptococcus species

Gram (+) rods

Corynebacterium species
Propionibacterium acnes

Gram (–) cocci

Moraxella
Neisseria species

Figure 2.2
Examples of bacteria that inhabit the conjunctival sac. [Note: Tears, which contain the antimicrobial enzyme lysozyme, help limit the bacterial population of the conjunctiva.]

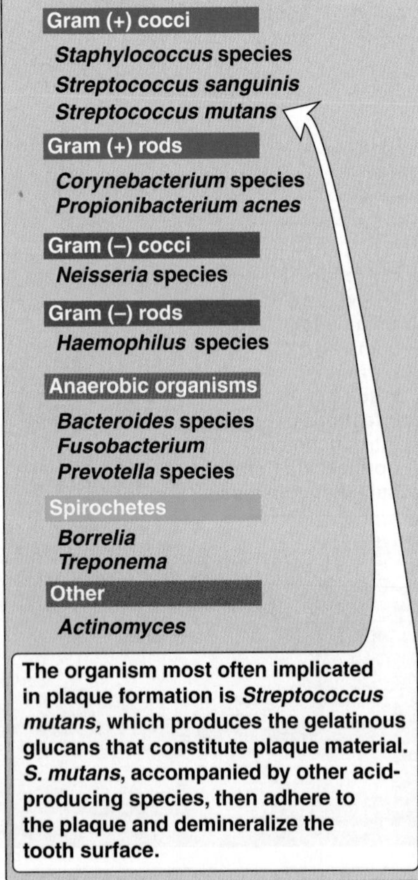

Gram (+) cocci
Staphylococcus species
Streptococcus sanguinis
Streptococcus mutans
Gram (+) rods
Corynebacterium species
Propionibacterium acnes
Gram (–) cocci
Neisseria species
Gram (–) rods
Haemophilus species
Anaerobic organisms
Bacteroides species
Fusobacterium
Prevotella species
Spirochetes
Borrelia
Treponema
Other
Actinomyces
The organism most often implicated in plaque formation is Streptococcus mutans, which produces the gelatinous glucans that constitute plaque material. S. mutans, accompanied by other acid-producing species, then adhere to the plaque and demineralize the tooth surface.

Figure 2.3
Examples of bacteria that inhabit the mouth.

III. DISTRIBUTION OF NORMAL FLORA IN THE BODY

The most common sites of the body inhabited by normal flora are, as might be expected, those in contact or communication with the outside world, namely, the skin, eye, and mouth as well as the upper respiratory, gastrointestinal, and urogenital tracts.

A. Skin

Skin can acquire any bacteria that happen to be in the immediate environment, but this transient flora either dies or is removable by washing. Nevertheless, the skin supports a permanent bacterial population (resident flora), residing in multiple layers of the skin (Figure 2.1). The resident flora regenerate even after vigorous scrubbing.

1. **Estimate of the skin microbiome using classical culture techniques:** *Staphylococcus epidermidis* and other coagulase-negative staphylococci (see p. 76) that reside in the outer layers of the skin appear to account for some 90 percent of the skin aerobes. Anaerobic organisms, such as *Propionibacterium acnes*, reside in deeper skin layers, hair follicles, and sweat and sebaceous glands. Skin inhabitants are generally harmless, although *S. epidermidis* can attach to and colonize plastic catheters and medical devices that penetrate the skin, sometimes resulting in serious bloodstream infections.

2. **Estimate of the skin microbiome using molecular sequencing techniques:** The estimate of the number of species present on skin bacteria has been radically changed by the use of the 16S ribosomal RNA gene sequence (see p. 28) to identify bacterial species present on skin samples directly from their genetic material. Previously, such identification had depended upon microbiological culture, upon which many varieties of bacteria did not grow and so were not detected. *Staphylococcus epidermidis* and *Staphylococcus aureus* were thought from culture-based research to be dominant. However DNA analysis research finds that, while common, these species make up only 5 percent of skin bacteria. The skin apparently provides a rich and diverse habitat for bacteria.

B. Eye

The conjunctiva of the eye is colonized primarily by *S. epidermidis*, followed by *S. aureus*, aerobic corynebacteria (diphtheroids), and *Streptococcus pneumoniae*. Other organisms that normally inhabit the skin are also present but at a lower frequency (Figure 2.2). Tears, which contain the antimicrobial enzyme lysozyme, help limit the bacterial population of the conjunctiva.

C. Mouth and nose

The mouth and nose harbor many microorganisms, both aerobic and anaerobic (Figure 2.3). Among the most common are diphtheroids (aerobic *Corynebacterium* species), *S. aureus*, and *S. epidermidis*. In addition, the teeth and surrounding gingival tissue are colonized by their own particular species, such as *Streptococcus mutans*. [Note: *S. mutans* can enter the bloodstream following dental surgery and colonize damaged or prosthetic heart valves, leading to potentially fatal infective endocarditis.] Some normal residents of the nasopharynx can also cause disease. For example, *S. pneumoniae*, found in the nasopharynx of many healthy individuals, can cause acute bacterial pneumonia, especially in older adults and those whose resistance is impaired. [Note: Pneumonia is frequently preceded by an upper or middle respiratory viral infection, which predisposes the individual to *S. pneumoniae* infection of the pulmonary parenchyma.]

D. Intestinal tract

In an adult, the density of microorganisms in the stomach is relatively low (10^3 to 10^5 per gram of contents) due to gastric enzymes and acidic pH. The density of organisms increases along the alimentary canal, reaching 10^8 to 10^{10} bacteria per gram of contents in the ileum and 10^{11} per gram of contents in the large intestine. Some 20 percent of the fecal mass consists of many different species of bacteria, more than 99 percent of which are anaerobes (Figure 2.4). *Bacteroides* species constitute a significant percentage of bacteria in the large intestine. *Escherichia coli*, a facultatively anaerobic organism, constitutes less than 0.1 percent of the total population of bacteria in the intestinal tract. However, this endogenous *E. coli* is a major cause of urinary tract infections.

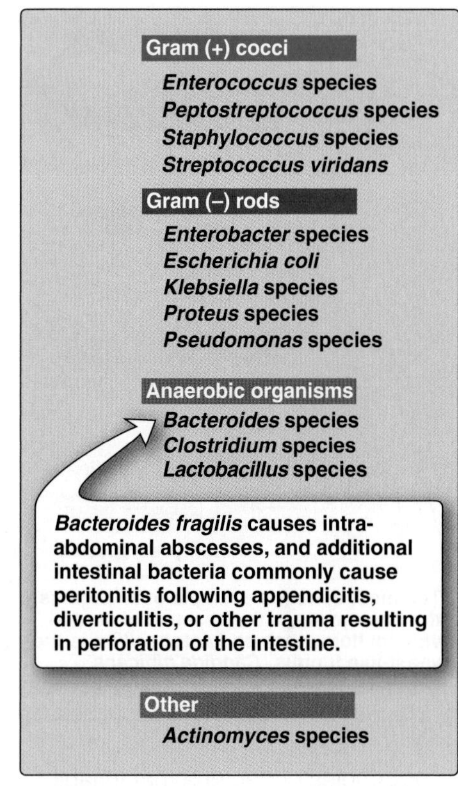

Figure 2.4
Examples of bacteria that inhabit the gastrointestinal tract.

E. Urogenital tract

The low pH of the adult vagina is maintained by the presence of *Lactobacillus* species, which are the primary components of normal flora. If the *Lactobacillus* population in the vagina is decreased (for example, by antibiotic therapy), the pH rises, and potential pathogens can overgrow. The most common example of such overgrowth is the yeast-like fungus, *Candida albicans* (see p. 213), which itself is a minor member of the normal flora of the vagina, mouth, and small intestine. The urine in the kidney and bladder is sterile but can become contaminated in the lower urethra by the same organisms that inhabit the outer layer of the skin and perineum (Figure 2.5).

IV. BENEFICIAL FUNCTIONS OF NORMAL FLORA

Normal flora can provide some definite benefits to the host. First, the sheer number of harmless bacteria in the lower bowel and mouth make it unlikely that, in a healthy person, an invading pathogen could compete for nutrients and receptor sites. Second, some bacteria of the bowel produce antimicrobial substances to which the producers themselves are not susceptible. Third, bacterial colonization of a newborn infant acts as a powerful stimulus for the development of the immune system. Fourth, bacteria of the gut provide important nutrients, such as vitamin K, and aid in digestion and absorption of nutrients. [Note: Although humans can obtain vitamin K from food sources, bacteria can be an important supplemental source if nutrition is impaired.]

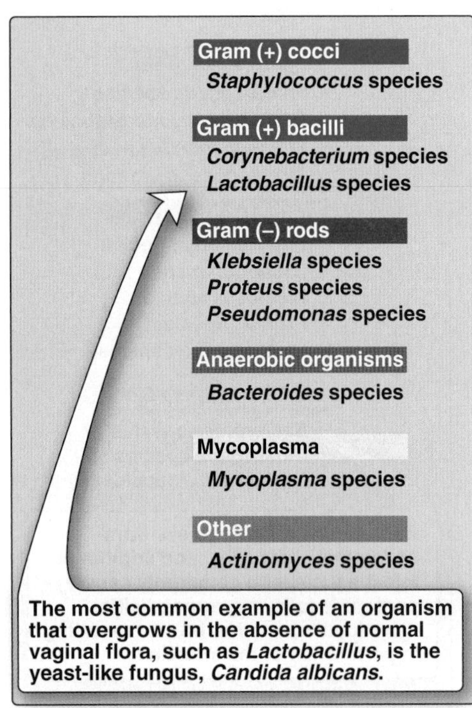

Gram (+) cocci
Staphylococcus species
Gram (+) bacilli
Corynebacterium species
Lactobacillus species
Gram (–) rods
Klebsiella species
Proteus species
Pseudomonas species
Anaerobic organisms
Bacteroides species
Mycoplasma
Mycoplasma species
Other
Actinomyces species
The most common example of an organism that overgrows in the absence of normal vaginal flora, such as Lactobacillus, is the yeast-like fungus, Candida albicans.

Figure 2.5
Examples of bacteria that inhabit the vagina.

V. HARMFUL EFFECTS OF NORMAL FLORA

Clinical problems caused by normal flora arise in the following ways: 1) The organisms are displaced from their normal site in the body to an abnormal site. An example already mentioned is the introduction of the normal skin bacterium, *S. epidermidis*, into the bloodstream where it can colonize catheters and heart valves, resulting in bacterial endocarditis. 2) Potential pathogens gain a competitive advantage due to diminished populations of harmless competitors. For example, when normal bowel flora are depleted by antibiotic therapy leading to overgrowth by the resistant *Clostridium difficile*, which can cause severe colitis. 3) Harmless, commonly ingested food substances are converted into carcinogenic derivatives by bacteria in the colon. A well-known example is the conversion by bacterial sulfatases of the sweetener cyclamate into the bladder carcinogen cyclohexamine. 4) When individuals are immunocompromised, normal flora can overgrow and become pathogenic. [Note: Colonization by normal, but potentially harmful, flora should be distinguished from the carrier state in which a true pathogen is carried by a healthy (asymptomatic) individual and passed to other individuals where it results in disease. Typhoid fever is an example of a disease that can be acquired from a carrier (see p. 116).]

Study Questions

Choose the ONE correct answer

2.1 The primary effect of lactobacilli in the adult vagina is to

A. maintain an alkaline environment.
B. maintain an acidic environment.
C. produce a protective mucus layer.
D. increase fertility.
E. keep the menstrual cycle regular.

Correct answer = B. Lactobacilli produce acid that, in turn, inhibits the growth of potential pathogenic bacteria and fungi. None of the other answers are known to be attributed to lactobacilli.

2.2 A patient presents with severe colitis associated with an overgrowth of *Clostridium difficile* in the lower bowel. The most likely cause of this condition is

A. botulinum food poisoning.
B. a stomach ulcer.
C. a compromised immune system.
D. antibiotic therapy.
E. mechanical blockage of the large intestine.

Correct answer = D. Antibiotic therapy can reduce normal flora in the bowel, allowing pathogenic organisms normally present in low numbers to overgrow. None of the other answers explains the overgrowth of *Clostridium difficile.*

2.3 The predominant bacterial species that colonizes the human skin is

A. *Lactobacillus.*
B. *Candida albicans.*
C. *Streptococcus pneumoniae.*
D. *Staphylococcus epidermidis.*
E. *Bacterioides fragilis.*

Correct answer = D. Human skin normally contains up to 10,000 *Staphylococcus epidermidis* per cm^2. Other colonizing bacteria may be present but in much lower numbers. *Candida albicans* is a yeast-like fungus, not a bacterium.

Pathogenicity of Microorganisms

3

I. OVERVIEW

A pathogenic microorganism is defined as one that is capable of causing disease. Some microorganisms are unequivocally pathogenic, whereas others (the majority) are generally harmless. An organism may invade an individual without causing infectious disease when the host's defense mechanisms are successful. The occurrence of such asymptomatic infections can be recognized by the presence of antibody against the organism in the patient's serum. Some infections result in a latent state, meaning that the organism is dormant but may be reactivated with the recurrence of symptoms. Moreover, some pathogens cause disease only under certain conditions (for example, being introduced into a normally sterile body site or infection of an immunocompromised host). Figure 3.1 summarizes some of the terms used to describe the diversity of infections.

Subclinical
- An infection with no detectable symptoms
- Example: asymptomatic gonorrhea

Latent
- An infection with the potential to become active at some time
- Examples: *Treponema pallidum* (syphilis) and *Mycobacterium tuberculosis* (tuberculosis)

Opportunistic
- An infection due to an organism that generally does not cause disease unless normal host defenses are compromised
- Example: *Pneumocystis* pneumonia in patients with HIV

Primary
- Infection by an organism that may become latent and later cause other disease manifestations
- Example: *Treponema pallidum* (syphilis)

Secondary
- a) Reactivation of a latent infection, or b) the second stage of an infection
- Examples: a) *Mycobacterium tuberculosis* (tuberculosis) b) *Treponema pallidum* (syphilis)

Mixed
- Two or more bacteria infecting the same tissue
- Example: Pelvic inflammatory disease may be initiated by infection with *N. gonorrhoeae* or *C. trachomatis* but other organisms including anaerobes play important roles in progression of the disease.

Pyogenic
- Pus forming
- Example: staphylococcal and streptococcal infections

Fulminant
- Infections that occur suddenly and intensely
- Example: Necrotizing fasciitis from *Streptococcus pyogenes*, also called "flesh-eating bacteria" [Note: fulminant is derived from the Latin word for lightning (fulmen).]

Figure 3.1
Terms used to describe infections.

II. BACTERIAL PATHOGENESIS

Although the mechanism of infectious process may vary among bacteria, the methods by which bacteria cause disease can, in general, be divided into several stages (Figure 3.2). Pathogenicity of a microorganism depends on its success in completing some or all of these stages. The terms "virulence" and "pathogenicity" are often used interchangeably. However, virulence can be quantified by how many organisms are required to cause disease in 50 percent of those exposed to the pathogen (ID_{50}, where I = Infectious and D = Dose), or to kill 50 percent of test animals (LD_{50}, where L = Lethal). The number of organisms required to cause disease varies greatly among pathogenic bacteria. For example, less than 100 *Shigella* cause diarrhea by infecting the gastrointestinal (GI) tract, whereas the infectious dose of *Salmonella* is approximately 100,000 organisms. The infectious dose of a bacterium depends primarily on its virulence factors. The probability that an infectious disease occurs is influenced by both the number and virulence of the infecting organisms and the strength of the host immune response opposing infection.

A. Virulence factors

Virulence factors are those characteristics of a bacterium that enhance its pathogenicity, that is, properties that enable a microorganism to establish itself and replicate on or within a specific host.

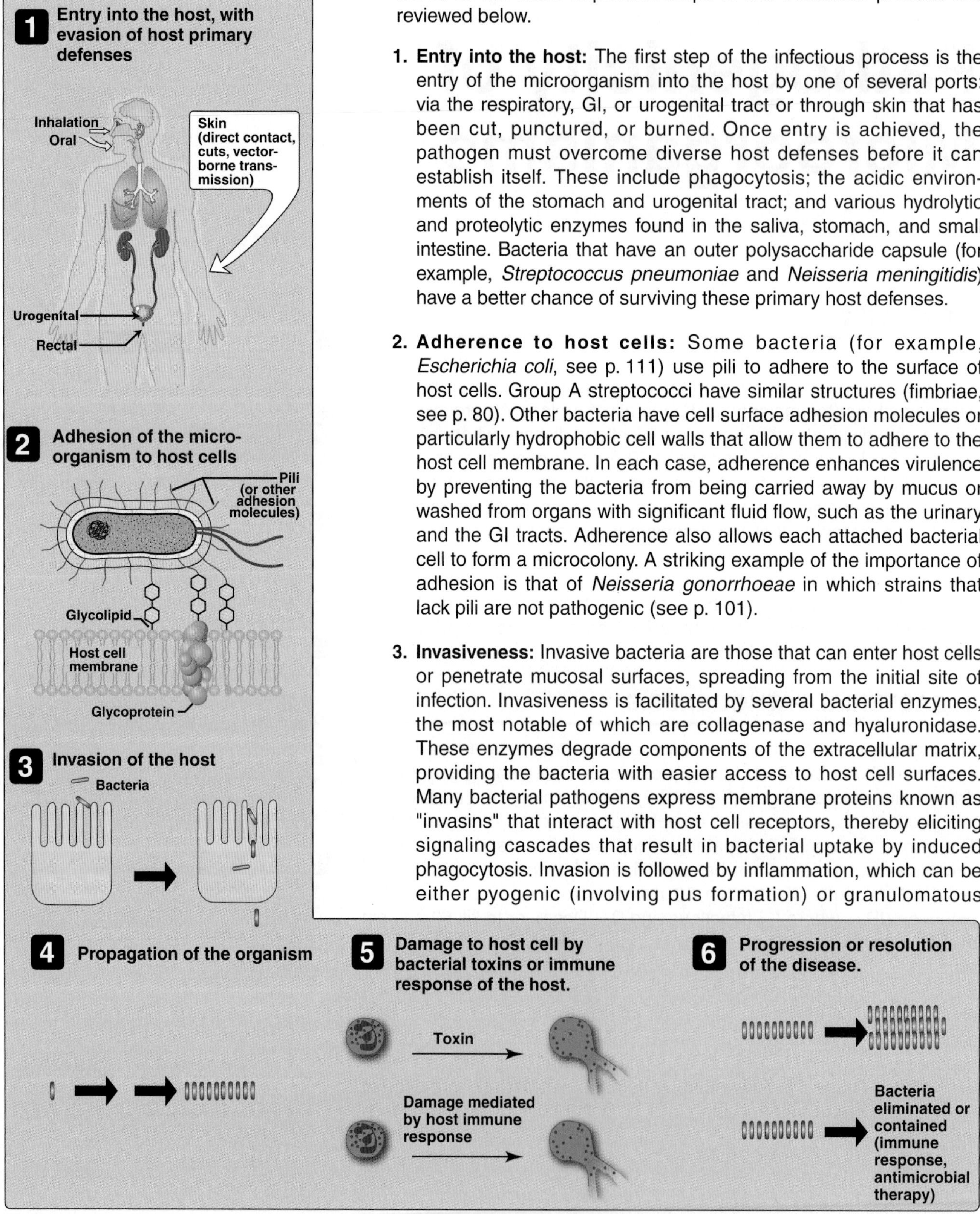

Figure 3.2
Mechanism of infectious process.

Some of the more important steps in the infectious process are reviewed below.

1. **Entry into the host:** The first step of the infectious process is the entry of the microorganism into the host by one of several ports: via the respiratory, GI, or urogenital tract or through skin that has been cut, punctured, or burned. Once entry is achieved, the pathogen must overcome diverse host defenses before it can establish itself. These include phagocytosis; the acidic environments of the stomach and urogenital tract; and various hydrolytic and proteolytic enzymes found in the saliva, stomach, and small intestine. Bacteria that have an outer polysaccharide capsule (for example, *Streptococcus pneumoniae* and *Neisseria meningitidis*) have a better chance of surviving these primary host defenses.

2. **Adherence to host cells:** Some bacteria (for example, *Escherichia coli*, see p. 111) use pili to adhere to the surface of host cells. Group A streptococci have similar structures (fimbriae, see p. 80). Other bacteria have cell surface adhesion molecules or particularly hydrophobic cell walls that allow them to adhere to the host cell membrane. In each case, adherence enhances virulence by preventing the bacteria from being carried away by mucus or washed from organs with significant fluid flow, such as the urinary and the GI tracts. Adherence also allows each attached bacterial cell to form a microcolony. A striking example of the importance of adhesion is that of *Neisseria gonorrhoeae* in which strains that lack pili are not pathogenic (see p. 101).

3. **Invasiveness:** Invasive bacteria are those that can enter host cells or penetrate mucosal surfaces, spreading from the initial site of infection. Invasiveness is facilitated by several bacterial enzymes, the most notable of which are collagenase and hyaluronidase. These enzymes degrade components of the extracellular matrix, providing the bacteria with easier access to host cell surfaces. Many bacterial pathogens express membrane proteins known as "invasins" that interact with host cell receptors, thereby eliciting signaling cascades that result in bacterial uptake by induced phagocytosis. Invasion is followed by inflammation, which can be either pyogenic (involving pus formation) or granulomatous

(having nodular inflammatory lesions), depending on the organism. The pus of pyogenic inflammations contains mostly neutrophils, whereas granulomatous lesions contain fibroblasts, lymphocytes, and macrophages.

4. **Iron sequestering:** Iron is an essential nutrient for most bacteria. To obtain the iron required for growth, bacteria produce iron-binding compounds, called siderophores. These compounds capture iron from the host by chelation, and then the ferrated siderophore binds to specific receptors on the bacterial surface. Iron is actively transported into the bacterium, where it is incorporated into essential compounds such as cytochromes. The pathogenic *Neisseria* species are exceptions in that they do not produce siderophores but instead utilize host iron-binding proteins, such as transferrin and lactoferrin, as iron sources. They do so by expressing dedicated receptors that bind to these host proteins and remove the iron for internalization.

5. **Virulence factors that inhibit phagocytosis:** The most important antiphagocytic structure is the capsule external to the cell wall, such as in *S. pneumoniae* and *N. meningitidis*. A second group of antiphagocytic factors are the cell wall proteins of gram-positive cocci, such as protein A of staphylococcus and M protein of group A streptococci (see pp. 70, 80).

6. **Bacterial toxins:** Some bacteria cause disease by producing toxic substances, of which there are two general types: exotoxins and endotoxin. Exotoxins, which are proteins, are secreted by both gram-positive and gram-negative bacteria. In contrast, endotoxin, which is synonymous with lipopolysaccharide (LPS), is not secreted but instead is an integral component of the cell walls of gram-negative bacteria.

   a. **Exotoxins:** These include some of the most poisonous substances known. It is estimated that as little as 1 µg of tetanus exotoxin can kill an adult human. Exotoxin proteins generally have two polypeptide components (Figure 3.3). One is responsible for binding the protein to the host cell, and one is responsible for the toxic effect. In several cases, the precise target for the toxin has been identified. For example, diphtheria toxin is an enzyme that blocks protein synthesis. It does so by attaching an adenosine diphosphate–ribosyl group to human protein elongation factor EF-2, thereby inactivating it (see p. 92). Most exotoxins are rapidly inactivated by moderate heating (60° C), notable exceptions being staphylococcal enterotoxin and *E. coli* heat-stable toxin (ST). In addition, treatment with dilute formaldehyde destroys the toxic activity of most exotoxins but does not affect their antigenicity. Formaldehyde-inactivated toxins, called toxoids, are useful in preparing vaccines (see p. 36). Exotoxin proteins are, in many cases, encoded by genes carried on plasmids or temperate bacteriophages. An example is the diphtheria exotoxin that is encoded by the *tox* gene of a temperate bacteriophage that can lysogenize *Corynebacterium diphtheriae*. Strains of *C. diphtheriae* that carry this phage are pathogenic, whereas those that lack the phage are nonpathogenic.

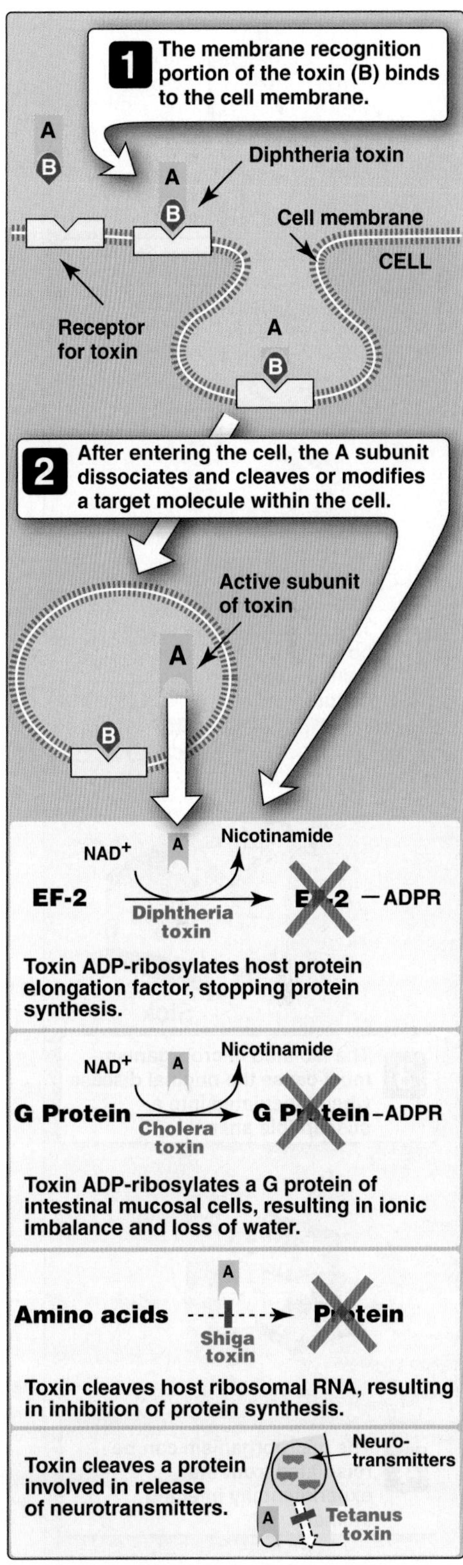

Figure 3.3
Action of exotoxins. ADP = adenosine diphosphate; ADPR = adenosine diphosphate ribose; NAD^+ = nicotinamide adenine dinucleotide.

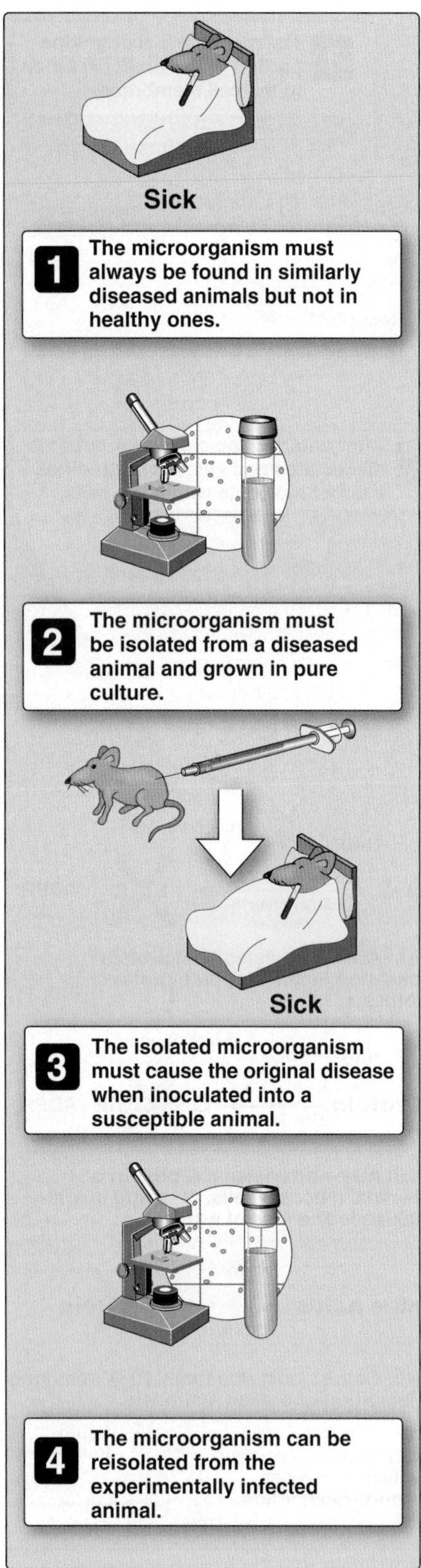

Sick
1 The microorganism must always be found in similarly diseased animals but not in healthy ones.
2 The microorganism must be isolated from a diseased animal and grown in pure culture.
Sick
3 The isolated microorganism must cause the original disease when inoculated into a susceptible animal.
4 The microorganism can be reisolated from the experimentally infected animal.

Figure 3.4
Koch's postulates.

b. Endotoxins: These are heat-stable, LPS components of the outer membranes of gram-negative (but not gram-positive) bacteria. They are released into the host's circulation following bacterial cell lysis. LPS consists of polysaccharide composed of repeating sugar subunits (O antigen), which protrudes from the exterior cell surface; a core polysaccharide; and a lipid component called lipid A that is integrated into the outer leaflet of the outer membrane. The lipid A moiety is responsible for the toxicity of this molecule. The main physiologic effects of LPS endotoxin are fever, shock, hypotension, and thrombosis, collectively referred to as septic shock. These effects are produced indirectly by macrophage activation, with the release of cytokines, activation of complement, and activation of the coagulation cascade. Death can result from multiple organ failure. Elimination of the causative bacteria with antibiotics can initially exacerbate the symptoms by causing sudden massive release of endotoxin into the circulation. Although gram-positive bacteria do not contain LPS, their cell wall peptidoglycan and teichoic acids can elicit a shock syndrome similar to that caused by LPS but usually not as severe.

B. Host-mediated pathogenesis

The pathogenesis of many bacterial infections is caused by the host response rather than by bacterial factors. Classic examples of host response–mediated pathogenesis are seen in diseases such as gram-negative bacterial sepsis, tuberculosis, and tuberculoid leprosy. The tissue damage in these infections is caused by various cytokines released from the lymphocytes, macrophages, and polymorphonuclear leukocytes at the site of infection or in the bloodstream. Often the host response is so intense that host tissues are destroyed, allowing remaining bacteria to proliferate.

C. Antigenic variation

A successful pathogen must evade the host's immune system that recognizes bacterial surface antigens. One important evasive strategy for the pathogen is to change its surface antigens. This is accomplished by several mechanisms. One mechanism, called phase variation, is the genetically reversible ability of certain bacteria to turn off and turn on the expression of genes coding for surface antigens. A second mechanism, called antigenic variation, involves the modification of the gene for an expressed surface antigen by genetic recombination with one of many variable unexpressed DNA sequences. In this manner, the expressed surface antigen can assume many different antigenic structures (see Figure 11.3).

D. Which is the pathogen?

Isolating a particular microorganism from infected tissue (for example, a necrotic skin lesion), does not conclusively demonstrate that it caused the lesion. The organism could, for example, be a harmless member of the normal skin flora (see p. 7) that happened to be in the vicinity. Alternatively, the organism may not be a natural resident of the skin but an opportunistic pathogen that secondarily infected the necrotic lesion. [Note: An opportunistic pathogen is an organism that is unable to cause disease in healthy, immunocompetent individuals but can infect people whose defenses have been impaired.] Robert Koch, a 19th century German microbiologist, recognized this dilemma and defined a series of criteria (Koch's postulates) to confirm the causative microbial agent of a disease (Figure 3.4). [Note: Although these criteria has been successful in establishing the etiology of most infections, it fails if the causative organism cannot be cultured *in vitro*.]

E. Infections in human populations

Bacterial diseases may be communicable from person to person or noncommunicable. For example, cholera is highly communicable (the disease-causing organism, *Vibrio cholerae*, is easily spread), whereas botulism is noncommunicable because only those people who ingest the botulinum exotoxin are affected. Highly communicable diseases, such as cholera, are said to be contagious and tend to occur as localized epidemics in which the disease frequency is higher than normal. When an epidemic becomes worldwide, it is called a pandemic. Pandemics, such as the 1918 influenza pandemic, arise because the human population has never been exposed to and, therefore, has no immunity against the specific strain of influenza virus.

III. VIRAL PATHOGENESIS

Viruses can replicate only inside living cells. Consequently, the first pathogenic manifestations of viral infection are seen at the cellular level. The course of events following initial exposure to some viruses may include rapid onset of observable symptoms, which is referred to as an acute infection. Alternatively, the initial infection by other viruses may be mild or asymptomatic. Following the initial infection, the most common outcome is that the virus is cleared completely from the body by the immune system. For some viruses, the initial infection is followed by either a persistent infection or a latent infection.

A. Viral pathogenesis at the cellular level

Cells show a variety of different responses to viral infection, depending on the cell type and virus. Many viral infections cause no apparent morphologic or functional changes in the cell. When changes do occur, several (potentially overlapping) responses can be recognized (Figure 3.5).

1. **Cell death:** A cell can be directly killed by the virus. In most cases, this is due to the inhibition of synthesis of cellular DNA, RNA, and protein. Some viruses have specific genes responsible for this inhibition. Dead or dying cells release a brood of progeny viruses that repeat the replication process. Examples of viruses that kill their host cells are adenovirus (see p. 250) and poliovirus (see p. 283).

2. **Transformation:** Some viruses transform normal cells into malignant cells. In many ways, this is the opposite of cell death, because malignant cells have less fastidious growth requirements

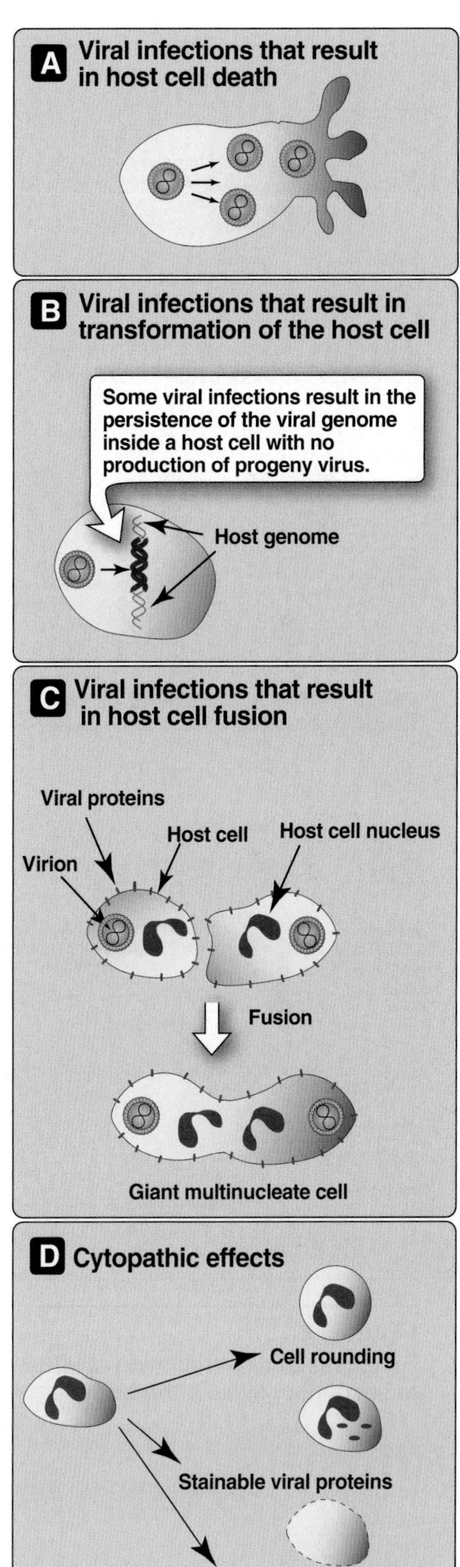

Figure 3.5
Types of viral pathogenesis at the cellular level.

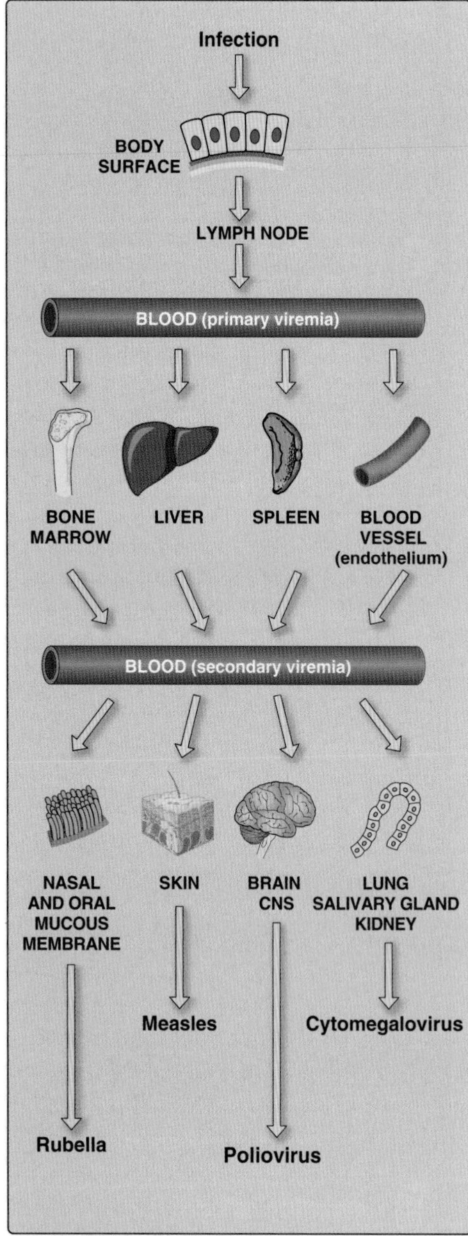

Figure 3.6
Examples of dissemination of virus to secondary sites in the body.

than do normal cells, and they have an indefinitely extended lifetime. Transformation is an irreversible genetic process caused by the integration of viral DNA into the host's DNA (see p. 243).

3. **Cell fusion:** Infection of cells with certain viruses causes the cells to fuse, producing giant, multinucleate cells. Viruses with this property include herpesviruses (see p. 257) and paramyxoviruses (see p. 312). The ability of infected cells to fuse is apparently due to virus-induced changes in the structure of the cell membrane.

4. **Cytopathic effect:** Cytopathic effect (CPE) is a catch-all term that refers to any visible change in appearance of an infected cell, for example, cell rounding, patches of stainable viral proteins inside the cell, and cell disintegration. Some viruses can be roughly identified by the time of onset and pattern of CPE in cell culture as well as by the types of cells in which these viruses cause CPE.

B. Initial infections

Following initial multiplication at the primary site of entry, the viral infection may remain localized or become disseminated. The infection may be asymptomatic (unapparent). Alternatively, typical symptoms of disease may occur, often in two temporally distinct forms: 1) early symptoms at the primary site of infection and 2) delayed symptoms due to dissemination from the primary site, causing infection of secondary sites. Virus transmission can occur before symptoms of the generalized illness are apparent, making it difficult to control the spread of viral diseases.

1. **Routes of entry and dissemination to secondary sites:** Common routes by which viruses enter the body are essentially the same as for bacterial infections (that is, through the skin or respiratory, GI, or urogenital tracts). In each case, some viruses remain localized and cause disease that is largely restricted to the primary site of infection. Other viruses undergo multiplication in cells at the primary site, which may be accompanied by symptoms, followed by invasion of the lymphatic system and the blood. [Note: The presence of virus in the blood is termed viremia.] Virus is disseminated throughout the body via the bloodstream and can infect cells at secondary sites characteristic for each specific virus type, thus causing the disease typically associated with that species (Figure 3.6).

2. **Typical secondary sites of localization:** Secondary sites of infection determine the nature of the delayed symptoms and, usually, the major characteristics associated with the resulting disease. Viruses frequently exhibit tropism for specific cell types and tissues. This specificity is usually caused by the presence of specific host cell surface receptors recognized by particular viruses. Although any tissue or organ system is a potential target for virus infection, the fetus represents an especially important site for secondary localization of virus infections. Virus from the maternal circulation infects cells of the placenta, thereby gaining access to the fetal circulation and, ultimately, to all tissues of the developing

fetus (Figure 3.7). Fetal death or developmental abnormalities are often the result. Neonatal infection can also occur during birth when the fetus comes into contact with infected genital secretions of the mother or after birth when the infant ingests infected breast milk.

3. **Virus shedding and mode of transmission:** The mode of transmission of a viral disease is largely determined by the tissues that produce progeny virus and/or the fluids into which they are released. These are not necessarily the secondary sites of infection but, in fact, are often the site of primary infection at a time before symptoms are apparent. The skin, respiratory and GI tracts, and bodily fluids are commonly sites of viral shedding.

4. **Factors involved in termination of acute infection:** In a typical, uncomplicated, acute infection, virus is totally eliminated from the host in 2 to 3 weeks. This outcome is primarily a function of the host's immune system, with involvement of both cell-mediated and humoral responses. The relative importance of these two responses depends on the virus and the nature of the disease.

   a. **Cell-mediated responses:** The earliest immune system response to virus infection is a generalized inflammatory response, accompanied by nonspecific killing of infected cells by natural killer cells. This latter activity, enhanced by interferon and other cytokines, begins well before the virus-specific immune response. Later, cytolysis by virus-specific cytotoxic T lymphocytes that recognize virus peptides displayed on the cell surface also eliminates infected cells. These cellular responses are especially significant in that they help limit the spread of the infection by killing infected cells before they have released progeny virus. Cell surface immunodeterminants recognized by T cells are often derived from nonstructural or internal proteins of the virus. Thus, this response complements the inactivation of free virus by humoral antibody, which is directed against capsid or envelope proteins.

   b. **Humoral response:** Although circulating antibodies may be directed against any virus protein, those that are of greatest significance in controlling an infection react specifically with epitopes on the surface of the virion and result in inactivation of the virus's infectivity. The process is called neutralization. This response is of primary importance in suppressing diseases that involve a viremic stage, but secretory antibodies (for example, immunoglobulin A) also play an important protective role in primary infections of the respiratory and GI tracts. Humoral antibodies also take part in killing infected cells by two mechanisms. The first is antibody-dependent, cell-mediated cytotoxicity, in which natural killer cells and other leukocytes bearing Fc receptors bind to the Fc portions of antibodies that are complexed to virus antigens on the surface of the infected cell and kill it. The second mechanism is complement-mediated lysis of infected cells to which virus-specific antibody has bound.

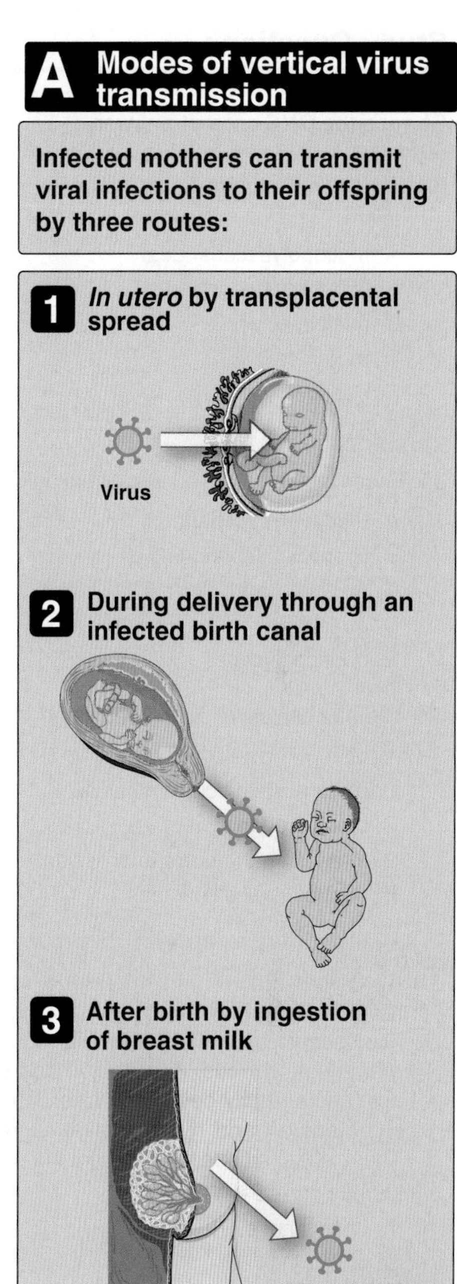

A Modes of vertical virus transmission
Infected mothers can transmit viral infections to their offspring by three routes:
1 In utero by transplacental spread
Virus
2 During delivery through an infected birth canal
3 After birth by ingestion of breast milk
Virus in milk
B Some viruses transmitted from mother to infant
Herpes simplex virus types 1 and 2
Human cytomegalovirus
Human immunodeficiency virus
Rubella virus

Figure 3.7
Mother-to-infant (vertical) transmission of viral infections.

Study Questions

Choose the ONE correct answer.

3.1 Endotoxin belongs to a class of biological molecules called

A. mucopolysaccharides.
B. lipopolysaccharides.
C. nucleic acids.
D. proteins.
E. peptidoglycans.

Correct answer = B. Endotoxin is an integral lipopolysaccharide constituent of the outer membrane of gram-negative bacteria. The peptidoglycans, present in large amounts in gram-positive bacteria can be toxic but are not considered endotoxin.

3.2 Exotoxins belong to a class of biologic molecules called

A. mucopolysaccharides.
B. lipopolysaccharides.
C. nucleic acids.
D. proteins.
E. peptidoglycans.

Correct answer = D. Exotoxins are secreted toxic proteins that, in many cases, have a well-defined cellular site of action.

3.3 The mechanism of action of diphtheria toxin is to

A. disrupt the cell membrane.
B. block nucleic acid synthesis.
C. block protein synthesis.
D. interfere with neurotransmission.
E. destroy the cell nucleus.

Correct answer = C. Diphtheria toxin inactivates the polypeptide elongation factor EF-2, blocking protein synthesis. Tetanus toxin interferes with neurotransmission.

3.4 A 48-year-old woman presented at the emergency room complaining of urinary urgency and flank pain. Microscopic examination of a urine sample revealed gram-negative rods. Prior to initiation of antibiotic therapy, she abruptly developed fever, chills, and delirium. Hypotension and hyperventilation rapidly followed. These observations suggest that the patient is responding to the release of bacterial

A. collagenase.
B. exotoxin.
C. hyaluronidase.
D. lipopolysaccharide.
E. peptidoglycan.

Correct answer = D. The patient is most likely suffering from septic shock. In two thirds of patients, septic shock results from infection with gram-negative bacteria, such as *Escherichia coli*, *Klebsiella*, *Enterobacter*, *Proteus*, *Pseudomonas*, and *Bacteroides*. Septicemia is more common in persons whose resistance is already compromised by an existing condition. The gram-negative bacteria release endotoxin or heat-stable, lipopolysaccharide (LPS) components of the outer membranes. The main physiologic effects of LPS endotoxin are fever, hypotension, and thrombosis, collectively referred to as septic shock. Death can result from multiple organ failure. Gram-positive bacteria release exotoxins that can elicit a shock syndrome, but response is usually not as severe as that of gram-negative septic shock.

Diagnostic Microbiology

4

I. OVERVIEW

Identifying the organism causing an infectious process is usually essential for effective antimicrobial and supportive therapy. Initial treatment may be empiric, based on the microbiologic epidemiology of the infection and the patient's symptoms. However, definitive microbiologic diagnosis of an infectious disease usually involves one or more of the following five basic laboratory techniques, which guide the physician along a narrowing path of possible causative organisms: 1) direct microscopic visualization of the organism, 2) cultivation and identification of the organism, 3) detection of microbial antigens, 4) detection of microbial DNA or RNA, and 5) detection of an inflammatory or host immune response to the microorganism (Figure 4.1).

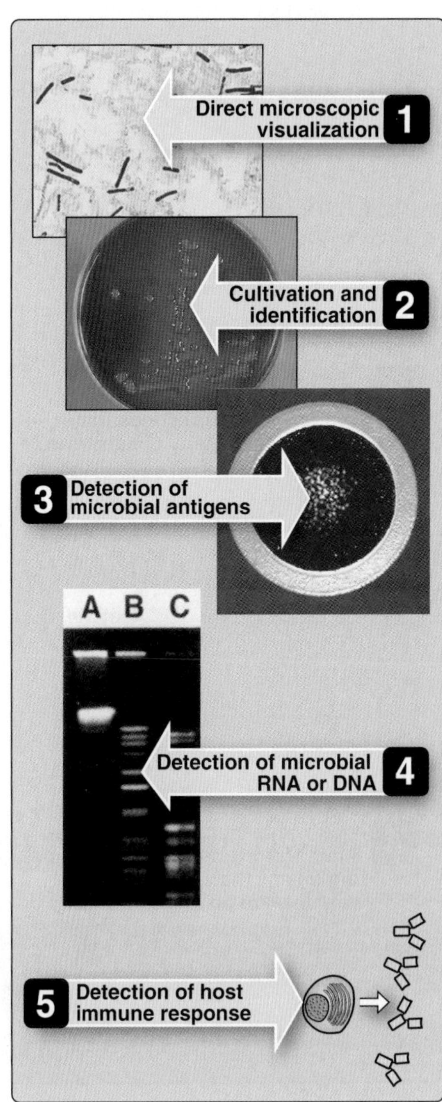

Figure 4.1
Laboratory techniques that are useful in diagnosis of microbial diseases.

II. PATIENT HISTORY AND PHYSICAL EXAMINATION

A clinical history is the most important part of patient evaluation. For example, a history of cough points to the possibility of respiratory tract infection, whereas dysuria (painful or difficult urination) suggests urinary tract infection. A history of travel to developing countries may implicate exotic organisms. For example, a patient who recently swam in the Nile has an increased risk of schistosomiasis. Patient occupations may suggest exposure to certain pathogens, such as brucellosis in a butcher or anthrax in farmers. Even the age of the patient can sometimes guide the clinician in predicting the identity of pathogens. For example, a gram-positive coccus in the spinal fluid of a newborn infant is unlikely to be *Streptococcus pneumoniae* (pneumococcus) but most likely to be *Streptococcus agalactiae* (group B). This organism is sensitive to penicillin G. By contrast, a gram-positive coccus in the spinal fluid of a 40-year-old patient is most likely to be *S. pneumoniae*. This organism is frequently resistant to penicillin G and requires treatment with a third-generation cephalosporin (such as cefotaxime or ceftriaxone) or vancomycin. The etiology implied by the patient's age may thus guide initial therapy. A physical examination often provides confirmatory clues to the presence and extent (localized or disseminated) of disease. For example, erythema migrans (a large skin lesion with a bright red outer border and partially clear central area; see p. 165) indicates early localized Lyme disease. Clues to the presence of bacteremia (a disseminated infection) may include chills, fever (or sometimes hypothermia), or cardiovascular instability heralding septic shock. Physical signs of pulmonary consolidation suggest pneumonia. If stupor and stiff neck are included in this constellation of findings, the organism causing the pneumonia may have spread to the meninges, warranting a further search for it in the cerebrospinal fluid (CSF). All laboratory studies must be directed by the patient's history and physical examination and then evaluated, taking into consideration the sensitivity and specificity of the test.

III. DIRECT VISUALIZATION OF THE ORGANISM

In many infectious diseases, pathogenic organisms (excluding viruses) can often be directly visualized by microscopic examination of patient specimens, such as sputum, urine, and CSF. The organism's microscopic morphology and staining characteristics can provide the first screening step in arriving at a specific identification. The organisms to be examined do not need to be alive or able to multiply. Microscopy yields rapid and inexpensive results and may allow the clinician to initiate treatment without waiting for the results of a culture, as noted in the spinal fluid example in the previous paragraph.

A. Gram stain

Because unstained bacteria are difficult to detect with the light microscope, most patient material is stained prior to microscopic evaluation. The most common and useful staining procedure is the Gram stain, which separates bacteria into two classifications according to their cell wall composition. If a clinical specimen on a microscope slide is treated with a solution of crystal violet and then iodine, the bacterial cells will stain purple. If the stained cells are then treated with a solvent, such as alcohol or acetone, gram-positive organisms retain the stain, whereas gram-negative species lose the stain, becoming colorless (Figure 4.2). Addition of the counterstain safranin stains the clear, gram-negative bacteria pink or red. Most, but not all, bacteria are stainable and fall into one of these two groups. [Note: Microorganisms that lack cell walls, such as mycoplasma, cannot be identified using the Gram stain.]

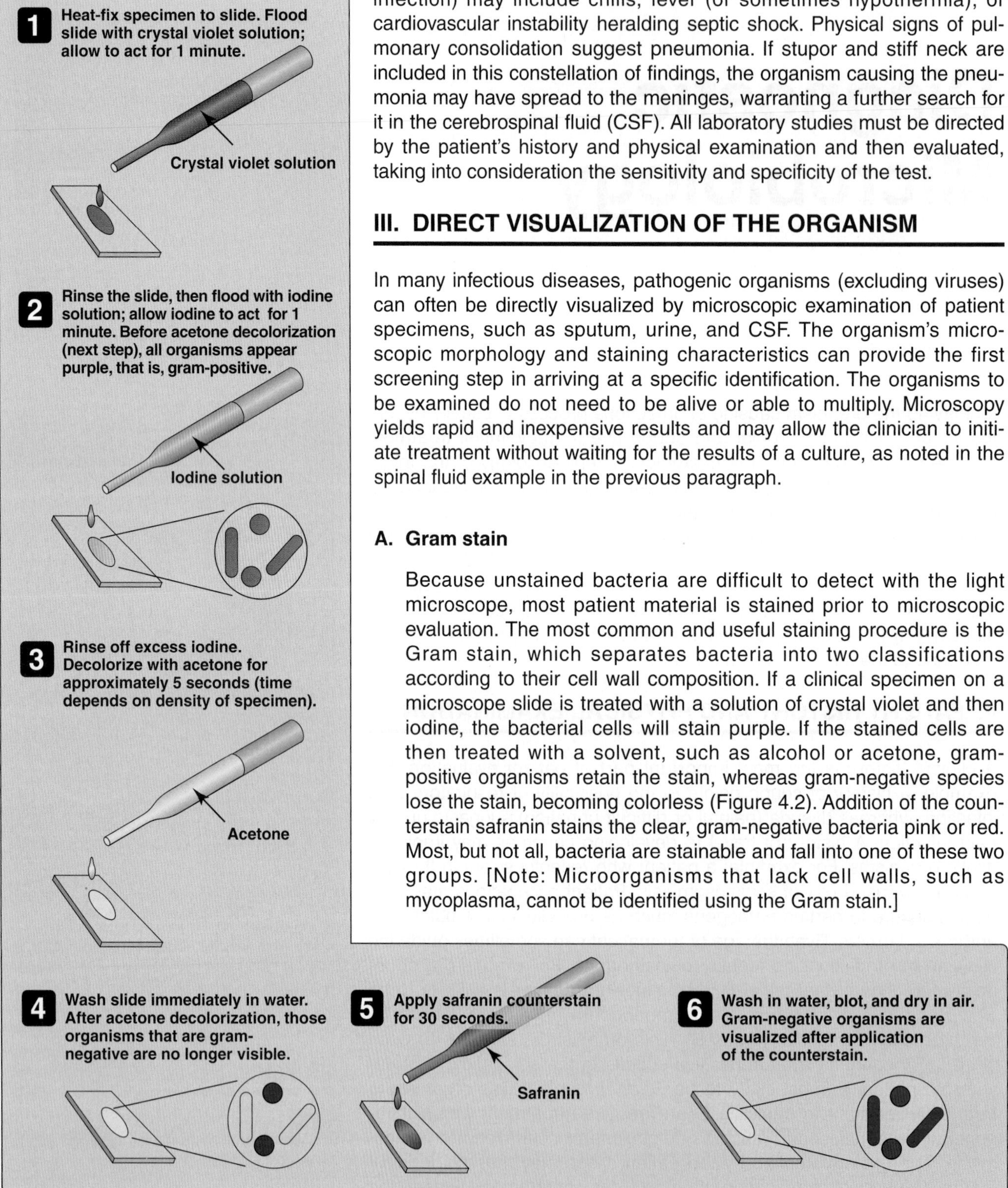

1 Heat-fix specimen to slide. Flood slide with crystal violet solution; allow to act for 1 minute.
Crystal violet solution
2 Rinse the slide, then flood with iodine solution; allow iodine to act for 1 minute. Before acetone decolorization (next step), all organisms appear purple, that is, gram-positive.
Iodine solution
3 Rinse off excess iodine. Decolorize with acetone for approximately 5 seconds (time depends on density of specimen).
Acetone
4 Wash slide immediately in water. After acetone decolorization, those organisms that are gram-negative are no longer visible.
5 Apply safranin counterstain for 30 seconds.
Safranin
6 Wash in water, blot, and dry in air. Gram-negative organisms are visualized after application of the counterstain.

Figure 4.2
Steps in Gram stain method.
Key: ● = Gram-positive violet. ▬ = Gram-negative red. ⬭ = Colorless.

1. **Gram stain applications:** The Gram stain is important therapeutically because gram-positive and gram-negative bacteria differ in their susceptibility to various antibiotics, and the Gram stain may, therefore, be used to guide initial therapy until the microorganism can be definitively identified. In addition, the morphology of the stained bacteria can sometimes be diagnostic. For example, gram-negative intracellular diplococci in urethral pus provide a presumptive diagnosis of gonorrhea. Gram stains of specimens submitted for culture are often invaluable aids in the interpretation of culture results. For example, a specimen may show organisms under the microscope but appear sterile in culture media. This discrepancy may suggest the presence of either fastidious organisms (bacteria with complex nutrient requirements) that are unable to grow on the culture media employed or fragile organisms, such as gonococcus or anaerobic organisms, that may not survive transport. In these cases, direct visualization with the Gram stain may provide the only clue to the nature, variety, and relative number of infecting organisms.

2. **Gram stain limitations:** The number of microorganisms required is relatively high. Visualization with the Gram stain requires greater than 10^4 organisms/mL. Liquid samples with low numbers of microorganisms (for example, in CSF), require centrifugation to concentrate the pathogens. The pellet is then examined after staining.

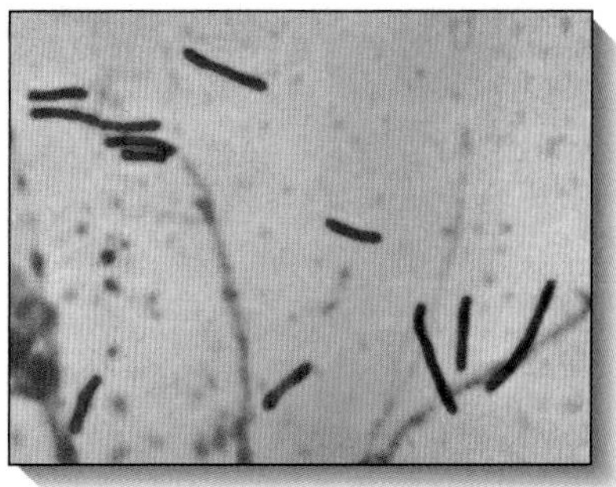

Figure 4.3
Mycobacterium tuberculosis stained with acid-fast stain.

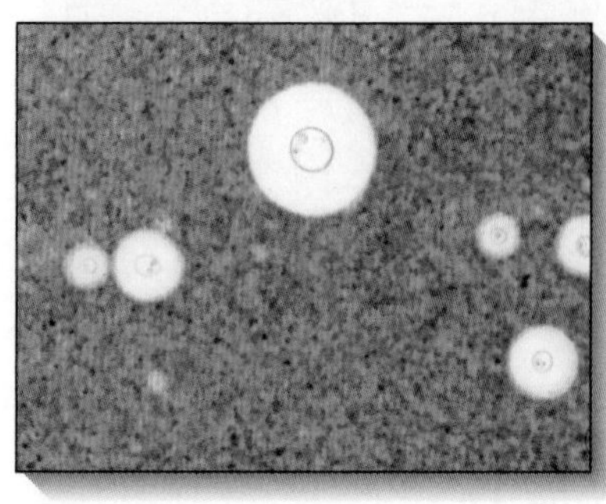

Figure 4.4
India ink preparation of *Cryptococcus neoformans* in cerebrospinal fluid. These yeast cells are identified by large transparent capsules that exclude the India ink particles.

B. Acid-fast stain

Stains such as Ziehl-Neelsen (the classic acid-fast stain) are used to identify organisms that have waxy material (mycolic acids) in their cell walls. Most bacteria that have been stained with carbolfuchsin can be decolorized by washing with acidic alcohol. However, certain acid-fast bacteria retain the carbolfuchsin stain after being washed with an acidic solution. The most clinically important acid-fast bacterium is *Mycobacterium tuberculosis*, which appears pink, often beaded, and slightly curved (Figure 4.3). Acid-fast staining is reserved for clinical samples from patients suspected of having mycobacterial infection.

C. India ink preparation

This is one of the simplest microscopic methods. It is useful in detecting *Cryptococcus neoformans* in CSF (Figure 4.4). One drop of centrifuged CSF is mixed with one drop of India ink on a microscope slide beneath a glass cover slip. Cryptococci are identified by their large, transparent capsules that displace the India ink particles.

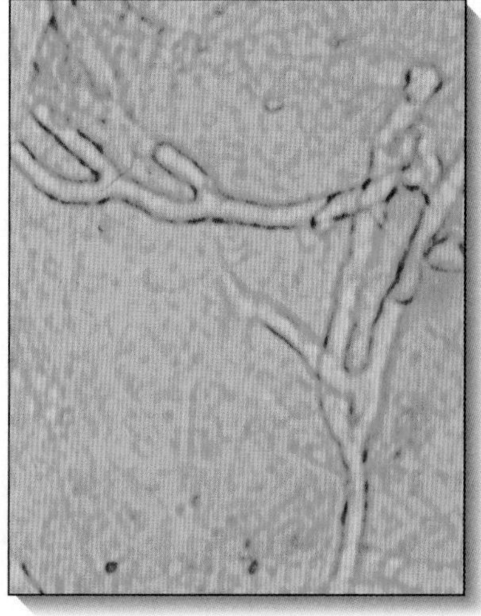

Figure 4.5
Fungi in unstained nasal sinus exudate, made distinct from other materials (such as cells) with potassium hydroxide.

D. Potassium hydroxide preparation

Treatment with potassium hydroxide (KOH) dissolves host cells and bacteria, sparing fungi (Figure 4.5). One drop of sputum or skin scraping is treated with 10 percent KOH, and the specimen is examined for fungal forms.

IV. GROWING BACTERIA IN CULTURE

Culturing is routine for most bacterial and fungal infections but is rarely used to identify helminths or protozoa. Culturing of many pathogens is straightforward, for example, streaking a throat swab onto a blood agar plate in search of group A β-hemolytic streptococcus. However, certain pathogens are very slow growing (for example, *M. tuberculosis*) or are cultured only with difficulty (for example, *Bartonella henselae*). Microorganisms isolated in culture are identified using such characteristics as colony size, shape, color, Gram stain, hemolytic reactions on solid media, odor, and metabolic properties. In addition, pure cultures provide samples for antimicrobial susceptibility testing (see p. 30). The success of culturing depends on appropriate collection and transport techniques and on selection of appropriate culture media, because some organisms may require special nutrients. Also, some media are used to suppress the growth of certain organisms in the process of identifying others (see p. 23)

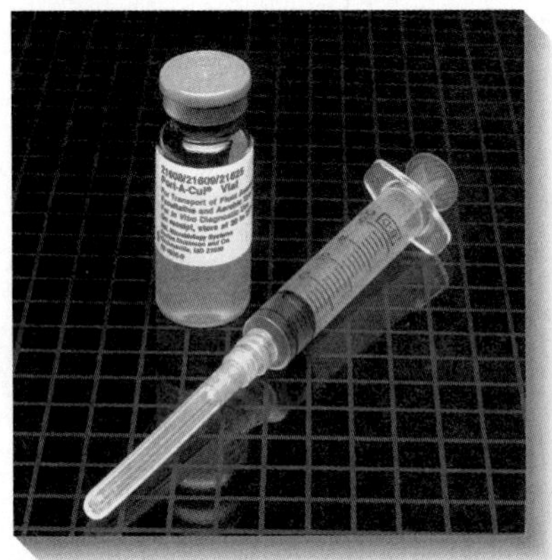

Figure 4.6
With anaerobic transport media containing a nonnutritive medium that retards diffusion of oxygen after addition of the specimen, microorganisms may remain viable for up to 72 hours. It is important to use an airless syringe for liquid specimens, such as pus, rather than a swab in a tube—especially when transport medium is not available. Also, if promptly transported in a syringe, the relative proportions of each morphology in mixed infections is visible.

A. Specimen collection

Many organisms are fragile and must be transported to the laboratory with minimal delay. For example, gonococci and pneumococci are very sensitive to heating and drying. Samples must be cultured promptly, or, if this is not possible, transport media must be used to extend the viability of the organism to be cultured. When anaerobic organisms are suspected, the patient's specimen must be protected from the toxic effect of oxygen (Figure 4.6).

B. Growth requirements

All clinically important bacteria are heterotrophs (that is, they require organic carbon for growth). Heterotrophs may have complex or simple requirements for organic molecules. [Note: Organisms that can reduce carbon dioxide and, therefore, do not require organic compounds for cell growth, are called autotrophs.] Most bacteria require varying numbers of growth factors, which are organic compounds required by the cell to grow, but which the organism cannot itself synthesize (for example, vitamins). Organisms that require either a large number of growth factors or must be supplied with very specific ones are referred to as fastidious.

C. Oxygen requirements

Bacteria can be categorized according to their growth responses in the presence and absence of oxygen. Strict aerobes cannot survive in the absence of oxygen and produce energy only by oxidative phosphorylation. Strict anaerobes generate energy by fermentation or by anaerobic respiration and are killed in the presence of oxygen. Facultative anaerobes can grow in the absence of oxygen but grow better in its presence. Aerotolerant anaerobes have mechanisms to protect themselves from oxygen (therefore, being able to grow in its presence or absence) but do not use oxygen in their metabolism. Finally, microaerophiles require oxygen for their metabolism but cannot survive at atmospheric levels of oxygen. Microaerophiles are found in lakes and wet soil where the oxygen concentration is within an acceptable range.

D. Media

Two general strategies are used to isolate pathogenic bacteria, depending on the nature of the clinical sample. The first method uses enriched media to promote the nonselective growth of any bacteria that may be present. The second approach employs selective media that only allow growth of specific bacterial species from specimens that normally contain large numbers of bacteria (for example, stool, genital tract secretions, and sputum). Isolation of a bacterium is usually performed on solid medium. Liquid medium is used to grow larger quantities of a culture of bacteria that have already been isolated as a pure culture.

1. **Enriched media:** Media fortified with blood, yeast extracts, or brain or heart infusions are useful in growing fastidious organisms. For example, sheep blood agar contains protein sources, sodium chloride, and 5 percent sheep blood and supports the growth of most gram-positive and gram-negative bacteria isolated from human sources (see p. 89). However, *Haemophilus influenzae* and *Neisseria gonorrhoeae*, among others, are highly fastidious organisms. They require chocolate agar, which contains red blood cells (RBCs) that have been lysed (see p. 130). This releases intracellular nutrients, such as hemoglobin, hemin ("X" factor), and nicotinamide adenine dinucleotide ("V" factor), required by these organisms. Enriched media are useful for culturing normally sterile body fluids, such as blood and CSF, in which the finding of any organisms provides reasonable evidence for infection by that organism. Failure to culture an organism may indicate that the culture medium is inadequate or that the incubation conditions do not support bacterial growth.

2. **Selective media:** The most commonly used selective medium is MacConkey agar (see p. 115), which supports the growth of most gram-negative rods, especially the Enterobacteriaceae, but inhibits growth of gram-positive organisms and some fastidious gram-negative bacteria, such as *Haemophilus* and *Neisseria* species. Growth on blood agar and chocolate agar but not MacConkey agar suggests a gram-positive isolate or a fastidious gram-negative species. In contrast, most gram-negative rods often form distinctive colonies on MacConkey agar. This agar is also used to detect organisms able to metabolize lactose (Figure 4.7). Clinical samples are routinely plated on blood agar, chocolate agar, and MacConkey agar. Hektoen enteric agar is also a selective medium that differentiates lactose/sucrose fermenters and nonfermenters as well as H_2S producers and nonproducers. It is often used to culture *Salmonella* and *Shigella* species. Thayer-Martin agar is another selective medium composed of chocolate agar supplemented with several antibiotics that suppress the growth of nonpathogenic *Neisseria* and other normal and abnormal flora. This medium is normally used to isolate gonococci. When submitting samples for culture, the physician must alert the laboratory to likely pathogens whenever possible, especially when unusual organisms are suspected. This allows inclusion of selective media that might not be used routinely. It also alerts the labo-

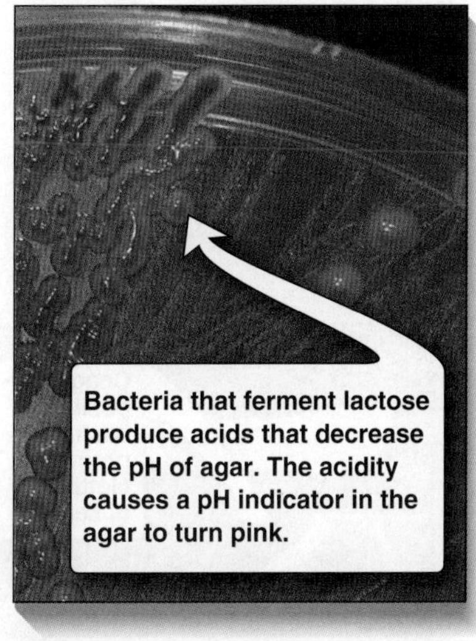

Bacteria that ferment lactose produce acids that decrease the pH of agar. The acidity causes a pH indicator in the agar to turn pink.

Figure 4.7
Lactose-fermenting, gram-negative rods produce pink colonies on MacConkey agar.

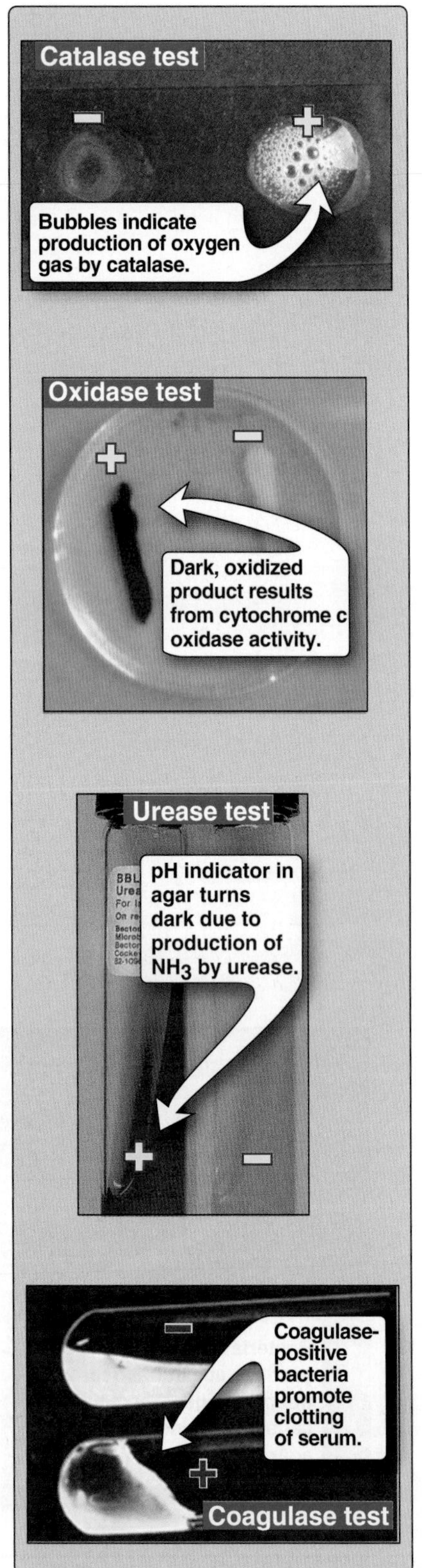

Figure 4.8
Tests commonly used in identifying bacteria.

ratory to hold specimens longer if a slow-growing organism, such as *Nocardia*, is suspected.

V. IDENTIFICATION OF BACTERIA

The most widely used identification scheme involves determining the morphologic and metabolic properties of the unknown bacterium and comparing these with properties of known microorganisms. Alternate identification schemes using nucleic acid–based methods are discussed on p. 29. Immunologic methods used in diagnosis are described on p. 25. It is essential to start identification tests with pure bacterial isolates grown from a single colony.

A. Single-enzyme tests

Different bacteria produce varying spectra of enzymes. For example, some enzymes are necessary for the bacterium's individual metabolism, and some facilitate the bacterium's ability to compete with other bacteria or establish an infection. Tests that measure single bacterial enzymes are simple, rapid, and generally easy to interpret. They can be performed on organisms already grown in culture and often provide presumptive identification.

1. **Catalase test:** The enzyme catalase catalyzes the degradation of hydrogen peroxide to water and molecular oxygen ($H_2O_2 \rightarrow H_2O + O_2$). Catalase-positive organisms rapidly produce bubbles when exposed to a solution containing hydrogen peroxide (Figure 4.8). The catalase test is key in differentiating between many gram-positive organisms. For example, staphylococci are catalase positive, whereas streptococci and enterococci are catalase negative. The production of catalase is an important virulence factor because H_2O_2 is antimicrobial, and its degradation decreases the ability of neutrophils to kill invading bacteria.

2. **Oxidase test:** The enzyme cytochrome c oxidase is part of electron transport and nitrate metabolism in some bacteria. The enzyme can accept electrons from artificial substrates (such as a phenylenediamine derivative), producing a dark, oxidized product (see Figure 4.8). This test assists in differentiating between groups of gram-negative bacteria. *Pseudomonas aeruginosa*, for example, is oxidase positive.

3. **Urease:** The enzyme urease hydrolyzes urea to ammonia and carbon dioxide ($NH_2CONH_2 + H_2O \rightarrow 2NH_3 + CO_2$). The ammonia produced can be detected with pH indicators that change color in response to the increased alkalinity (see Figure 4.8). The test helps to identify certain species of Enterobacteriaceae, *Corynebacterium urealyticum*, and *Helicobacter pylori*.

4. **Coagulase test:** Coagulase is an enzyme that causes a clot to form when bacteria are incubated with plasma (see Figure 4.8). The test is used to differentiate *Staphylococcus aureus* (coagulase positive) from coagulase-negative staphylococci.

B. Automated systems

Microbiology laboratories are increasingly using automated methods to identify bacterial pathogens. For example, in the Vitek System, small plastic reagent cards containing microliter quantities of various biochemical test media in 30 wells provide a biochemical profile that allows for organism identification (Figure 4.9). An inoculum derived from cultured samples is automatically transferred into the card, and a photometer intermittently measures color changes in the card that result from the metabolic activity of the organism. The data are analyzed, stored, and printed in a computerized database. There are many commercial variants of these automated systems and several can be used for simultaneous identification and antimicrobial susceptibility determination.

C. Tests based on the presence of metabolic pathways

These tests measure the presence of metabolic pathways in a bacterial isolate, rather than a single enzyme. Commonly used assays include those for oxidation and fermentation of different carbohydrates, the ability to degrade amino acids, and use of specific substrates. A widely used manual system for rapid identification of members of the family Enterobacteriaceae and other gram-negative bacteria makes use of twenty microtubes containing substrates for various biochemical pathways. The test substrates in the microtubes are inoculated with the bacterial isolate to be identified, and, after 5 hours incubation, the metabolic profile of the organism is constructed from color changes in the microtubes. These color changes indicate the presence or absence of the bacteria's ability to metabolize a particular substrate. The results are compared with a data bank containing test results from known bacteria (Figure 4.10). The probability of a match between the test organism and known pathogens is then calculated.

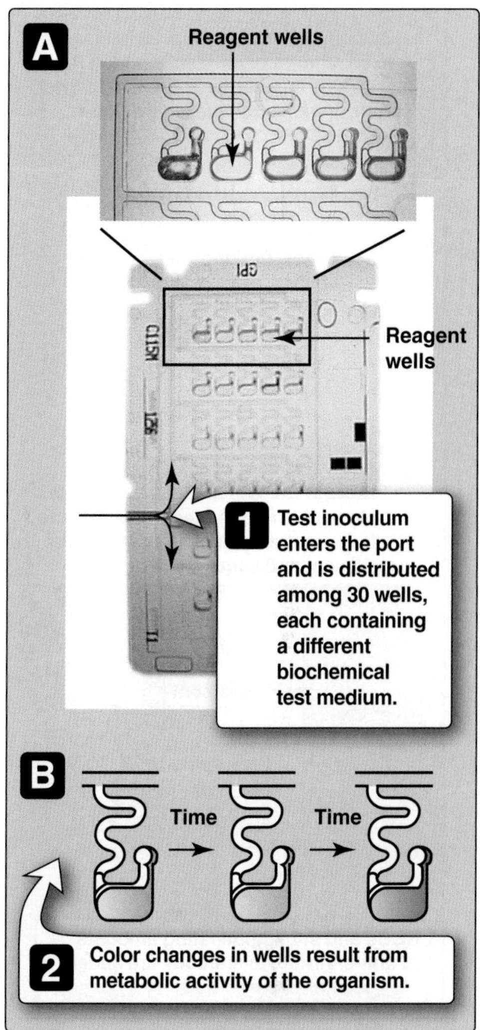

Figure 4.9
A. Vitek test card containing test wells.
B. Color of well changes with time.

VI. IMMUNOLOGIC DETECTION OF MICROORGANISMS

In the diagnosis of infectious diseases, immunologic methods take advantage of the specificity of antigen–antibody binding. For example,

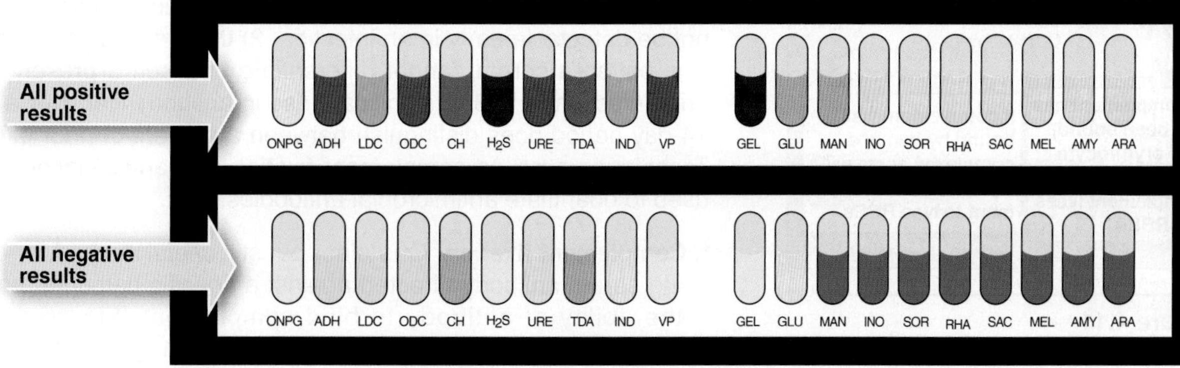

Figure 4.10
Rapid manual biochemical system for bacterial identification. Different appearances of the upper and lower pairs of wells indicate the positive or negative ability of a bacterium to utilize each substrate.

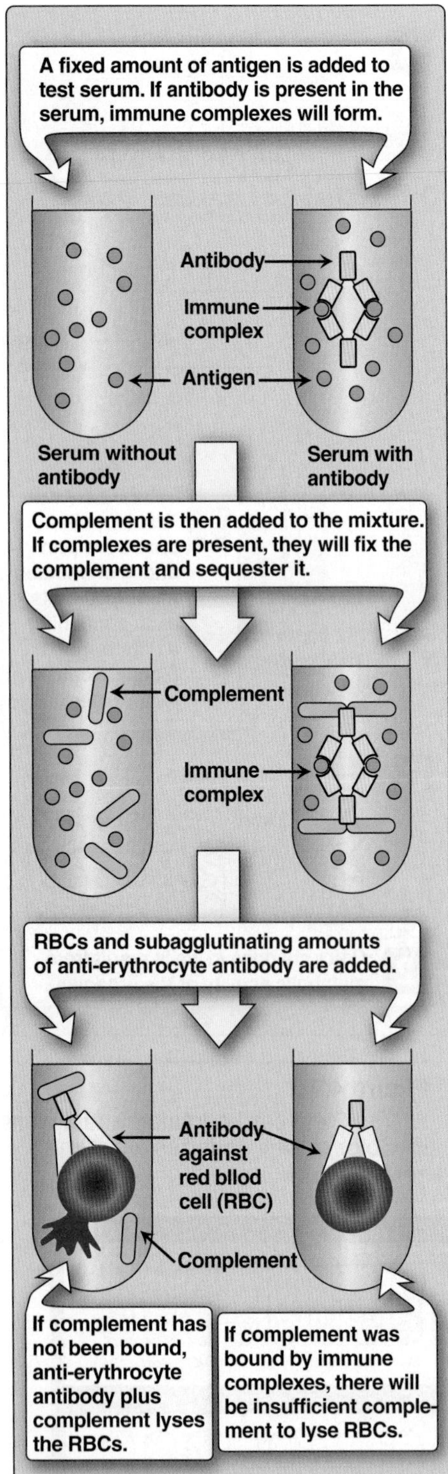

Figure 4.11
Complement fixation.

known antigens and antibodies are used as diagnostic tools in identifying microorganisms. In addition, serologic detection of a patient's immune response to infection, or antigenic or nucleic acid evidence of a pathogen in a patient's body fluids, is frequently useful. Immunologic methods are useful when the infecting microorganism is difficult or impossible to isolate or when a previous infection needs to be documented. Most methods for determining whether antibodies or antigens are present in patients' sera or other body fluids require some type of immunoassay procedure such as those described in this section.

A. Detection of microbial antigen with known antiserum

These methods of identification are often rapid and show favorable sensitivity and specificity. However, unlike microbial culturing techniques, these immunologic methods do not permit further characterization of the microorganism, such as determining its antibiotic sensitivity or characteristic metabolic patterns.

1. **Quellung reaction:** Some bacteria having capsules can be identified directly in clinical specimens by a reaction that occurs when the organisms are treated with serum containing specific antibodies (see Figure 9.10). The Quellung reaction makes the capsule more refractile and thus more visible, but the capsule does not actually swell. This method can be used for all serotypes of *S. pneumoniae*, *H. influenzae* type b, and *Neisseria meningitidis* groups A and C.

2. **Slide agglutination test:** Some microorganisms, such as *Salmonella* and *Shigella* species, can be identified by agglutination (clumping) of a suspension of bacterial cells on a microscopic slide. Agglutination occurs when a specific antibody directed against the microbial antigen is added to the suspension, causing cross-linking of the bacteria.

B. Identification of serum antibodies

Detection in a patient's serum of antibodies that are directed against microbial antigens provides evidence for a current or past infection with a specific pathogen. A discussion of the general interpretation of antibody responses includes the following rules: 1) antibody may not be detectable early in an infection, 2) the presence of antibodies in a patient's serum cannot differentiate between a present and a prior infection, and 3) a significant rise in antibody titer over a 10 to-14-day period does distinguish between a present or prior infection. Techniques such as complement fixation and agglutination can be used to quantitate antimicrobial antibodies.

1. **Complement fixation:** One older but still useful method for detecting serum antibody directed against a specific pathogen employs the ability of antibody to bind complement (Figure 4.11). A patient's serum is first incubated with antigen specific for the suspected infectious agent, followed by the addition of complement. If the patient's serum does contain immunoglobulin (Ig) G or IgM antibodies that target the specific antigen (indicating past or current infection), then the added complement will be sequestered in

an antigen–antibody–complement complex ("complement fixation"). Next, sensitized (antibody-coated) indicator sheep RBCs are added to the solution. If complement has been fixed (because the patient's serum contained antibodies against the added antigen), then little complement will be available to bind to the antibody–RBC complexes, and the cells will not lyse. If complement has not been depleted by initial antigen–antibody complexes (because the patient's serum does not contain antibodies to the specific antigen), the complement will bind to the antibody–RBC complexes, causing the cells to lyse. As hemolyzed RBCs release hemoglobin, the reaction can be monitored with a spectrophotometer.

2. **Direct agglutination:** Direct bacterial agglutination testing is sometimes ordered when a suspected pathogen is difficult or dangerous to culture in the laboratory. This test measures the ability of a patient's serum antibody to directly agglutinate specific killed (yet intact) microorganisms. This test is used to evaluate patients suspected of being infected by *Brucella abortus* or *Francisella tularensis*, among others.

3. **Direct hemagglutination:** Antibodies directed against RBCs can arise during the course of various infections. For example, such antibodies are typically found during infectious mononucleosis caused by Epstein-Barr virus (see p. 267). When uncoated (native) animal or human RBCs are used in agglutination reactions with serum from a patient infected with such an organism, antibodies to RBC antigens can be detected. The patient's antibodies cause the RBCs to clump. This test is, therefore, a direct hemagglutination reaction. In the case of some diseases, including pneumonia caused by *Mycoplasma pneumoniae*, IgM autoantibodies may develop that agglutinate human RBCs at 4°C but not at 37°C. This is termed the "cold agglutinins" test.

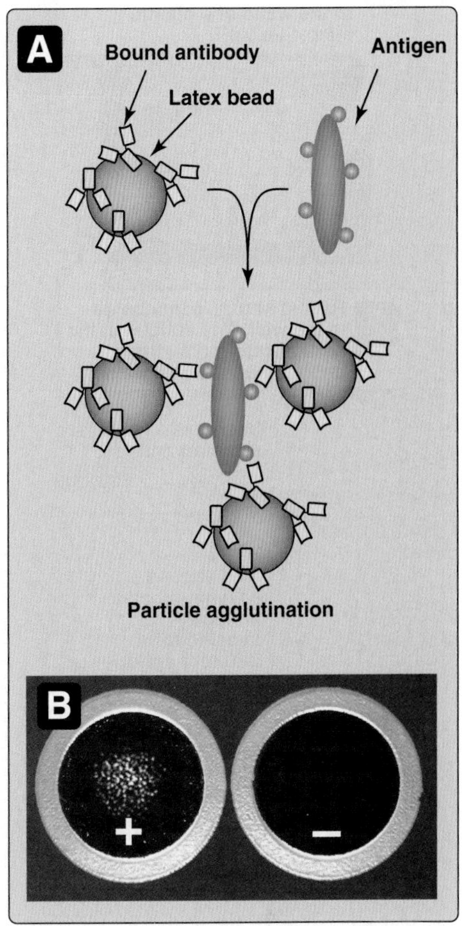

Figure 4.12
A. Schematic representation of antigens agglutinating latex beads with bound antibody. B. Photograph of agglutination reaction.

C. Other tests used to identify serum antigens or antibodies

1. **Latex agglutination test:** Latex and other particles can be readily coated with either antibody (for antigen detection) or antigen (for antibody detection). Addition of antigen to antibody-coated latex beads causes agglutination that can be visually observed (Figure 4.12). For example, such methods are used to rapidly test CSF for antigens associated with common forms of bacterial or fungal meningitis. When antigen is coated onto the latex bead, antibody from a patient's serum can be detected. Latex agglutination tests are widely used for the identification of β-hemolytic streptococci group A.

2. **Enzyme-linked immunosorbent assay:** Enzyme-linked immunosorbent assay (ELISA) is a diagnostic technique in which antibody specific for an antigen of interest is bound to the walls of a plastic microtiter well (Figure 4.13). Patient serum is then incubated in the wells, and any antigen in the serum is bound by the antibody on the well walls. The wells are then washed, and a second antibody is added. This one is also specific for the antigen but

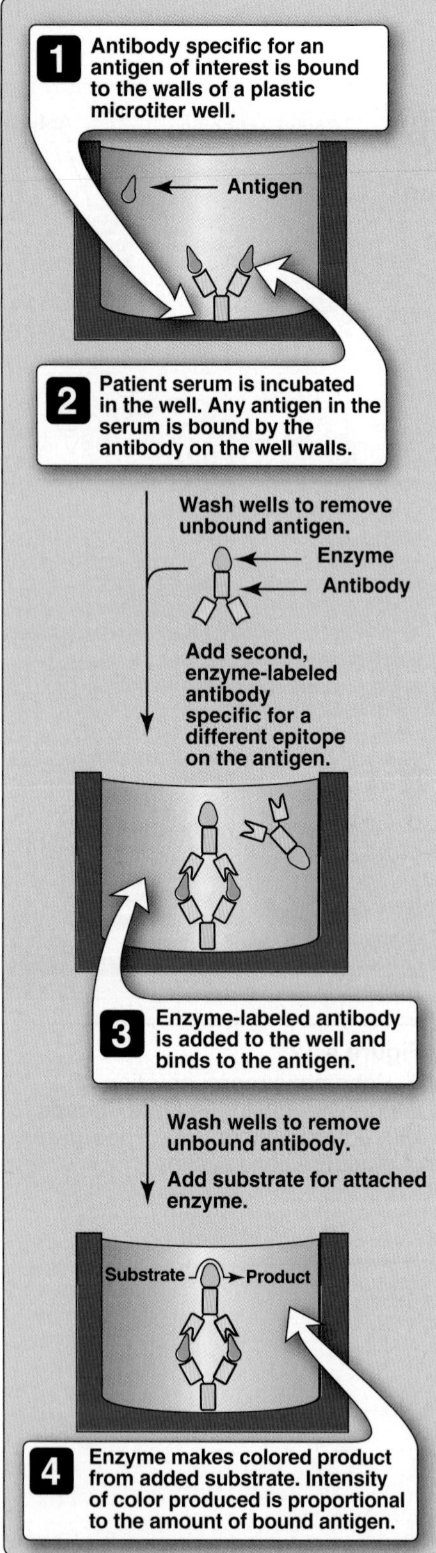

1
Antibody specific for an antigen of interest is bound to the walls of a plastic microtiter well.
Antigen
2
Patient serum is incubated in the well. Any antigen in the serum is bound by the antibody on the well walls.
Wash wells to remove unbound antigen.
Enzyme
Antibody
Add second, enzyme-labeled antibody specific for a different epitope on the antigen.
3
Enzyme-labeled antibody is added to the well and binds to the antigen.
Wash wells to remove unbound antibody.
Add substrate for attached enzyme.
Substrate
Product
4
Enzyme makes colored product from added substrate. Intensity of color produced is proportional to the amount of bound antigen.

Figure 4.13
Principle of enzyme-linked immunosorbent assay (ELISA).

recognizes epitopes different from those bound by the first antibody. After incubation, the wells are again washed, removing any unattached antibody. Attached to the second antibody is an enzyme, which, when presented with its substrate, produces a colored product, the intensity of the color produced being proportional to the amount of bound antigen. ELISAs can also be used to detect or quantitate antibody in a patient's serum. In this instance, the wells are coated with antigen specific for the antibody in question. The patient's serum is allowed to react with the bound antigen, the wells are washed, and a secondary antibody (that recognizes the initial antibody) conjugated to a color product–producing enzyme is added to the well. After a final washing, substrate for the bound enzyme is added to the well, and the intensity of the colored product can be measured.

3. **Fluorescent-antibody tests:** Organisms in clinical samples can be detected directly by specific antibodies coupled to a fluorescent compound such as fluorescein. In the direct immunofluorescence antibody technique, a sample of concentrated body fluid (for example, CSF or serum), tissue scraping (for example, skin), or cells in tissue culture is incubated with a fluorescein-labeled antibody directed against a specific pathogen. The labeled antibody bound to the microorganism absorbs ultraviolet light and emits visible fluorescence that can be detected using a fluorescence microscope. A variation of the technique, the indirect immunofluorescence antibody technique, involves the use of two antibodies. The first is unlabeled antibody (the target antibody), which binds a specific microbial antigen in a sample such as those described above. This clinical sample is subsequently stained with a fluorescent antibody that recognizes the target antibody. Because a number of labeled antibodies can bind to each target antibody, the fluorescence from the stained microorganism is intensified.

VII. NUCLEIC ACID–BASED TESTS

The most widely used methods for detecting microbial DNA fall into three categories: 1) direct hybridization (nonamplified assay), 2) amplification methods using the polymerase chain reaction (PCR)[1] or one its variations, and 3) DNA microarrays. Although not likely to completely replace culture techniques in the near future, nucleic acid–based tests for the diagnosis of infectious diseases are gaining wider acceptance as more products approved by the Food and Drug Administration become commercially available.

A. Direct detection of pathogens without target amplification

This highly specific method of pathogen detection involves identification of the DNA of the pathogen in a patient sample or, more commonly, organisms isolated in culture. The basic strategy is to detect a relatively short sequence of nucleotide bases of DNA (target

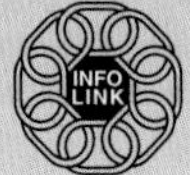

[1]See Chapter 33 ***Lippincott's Illustrated Reviews: Biochemistry*** for a more detailed presentation of the techniques used in molecular biology.

sequence) that is unique to the pathogen. This is done by hybridization with a probe, a single-stranded piece of DNA (usually labeled with a fluorescent molecule) containing a complementary sequence of bases. [Note: In bacteria, DNA sequences coding for 16S ribosomal RNA sequences (rRNA) are commonly used targets because each microorganism contains multiple copies of its specific 16S rRNA gene, thereby increasing the sensitivity of the assay.] When the probe is bound to the target, the label will give off a signal after the free probe is washed away. A limitation of standard direct probe hybridization is the requirement for a 10^4 or greater number of copies of target nucleic acid for detection.

B. Nucleic acid amplification for diagnosis

Nucleic acid amplification overcomes the principal limitation of direct detection with nucleic acid probes by selectively amplifying specific DNA targets present in low concentrations. The bacterial 16S rRNA gene has emerged as the most useful marker for microbial detection and identification. Ribosomal DNA genes contain highly conserved areas (that are used as targets for primers) separated by internal transcribed sequences containing variable, species-specific regions. These sequences are like fingerprints. Comparing certain locations on a 16s rRNA gene with a database of known organisms allows the identification of organisms. For virus detection, primers are constructed to target highly conserved DNA or RNA sequences unique to the pathogen. Amplification and detection of the viral genomes are highly sensitive and are especially valuable when the viral load is too low to be detected by culture or when results are needed rapidly.

1. **Conventional polymerase chain reaction:** In this method, DNA polymerase repetitively amplifies targeted portions of DNA (ideally sequences that are highly conserved and unique to the pathogen). Each cycle of amplification doubles the amount of DNA in the sample, leading to an exponential increase in DNA with repeated cycles of amplification. The amplified DNA sequence can then be analyzed by gel electrophoresis, Southern blotting, or direct sequence determination.

2. **Real-time polymerase chain reaction**: This variant of PCR combines nucleic acid amplification and fluorescent detection of the amplified product in the same closed automated system. Real-time PCR limits the risk of contamination and provides a rapid (30–40 minutes) diagnosis. Real-time PCR is a quantitative method and allows the determination of the concentrtion of pathogens in various samples.

3. **Advantages of polymerase chain reaction:** Methods employing nucleic acid–amplification techniques have a major advantage over direct detection with nucleic acid probes because amplification methods allow specific DNA or RNA target sequences of the pathogen to be amplified millions of times without having to culture the microorganism itself for extended periods. PCR also permits identification of noncultivatable or slow-growing microorganisms, such as mycobacteria, anaerobic bacteria, and viruses. Nucleic acid–amplification methods are sensitive, specific

ORGANISM
Bacillus anthracis
Bordetella pertussis
Chlamydia trachomatis
Cytomegalovirus
Enterovirus
Epstein-Barr virus
Hepatitis B virus
Hepatitis C virus
Herpes simplex virus
Human immunodeficiency virus
Human papilloma virus
Methicillin-resistant *Staphylococcus aureus*
Mycobacterium tuberculosis
Neisseria gonorrhoeae
SARS coronavirus
Vancomycin-resistant enterococci
Varicella zoster virus
Variola virus
West Nile virus

Figure 4.14
Commercial nucleic acid–amplification systems for diagnosis of infectious diseases. The table is not intended to be all inclusive.

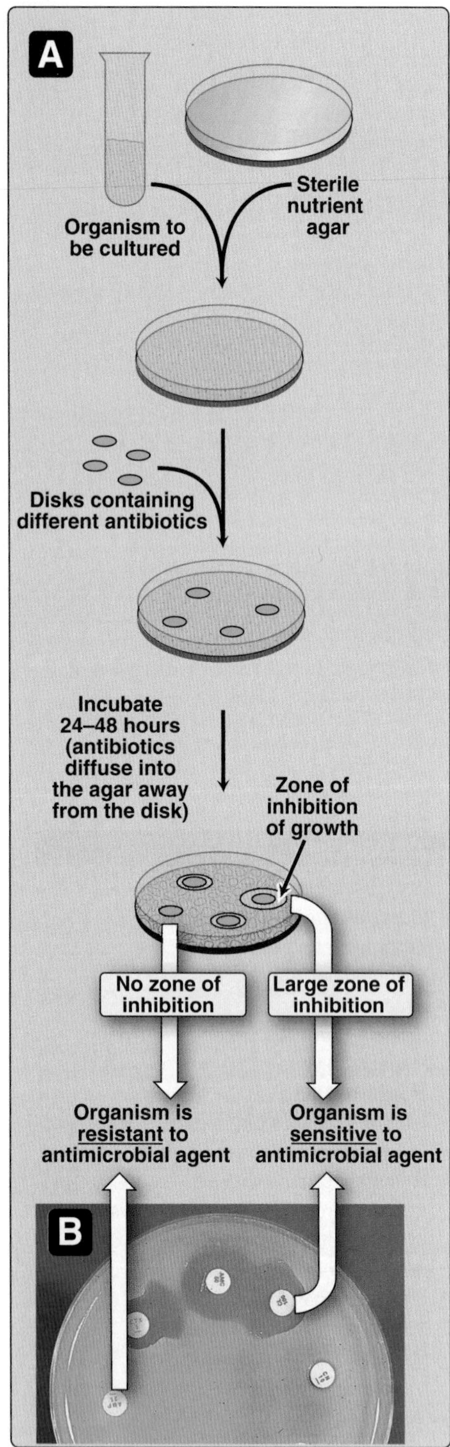

Figure 4.15
A. Outline of disk-diffusion method for determining the sensitivity of bacteria to antimicrobial agents.
B. Photograph of culture plate with antibiotic-impregnated disks.

for the target organism, and are unaffected by the prior administration of antibiotics.

4. **Applications:** Nucleic acid–amplification techniques are generally quick, easy, and accurate. A major use of these techniques is for the detection of organisms that cannot be grown *in vitro* or for which current culture techniques are insensitive. Moreover, they are useful in the detection of organisms that require complex media or cell cultures and/or prolonged incubation times (Figure 4.14).

5. **Limitations:** PCR amplification is limited by the occurrence of spurious false-positives due to cross-contamination with other microorganisms' nucleic acid. PCR tests are often costly and require skilled personnel.

C. DNA microarrays

Although microarrays are now routinely used to measure gene expression, the technique is an emerging technology in the diagnostic microbiology laboratory. Microarrays have the unprecedented potential to simultaneously detect and identify many pathogens from the same specimen. For example, an oligonucleotide microarray targeting the 16S rRNA gene has been developed for the detection of a panel of forty predominant human intestinal bacterial pathogens in human fecal samples.

1. **Diagnostic use of microarrays:** A DNA microarray consists of microscopic spots of immobilized DNA oligonucleotides, each containing specific DNA sequences, known as probes. The probes are constructed to be complementary to specific gene sequences of interest in suspected pathogens. DNA of the microorganism obtained from a clinical specimen, known as the target, is extracted and amplified using PCR and fluorescent labeling techniques. The target DNA is exposed to the probe microarray. If the labeled DNA from the microorganism and the immobilized probe have a complementary base sequence, they will hybridize, thereby increasing fluorescence intensity. After washing off of nonspecific bonding sequences, only strongly paired strands will remain hybridized and fluoresce. The intensity of fluorescence at each spot is a measure of the amount of that particular microbial DNA in the sample. Correlating fluorescence with the identity of the probe allows for the detection and quantitation of specific pathogens.

VIII. SUSCEPTIBILITY TESTING

After a pathogen is cultured, its sensitivity to specific antibiotics serves as a guide in choosing antimicrobial therapy. Some pathogens, such as *Streptococcus pyogenes* and *N. meningitidis*, usually have predictable sensitivity patterns to certain antibiotics. In contrast, most gram-negative bacilli, enterococci, and staphylococcal species show unpredictable sensitivity patterns to various antibiotics and require susceptibility testing to determine appropriate antimicrobial therapy.

A. Disk-diffusion method

The classic qualitative method to test susceptibility to antibiotics has been the Kirby-Bauer disk-diffusion method, in which disks with exact amounts of different antimicrobial agents are placed on culture dishes inoculated with the microorganism to be tested. The organism's growth (resistance to the drug) or lack of growth (sensitivity to the drug) is then monitored (Figure 4.15). In addition, the size of the zone of growth inhibition is influenced by the concentration and rate of diffusion of the antibiotic on the disk. The disk-diffusion method is useful when susceptibility to an unusual antibiotic, not available in automated systems, is to be determined.

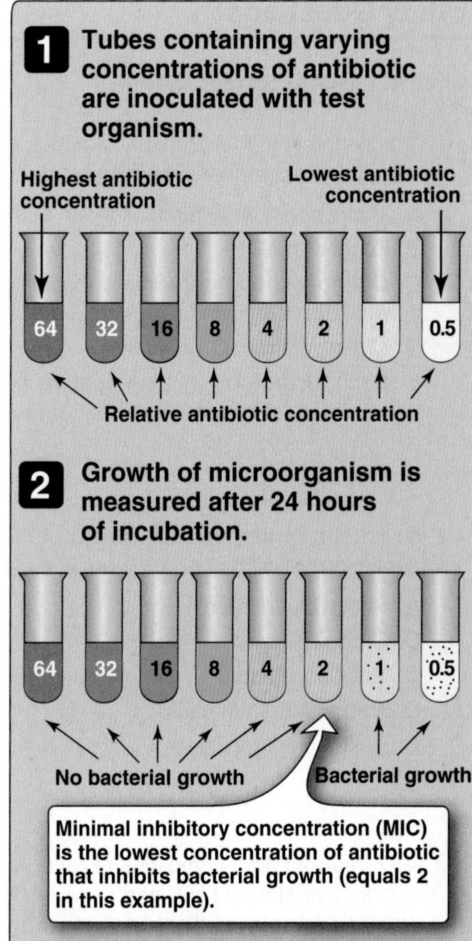

Figure 4.16
Determination of minimal inhibitory concentration (MIC) of an antibiotic.

B. Minimal inhibitory concentration

Quantitative testing uses a dilution technique in which tubes containing serial dilutions of an antibiotic are inoculated with the organism whose sensitivity to that antibiotic is to be tested. The tubes are incubated and later observed to determine the minimal inhibitory concentration (MIC) of the antibiotic necessary to prevent bacterial growth (Figure 4.16). [Note: MICs are now automated and often done simultaneously with automated biochemical identifications.] To provide effective antimicrobial therapy, the clinically obtainable antibiotic concentration in body fluids should be greater than the MIC. Quantitative susceptibility testing may be necessary for patients who either fail to respond to antimicrobial therapy or who relapse during therapy. In some clinical cases, the minimal bactericidal concentration may need to be determined. This is the lowest concentration of antibiotic that kills 100 percent of the bacteria, rather than simply inhibiting growth.

C. Bacteriostatic versus bactericidal drugs

As noted above, antimicrobial drugs may be bacteriostatic or bactericidal. Bacteriostatic drugs arrest the growth and replication of bacteria at serum levels achievable in the patient, thereby limiting the spread of infection while the body's immune system attacks, immobilizes, and eliminates the pathogens. If the drug is removed before the immune system has scavenged the organisms, enough viable organisms may remain to begin a second cycle of infection. For example, Figure 4.17 shows a laboratory experiment in which the growth of bacteria is arrested by the addition of a bacteriostatic agent. Note that viable organisms remain even in the presence of the bacteriostatic drug. By contrast, addition of a bactericidal agent kills bacteria, and the total number of viable organisms decreases. Although practical, this classification may be too simplistic because it is possible for an antibiotic to be bacteriostatic for one organism and bactericidal for another (for example, chloramphenicol is bacteriostatic against gram-negative rods and bactericidal against pneumococci).

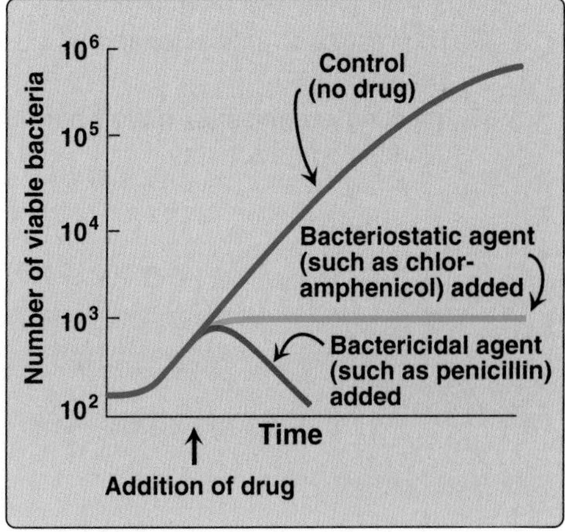

Figure 4.17
Effects of bactericidal and bacteriostatic drugs on the growth of bacteria *in vitro*.

Study Questions

Choose the ONE correct answer.

4.1 Choose the item that correctly matches the microorganism with an appropriate stain or preparation.

A. *Mycobacterium tuberculosis* with India ink
B. Fungi with KOH
C. *Cryptococcus neoformans* in cerebrospinal fluid with Ziehl-Neelsen (classic acid-fast stain)
D. *Chlamydia* with Gram stain
E. *Escherichia coli* (gram-negative bacterium) with crystal violet followed by treatment with acetone

Correct answer = B. Treatment with KOH dissolves host cells and bacteria, allowing fungi to be visualized. *Mycobacterium tuberculosis* is stained by the Ziehl-Neelsen stain (the classic acid-fast stain). *Cryptococcus neoformans* in cerebrospinal fluid is visualized with India ink. Organisms that are intracellular, such as *Chlamydia*, or that lack a cell wall, such as *Mycoplasma* or *Ureaplasma*, are not readily detected by Gram stain. Most bacteria stain purple with crystal violet and iodine. If the stained cells are then treated with acetone, gram-positive organisms retain the stain, whereas gram-negative species, such as *Escherichia coli,* lose the stain, becoming colorless. Visualization of *E. coli* requires the addition of the counterstain safranin, which stains gram-negative bacteria pink or red.

4.2 Which one of the following media is most suitable for identifying *Neisseria gonorrhoeae* in a cervical swab?

A. Sheep blood agar
B. Chocolate agar
C. MacConkey agar
D. Thayer-Martin medium
E. Hektoen enteric agar

Correct answer = D. Thayer-Martin medium, which is composed of chocolate agar supplemented with several antibiotics, suppresses the growth of nonpathogenic *Neisseria* and other normal and abnormal flora, but permits the growth of gonococcus. Sheep blood agar supports the growth of most bacteria, both gram-positive and gram-negative. Chocolate agar provides the growth requirements for fastidious organisms such as *Haemophilus influenzae* or *Neisseria gonorrhoeae*, as well as for most other less-fastidious bacteria. MacConkey agar supports most gram-negative rods, especially the Enterobacteriaceae, but inhibits growth of gram-positive organisms and some fastidious gram-negative bacteria, such as *Haemophilus* and *Neisseria* species. Hektoen enteric agar is also a selective medium often used to culture *Salmonella* and *Shigella* species.

4.3 A 57-year-old man complains of fever, headache, confusion, aversion to light, and neck rigidity. A presumptive diagnosis of bacterial meningitis is made. Antimicrobial therapy should be initiated after which one of the following occurrences?

A. Fever is reduced with antipyretic drugs.
B. Samples of blood and cerebrospinal fluid have been taken.
C. A Gram stain has been performed.
D. The results of antibacterial drug susceptibility tests are available.
E. Infecting organism(s) have been identified by the microbiology laboratory.

Correct answer = B. Bacterial meningitis is a medical emergency that requires immediate diagnosis and treatment. Specimens for possible microbial identification must be obtained before drugs are administered whenever possible. Therapy should not be delayed until laboratory results are available.

Vaccines and Antimicrobial Agents

5

I. OVERVIEW

A vaccine is a biological preparation that enhances immunity to a particular disease. A vaccine typically contains an agent that resembles a disease-causing microorganism and is often made from weakened or killed forms of the microbe, its toxins, or one of its surface proteins. The agent stimulates the body's immune system to produce specific antibodies or a cellular immune response that destroys or neutralizes the microorganism or its toxins. Immunization against hepatitis A and B, diphtheria, tetanus, pertussis, *Haemophilus influenzae* type b (Hib), polio, rotavirus, measles, mumps, rubella, varicella-zoster virus (VZV), pneumococcus, influenza, meningococcus, and human papillomavirus is considered the standard for the United States. [Note: The reader is reminded of the common names for some childhood diseases discussed in this chapter: pertussis = whooping cough; rubella = German measles; rubeola = measles; varicella = chickenpox.] The availability of vaccines has resulted in the global eradication of smallpox and the virtual elimination of poliomyelitis, tetanus, and diphtheria in the United States (Figure 5.1). Protection of individuals from disease by vaccination can take two forms: passive or active immunization.

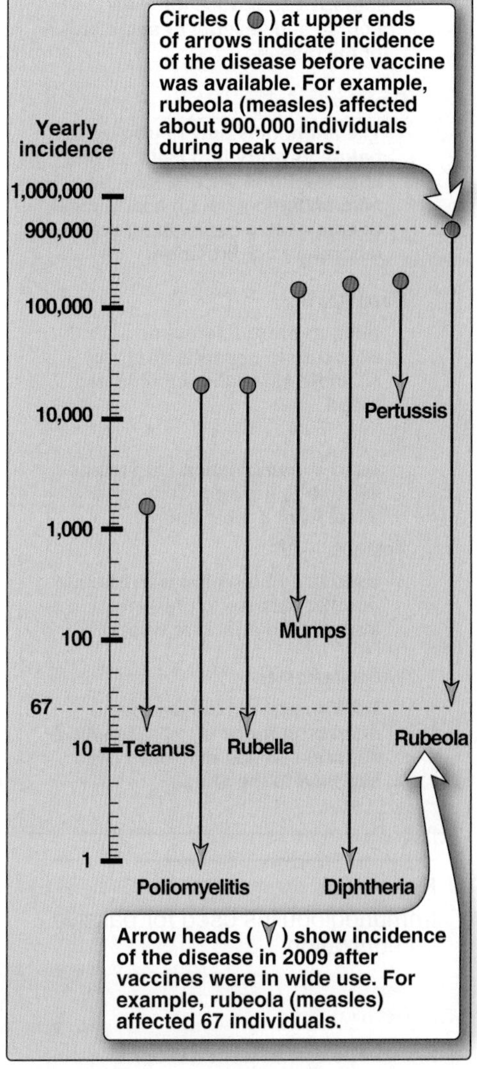

Figure 5.1
Incidence of vaccine-preventable diseases in the United States at their highest incidence and in 2009. [Note: Y axis is a logarithmic scale.]

II. PASSIVE IMMUNIZATION

Passive immunization is achieved by injecting a recipient with preformed immunoglobulins (Igs) obtained from human (or, occasionally, equine) serum. Passive immunization provides immediate protection to individuals who have been exposed to an infectious organism and who lack active immunity to that pathogen. Because passive immunization does not activate the immune system, it generates no memory response. Passive immunity dissipates after a few weeks to months as the Igs are cleared from the recipient's serum. Two basic formulations of prepared Igs have been developed: one from the serum of pooled human donors and one from serum obtained from hyperimmune donors (Figure 5.2).

III. ACTIVE IMMUNIZATION

Active immunization is achieved by injection of viable or nonviable pathogens, or purified pathogen product, prompting the immune system to respond as if the body were being attacked by an intact infectious

STANDARD HUMAN IMMUNOGLOBULINS

Hepatitis A or measles

Used in individuals who may have been exposed to these viruses.

HYPERIMMUNE HUMAN IMMUNOGLOBULINS

Botulism

Depending on the time lapse between exposure to the toxin and administration of the antitoxin, therapy can reduce the time course and severity of symptoms of the disease.

Diphtheria

The antibodies only neutralize toxin before its entry into cells, so it is important that the antitoxin be administered as soon as a clinical diagnosis has been made, before laboratory confirmation.

Hepatitis B

Used to prevent infection after exposure to hepatitis virus, for example, through contaminated blood.

Rabies

Used in combination with rabies vaccine to prevent rabies after a bite from a rabid animal.

Tetanus

Used in combination with tetanus booster vaccine to prevent tetanus after a deep puncture wound.

Varicella zoster

Used to prevent disseminated disease in those who are immunosuppressed and may have been exposed to the virus.

Figure 5.2
Immunoglobulins used for passive immunization.

microorganism. Whereas passive immunization provides immediate protection, active immunization may require several days to months to become effective. Active immunization leads to prolonged immunity and is generally preferred over the short-term immunity provided by passive immunization with preformed Igs. Simultaneous administration of active and passive immunizations may be required after exposure to certain infections such as hepatitis B.

A. Formulations for active immunization

Vaccines are 1) live, attenuated microorganisms; 2) killed microorganisms; 3) microbial extracts; 4) vaccine conjugates; or 5) inactivated toxins (toxoids). Both bacterial and viral pathogens are targeted by these diverse means.

1. **Live pathogens:** When live pathogens are used, they are attenuated (weakened) to preclude clinical consequences of infection. Attenuated microbes reproduce in the recipient, typically leading to a more robust and long-lasting immune response than can be obtained through vaccination with killed organisms. However, with live, attenuated vaccines, there is a possibility that the attenuated vaccine strain will revert to an active pathogen after administration to the patient. For example, vaccine-associated poliomyelitis occurs following administration of approximately 1 of every 2.4 million doses of live polio vaccine. All recent cases of polio in the United States are vaccine associated. Also, live, attenuated vaccines should not be given to immunocompromised individuals because there is the potential for a disseminated infection.

2. **Killed microorganisms:** Killed vaccines have the advantage over attenuated microorganisms in that they pose no risk of vaccine-associated infection. As noted above, killed organisms often provide a weak or short-lived immune response. Some vaccines, such as polio and typhoid vaccines, are available both in live and killed versions.

3. **Microbial extracts:** Instead of using whole organisms, vaccines can be composed of antigen molecules (often those located on the surface of the microorganism) extracted from the pathogen or prepared by recombinant DNA techniques. The efficacy of these vaccines varies. In some instances, the vaccine antigen is present on all strains of the organism, and the vaccine, thus, protects against infection by all strains. With other pathogens, such as pneumococcus, protective antibody is produced against only a specific capsular polysaccharide, one among more than 80 distinct types. Immunity to one polysaccharide type does not confer immunity to any other type. For this reason, the pneumococcal vaccine is composed of 23 different polysaccharides, comprising the antigens produced by the most common types of disease-causing pneumococci. Some pathogens, such as influenza virus, frequently change their antigenic determinants. Therefore, influenza virus vaccines must also change regularly to counter the different antigens of influenza A and B virus strains in circulation. In the case of rhinovirus infections (the leading cause of the common cold) at least 100 types of the virus are known. It is not

feasible to develop a vaccine that confers protection to this large number of antigenic types.

4. **Vaccine conjugates:** Vaccines can produce humoral immunity through B cell proliferation leading to antibody production, which may or may not involve helper T cells. For example, pneumococcal polysaccharide and the polysaccharide of Hib induce B-cell type-specific protective antibody without involvement of helper T cells. These T cell–independent responses are characterized by low antibody titers, particularly in children younger than age 18 months. Thus, conventional *H. influenzae* polysaccharide vaccine does not provide protection for children ages 3 to 18 months. Consequently, this organism has, in the past, produced severe infections in this age group. However, by covalently conjugating the *Haemophilus* polysaccharide to a protein antigen, such as diphtheria toxoid, *H. influenzae* vaccines produce a robust T cell–dependent antibody response even in 3-month-old infants. Figure 5.3 shows the decreased incidence of *H. influenzae* disease following introduction of conjugated vaccine. Conjugate vaccines are also currently available for *Streptococcus pneumoniae* and *Neisseria meningitidis.* Figure 5.4 shows the favorable antibody response to conjugated polysaccharide obtained from *N. meningitidis*.

5. **Toxoids:** These are derivatives of bacterial exotoxins produced by chemically altering the natural toxin or by engineering bacteria to produce harmless variants of the toxin. Vaccines containing toxoid are used when the pathogenicity of the organism is a result of the secreted toxin. Depending on the specific vaccine, administration is generally via intramuscular or subcutaneous routes. Figure 5.5 shows the formulation of some of the vaccines currently licensed in the United States. Details of the various vaccines are presented in the chapters in which the target microorganisms are discussed.

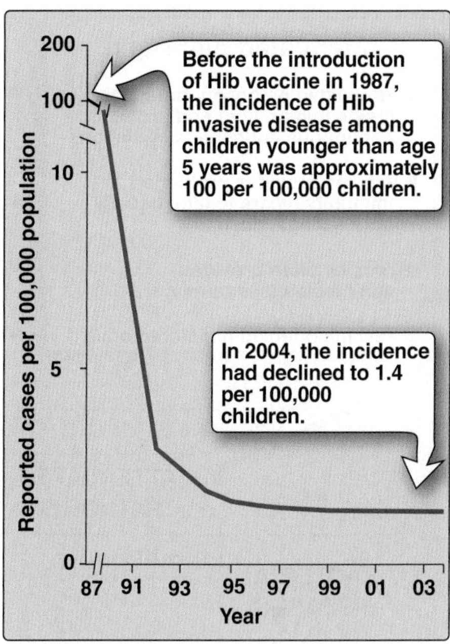

Figure 5.3
Incidence of infection in children due to *Haemophilus influenzae* type b (Hib) following introduction of conjugate vaccine in 1987.

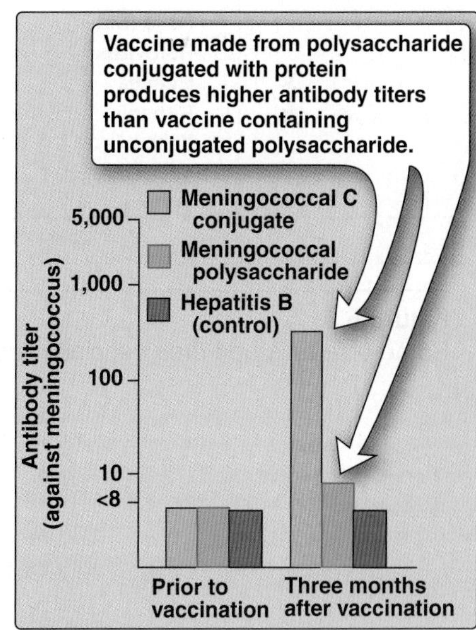

Figure 5.4
Serum bactericidal antibody response to vaccination with meningococcal C conjugate, meningococcal polysaccharide, and hepatitis B vaccine (control) in children ages 15 to 23 months.

B. Types of immune response to vaccines

Vaccines containing killed pathogens (such as hepatitis A or the Salk polio vaccine) or antigenic components of pathogens (such as hepatitis B subunit vaccine) do not enter host cells, thereby eliciting a primary B cell–mediated humoral response. These antibodies are ineffective in attacking intracellular organisms. By contrast, attenuated live vaccines (usually viruses) do penetrate cells. This results in the production of intracellular antigens that are displayed on the surface of the infected cell, prompting a cytotoxic T-cell response, which is effective in eliminating intracellular pathogens.

C. Effect of age on efficacy of immunization

1. **Passive immunity from mother:** Newborns receive serum IgG antibodies from their mothers, which gives them temporary protection against those diseases to which the mother was immune. In addition, maternal milk also contains secretory antibodies that provide some protection against gastrointestinal (GI) and respiratory tract infections.

Attenuated pathogen

- Attenuated pathogen multiplies inside human host and provides continuous antigenic stimulation.
- Vaccine provides prolonged immunity (years to life), usually after a single dose.
- Vaccine often provides cell-mediated immunity.
- Vaccine often administered orally.

Killed pathogen

- Killed pathogen does not multiply in the human host; the immune response is determined by the antigen content of the vaccine.
- Multiple doses of vaccine are required, with subsequent booster doses.
- Vaccine provides little cell-mediated immunity.
- Vaccine is administered by injection.

Microbial extracts or products of pathogens

- Instead of using whole organisms, vaccines can be composed of antigenic molecules extracted from the pathogen, from an acellular (noninfectious) filtrate of the culture medium in which the organism was grown, or produced by recombinant DNA techniques.
- Vaccines can be prepared against toxoids (derivatives of exotoxins). These are used when the pathogenicity of the organism is the result of the secreted toxin.

	DISEASE OR VACCINE COMPONENTS		
	ATTENUATED PATHOGEN	KILLED PATHOGEN	MICROBIAL EXTRACTS OR PRODUCTS OF PATHOGENS
BACTERIAL DISEASES	Typhoid fever	Cholera Pertussis Plague Q Fever Typhoid fever	Anthrax (noninfectious culture filtrate) Diphtheria (toxoid) *Haemophilus influenzae* type b meningitis (capsule) Meningococcal meningitis (capsule) Pertussis (acellular *Bordetella pertussis* antigen) Pneumococcal pneumonia (capsule) Tetanus (toxoid)
VIRAL DISEASES	Adenovirus infections Measles Mumps Polio (Sabin) Rotovirus Rubella Rubeola Yellow fever Varicella zoster Variola	Hepatitis A Influenza (whole virus) Japanese encephalitis Polio (Salk) Rabies	Hepatitis B (inactivated surface antigen; recombinant antigen)

Conjugated polysaccharide vaccines

- Covalent binding (conjugation) of an antigenic polysaccharide to a protein enhances the immune response to these vaccines, particularly in children younger than age 2 years.

Figure 5.5
Some diseases and their vaccines licensed for use in humans in the United States.

2. **Active immunization:** The infant's antibody-producing capacity develops slowly during the first year of life. Although the immune system is not fully developed, it is desirable to begin immunization at age 2 months because diseases are common in this age group and can be particularly severe (for example, pertussis, *H. influenzae* meningitis). As with infants, older adults have a reduced antibody response to vaccines.

D. Adverse reactions to active vaccination

Adverse consequences of vaccinations range from mild to severe and even life threatening (Figure 5.6). Symptoms vary among individuals and with the nature of the vaccination. Among the most common and mildest consequences of immunization are tenderness and swelling at the site of injection and a mild fever.

IV. BACTERIAL VACCINES

Vaccines against commonly encountered bacterial pathogens are summarized in Figure 5.7. A complete description of the vaccine schedule is available on the Centers for Disease Control Web site, www.cdc.gov. Vaccines with more specialized indications are described below.

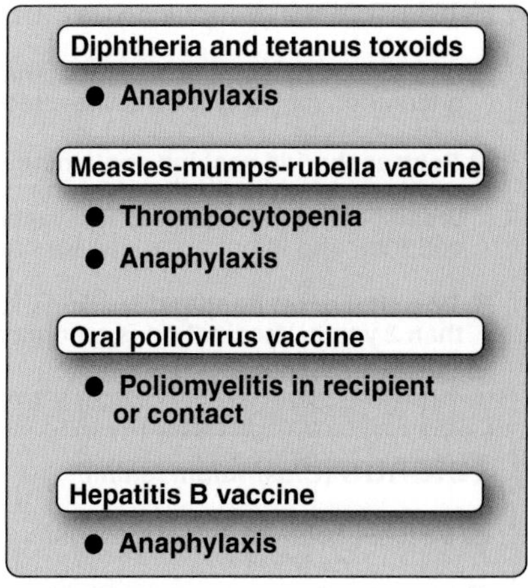

Figure 5.6
Rare adverse effects associated with childhood vaccines.

A. Less common bacterial pathogens

1. **Anthrax (*Bacillus anthracis*):** Anthrax vaccine consists of a non-infectious sterile filtrate from the culture of an attenuated strain of *B. anthracis* that contains no dead bacteria. The filtrate is adsorbed to an adjuvant, aluminum hydroxide. [Note: Adjuvants are substances that when injected with an antigen, serve to enhance the immunogenicity of that antigen.] The incidence of all forms of naturally occurring anthrax is low, particularly the inhalation form of the disease. Thus, there is no opportunity to conduct field trials of the vaccine against inhalation anthrax, the form most likely to be used in a biologic attack. Safety and efficacy of the vaccine are supported by studies in nonhuman primates in which efficacy was close to 100 percent. The vaccine is recommended for goat hair and wool mill workers, veterinarians, laboratory workers, and livestock handlers who are at risk as a result of occupational exposure. Military personnel are vaccinated against anthrax as well.

2. **Cholera (*Vibrio cholerae*):** The vaccine contains killed bacteria and is given to individuals traveling to areas with increased risk of acquiring cholera.

3. **Typhoid fever (*Salmonella typhi*):** The most commonly used vaccine contains an attenuated recombinant strain of *S. typhi*. It is given to individuals living in or traveling to high-risk areas and to members of the military.

4. **Plague (*Yersinia pestis*):** The vaccine contains killed bacteria and is given to high-risk individuals.

V. VIRAL VACCINES

Immunity to viral infection requires an immune response to antigens located on the surface of the viral particles or on virus-infected cells. For enveloped viruses, these antigens are often surface glycoproteins. The main limitation of viral vaccines occurs with viruses that show a genetically unstable antigenicity (that is, they display antigenic determinants that continuously vary, such as with influenza viruses or the human immunodeficiency virus [HIV]). Common viral pathogens for which there are vaccines include the following.

A. Hepatitis A

Formalin-inactivated whole virus vaccine produces antibody levels in adults similar to those observed following natural infection and

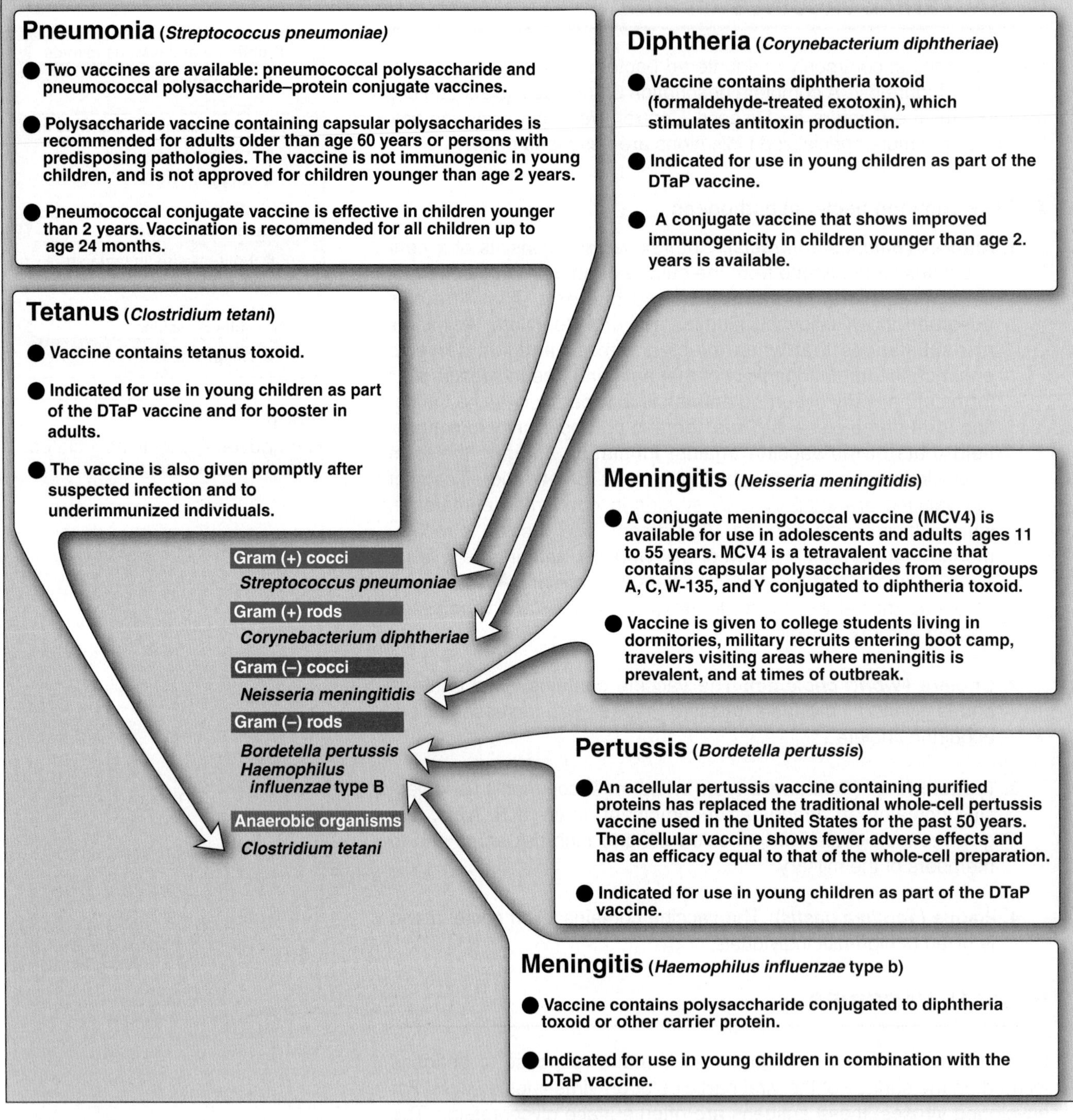

Pneumonia (Streptococcus pneumoniae)
Two vaccines are available: pneumococcal polysaccharide and pneumococcal polysaccharide–protein conjugate vaccines.
Polysaccharide vaccine containing capsular polysaccharides is recommended for adults older than age 60 years or persons with predisposing pathologies. The vaccine is not immunogenic in young children, and is not approved for children younger than age 2 years.
Pneumococcal conjugate vaccine is effective in children younger than 2 years. Vaccination is recommended for all children up to age 24 months.
Diphtheria (Corynebacterium diphtheriae)
Vaccine contains diphtheria toxoid (formaldehyde-treated exotoxin), which stimulates antitoxin production.
Indicated for use in young children as part of the DTaP vaccine.
A conjugate vaccine that shows improved immunogenicity in children younger than age 2. years is available.
Tetanus (Clostridium tetani)
Vaccine contains tetanus toxoid.
Indicated for use in young children as part of the DTaP vaccine and for booster in adults.
The vaccine is also given promptly after suspected infection and to underimmunized individuals.
Gram (+) cocci
Streptococcus pneumoniae
Gram (+) rods
Corynebacterium diphtheriae
Gram (–) cocci
Neisseria meningitidis
Gram (–) rods
Bordetella pertussis
Haemophilus influenzae type B
Anaerobic organisms
Clostridium tetani
Meningitis (Neisseria meningitidis)
A conjugate meningococcal vaccine (MCV4) is available for use in adolescents and adults ages 11 to 55 years. MCV4 is a tetravalent vaccine that contains capsular polysaccharides from serogroups A, C, W-135, and Y conjugated to diphtheria toxoid.
Vaccine is given to college students living in dormitories, military recruits entering boot camp, travelers visiting areas where meningitis is prevalent, and at times of outbreak.
Pertussis (Bordetella pertussis)
An acellular pertussis vaccine containing purified proteins has replaced the traditional whole-cell pertussis vaccine used in the United States for the past 50 years. The acellular vaccine shows fewer adverse effects and has an efficacy equal to that of the whole-cell preparation.
Indicated for use in young children as part of the DTaP vaccine.
Meningitis (Haemophilus influenzae type b)
Vaccine contains polysaccharide conjugated to diphtheria toxoid or other carrier protein.
Indicated for use in young children in combination with the DTaP vaccine.

Figure 5.7
Summary of common vaccines against bacterial diseases. DTaP = diphtheria and tetanus toxoids and acellular pertussis vaccine.

approximately 15 times those achieved by passive injection of immunoglobulin. Projections indicate that immunity to hepatitis A virus will probably last for approximately 10 years after two doses of vaccine. The vaccine is indicated for travelers to endemic areas, men who have sex with men, injecting drug users, and daycare workers. Currently in the United States, hepatitis A virus vaccination is not recommended for children younger than age 2 years because residual anti-hepatitis A passively acquired from the mother may interfere with vaccine immunogenicity.

B. Hepatitis B

The current vaccine contains recombinant hepatitis surface antigen. Efficacy is 95 to 99 percent in healthy infants, children, and young adults. Its use is indicated for healthcare workers in contact with blood and persons residing in an area with a high rate of endemic disease. Igs obtained from hyperimmunized humans can provide passive immunity after accidental exposure (for example, from a needlestick or for the neonate of an infected mother). Active and passive treatments can be administered into different sites at the same time. Recommended uses of hepatitis A and B vaccines are shown in Figure 5.8.

HEPATITIS A VACCINE

Routine immunization

- Children living in communities with high hepatitis A rates and periodic disease outbreaks

Increased risk of hepatitis A

- International travelers to regions of endemic disease
- Men who have sex with men
- Users of illicit injectable drugs

HEPATITIS B VACCINE

Routine immunization

- All infants and previously unvaccinated children by the age 11 years

Increased risk of hepatitis B

- People with multiple sexual partners
- Sexual partners or household contacts of HBsAG-positive people
- Men who have sex with men
- Users of illicit injectable drug
- Travelers to region of endemic disease
- People occupationally exposed to blood or body fluids
- Patients with renal failure
- Patient receiving clotting-factor concentrates

Figure 5.8
Candidates for hepatitis immunization. HBsAg = hepatitis B surface antigen.

C. Varicella zoster

This vaccine contains live, attenuated, temperature-sensitive varicellazoster virus. Its efficacy in preventing chickenpox is approximately 85 to 100 percent in children, and this immunity is persistent. Anti–varicella-zoster Ig provides passive immunity for immunocompromised individuals at risk of infection. A live, attenuated chickenpox vaccine that was approved in 1995 for use in the United States by children age 1 year or older is now recommended as one of the routine childhood vaccines. Mild, breakthrough cases of chickenpox have been reported as a side effect of vaccine administration. The vaccine is also indicated for nonimmune adults at risk of being exposed to contagious individuals. Zostavax is a high-potency version of the chickenpox vaccine, which also contains live, attenuated virus. Zostavax has been approved by the Food and Drug Administration for use in adults over age 50 years for prevention of zoster and, with it, the debilitating effects of postherpetic neuralgia.

D. Polio

Vaccination is the only effective method of preventing poliomyelitis. Both the inactivated polio vaccine and the live, attenuated, orally administered polio vaccine have established efficacy in preventing poliovirus infection and paralytic poliomyelitis (see p. 284).

1. **Inactivated poliovirus (Salk) vaccine:** Because the inactivated vaccine cannot cause poliomyelitis, it is safe for use in immunocompromised persons and their contacts. The disadvantages of this inactivated vaccine are: 1) administration is by injection only, and 2) it provides less GI immunity, resulting in the possibility of asymptomatic infection of the GI tract with wild poliovirus, which could be transmitted to other persons. To eliminate the risk for vaccine-associated paralytic poliomyelitis (see next section), an all-inactivated poliovirus vaccine schedule is recommended for routine childhood vaccinations in the United States.

2. **Attenuated live poliovirus (Sabin) vaccine:** Advantages of this vaccine include: 1) it can be administered orally, 2) it provides lifelong protection from poliovirus for more than 95 percent of recipi-

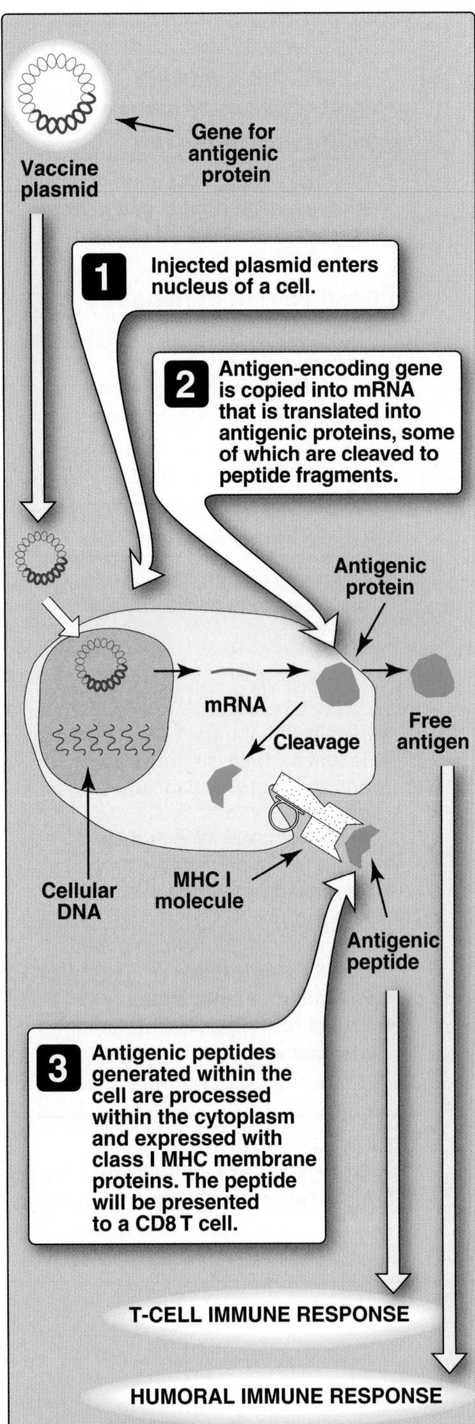

Figure 5.9
DNA vaccines produce antigen needed to generate immunity. MHC = major histocompatibility complex.

ents after the primary three-dose series, and 3) it provides early GI immunity. The main disadvantage of attenuated live virus vaccine is a small risk of clinical disease, estimated to be 1 per 2.4 million doses.

E. Influenza

The traditional "flu shot" vaccine contains formalin-inactivated virus. A live, attenuated influenza vaccine is administered intranasally. The vaccine provides peak protection about 2 weeks after its administration. Vaccine efficacy of 70 to 90 percent is generally achieved in young adults. The vaccine is recommended for adults older than age 65, high-risk persons age 6 months or older, and those who might transmit the virus to persons at high risk. Antigenic drift requires that individuals be vaccinated against influenza annually prior to the winter flu season.

F. Measles, mumps, and rubella

This combination vaccine contains live, attenuated virus and should be administered to young children prior to entering school. Measles vaccine should also be administered to individuals traveling in endemic areas.

J. Human papillomavirus vaccine

Human papillomavirus (HPV) vaccine is recommended for routine administration in all children beginning at ages 11 to 12 years. Quadrivalent HPV vaccine is the only vaccine approved for males for protection against genital warts, and either quadrivalent or bivalent vaccine may be used in females for the protection against cervical cancer and reducing the incidence of genital warts.

VI. DNA VACCINES

DNA vaccines represent a new approach to vaccination. The proposed mechanism for these vaccines is that the gene for the antigen of interest is cloned into a bacterial plasmid, which is engineered to increase the expression of the inserted gene in mammalian cells (Figure 5.9). After being injected, the plasmid enters a host cell where it remains in the nucleus as an episome (that is, it is not integrated into the cell's DNA). Using the host cell's protein synthesis machinery, the plasmid DNA in the episome directs the synthesis of the protein it encodes. This antigenic microbial protein may leave the cells and interact with T helper and B cells, or it may be cleaved into fragments and presented as major histocompatiblity complex I antigen complex on the cell surface, resulting in activation of killer T cells. To date, the potency of DNA vaccines in humans has been disappointing.

VII. OVERVIEW OF ANTIMICROBIAL AGENTS

Antimicrobial drugs are effective in the treatment of infections because of their selective toxicity (that is, they have the ability to kill or inhibit the growth of an invading microorganism without harming the cells of the host). In most instances, the selective toxicity is relative, rather than absolute, requiring that the concentration of the drug be carefully controlled to attack the microorganism while still being tolerated by the host. Selective antimicrobial therapy takes advantage of the biochemical differences that exist between microorganisms and human beings.

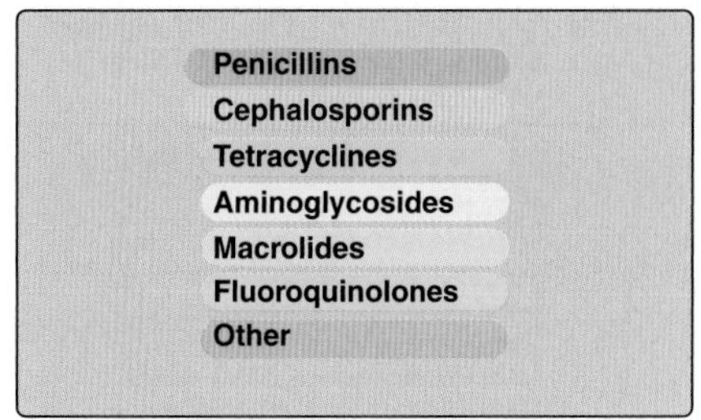

Figure 5.10
Bar chart showing the most commonly used drug families. The group labeled "Other" represents drugs not included in one of the six drug families.

VIII. AGENTS USED TO TREAT BACTERIAL INFECTIONS

In this book, the clinically useful antibacterial drugs are organized into six families: penicillins, cephalosporins, tetracyclines, aminoglycosides, macrolides, and fluoroquinolones, plus a seventh group labeled "other" used to represent any drug not included in one of the other six drug families. Here and throughout the book, these seven groups are graphically presented as a bar chart (Figure 5.10). The drug(s) of choice within each family that is/are used for treating a specific bacterial infection are indicated. [Note: As was introduced in Chapter 1 (see p. 5), the clinically important bacteria are also organized into groups based on Gram stain, morphology, and biochemical or other characteristics.] This chapter illustrates the spectra of bacteria for which a particular class of antibiotics is therapeutically effective. The general mechanisms of action and antibacterial spectra of the major groups of antibiotics are presented below.

A. Penicillins

Penicillins are β-lactam antibiotics, named after the β-lactam ring that is essential to their activity. Penicillins selectively interfere with the synthesis of the bacterial cell wall (see p. 57), a structure not found in mammalian cells. Penicillins are inactive against organisms devoid of a peptidoglycan cell wall, such as mycoplasma, protozoa, fungi, and viruses. To be maximally effective, penicillins require actively proliferating bacteria, and they have little or no effect on bacteria that are not dividing. Their action is usually bactericidal (see p. 31). Penicillins are the most widely effective antibiotics. For example, penicillin G is the cornerstone of therapy for infections caused by several different types of bacteria (Figure 5.11). The major adverse reaction to penicillins is hypersensitivity. Unfortunately, many bacteria have developed resistance to these drugs.

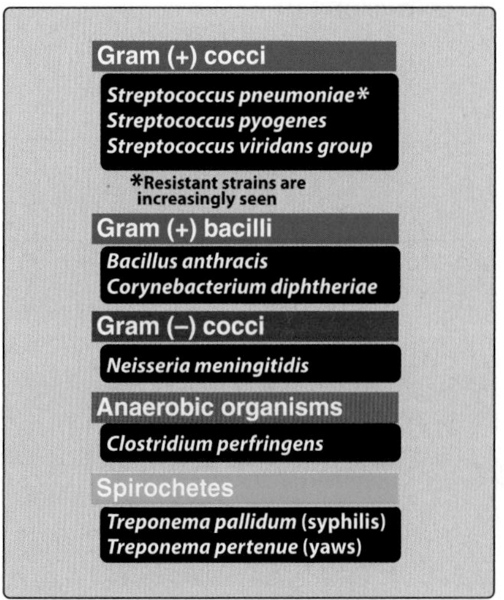

Figure 5.11
Summary of therapeutic applications of penicillin G.

B. Cephalosporins

Cephalosporins are β-lactam antibiotics that are closely related both structurally and functionally to the penicillins, and they are also bactericidal. Cephalosporins have the same mode of action as the penicillins, but they tend to be more resistant than the penicillins to inactivation by β-lactamases produced by some bacteria. Cephalosporins are classified as first, second, or third generation, largely on the basis of bacterial susceptibility patterns and resistance to β-lactamases (Figure 5.12). In this classification system, first-generation agents are active primarily against gram-positive organisms, including methicillin-sensitive *Staphylococcus aureus*, and have limited activity against gram-negative bacilli. Second-gen-

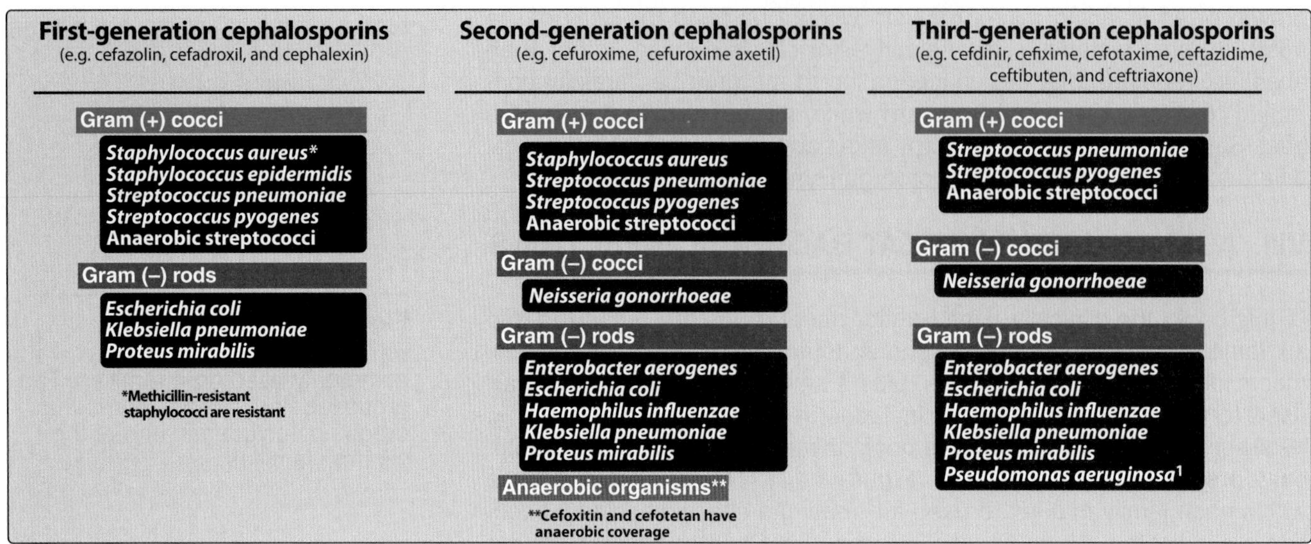

Figure 5.12
Summary of therapeutic applications of cephalosporins. [Note: Not shown is cefepime (a fourth-generation cephalosporin) and ceftobiprole (a fifth-generation cephalosporin), which offer potential advantages over third-generation agents, particularly against organisms with inducible, chromosomal resistance.] [1][Note: *Pseudomonas aeruginosa* is not susceptible to ceftriaxone.]

eration agents have increased activity against gram-negative bacilli and variable activity against gram-positive cocci. Third-generation agents have significantly increased activity against gram-negative bacilli, with some of these agents active against *Pseudomonas aeruginosa*. [Note: Cefepime has been classified by some as fourth-generation because of its extended spectrum of activity against both gram-positive and gram-negative organisms that include *P. aeruginosa*.]

C. Tetracyclines

A number of antibiotics, including tetracyclines, aminoglycosides, and macrolides, exert antimicrobial effects by targeting the bacterial ribosome, which has components that differ structurally from those of the mammalian cytoplasmic ribosomes. Binding of tetracyclines to the 30S subunit of the bacterial ribosome is believed to block access of the amino acyl-tRNA to the mRNA-ribosome complex at the acceptor site, thereby inhibiting bacterial protein synthesis. Tetracyclines are broad-spectrum antibiotics (that is, many bacteria are sensitive to these drugs, Figure 5.13). Tetracyclines are generally bacteriostatic (see p. 31).

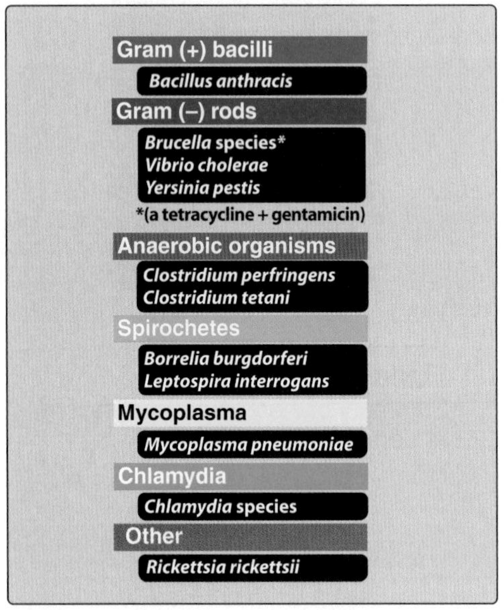

Figure 5.13
Summary of therapeutic applications of tetracyclines.

D. Aminoglycosides

Aminoglycosides inhibit bacterial protein synthesis. Susceptible organisms have an oxygen-dependent system that transports the antibiotic across the cell membrane. All aminoglycosides are bactericidal. They are effective only against aerobic organisms because anaerobes lack the oxygen-requiring transport system. Gentamicin is used to treat a variety of infectious diseases including those caused by many of the Enterobacteriaceae (Figure 5.14) and, in combination with penicillin, endocarditis caused by viridans-group streptococci.

E. Macrolides

Macrolides are a group of antibiotics with a macrocyclic lactone structure. Erythromycin was the first of these to find clinical application, both as the drug of first choice and as an alternative to penicillin in individuals who are allergic to β-lactam antibiotics. Newer macrolides, such clarithromycin and azithromycin, offer extended activity against some organisms and less severe adverse reactions. The macrolides bind irreversibly to a site on the 50S subunit of the bacterial ribosome, thereby inhibiting the translocation steps of protein synthesis. Generally considered to be bacteriostatic (see p. 31), they may be bactericidal at higher doses (Figure 5.15).

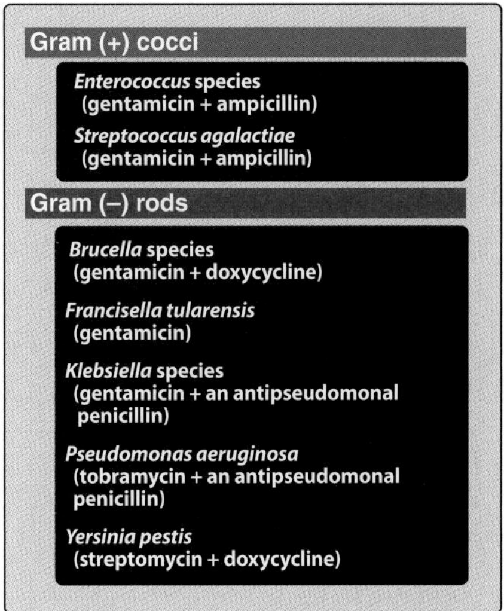

Figure 5.14
Summary of therapeutic applications of aminoglycosides.

F. Fluoroquinolones

Fluoroquinolones uniquely inhibit the replication of bacterial DNA by interfering with the action of DNA gyrase (topoisomerase II) during bacterial growth. Binding quinolone to both the enzyme and DNA to form a ternary complex inhibits the rejoining step, and, thus, can cause cell death by inducing cleavage of the DNA. Because DNA gyrase is a distinct target for antimicrobial therapy, cross-resistance with other more commonly used antimicrobial drugs is rare but is increasing with multidrug-resistant organisms. All of the fluoroquinolones are bactericidal. Figure 5.16 shows some of the applications of the fluoroquinolone ciprofloxacin.

G. Carbapenems

Carbapenems are synthetic β-lactam antibiotics that differ in structure from the penicillins. Imipenem, meropenem, doripenem, and ertapenem are the drugs of this group currently available. Imipenem is compounded with cilastatin to protect it from metabolism by renal dehydropeptidase. Imipenem resists hydrolysis by most β-lactamases. This drug plays a role in empiric therapy because it is active against β-lactamase–producing gram-positive and gram-negative organisms, anaerobes, and *P. aeruginosa* (Figure 5.17). Meropenem and doripenem have antibacterial activity similar to that of imipenem. However, ertapenem is not an alternative for *P. aeruginosa* coverage because most strains exhibit resistance. Ertapenem also lacks coverage against *Enterococcus* species and *Acinetobacter* species.

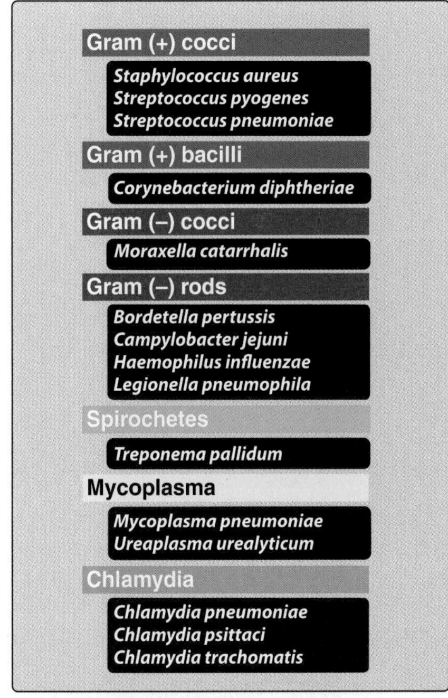

Figure 5.15
Summary of therapeutic applications of macrolides.

H. Other important antibacterial agents

1. **Vancomycin:** Vancomycin is a tricyclic glycopeptide that has become increasingly medically important because of its effectiveness against multidrug-resistant organisms such as methicillin-resistant staphylococci. Vancomycin inhibits synthesis of bacterial cell wall phospholipids as well as peptidoglycan polymerization at a site earlier than that inhibited by β-lactam antibiotics. Vancomycin is useful in patients with serious allergic reactions to β-lactam antibiotics and who have gram-positive infections. Vancomycin is also used for potentially life-threatening antibiotic-associated colitis caused by *Clostridium difficile* or staphylococci. To curtail the increase in vancomycin-resistant bacteria, use of this agent should be restricted to the treatment of serious infec-

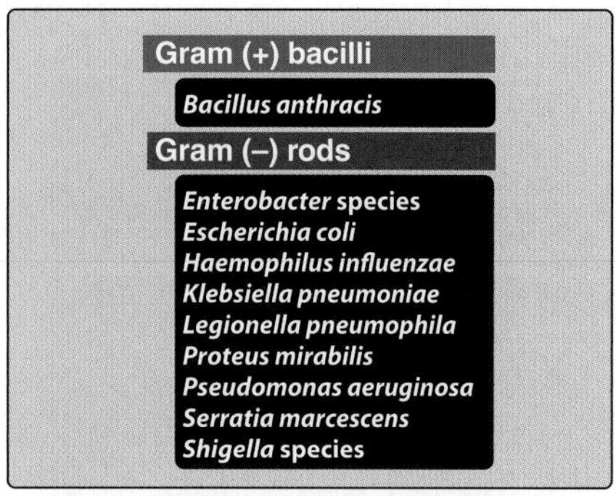

Figure 5.16
Typical therapeutic applications of ciprofloxacin.

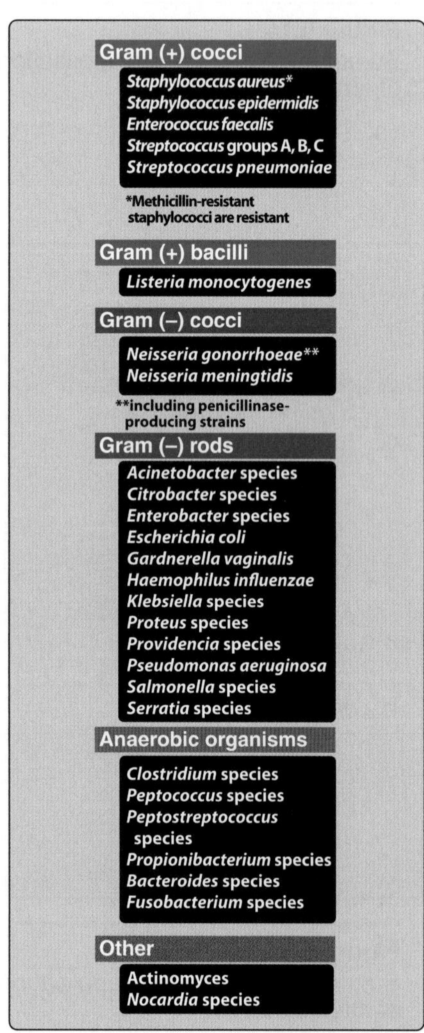

Figure 5.17
Antimicrobial spectrum of imipenem.

tions caused by β-lactam–resistant gram-positive microorganisms. Vancomycin is ineffective against gram-negative bacteria.

2. **Trimethoprim-sulfamethoxazole**: A combination called co-trimoxazole shows greater antimicrobial activity than equivalent quantities of either drug used alone. The synergistic antimicrobial activity of co-trimoxazole results from its inhibition of two sequential steps in the synthesis of tetrahydrofolic acid: sulfamethoxazole inhibits incorporation of PABA into folic acid, and trimethoprim prevents reduction of dihydrofolate to tetrahydrofolate. It is effective in treating urinary tract infections and respiratory tract infections as well as in *Pneumocystis jiroveci* pneumonia and ampicillin- and chloramphenicol-resistant systemic *Salmonella* infections. It has activity versus methicillin-resistant *S. aureus* and can be particularly useful for community acquired skin and soft tissue infections caused by this organism.

IX. DRUG RESISTANCE

Bacteria are said to be resistant to an antimicrobial drug if the maximal level of the agent that can be achieved *in vivo* or tolerated by the host does not halt their growth. Some organisms are inherently resistant to an antibiotic, for example, because they lack the target of the antimicrobial agent. However, microbes that are normally responsive to a particular drug may develop resistance through spontaneous mutation or by acquisition of new genes followed by selection. Some strains may even become resistant to more than one antibiotic by acquisition of genetic elements that encode multiple resistance genes.

A. Genetic alterations leading to drug resistance

Acquired antibiotic resistance involves mutation of existing genes or the acquisition of new genes.

1. **Spontaneous mutations in DNA:** Chromosomal alteration may occur by insertion, deletion, or substitution of one or more nucleotides within the genome. The resulting mutation may persist, be corrected by the organism, or be lethal to the cell. If the cell survives, it can replicate and transmit its mutated properties to progeny cells. Mutations that produce antibiotic-resistant strains can result in organisms that proliferate under selective pressures such as in the presence of the antimicrobial agent. An example is the emergence of rifampin-resistant *Mycobacterium tuberculosis* when rifampin is used as a single antibiotic.

2. **DNA transfer of drug resistance:** Of particular clinical concern is resistance acquired due to DNA transfer from one bacterium to another. Resistance properties are often encoded on extrachromosomal plasmids, known as R, or resistance, factors. DNA can be transferred from donor to recipient cell by processes including transduction (phage mediated), transformation, or bacterial conjugation.

B. Altered expression of proteins in drug-resistant organisms

Drug resistance may be mediated by several different mechanisms, including an alteration in the antimicrobial drug target site, decreased uptake of the drug due to changes in membrane permeability, increased efflux of the drug, or the presence of antibiotic-inactivating enzymes.

1. **Modification of target sites:** Alteration of an antimicrobial agent's target site through mutation can confer resistance to one or more related antibiotics. For example, *S. pneumoniae* resistance to β-lactam drugs involves alterations in one or more of the major bacterial penicillin-binding proteins, resulting in decreased binding of the antimicrobial to its target.

2. **Decreased accumulation:** Decreased uptake or increased efflux of an antimicrobial agent can confer resistance because the drug is unable to attain access to the site of its action in sufficient concentrations to inhibit or kill the organism. For example, gram-negative organisms can limit the penetration of certain agents, including β-lactam antibiotics, tetracyclines, and chloramphenicol, as a result of an alteration in the number and structure of porins (channels) in the outer membrane. Also, expression of an efflux pump can limit levels of a drug that accumulate in an organism. For example, transmembrane proteins located in the cytoplasmic membrane actively pump intracellular antibiotic molecules out of the microorganism (Figure 5.18). These drug efflux pumps for xenobiotic compounds have a broad substrate specificity and are responsible for decreased drug accumulation in multidrug-resistant cells. The efflux pumps may be encoded on chromosomes and plasmids, thus contributing to both intrinsic (natural) and acquired resistance, respectively. As an intrinsic mechanism of resistance, efflux pump genes allow bacteria expressing them to survive a hostile environment (for example, in the presence of antibiotics), which allows for the selection of mutants that overexpress these genes. Being located on transmissible genetic elements as plasmids or transposons is also advantageous for the microorganism insofar as it allows for the easy spread of efflux genes between distinct species.

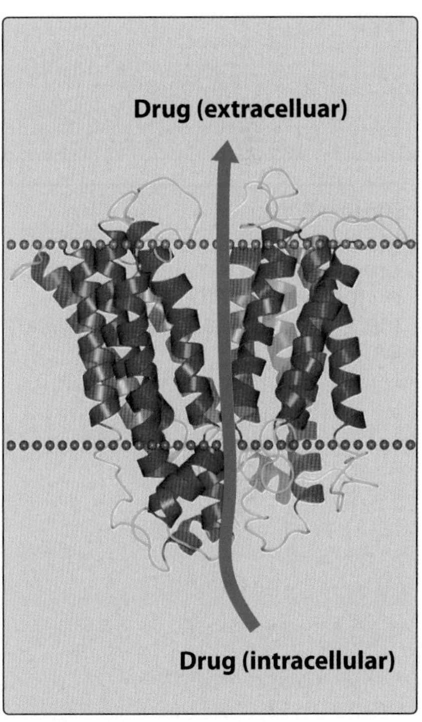

Figure 5.18
Schematic representation of an efflux pump.

3. **Enzymatic inactivation:** The ability to destroy or inactivate the antimicrobial agent can also confer resistance to microorganisms. Examples of antibiotic-inactivating enzymes include 1) β-lactamases that hydrolytically inactivate the β-lactam ring of penicillins, cephalosporins, and related drugs; 2) acetyltransferases that transfer an acetyl group to the antibiotic, inactivating chloramphenicol or aminoglycosides; and 3) esterases that hydrolyze the lactone ring of macrolides.

X. AGENTS USED TO TREAT VIRAL INFECTIONS

When viruses reproduce, they use much of the host's own metabolic machinery. Therefore, few drugs are selective enough to prevent viral repli-

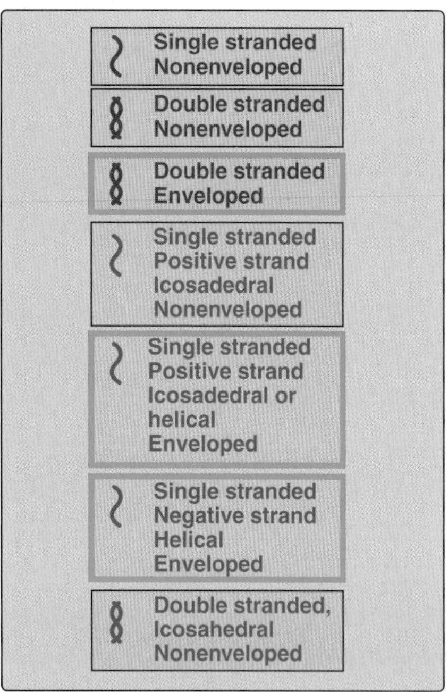

Figure 5.19
Medically important viruses organized into similar groups based on the nature of the genome and the presence or absence of a lipid envelope.

cation without injury to the host. Viruses are also not affected by antibacterial agents. Nevertheless, some drugs sufficiently discriminate between cellular and viral reactions to be effective and yet relatively nontoxic. For example, efficient management strategies are available for infections due to herpes simplex virus, varicella-zoster virus, cytomegalovirus, influenza A and B viruses, and chronic hepatitis B and C and HIV.

A. Organization of viruses

The clinically important viruses can be conveniently divided into seven groups based on the nature of their genome, symmetry of organization, and the presence or absence of a lipid envelope (Figure 5.19). The therapeutic applications of selected antiviral agents are shown in Figure 5.20.

B. Treatment of herpesvirus infections

Most antiviral agents used in treating herpesvirus infections are nucleoside analogues that require conversion to mono-, di-, and triphosphate forms by cellular kinases, viral kinases, or both to selectively inhibit viral DNA synthesis. This class of antiviral agents includes acyclovir, cidofovir, famciclovir, ganciclovir, penciclovir, valacyclovir, valganciclovir, fomivirsen and vidarabine. A second class of antiviral drugs with action against herpesviruses is represented by the pyrophosphate analogue, foscarnet. Most antiviral agents, including nucleoside analogues and foscarnet, exert their actions during the acute phase of viral infections and are without effect in the latent phase.

C. Treatment of acquired immunodeficiency syndrome

Antiretroviral drugs are divided into five main classes based on their mode of inhibition of viral replication. The first class represents nucleoside analogs that inhibit the viral RNA–dependent DNA polymerase (reverse transcriptase) of HIV. A second class of reverse transcriptase inhibitors includes nonnucleoside analogs. The third class includes protease inhibitors. The fourth class is a fusion inhibitor that prevents HIV from entering the host cell. The fifth class, integrase inhibitors, blocks the action of integrase, a viral enzyme that inserts the viral genome into the DNA of the host cell. Therapy with these antiretroviral agents, usually in combinations (a “cocktail” of drugs referred to as highly active antiretroviral therapy, or HAART), is beneficial to prolong survival, to reduce the incidence and severity of opportunistic infections in patients with advanced HIV disease (by allowing at least partial recovery of CD4 lymphocyte populations), and to delay disease progression in asymptomatic HIV-infected patients.

D. Treatment of viral hepatitis

Prolonged (months) treatment with interferon-α has succeeded in reducing or eliminating indicators of hepatitis B virus replication in about one third of patients. However, recurrence of indications of the infection may occur after therapy cessation. Lamivudine, an oral nucleoside analogue, is an effective treatment in patients with previ-

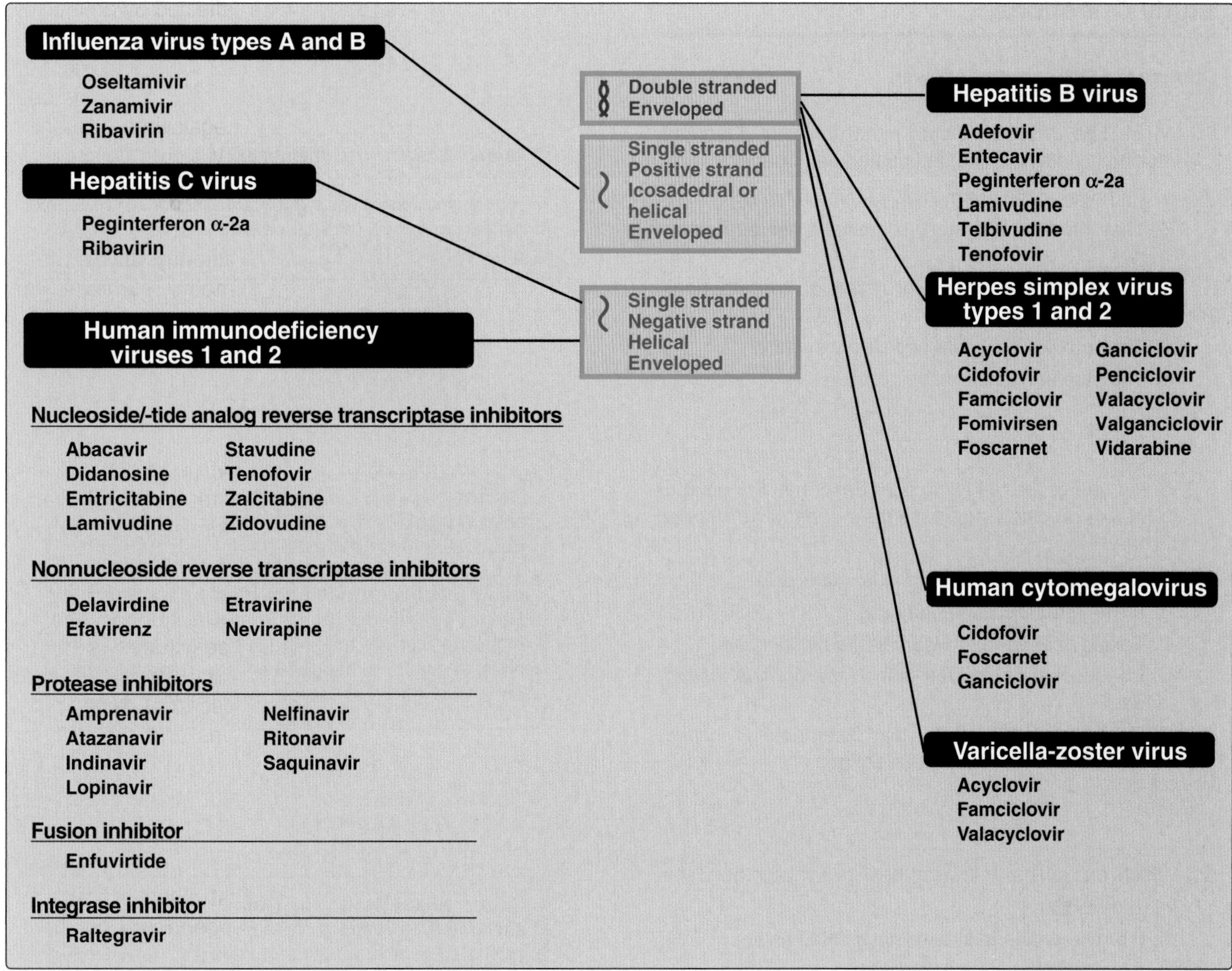

Figure 5.20
Summary of therapeutic applications of selected antiviral agents.

ously untreated chronic hepatitis B. However, only a minority of patients is cured or remains in remission after lamivudine therapy is withdrawn. Maintenance therapy may be indicated, but long-term use of lamivudine is limited by the appearance of viral polymerase gene mutants, which leads to reemergence of disease. The therapy of choice for hepatitis C is interferon-α in combination with ribavirin. The overall rate of response to this drug combination is three times greater than that seen with interferon-α monotherapy. However, anemia is a common adverse effect induced by ribavirin.

E. Treatment of influenza

Zanamivir and oseltamivir are effective against influenza A and B. They inhibit viral neuraminidase, thereby preventing the release of virus from infected cells.

Study Questions

Choose the ONE correct answer.

5.1 Which one of the following most correctly describes vaccines containing live, attenuated pathogens?

A. Pathogen does not multiply in human hosts.
B. They provide extended, sometimes life-long immunity.
C. There is no possibility for reversion to pathogenic form.
D. They provide little cell-mediated immunity.
E. They are administered by injection.

Correct answer = B. Attenuated microbes reproduce in the recipient, typically leading to a more robust and longer-lasting immune response than can be obtained through vaccination with killed organisms.

5.2 Which one of the following best describes the components of vaccines against *Haemophilus influenzae* disease?

A. Live, attenuated *Haemophilus influenzae*
B. Killed *Haemophilus influenzae*
C. Toxoid derived from *Haemophilus influenzae*
D. Polysaccharide derived from *Haemophilus influenzae*
E. Polysaccharide derived from *Haemophilus influenzae* conjugated to a protein antigen

Correct answer = E. Covalent conjugates of capsular polysaccharide with diphtheria protein have been developed for *Haemophilus influenzae*. Unconjugated polysaccharide is weakly immunogenic in children younger than age 2 years. However, the conjugated vaccine produces higher of titers of antibody, superior responsiveness in children younger than age 2 years, and enhanced efficacy of booster administrations.

5.3 Which one of the following best describes the Sabin polio vaccine?

A. It provides little gastrointestinal immunity.
B. It is prepared with inactive virus.
C. It is administered by injection.
D. It carries a small risk of causing disease.
E. It is an example of passive immunity.

Correct answer = D. The main disadvantage of attenuated live virus is the small risk of disease, estimated to be 1 per 2.4 million doses.

5.4 A 25-year-old woman whose blood tested positive for hepatitis B surface antigen gave birth to a full-term child. Which of the following therapies would be most likely to minimize the transmission of hepatitis B to the neonate?

A. Administer hepatitis B immunoglobulin.
B. Administer hepatitis B vaccine.
C. Administer hepatitis B immunoglobulin and hepatitis B vaccine.
D. Bottle-feed the neonate.

Correct answer = C. Infants born to infected mothers are given hepatitis B immunoglobulin plus hepatitis B vaccine at birth, followed by additional doses of vaccine at ages 1 and 6 months. [Note: The two injections must be given at separate anatomical sites to prevent injected hepatitis B immunoglobulin from neutralizing the injected vaccine.] Perinatal infection of the neonate occurs at the time of delivery and is not related to consumption of breast milk.

UNIT II:
Bacteria

Bacterial Structure, Growth, and Metabolism

6

I. OVERVIEW

The cellular world is divided into two major groups, based on whether or not the cells have a nucleus (that is, an internal membrane-enclosed region that contains the genetic material). Cells that have a well-defined nucleus are called eukaryotic, whereas cells that lack a nucleus are called prokaryotic. All bacteria are prokaryotes. In addition, bacterial DNA is not organized into the elaborate multichromosomal structures of the eukaryotes, but typically is a single double-stranded molecule of DNA. Prokaryotes and eukaryotes employ very similar metabolic pathways to achieve cell growth and maintain viability. However, prokaryotes synthesize substances and structures that are unique to bacteria, for example, peptidoglycan. A generalized prokaryotic cell is shown in Figure 6.1.

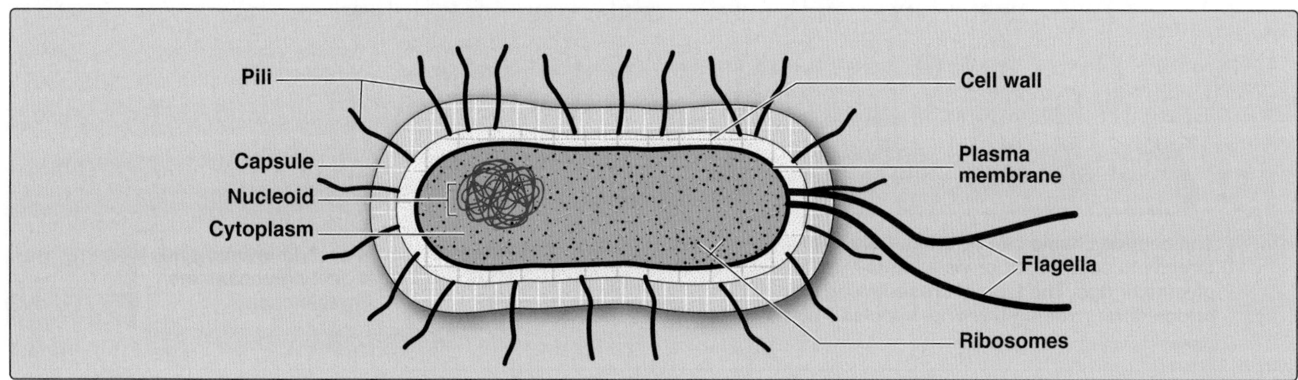

Figure 6.1
Generalized structure of a bacterial cell.

II. THE CELL ENVELOPE

The bacterial "cell envelope" is a term applied to all material external to and enclosing the cytoplasm. It consists of several chemically and functionally distinct layers, the most prominent of which are the cell wall and the cytoplasmic membrane. The cell envelope also includes the capsule or glycocalyx, if present.

A. Cytoplasmic membrane

The cell membrane is composed of phospholipid, the molecules of which form two parallel surfaces (called a lipid bilayer) such that the polar phosphate groups are on the outside of the bilayer and the nonpolar lipid chains are on the inside. The membrane acts as a permeability barrier, restricting the kind and amount of molecules that enter and leave the cell.

B. Peptidoglycan

The peptidoglycan layer determines the shape of the cell. It is composed of a cross-linked polymeric mesh (Figure 6.2.) The glycan portion is a linear polymer of alternating monosaccharide subunits:

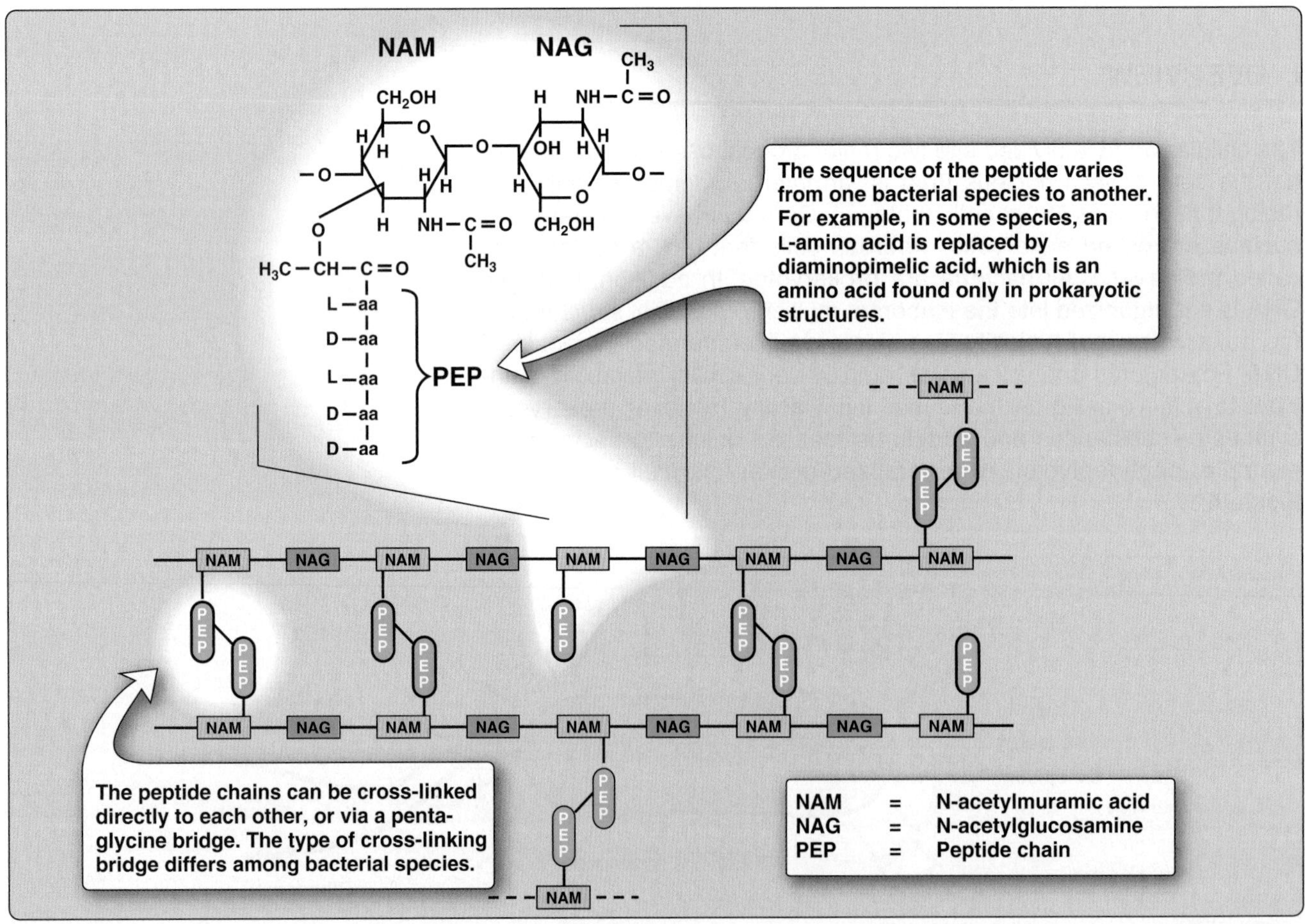

NAM
NAG
PEP
The sequence of the peptide varies from one bacterial species to another. For example, in some species, an L-amino acid is replaced by diaminopimelic acid, which is an amino acid found only in prokaryotic structures.
The peptide chains can be cross-linked directly to each other, or via a pentaglycine bridge. The type of cross-linking bridge differs among bacterial species.
NAM = N-acetylmuramic acid
NAG = N-acetylglucosamine
PEP = Peptide chain

Figure 6.2
Structure of peptidoglycan, the major polymer of bacterial cell walls.

N-acetylglucosamine (NAG) and N-acetylmuramic acid (NAM). This polymer is the carbohydrate "backbone" of the mesh. The "peptido" portion of the polymer is a short string of amino acids that serves to cross-link adjacent polysaccharide strands at the NAM subunits of the backbone, forming a network with high tensile strength (see Figure 6.2). [Note: The presence of D-amino acids helps render the bacterial wall resistant to host peptidases such as those in the intestine.] A discussion of cell wall synthesis is presented on p. 55.

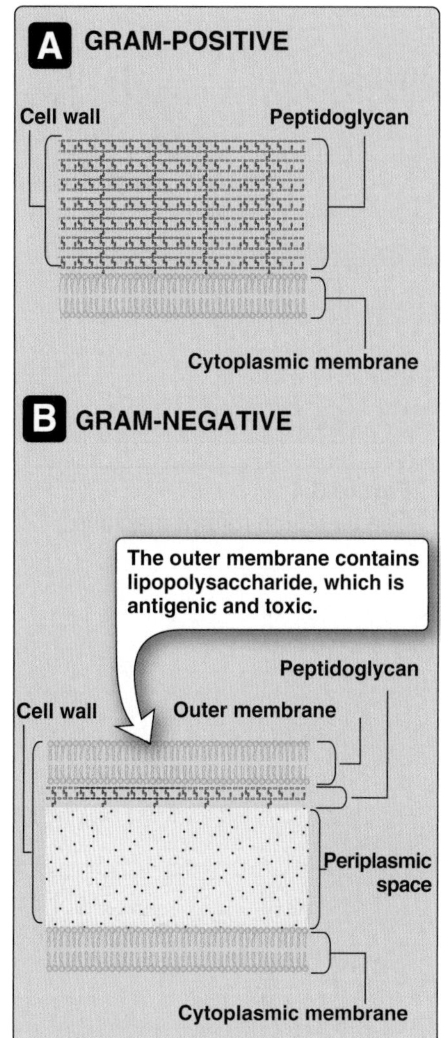

Figure 6.3
Comparison of gram-positive and gram-negative bacterial cell walls.

C. Differences between gram-positive and gram-negative cell walls

The molecular details of the cell walls of gram-positive and gram-negative bacteria are shown in Figure 6.3. Additional surface layers, such as a capsule or glycocalyx, can be found outside of the cell wall in some species of gram-positive and gram-negative bacteria.

1. **Gram-positive organisms:** Gram-positive bacteria have thick, multilayered, peptidoglycan cell walls that are exterior to the cytoplasmic membrane. The peptidoglycan in most gram-positive species is covalently linked to teichoic acid, which is essentially a polymer of substituted glycerol units linked by phosphodiester bonds. The teichoic acids are major cell surface antigens. Teichoic acids are integrated into the peptidoglycan layers but not tethered to the cytoplasmic membrane. Lipoteichoic acids are lipid modified and integrated by this moiety into the outer leaflet of the cytoplasmic membrane.

2. **Gram-negative organisms:** Gram-negative bacteria have a more complex cell wall structure composed of two membranes (an outer membrane and an inner, that is, cytoplasmic, membrane). The two membranes are separated by the periplasmic space, which contains the peptidoglycan layer. The periplasmic space also contains degradative enzymes and transport proteins. In contrast to gram-positive cells, the peptidoglycan layer of gram-negative cells is thin, and the cells are consequently more susceptible to physical damage. The outer membrane is distinguished by the presence of embedded lipopolysaccharide (LPS) that is the major constituent of the outer leaflet of the outer membrane. The polysaccharide portion of LPS (O-polysaccharide) is antigenic and can, therefore, be used to identify different strains and species. The lipid portion (called lipid A) is imbedded in the membrane and is toxic to humans and animals. Because lipid A is an integral part of the membrane, it is called endotoxin, as opposed to exotoxins, which are secreted substances. Do not confuse endotoxin or exotoxins with enterotoxins, which are exotoxins that are toxic for the mucosal membrane of the intestine. "Enterotoxin" denotes the site of action, rather than its origin.

D. The external capsule and glycocalyx

Many bacteria secrete a sticky, viscous material that forms an extracellular coating around the cell. The material is usually a polysaccharide. However, in the case of pathogenic *Bacillus anthracis*, the capsule is composed of poly-D-glutamic acid. If the material is tightly bound to the cell and has an organized structure, it is called a cap-

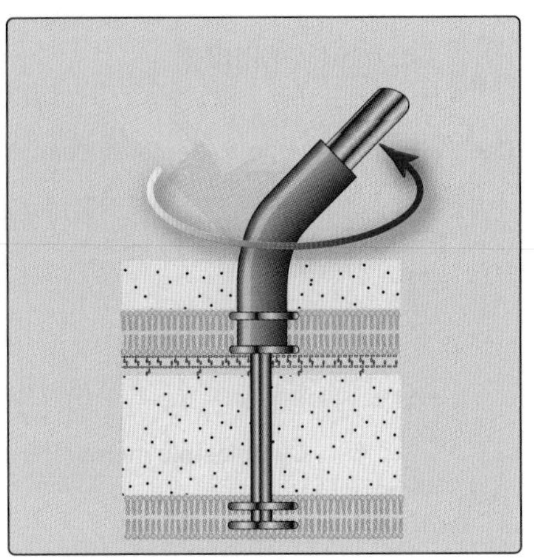

Figure 6.4
The flagellum rotator machine.

sule (see Figure 6.1). If the material is loosely bound and amorphous, it is called a slime layer, or glycocalyx. The capsule or glycocalyx allow cells to adhere to surfaces, protect bacteria from antibodies and phagocytosis, and act as diffusion barriers against some antibiotics, thus contributing to the organisms' pathogenicity. Capsules can also protect bacteria against dessication, or drying, which facilitates transmission.

E. Appendages

Many bacteria have hairlike appendages that project from the cell wall. There are of two kinds of appendages: flagella (singular, flagellum) and pili (singular, pilus).

1. **Flagella:** Prokaryotic flagella are long, semirigid, helical, hollow tubular structures composed of several thousand molecules of the protein flagellin. They enable bacteria to move in a directed fashion, for example, in response to a chemotactic stimulus. Flagella are anchored in the cell membranes by a basal body, which is a complex molecular machine that rotates the flagellum like the screw propeller of a ship (Figure 6.4). Cells may have one or many flagella. Flagella are highly antigenic. Bacteria that have flagella often do not form compact colonies on an agar surface, but instead swarm over the surface of the agar if it is sufficiently wet, producing a scumlike mat.

2. **Pili:** Pili (sometimes called fimbriae) are shorter and thinner than flagella and function as attachment structures that promote specific cell-to-cell contact (see Figure 6.1). The attachment can be between the bacterial cell and the host eukaryotic cell or between one bacterial cell and another.

F. Antigenic variation

Antigenic variation is the expression of various alternative forms of antigen on the cell surface. Most surface structures are subject to antigenic variation, including LPS, capsules, lipoteichoic acids, pili, and flagella. This variation is important for immune evasion by the pathogen. For example, in *Neisseria* species, antigenic variation by gene conversion (p. 101) allows the organism to produce antigenically different pilin molecules at high frequency. Variation in the surface structures between strains of the same species is detected by serology.

III. SPORES AND SPORULATION

To enhance survival during periods of environmental hostility (such as nutritional deprivation), some gram-positive rods undergo profound structural and metabolic changes. These result in the formation of a dormant cell called an endospore inside the original cell. Endospores can be released from the original cell as free spores (Figure 6.5). Spores are the most resistant life forms known. They are remarkably resistant to heat (they survive boiling), desiccation, ultraviolet light, and bactericidal chemical agents. In fact, sterilization procedures are assessed by their ability to inactivate spores.

A. Sporulation

Sporulation can be thought of as repackaging a copy of bacterial DNA into a new form that contains very little water, has no metabolic activity, does not divide, and has a restructured, highly impermeable, multilayered envelope. Spore formation begins with the invagination of the parent cell membrane, producing a double membrane that encapsulates and isolates a copy of the bacterial DNA in what will become the core of the spore. The mature spore retains the complete machinery for protein synthesis, and new spore-specific enzymes are synthesized in the core of the spore. The core also has high levels of a unique compound called calcium dipicolinate, which is thought to be important for protection of the spore DNA from environmental damage. Many enzymes of the original vegetative (nondividing) cell are degraded. When the endospore is completed, the parent cell lyses, releasing the spore.

B. Spore germination

To return to the vegetative state, spores must first be subjected to a treatment that weakens the spore coat (such as heat or extremes of pH), thus allowing germination to occur. If the activated spore is in a nutritious environment, which it senses by monitoring various key metabolites, it begins to germinate. This process involves destruction of the cortex by lytic enzymes, followed by uptake of water, and release of calcium dipicolinate from the cell.

C. Medical significance of sporulation

Some of the most notorious pathogens are spore-formers, including *B. anthracis* (anthrax, see p. 94), *Bacillus cereus* (gastroenteritis, see p. 118), *Clostridium tetani* (tetanus, see p. 155), *Clostridium botulinum* (botulism, see p. 153), *Clostridium perfringens* (gas gangrene, see p. 150), and *Clostridium difficile* (see page 157). Spores of these organisms can remain viable for many years and are generally not killed by boiling, but they can be killed by autoclaving (that is, subjecting the spores to temperatures above 120°C at elevated pressure). In the absence of an autoclave, spores can be largely eliminated by a primary boiling to activate germination and, after a short period of vegetative growth, a second boiling.

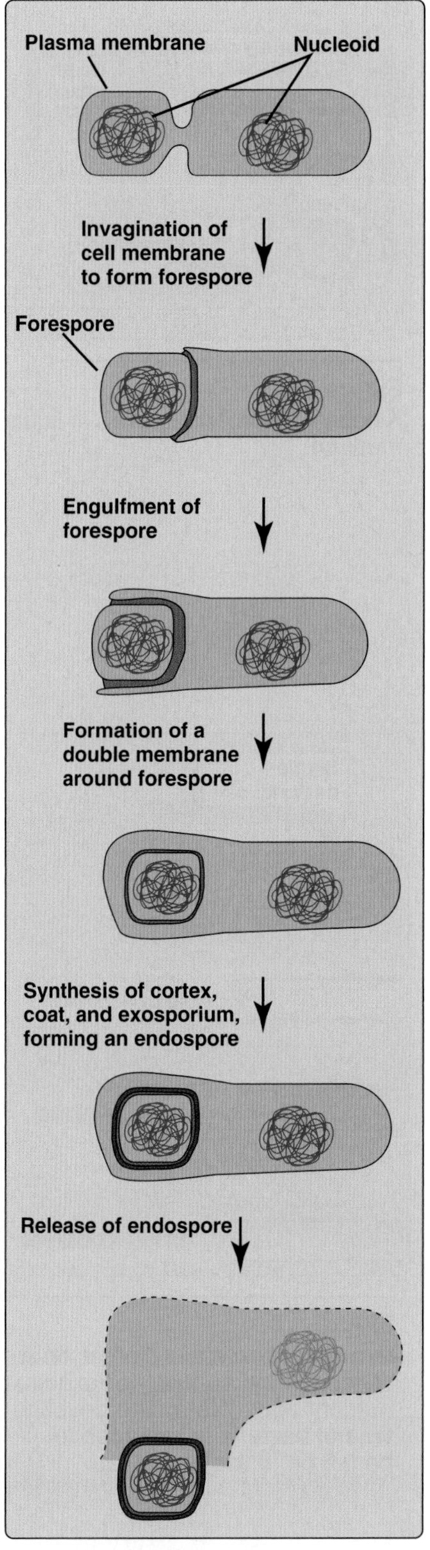

Figure 6.5
Formation of an endospore.

IV. GROWTH AND METABOLISM

All cells must accomplish certain metabolic tasks to grow and divide. All cells, whether bacterial or human, accomplish these metabolic tasks by similar pathways. There are, however, some important differences that set bacteria apart metabolically from eukaryotic cells, and these differences can often be exploited in the development of antibacterial therapies.

A. Characteristics of bacterial growth

If bacterial cells are suspended in a liquid nutrient medium, the increase in cell number or mass can be measured in several ways. Techniques include microscopically counting the cells in a given volume using a ruled slide, counting the number of appropriately

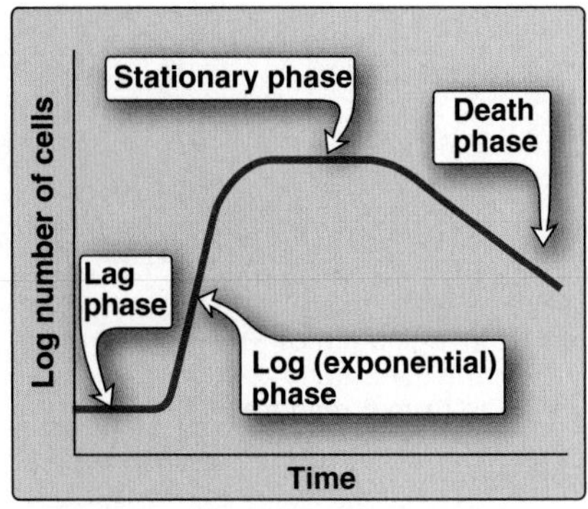

Figure 6.6
Kinetics of bacterial growth in liquid medium.

diluted cells that are able to form colonies following transfer to a solid nutrient (agar) surface, or quantitating the turbidity—which is proportional to the cell mass—of a culture in liquid medium.

1. **Stages of the bacterial growth cycle:** Because bacteria reproduce by binary fission (one becomes two, two become four, four become eight, etc.), the number of cells increases exponentially with time (the exponential, or log, phase of growth). Depending on the species, the minimum doubling time can be as short as 10 minutes or as long as several days. For example, for a rapidly growing species such as *Escherichia coli* in a nutritionally complete medium, a single cell can give rise to some 10 million cells in just 8 hours. Eventually, growth slows and ceases entirely (stationary phase) as nutrients are depleted, and toxic waste products accumulate. Most cells in a stationary phase are not dead, however. If they are diluted into fresh growth medium, exponential growth will resume after a lag phase. The phases of the growth cycle are illustrated in Figure 6.6.

2. **Surface growth:** If a single bacterial cell is placed on a solid nutrient agar surface, the progeny of this cell remain close to the site of deposition and eventually form a compact macroscopic mass of cells called a colony (Figure 6.7). For rapidly growing species, overnight incubation at 30°C to 37°C is sufficient to produce visible colonies, each containing millions of cells. The gross characteristics of colonies (for example, color, shape, adherence, smell, and surface texture) can be useful guides for identification of the species of bacterium. Some species do not form compact circular colonies because the cells are capable of movement and swarm over the agar surface, especially if the surface is moist. Other species, particularly the actinomycetes, grow as long filaments of cells (mycelial growth).

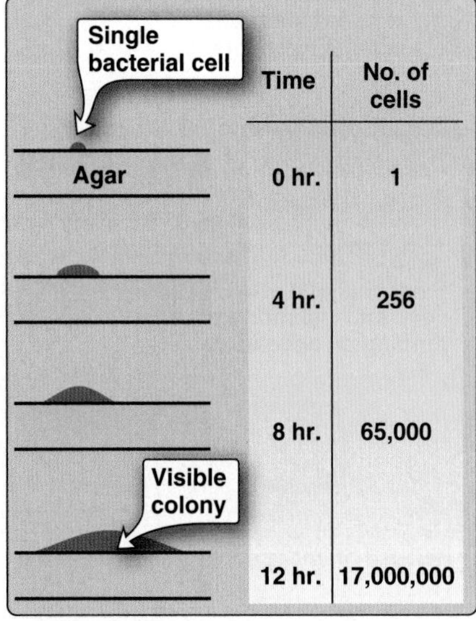

Figure 6.7
Growth of bacterial colonies on a solid, nutrient surface, for example, nutrient agar. [Note: The doubling time of bacteria is assumed to be 0.5 hr. in this example]

B. Energy production

A distinctive feature of bacterial metabolism is the variety of mechanisms used to generate energy from carbon sources. Depending on the biochemical mechanism used, bacterial metabolism can be categorized into three types: aerobic respiration, anaerobic respiration, and fermentation (Figure 6.8).

1. **Aerobic respiration** is the metabolic process in which molecular oxygen serves as the terminal electron acceptor of the electron transport chain. In this process, oxygen is reduced to water. Respiration is the energy-generating mode used by all aerobic bacteria.

2. **Anaerobic respiration** is the metabolic process in which inorganic compounds other than molecular oxygen serve as the terminal electron acceptors. Depending on the species, acceptors can be molecules such as nitrate or sulfate. Anaerobic respiration can be used as an alternative to aerobic respiration in some species (facultative organisms), but is obligatory in other species (some obligate

anaerobes). [Note: Other obligate anaerobes use fermentation as the main mode of energy metabolism. This is particularly true among the anaerobic bacteria of medical importance.]

3. **Fermentation** is an anaerobic process utilized by some bacterial species. It is the metabolic process by which an organic metabolic intermediate derived from a "fermentable" substrate serves as the final electron acceptor. The substrates that can be fermented and the final endproducts depend on the species. Regardless of the bacterium and the fermentation pathway, several unifying concepts are common to fermentation. By comparison to aerobic and anaerobic respiration, fermentation yields very little energy. The purpose of fermentation is to recycle nicotinamide adenine dinucleotide hydrogen (NADH) back to NAD. The reducing power that can be converted to energy via respiration is unrealized. The terminal electron acceptor in fermentation is pyruvate or a pyruvate derivative. Beyond these commonalities, the pathways and endproducts of fermentation are incredibly varied. These endproducts can be measured and are sometimes diagnostic for a given species. In addition, some fermentation endproducts can result in host toxicity and tissue damage.

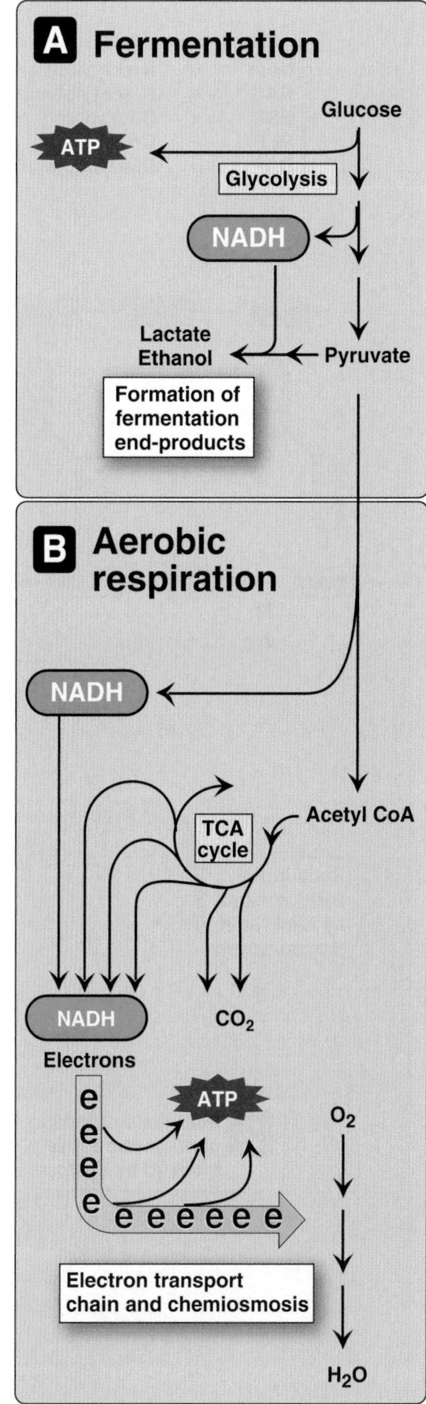

Figure 6.8
Overview of respiration, fermentation, and energy production in bacteria. [Note: Compounds other than oxygen, such as nitrate and sulfate, can be used as terminal electron acceptors in anaerobic respiration.]

C. Peptidoglycan synthesis

The bacterial peptidoglycan polymer is constructed on the surface of the cell membrane and is composed of a repeating carbohydrate backbone subunit, which is NAG–NAM (see p. 50). These backbone chains are cross-linked by short peptides (PEP) to form a rigid meshwork (Figure 6.9). Peptidoglycan biosynthesis occurs via the following series of steps.

1. **Activation of carbohydrate subunits:** As in all biologic polymerizations, NAM and NAG subunits are activated by attachment to a carrier molecule, which in this case is the nucleotide uridine diphosphate (UDP).

2. **Synthesis of the linking peptide:** A pentapeptide is added to UDP–NAM by sequential transfer of amino acids, with the two terminal alanine residues added as a dipeptide. This pentapeptide may contain some nonstandard amino acids, including, for example, diaminopimelic acid ([DAP] a metabolic precursor of lysine), and D-amino acids. The sequence of the pentapeptide is not dictated by an RNA template, but rather the specificity of the enzymes that form the peptide bonds.

3. **Transfer of the peptidoglycan unit to bactoprenol phosphate:** The NAM–PEP moiety is transferred from the UDP carrier to another carrier, bactoprenol phosphate (BPP), located on the inner surface of the cell membrane. At this point, UDP–NAG transfers NAG to NAM–PEP, completing the peptidoglycan repeat unit, NAG–NAM–PEP, which is now attached to the carrier BPP.

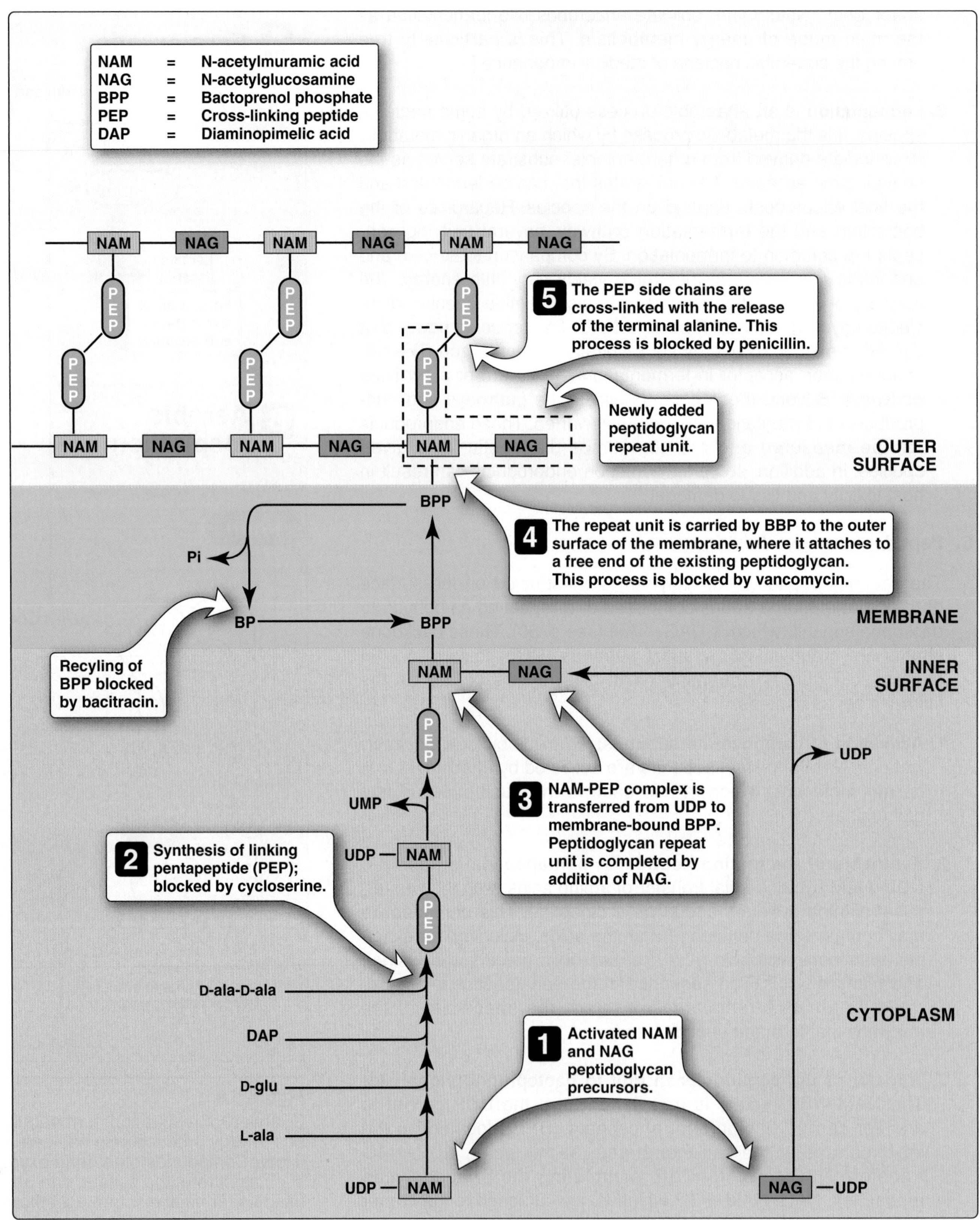

Figure 6.9
Synthesis of a bacterial cell wall.

4. **Addition of the repeat unit to the existing peptidoglycan:** BPP carries the NAG–NAM–PEP repeat unit through the cell membrane to the outside surface where the peptidoglycan of the existing cell wall is located. The repeat unit is added to a free end of the existing peptidoglycan, increasing the length of the polymer by one repeat unit. Presumably, free ends are created by a limited hydrolytic loosening of the preexisting peptidoglycan.

5. **Cross-linking of the pentapeptide to the peptidoglycan backbone:** Although the N–terminal end of the pentapeptide is attached to the NAM moieties of the backbone, the C–terminal end is dangling free. Cross-linking is brought about by a transpeptidation reaction that bonds DAP of the peptide in one chain to the alanine (ala) at position four of the peptide in an adjacent chain, causing the release of the terminal ala. This mode of direct cross-linking is characteristic of *E. coli* and many other gram-negative species. By contrast, in gram-positive bacteria, such as *Staphylococcus aureus*, a glycine pentapeptide is usually interposed between the lysine (lys) at position three of one PEP and the ala at position four of the PEP to which the linkage is to be made (Figure 6.10).

6. **Peptidoglycan biosynthesis as a target of some antibacterial agents:** Because many of the reactions involved in the synthesis of peptidoglycan are unique to bacteria, cell wall synthesis is an ideal target for some highly specific antibacterial agents, particularly the β-lactam antibiotics.

   a. **β-Lactam antibiotics:** Penicillins and cephalosporins inhibit the enzymes that catalyze transpeptidation and carboxypeptidation reactions of cell wall assembly. These enzymes are called penicillin-binding proteins (PBPs) because they all have active sites that bind β-lactam antibiotics. No single PBP species is the target of β-lactam antibiotics. Rather, their lethal effect on bacteria is the result of inactivation of multiple species of PBPs. Most PBPs are involved in bacterial cell wall synthesis. Acquired resistance to β-lactam antibiotics may result from genetic modifications that result in production of new PBPs that have a lower affinity for β-lactam antibiotics (see p. 64).

   b. **Bacitracin, cycloserine, and vancomycin:** Other antibiotics that interfere with peptidoglycan synthesis include bacitracin, which inhibits the recycling of bactoprenol phosphate; cycloserine, which inhibits synthesis of the D–ala–D–ala dipeptide that provides the two terminal residues of the pentapeptide; and vancomycin, which blocks incorporation of the NAG–NAM–PEP repeat unit into the growing peptidoglycan chain (see Figure 6.9). Because vancomycin binds to the terminat D-ala-D-ala dipeptide, this antibacterial agent also prevents transpeptidation.

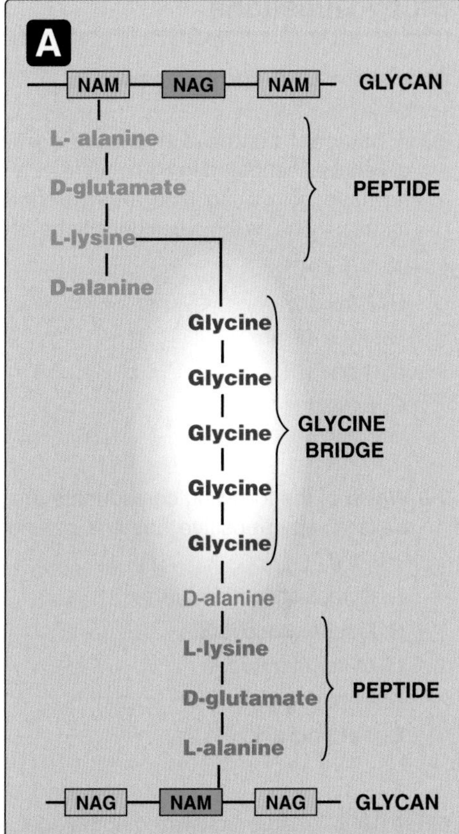

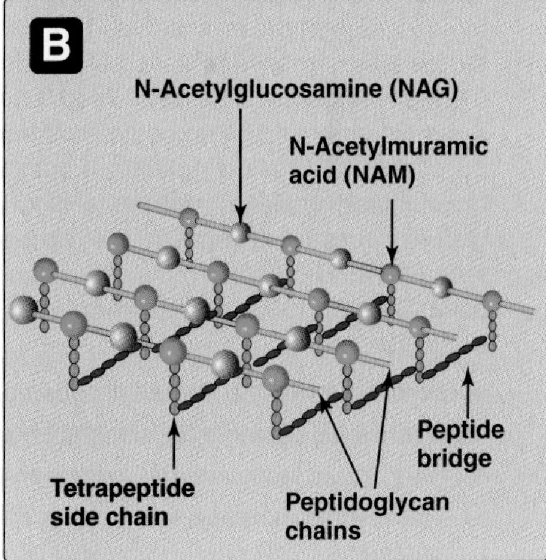

Figure 6.10
A. Glycine bridge in the peptidoglycan of *Staphylococcus aureus*.
B. Organization of peptidoglycan layer in gram-positive cells.

Study Questions

Choose the ONE correct answer.

6.1 A bacterial culture with a starting density of 1×10^3 cells/ml is incubated in liquid nutrient broth. If the bacteria have both a lag time and a generation time of 10 minutes, what will the cell density be at 30 minutes?

A. 1.0×10^3
B. 2.0×10^3
C. 3.0×10^3
D. 4.0×10^3
E. 6.0×10^3

Correct answer = D. After a 10-minute lag, the bacteria will double in number at 20 minutes and double again by 30 minutes.

6.2 Which of the following components are found in the cell walls of gram-positive bacteria but not gram-negative bacteria?

A. Cytoplasmic membrane
B. Lipopolysaccharide
C. Outer membrane
D. Peptidoglycan
E. Teichoic acid

Correct answer = E. Gram-positive bacteria have thick, multilayered, peptidoglycan cell walls that are exterior to the membrane. The peptidoglycan in most gram-positive species is covalently linked to teichoic acid, which is essentially a polymer of substituted glycerol units linked by phosphodiester bonds. All gram-positive species also have lipoteichoic acid in their membranes, where it is covalently linked to glycolipid. Teichoic acids are major cell surface antigens. Gram-negative bacteria have two membranes—an outer membrane and an inner (cytoplasmic) membrane. Their peptidoglycan layer is located between the two membranes in the periplasmic space. The periplasmic space also contains enzymes and various other substances. The outer membrane is distinguished by the presence of various lipopolysaccharides.

6.3 In 1998, a large botulism outbreak occurred in El Paso, Texas. The foodborne illness was shown to be caused by foil-wrapped baked potatoes that were held at room temperature for several days before their use in dips at a Greek restaurant. The dip yielded botulinum toxin type A, as did stool and, in some cases serum samples from 18 of the 30 affected patients. Four patients required mechanical ventilation, but none died. What would be the expected outcome if the potatoes had been reheated to 100°C for 10 minutes before being served? [Hint: See pp. 153–154 for properties of *Clostridium botulinum* toxin.]

A. Heat would kill the spores of *Clostridium botulinum.*
B. Heat would promote the vegetative state.
C. Heat would inactivate the toxin in the potato dip.
D. Heat would increase the number of toxin-producing bacteria.
E. Heat would not alter the outcome.

Correct answer = C. *Clostridium botulinum* spores are commonly found on raw potatoes and generally are not killed if the potatoes are baked in foil, which holds in moisture and, thus, keeps the potatoes' surface temperature at 100°C (below the temperature required for spore killing of >120°C). During storage at room temperature in the anaerobic environment provided by the foil, spores germinate, and toxin forms. Heating at 100°C would kill most *C. botulinum* because the bacterium is in its vulnerable, vegetative state. Heat would also inactivate toxin produced during room-temperature storage. However, any remaining spores would not be killed.

Bacterial Genetics

7

I. OVERVIEW

Because a single type of molecule, DNA, is the genetic material of all cellular organisms from bacteria to humans, basic genetic phenomena (that is, gene mutation, gene replication, and gene recombination) are much the same for all life forms. The prototypic organism used in microbial genetic studies for the past 50 years is the enteric, gram-negative *Escherichia coli* (see p. 111). An aspect of microbial genetics of great clinical importance is the ability of bacteria to transfer genes, especially genes for antibiotic resistance, to other bacteria both within and between species. Such transfer allows the flow of antibiotic resistance genes from nonpathogenic bacterial populations to pathogenic populations, as well as between pathogens, with potentially dire consequences for public health.

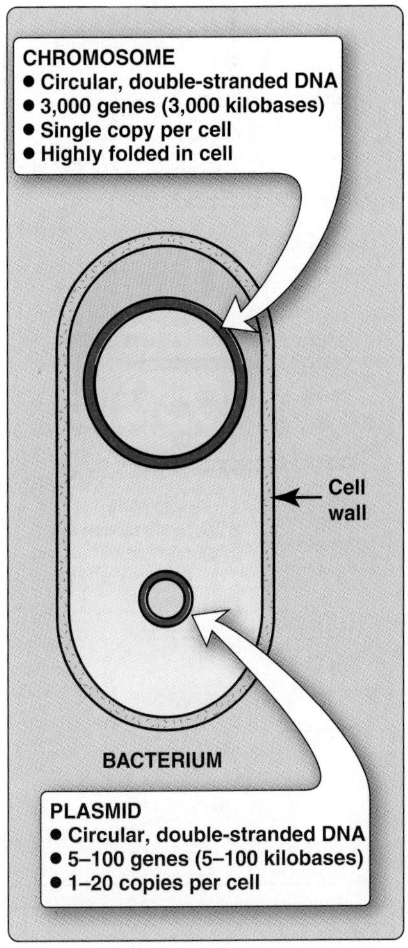

Figure 7.1
The bacterial genome. [Note: Helical double-stranded DNA is shown as two concentric circles.]

II. THE BACTERIAL GENOME

The genome of an organism is defined as the totality of its genetic material. For bacteria, the genome often consists of a single chromosome that carries all of the essential genes and one or more varieties of plasmid that generally carry nonessential genes (Figure 7.1).

A. The chromosome

All of the essential genes and many nonessential genes of the bacterium are generally carried on a single, long piece of circular, double-stranded DNA. This molecular structure is called the "chromosome" by analogy with the heredity-carriers of eukaryotic cells. Most bacteria have chromosomes that contain 2,000 to 4,000 genes.

B. Pathogenicity islands

Pathogenicity islands are discrete genetic elements that encode virulence factors, such as toxins, adhesins, secretion systems, and iron transport proteins. These islands, which range in size from 10 to

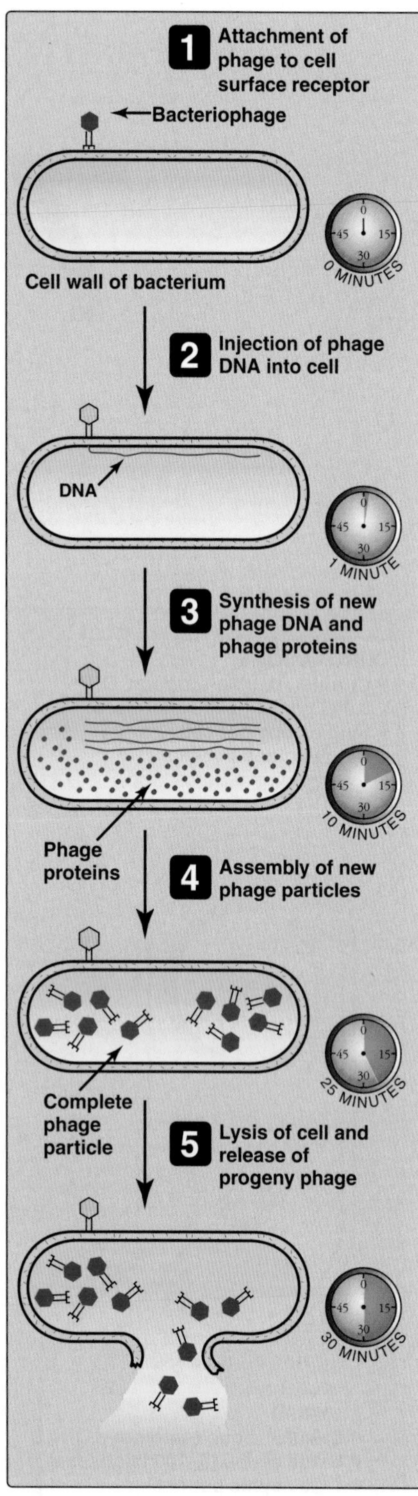

Figure 7.2
Bacteriophage replication. Clock indicates total elapsed time starting with attachment at t = 0. [Note: Bacterial chromosome and plasmid are not shown.]

200 kB, can be horizontally transferred between bacteria, resulting in enhanced virulence and fitness in the recipient. [Note: Horizontal gene transfer is any process (such as transformation, transduction, or bacterial conjugation) in which an organism incorporates genetic material from another organism without being the progeny of that organism. By contrast, vertical transfer occurs when an organism receives genetic material from its ancestor, for example, a species from which it has evolved.] Pathogenicity islands differ from the rest of the chromosome in G+C content and are usually flanked in the recipient's chromosome by repeated sequence elements or genes that encode tRNAs.

C. Plasmids

Typically, bacteria contain small DNA circles (plasmids), which range in size from 1.5 kilobase (kb) pairs to 120 kb pairs (less than one tenth the size of the bacterial chromosome). Plasmids replicate independently of the chromosome and can exist in the cell as one copy or as many copies. Plasmids can carry genes that encode toxins or proteins that promote the transfer of the plasmid to other cells but usually do not include genes that are essential for cell growth or replication. Many plasmids contain mobile DNA sequences (transposons) that can move between plasmids and between plasmids and the chromosome (see pp. 63–64). Transposons, the repository for many antibiotic resistance genes, are responsible for the ability of some plasmids to integrate into the chromosome.

III. BACTERIOPHAGE

A bacteriophage (phage) is a virus that replicates inside a bacterial cell. It consists of nothing more than a piece of nucleic acid encapsulated in a protective protein coat. Depending on the phage, the nucleic acid can be DNA or RNA, double stranded or single stranded, and range in size from about 3,000 bases (3 genes) to about 200,000 bases (200 genes). The typical replicative cycle (Figure 7.2) begins with attachment of the phage to receptors on the cell surface, followed by injection of the nucleic acid into the bacterial cell, leaving all or most of the protein outside the cell. [Note: This is in contrast to viral infection of vertebrate cells, in which the entire virus is taken up by the cell, and its nucleic acid released intracellularly (see pp. 236–237).] The phage nucleic acid encodes proteins that take over the cell's biosynthetic machinery to replicate the phage's own genetic material and to synthesize phage-specific proteins. When sufficient coat proteins and new phage DNA have accumulated, these components self-assemble into mature phage particles, with the DNA encapsulated by the phage coat. Release of new phage particles is accomplished by a phage-specific enzyme (lysozyme) that dissolves the bacterial cell wall. The number of phage particles in a sample can be determined by a simple and rapid plaque assay. If a single phage particle is immobilized in a confluent bacterial lawn growing on a nutrient agar surface, this phage, within a few hours, will produce millions of progeny at the expense of neighboring bacterial cells, leaving a visible "hole" or plaque in the otherwise opaque lawn (Figure 7.3). Phage are classified as virulent or temperate, depending on the nature of their relationship to the host bacterium.

A. Virulent phage

Infection of a bacterium with a virulent phage inevitably results in the death of the cell by lysis, with release of newly replicated phage particles. Under optimal conditions, a bacterial cell infected with only one phage particle can produce hundreds of progeny in 20 minutes. [Note: Generally, phage that attack one bacterial species do not attack other bacterial species.]

B. Temperate phage

A bacterium infected with a temperate phage can have the same fate as a bacterium infected with a virulent phage (lysis rapidly following infection). However, an alternative outcome is also possible: Namely, after entering the cell, the phage DNA, rather than replicating autonomously, can integrate into the chromosome of the host cell. In this state (prophage), the expression of phage genes is repressed indefinitely by a regulatory protein encoded within the phage genome. No new phage particles are produced, the host cell survives, and the phage DNA replicates as part of the host's chromosome.

C. Lysogenic bacteria

Lysogenic bacteria carry a prophage. This phenomenon is termed "lysogeny," and the bacterial cell is said to be "lysogenized." Nonlysogenic bacteria can be made lysogenic by infection with a temperate phage. The association of prophage and bacterial cell is highly stable but can be destabilized by various treatments, such as exposure to ultraviolet light, that damage the host DNA. When DNA damage occurs, repression of phage genes is lifted, and the prophage excises from the host chromosome, replicates autonomously, and produces progeny phage particles. The host cell is lysed just as with a virulent phage. The emergence of the virus from its latent prophage state is called induction. The acquisition by bacteria of properties due to the presence of a prophage is called lysogenic conversion.

IV. GENE TRANSFER

Genes can be transferred from one bacterial cell to another by three distinct mechanisms: conjugation, transduction, and transformation. Because some types of transferred DNA do not contain an origin of replication, these genes will only be passed on to succeeding generations if the transferred DNA becomes incorporated into the recipient chromosome, which has an origin of replication. Plasmids contain their own origin of replication and can, therefore, be maintained in a host through subsequent generations without being integrated into the chromosome.

A. Conjugation

Conjugation is the process by which bacteria transfer genes from one cell to another by cell-to-cell contact. The donor (male) and recipient (female) cells must have the proper genetic constitution to adhere to each other, and they form a cytoplasmic bridge between

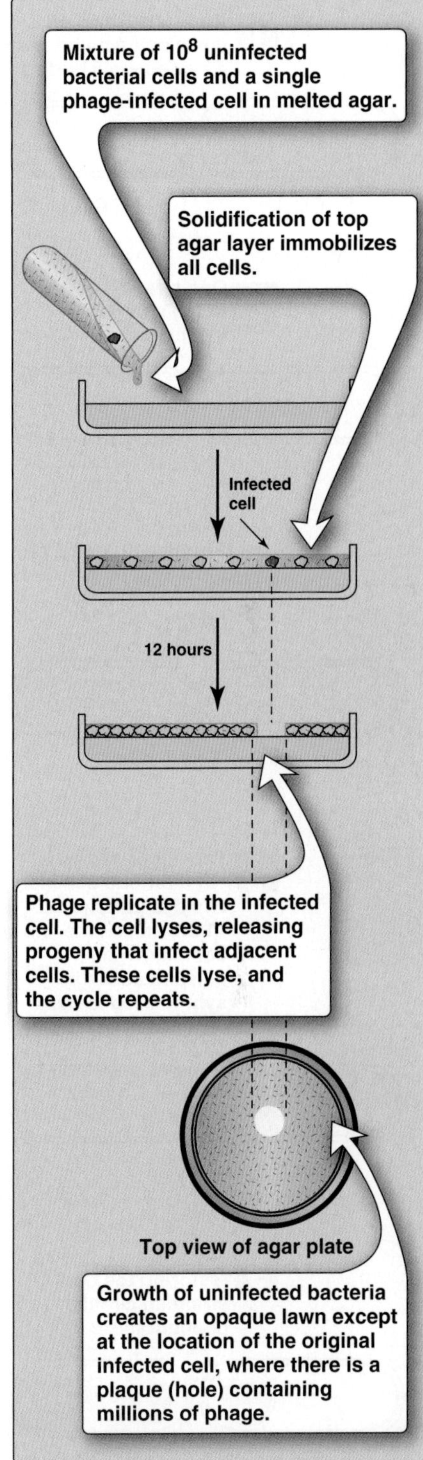

Mixture of 10^8 uninfected bacterial cells and a single phage-infected cell in melted agar.
Solidification of top agar layer immobilizes all cells.
Infected cell
12 hours
Phage replicate in the infected cell. The cell lyses, releasing progeny that infect adjacent cells. These cells lyse, and the cycle repeats.
Top view of agar plate
Growth of uninfected bacteria creates an opaque lawn except at the location of the original infected cell, where there is a plaque (hole) containing millions of phage.

Figure 7.3
Visual detection of bacteriophage by the plaque method.

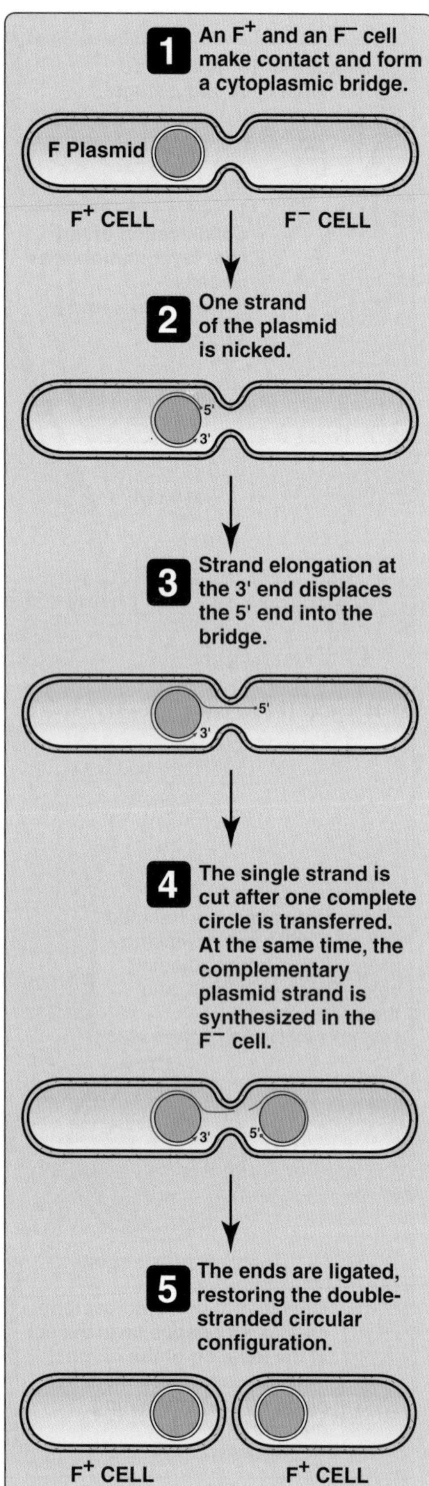

1 An F+ and an F− cell make contact and form a cytoplasmic bridge.
F Plasmid
F+ CELL
F− CELL
2 One strand of the plasmid is nicked.
5'
3'
3 Strand elongation at the 3' end displaces the 5' end into the bridge.
5'
3'
4 The single strand is cut after one complete circle is transferred. At the same time, the complementary plasmid strand is synthesized in the F− cell.
3'
5'
5 The ends are ligated, restoring the double-stranded circular configuration.
F+ CELL
F+ CELL

Figure 7.4
Cell-to-cell transfer of a conjugative plasmid (chromosomal DNA is not shown).

the cells through which DNA can pass. Specifically, the process requires the presence on the donor cell of a hairlike projection called a sex pilus that makes contact with a specific receptor site on the surface of the recipient cell. This contact results in the formation of a relatively stable cell pair and the initiation of DNA transfer (Figure 7.4).

B. Transduction

Transduction refers to transfer of genes from one cell to another via a phage vector without cell-to-cell contact. There are two ways in which this can occur: generalized transduction and specialized transduction. In each case, the transducing phage is a temperate phage, so that the recipient cell survives the phage infection.

1. **Generalized transduction:** In generalized transduction, a random fragment of bacterial DNA is accidentally encapsulated in a phage protein coat in place of the phage DNA (Figure 7.5A). When this rare phage particle infects a recipient cell, it injects the bacterial DNA fragment into the cell. If this fragment becomes integrated into the recipient chromosome by recombination, the recipient cell will be stably transduced.

2. **Specialized transduction:** In specialized transduction, only certain bacterial genes, located on the bacterial chromosome in close proximity to the prophage insertion site of the transducing phage, are transduced (Figure 7.5B). The phage acquires the bacterial genes by a rare, abnormal excision from the bacterial chromosome. A specialized transducing phage particle contains both phage and bacterial DNA joined together as a single molecule. After infecting another cell, this joint molecule integrates into the recipient chromosome just as phage DNA normally does in the process of becoming a prophage.

C. Transformation

Transformation is the transfer of genes from one cell to another by means of naked DNA. The discovery of transformation in 1928, one of the most important in all of biology, led eventually to the identification of DNA as the genetic material. Studies of the transformation phenomenon itself revealed that the ability of a cell to be transformed (called competence) depends on a physiologic state of the cell that allows DNA to cross the cell membrane. As free, double-stranded DNA enters the recipient cell, one of the two strands is destroyed by nucleases. The remaining single strand invades the resident chromosome, seeking a region of sequence homology. If such a sequence is found, the invading strand replaces one of the two resident strands by a complex cut-and-paste process.

V. GENETIC VARIATION

Although all of the cells in a "pure" bacterial culture are derived from a single original cell, the culture typically contains rare cells that differ from the originating cell. The majority of such variants (mutants) are due to changes (mutations) in their DNA.

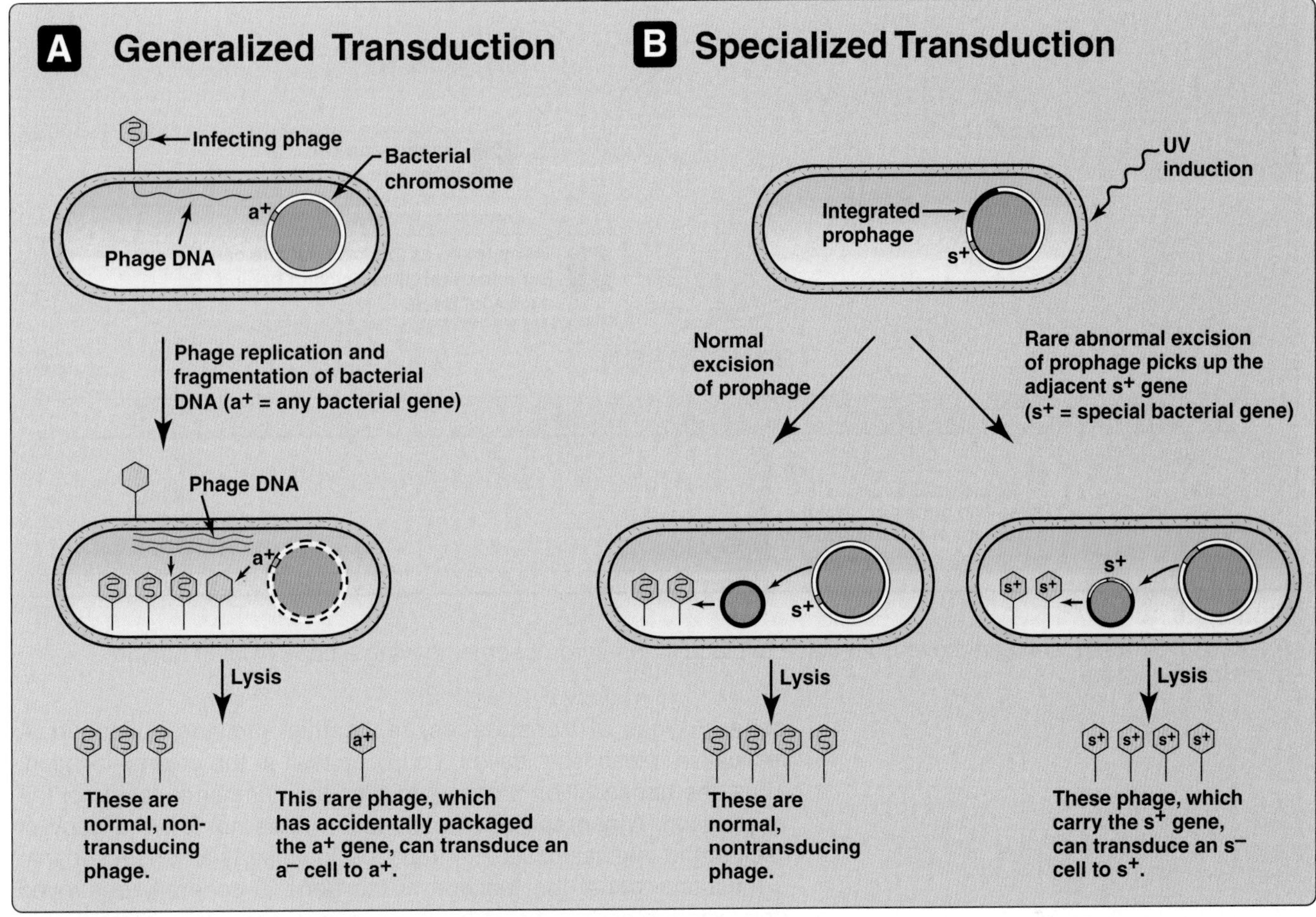

Figure 7.5
Certain phage can package bacterial genes and transfer them to other bacteria (transduction). By one mechanism (A) any bacterial gene can be transferred. By a second mechanism (B) only certain genes can be transferred, namely those in close proximity to a prophage.

A. Mutations

Strictly speaking, any change in the structure of genetic material or, more specifically, any change in the base sequence of DNA, is called a mutation. Some mutations are unstable (that is, they frequently revert back to their original state), and others do not noticeably affect the organism. Mutations that come under study are usually those that are stable and that cause some change in the characteristics of the organism. Mutations can be classified according to the kind of chemical change that occurs in the DNA or, when the mutation affects a protein-coding gene, by the effect the mutation has on the translation of the message.

B. Mobile genetic elements

In recent years, it has been recognized that the arrangement of genes in the genome of bacteria (and probably all organisms) is not entirely static. Certain DNA segments, called transposons, have the ability to move from place to place on the chromosome and into and out of plasmids. Transposons do not exist as segments free of the genome but only as segments within the genome. There are two

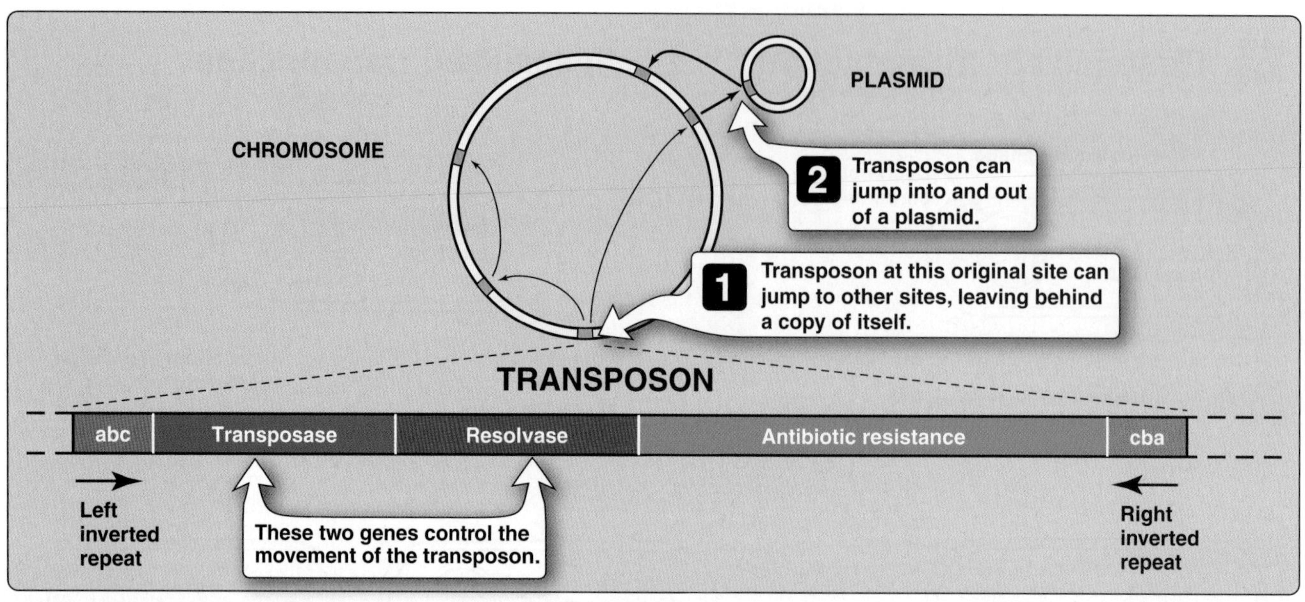

Figure 7.6
A replicative transposon can move from place to place in the chromosome, leaving a copy of itself behind at the previous site.

general types of transposons: replicative and nonreplicative. A replicative transposon leaves a copy of itself at the original location. Thus, the transposition process doubles the number of copies of the transposon. A nonreplicative transposon does not leave a copy of itself at the original location. If transposition inserts a transposon into a functional gene, the function of the gene is generally destroyed (this was the original basis by which transposons were discovered). Transposons can, thus, be viewed as internal mutagenic agents. The transposition process and the structure of a typical replicative transposon are shown in Figure 7.6. This transposon has three genes and a length of about five kilobases. The transposase and resolvase genes code for enzymes involved in the transposition process, whereas the antibiotic resistance gene is a "passenger." The transposon is bounded by short (about 50 bases), inverted repeats. These inverted repeats are the elements recognized by the transposase as it initiates the transposition. Mobile genetic elements are probably responsible for most of the genetic variability in natural bacterial populations and for the spread of antibiotic resistance genes.

C. Mechanisms of acquired antibiotic resistance

Acquired antibiotic resistance requires a temporary or permanent gain or alteration of bacterial genetic information. Although most resistance genes are plasmid mediated, plasmid-mediated traits can interchange with chromosomal elements. Transfer of genetic material from plasmid to chromosome can occur by simple recombinational events, but the process is greatly facilitated by transposons. Many resistance genes, such as plasmid-mediated β-lactamases, tetracycline-resistance genes, and aminoglycoside-modifying enzymes, are organized on transposons. Resistance to antibiotics is accomplished by five principal mechanisms, three of which are shown in Figure 7.7.

1. **Decreased uptake of antibiotic:** Gram-negative organisms can limit the penetration of certain agents, including β-lactam antibiotics, tetracyclines, and chloramphenicol, as a result of alteration in the number and structure of porins (proteins that form channels) in the outer membrane.
2. **Antibiotic efflux:** Some gram-negative organisms encode multi-component membrane-imbedded efflux systems that recognize and pump out diverse, toxic substances, including detergents and antibiotics. Expression of these systems is generally tightly regulated and often induced by the presence of substrates recognized by the pump.
3. **Alteration of the target site for antibiotic:** *Streptococcus pneumoniae* resistance to β-lactam antibiotics, for example, involves alterations in one or more of the major bacterial penicillin-binding proteins (see p. 75), which results in decreased binding of the antibiotic to its target.
4. **Acquisition of the ability to destroy or modify the antibiotic:** Examples of antibiotic inactivating enzymes include: 1) β-lactamases that hydrolytically inactivate the β-lactam ring of penicillins, cephalosporins, and related drugs; 2) acetyltransferases that transfer an acetyl group to the antibiotic, inactivating chloramphenicol or aminoglycosides; and 3) esterases that hydrolyze the lactone ring of macrolides.
5. **Acquisition of a new target:** Some *Staphylococcus aureus* isolates, for example, are vancomycin resistant due to expression of newly acquired genes that modify the D-ala-D-ala (the target of vancomycin) residues on the stem peptide, converting them instead to D-ala-D-lac. Although this new target is effectively polymerized to form a peptidoglycan network with sufficient stability, D-ala-D-lac is not bound by vancomycin, and, therefore, the antimicrobial agent is no longer effective.

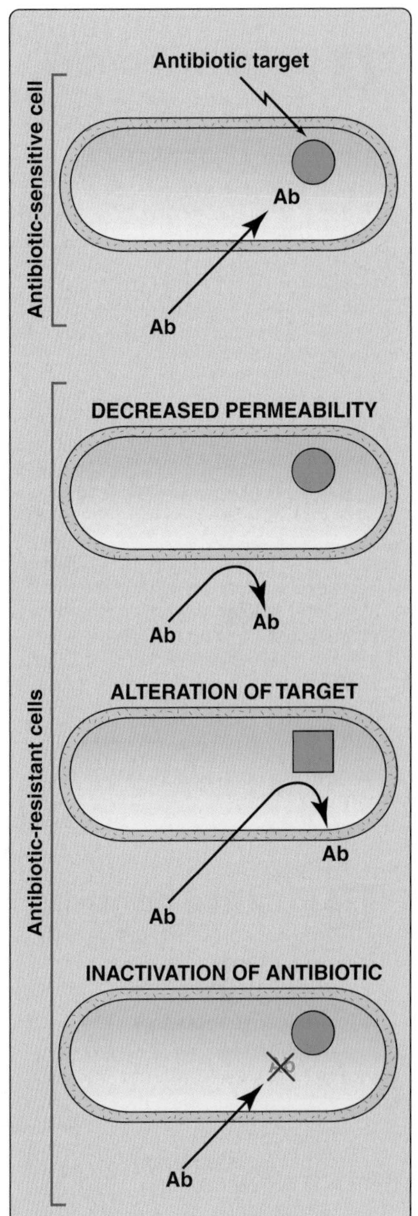

Figure 7.7
Three common mechanisms of antibiotic resistance.

VI. GENE REGULATION

Many bacteria can manufacture most of the organic compounds (such as amino acids, nucleotides, carbohydrates, lipids) that they need, and, in this regard, they are more versatile than higher organisms. This metabolic resourcefulness is a distinct advantage when the organism is in a nutritionally poor environment but is extremely wasteful in a nutritious environment if the bacterium must keep all of the unneeded biosynthetic enzymes ready. Therefore, bacteria have evolved various mechanisms for producing certain metabolic enzymes only when they are needed. Most regulation in bacteria involves control of transcription, rather than control of translation of the mRNA into protein. The following classical example describes the mechanisms that regulate expression of the lac operon in *E. coli*.

A. Negative control (repression)

Lactose is a disaccharide composed of glucose and galactose. The first step in lactose metabolism is cleavage into monosaccharide units, a job performed by the enzyme β-galactosidase. To avoid being

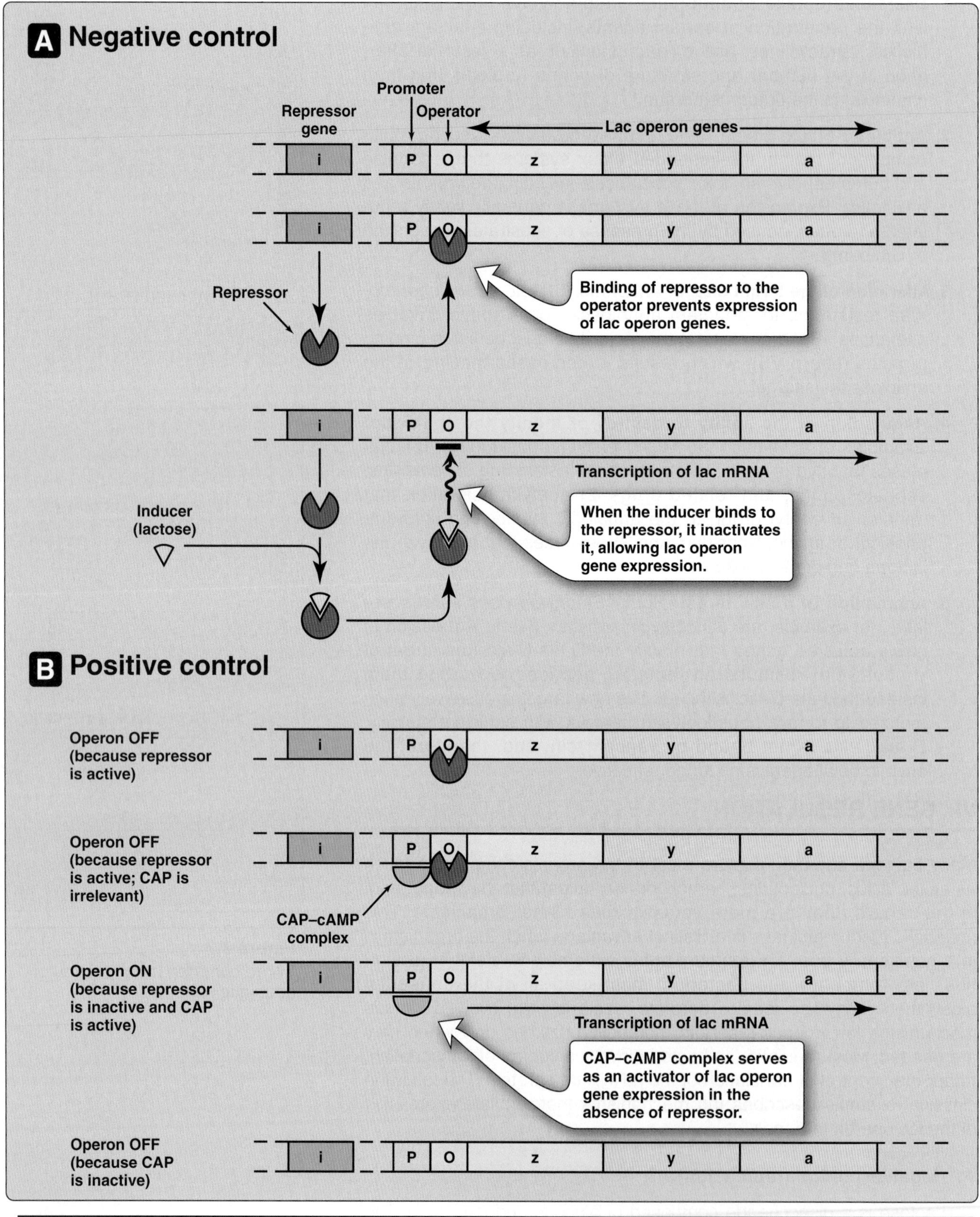

Figure 7.8
Bacterial genes can be controlled negatively by repressors or positively by activators. CAP = catabolite activator protein; cAMP = cyclic adenosine monophosphate.

wasteful, bacteria synthesize β-galactosidase only when lactose is present in the growth medium. Bacteria accomplish this control by producing a repressor protein that, when lactose is absent, binds to a specific site on the DNA (operator site) near the start of the β-galactosidase gene (Figure 7.8A). When repressor is bound, RNA polymerase, which recognizes the promoter region that is upstream from the operator site, is blocked from initiating transcription of the genes. When lactose is present, it binds to the repressor protein, preventing the repressor from binding to the DNA, and allowing transcription of the genes. The β-galactosidase gene is actually one of a set of three contiguous genes. The other two are a lactose permease and β-galactoside transacetylase. Together, these three genes, all of which are controlled by the same repressor, comprise the lac operon. This mechanism is called negative control because the controlling element (that is, the repressor) acts to prevent transcription. In this example, lactose is an inducer of the lac operon. [Note: In other cases, the free repressor does not repress unless it binds to another compound (corepressor). For example, the repressor for the tryptophan operon is active only when it binds to tryptophan.]

B. Positive control (activation)

If bacteria are grown in medium containing glucose and another sugar, the bacteria use glucose exclusively as an energy source. This is because transcription of all of the operons for use of sugars other than glucose fails to occur, even though the inducing sugars are present. The reason for this failure is that the sugar-utilization operons (for example, the lac operon), must be activated by a specific protein called catabolite activator protein (CAP), which, in turn, is only functional as an activator when complexed with cyclic adenosine monophosphate (cAMP). [Note: CAP is also called CRP (cAMP receptor protein).] Glucose, in turn, regulates CAP activity by regulating the level of cAMP. When glucose is present at a high level, cAMP is at a low level, and sugar-utilization operons are not activated. When glucose is absent or at a low level, cAMP is at a high level, and sugar utilization operons are activated (Figure 7.8B). Although this process is technically activation, it is more often referred to as "catabolite repression." Catabolite repression is a global regulatory mechanism by which many operons, each under individual control, are coordinately regulated by a single activator protein.

C. Modifications of RNA polymerase specificity

Microorganisms are often compelled to switch on or off large groups of genes in response to stressful environmental conditions. For example, under starvation conditions, many species sporulate, a process that requires major changes in metabolic pathways. Similarly, sudden exposure to elevated temperature ("heat shock") elicits formation of many new proteins. In both cases, the shift in gene expression results from a modification of the RNA polymerase, specifically, a replacement of the normal σ (sigma) subunit with an alternative subunit that recognizes a different set of promoters.

Study Questions

Choose the ONE correct answer

7.1 A lysogenic bacterium

A. carries a prophage.
B. causes lysis of other bacteria on contact.
C. cannot support the replication of a virulent phage.
D. is often a human pathogen.
E. is usually not capable of conjugal genetic transfer.

Correct answer = A. A lysogenic bacterium can generate phage because it carries phage genes in a latent state (prophage). Lysogeny does not impart any special lytic properties to the bacterium nor, in general, does it affect conjugal transfer or the ability to support the replication of other unrelated phage. The presence of a prophage can convert certain bacteria to human pathogens, but such cases are rare.

7.2 Which one of the following statements concerning plasmids is true?

A. All plasmids can be transfered between bacteria by conjugation.
B. Much of the information coded in the plasmid is essential to the survival of the bacteria cell.
C. Resistance plasmids carry genes for antibiotic resistance.
D. Resistance plasmids cannot be transferred to other bacterial cells.
E. Plasmids lack an origin of replication.

Correct answer = C. Plasmids are small, circular, supercoiled DNA molecules found in some bacteria. They usually do not carry essential genes, but some plasmids, such as R (resistance) plasmids, carry genes coding for antibiotic resistance. All plasmids have their own origin of replication, so that they are replicated along with the host chromosome and passed along to progeny cells. Only some plasmids possess genes that allow for transmittal to other bacteria by the process of conjugation.

7.3 What occurs when a temperate bacteriophage enters a state called "lysogeny"?

A. Most viral genes are expressed.
B. The bacterial cell is lysed.
C. Many new viruses are produced.
D. Most normal bacterial functions are turned off.
E. The virus may become integrated into the host genome.

Correct answer = E. There are two types of bacteriophages: lytic and temperate. The distinction is made according to the life cycle of the bacteriophage. On entering a bacterium, lytic phages produce phage nucleic acids and proteins, assemble many new phage particles, lyse the cell, and release the progeny phage. Temperate phages, however, can penetrate the bacterium and enter a dormant state called lysogeny, in which most viral genes are repressed. Bacterial functions remain active and the bacterium is not harmed. Some dormant phages replicate as plasmids; others, such as phage λ (lambda), become integrated into the host genome as prophages. The prophage DNA is replicated along with the host DNA as the bacterium grows and divides.

7.4 A virulence factor can be transferred from one strain of bacteria to another in a genetic process that is independent of cell-to-cell contact between the donor and the recipient. Addition of DNase does not interfere with the transfer of the virulence factor either. From these characteristics, which of the following processes is involved in this genetic transfer?

A. Conjugation
B. Transformation
C. Transduction
D. Transposition
E. Transversion

Correct answer = C. Transduction is the process by which genetic material is transferred from donor to recipient within a bacteriophage. This process does not require cell-to-cell contact and is resistant to DNase. Conjugation requires cell-to-cell contact between the donor and receipient cells. Transformation involves the exchange of naked DNA between donor and recipient in the absence of cell-to cell contact. However, DNA transformation is sensitive to DNase treatment. Transposition is the process in which a transposon excises from one location and integrates in another location within the same bacterial cell. Thus this process would not explain the transfer of a genetic marker between different bacterial cells. Transversion is not a means of genetic exchange.

Staphylococci

8

I. OVERVIEW

Staphylococci and streptococci (see Chapter 9) constitute the main groups of medically important gram-positive cocci. Staphylococcal infections range from the trivial to the rapidly fatal. They can be very difficult to treat, especially those contracted in hospitals, because of the remarkable ability of staphylococci to become resistant to antibiotics. Staphylococci are ubiquitous in nature, with about a dozen species occurring as part of human flora. The most virulent of the genus, *Staphylococcus aureus*, is one of the most common causes of bacterial infections, and is also an important cause of food poisoning and toxic shock syndrome. Among less virulent staphylococcal species, *Staphylococcus epidermidis* is an important cause of prosthetic implant infections, whereas *Staphylococcus saprophyticus* causes urinary tract infections, especially cystitis in women. Figure 8.1 summarizes the staphylococci described in this chapter.

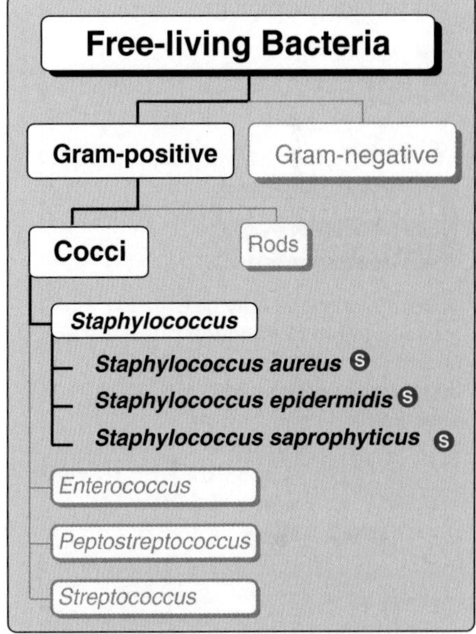

Figure 8.1
Classification of Staphylococci.
S See pp. 349–350 for summaries of these organisms.

II. GENERAL FEATURES

Staphylococci generally stain darkly gram positive (Figure 8.2). They are round rather than oval and tend to occur in bunches like grapes. Because growth of staphylococci requires supplementation with various amino acids and other growth factors, they are routinely cultured on enriched media containing nutrient broth and/or blood (see p. 23). Staphylococci are facultatively anaerobic organisms. They produce catalase, which is one feature that distinguishes them from the catalase-negative streptococci. The most virulent species of staphylococcus is *S. aureus*, almost all isolates of which secrete coagulase, an enzyme that causes citrated plasma to clot. Other species that occasionally cause disease and lack coagulase are often referred to as coagulase-negative staphylococci. Staphylococci are hardy, being resistant to heat and drying, and thus can persist for long periods on fomites (inanimate objects), which can then serve as sources of infection. Frequent handwashing before and after contact with food or potentially infected individuals decreases the transmission of staphylococcal disease.

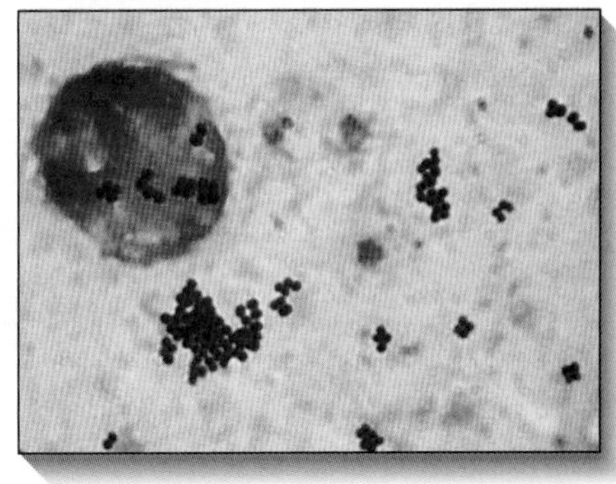

Figure 8.2
Gram stain of *Staphylococcus aureus*.

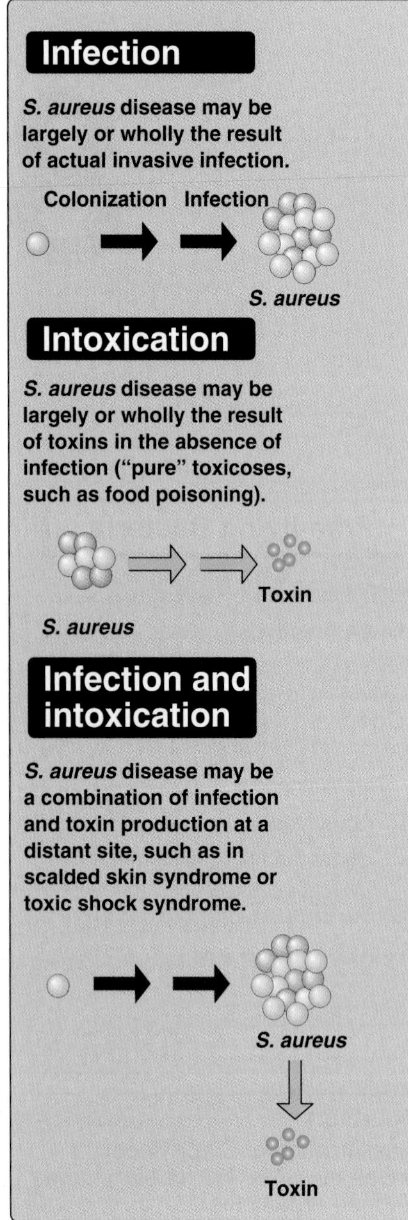

Figure 8.3
Causes of disease resulting from infection with *Staphylococcus aureus.*

III. STAPHYLOCOCCUS AUREUS

Generally, significant host compromise is required for *S. aureus* infection, such as a break in the skin or insertion of a foreign body (for example, wounds, surgical infections, or central venous catheters), an obstructed hair follicle (folliculitis), or a compromised immune system. *S. aureus* disease may be: 1) largely or wholly the result of actual invasive infection, overcoming host defense mechanisms, and the production of extracellular substances which facilitate invasion; 2) a result of toxins in the absence of invasive infection ("pure" toxinoses); or 3) a combination of invasive infection and intoxication (Figure 8.3).

A. Epidemiology

S. aureus is frequently carried by healthy individuals on the skin and mucous membranes. Carriers serve as a source of infection to themselves and others; for example, by direct contact, by contamination of fomites (objects such as a doorknob, which in turn can be a source of infection) or contamination of food, which can then result in food poisoning.

B. Pathogenesis

Virulence factors are the genetic, biochemical, or structural features that enable an organism to produce disease. The clinical outcome of an infection depends on the virulence of the pathogen and the opposing effectiveness of the host defense mechanisms. *S. aureus* expresses many potential virulence factors (Figure 8.4). [Note: Coagulase activity results in localized clotting, which restricts access by polymorphonuclear neutrophils (PMNs) and other immune defenses. This would make coagulase a virulence factor, even though mutants lacking the ability to make this factor remain virulent in animal models]. For the majority of diseases caused by *S. aureus*, pathogenesis depends on the combined actions of several virulence factors, so it is difficult to determine precisely the role of any given factor.

1. Cell wall virulence factors:

a. Capsule: Most clinical isolates express a polysaccharide "microcapsule" of Types 5 or 8. The capsule layer is very thin but has been associated with increased resistance to phagocytosis. Clinical isolates produce capsule but expression is rapidly lost upon *in vitro* cultivation.

b. Protein A: Protein A is a major component of the *S. aureus* cell wall. It binds to the Fc region of IgG, exerting an anti-opsonin (and therefore strongly antiphagocytic) effect.

c. Fibronectin-binding protein: Fibrinectin-binding protein (FnBP) and other staphylococcal surface proteins promote binding to mucosal cells and tissue matrices.

d. Clumping factor: This FnBP enhances clumping of the organisms in the presence of plasma.

2. **Cytolytic exotoxins:** α, β, γ, and δ Toxins attack mammalian cell (including red blood cell) membranes, and are often referred to as hemolysins. α Toxin is the best studied, and is chromosomally encoded. It polymerizes into tubes that pierce membranes, resulting in the loss of important molecules and, eventually, in osmotic lysis.

3. **Panton-Valentine leukocidin:** This pore-forming toxin lyses PMNs. Production of this toxin makes strains more virulent. This toxin is produced predominantly by community-acquired methicillin-resistant *S. aureus* (MRSA) strains (see p. 74).

4. **Superantigen exotoxins:** These toxins have an affinity for the T-cell receptor–major histocompatibility complex Class II antigen complex. They stimulate enhanced T-lymphocyte response (as many as 20 percent of T cells respond, compared with 0.01 percent responding to the usual processed antigens). This difference is a result of their ability to recognize a relatively conserved region of the T-cell receptor. This major T-cell activation can cause toxic shock syndrome, primarily by release into the circulation of inordinately large amounts of T-cell cytokines, such as interleukin-2 (IL-2), interferon-γ (IFN-γ), and tumor necrosis factor-α (TNF-α).

   a. **Enterotoxins:** Enterotoxins (six major antigenic types: A, B, C, D, E, and G) are produced by approximately half of all *S. aureus* isolates. When these bacteria contaminate food and are allowed to grow, they secrete enterotoxin, ingestion of which can cause food poisoning. [Note: The toxin stimulates the vomiting center in the brain by binding to neural receptors in the upper gastrointestinal (GI) tract.] Enterotoxins are superantigens that are even more heat-stable than *S. aureus*. Therefore, organisms are not always recovered from incriminated food but the toxin may be recovered.

   b. **Toxic shock syndrome toxin (TSST–1):** This is the classic cause of toxic shock syndrome (TSS). Because of similarities in molecular structure, it is sometimes referred to as staphylococcal enterotoxin F, although it does not cause food poisoning when ingested.

   c. **Exfoliatin (exfoliative toxin, ET)** is also a superantigen. It causes scalded skin syndrome in children. The toxin cleaves desmoglein 1, which is a component of desmosomes (cell structures specialized for cell-to-cell adhesion). Cleavage results in loss of the superficial skin layer.

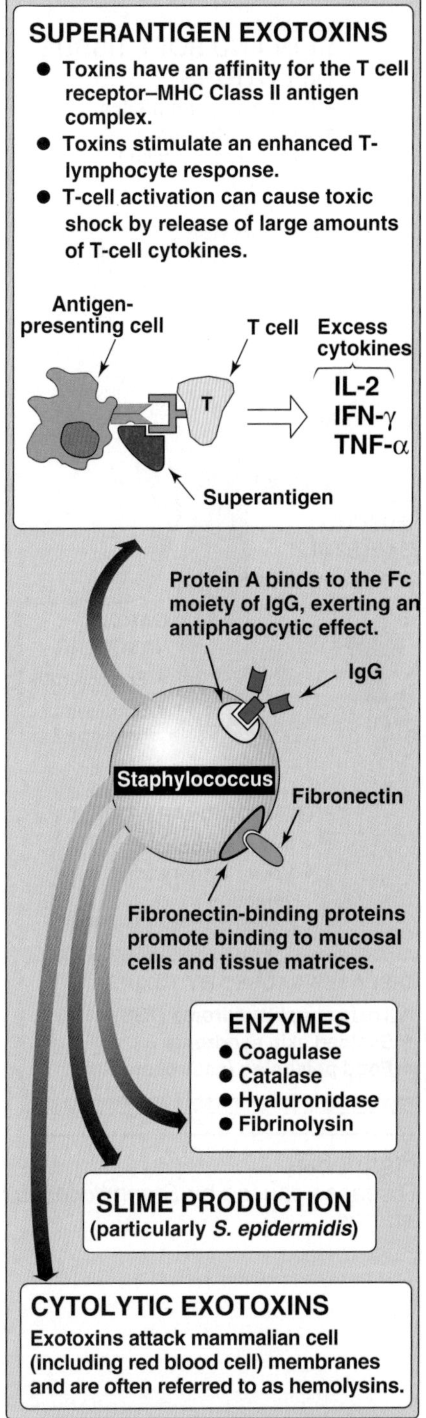
SUPERANTIGEN EXOTOXINS
• Toxins have an affinity for the T cell receptor–MHC Class II antigen complex.
• Toxins stimulate an enhanced T-lymphocyte response.
• T-cell activation can cause toxic shock by release of large amounts of T-cell cytokines.
Antigen-presenting cell
T cell
Excess cytokines
T
IL-2
IFN-γ
TNF-α
Superantigen
Protein A binds to the Fc moiety of IgG, exerting an antiphagocytic effect.
IgG
Staphylococcus
Fibronectin
Fibronectin-binding proteins promote binding to mucosal cells and tissue matrices.
ENZYMES
• Coagulase
• Catalase
• Hyaluronidase
• Fibrinolysin
SLIME PRODUCTION
(particularly S. epidermidis)
CYTOLYTIC EXOTOXINS
Exotoxins attack mammalian cell (including red blood cell) membranes and are often referred to as hemolysins.

Figure 8.4
Virulence factors that may play a role in the pathogenesis of staphylococcal infections. MHC = major histocompatibility complex; IL = interleukin; IFN = interferon; TNF = tumor necrosis factor; IgG = immunoglobulin G.

C. Clinical significance

S. aureus causes disease by infecting tissues, typically creating abscesses and/or by producing toxins (Figure 8.5). A common entry point into the body is a break in the skin, which may be a minute needlestick or a surgical wound. Another portal of entry is the respiratory tract. For example, staphylococcal pneumonia is a important

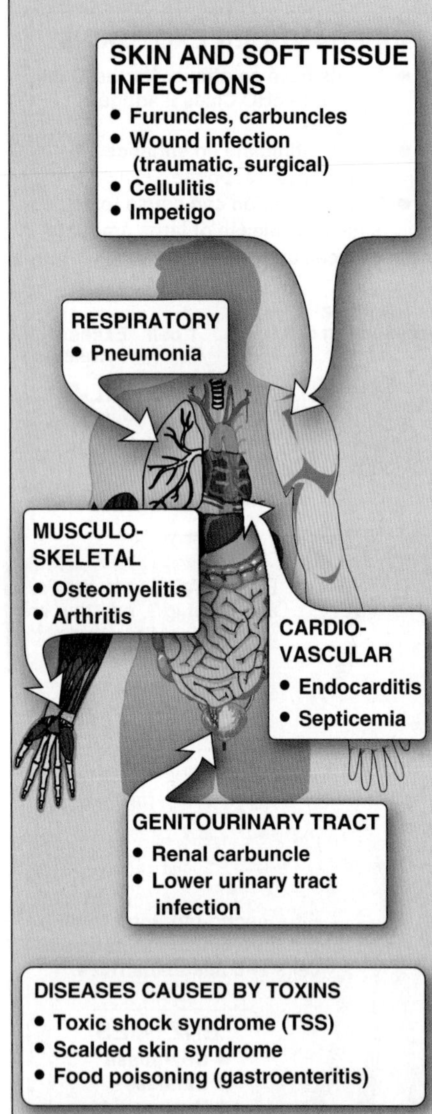

Figure 8.5
Diseases caused by *Staphylococcus aureus*.

complication of influenza. The localized host response to staphylococcal infection is inflammation, characterized by swelling, accumulation of pus, and necrosis of tissue. Fibroblasts and their products may form a wall around the inflamed area, which contains bacteria and leukocytes. This creates a characteristic pus-filled boil or abscess. Serious consequences of staphylococcal infections occur when the bacteria invade the bloodstream. The resulting septicemia (the presence and persistence of pathogenic microorganisms or their toxins in the blood) may be rapidly fatal. Bacteremia (the presence of viable bacteria circulating in the bloodstream) may result in seeding internal abscesses, skin lesions, or infections in the lung, kidney, heart, skeletal muscle, or meninges.

1. **Localized skin infections:** The most common *S. aureus* infections are small, superficial abscesses involving hair follicles (folliculitis) or sweat or sebaceous glands (see Figure 8.12). For example, the common sty (external hordeolum) is created by infection of an eyelash follicle. Subcutaneous abscesses called furuncles (boils) often form around foreign bodies such as splinters. These generally respond to local therapy, that is, removal of the foreign body, soaking, and drainage as indicated. Carbuncles are larger, deeper, multiloculated skin infections that can lead to bacteremia and require antibiotic therapy and debridement. Impetigo is usually a localized, superficial, spreading crusty skin lesion generally seen in children. It can be caused by *S. aureus*, although more commonly by *Streptococcus pyogenes* (see p. 80), or both organisms together. Human staphylococcal infections usually remain localized at the portal of entry by normal host defenses.

2. **Deep, localized infections:** These may be metastatic from superficial infections or skin carriage or may result from trauma. *S. aureus* is the most common cause of acute and chronic infection of bone marrow. *S. aureus* is also the most common cause of acute infection of joint space in children (septic joint). [Note: Septic joints are medical emergencies because pus can rapidly cause irreparable cartilage damage. They must be treated promptly with drainage and an antibiotic.]

3. **Acute endocarditis**: Generally associated with intravenous drug abuse, acute endocarditis is caused by injection of contaminated preparations or by needles contaminated with *S. aureus*. *S. aureus* also colonizes the skin around the injection site, and if the skin is not sterilized before injection, the bacteria can be introduced into soft tissues and the bloodstream, even when a sterilized needle is used. An abscess in any organ or tissue is cause to suspect *S. aureus,* although many other bacteria can cause abscesses.

4. **Septicemia** is a generalized infection with sepsis or bacteremia that may be associated with a known focus (for example, a septic joint) or not (an occult focus).

5. **Pneumonia:** *S. aureus* is a cause of severe, necrotizing pneumonia.

6. **Nosocomial infections:** *S. aureus* is one of the most common causes of hospital-associated infections, often of wounds (surgical, decubital) or bacteremia associated with catheters (see Figure 8.10). Progression to septicemia is often a terminal event.

7. **Toxinoses:** These are diseases caused by the action of a toxin, frequently when the organism that secreted the toxin is undetectable. Toxinoses caused by *S. aureus* include:

   a. **Toxic shock syndrome**: TSS results in high fever, rash (resembling a sunburn, with diffuse erythema followed by desquamation), vomiting, diarrhea, hypotension, and multiorgan involvement (especially GI, renal, and/or hepatic damage). An outbreak of TSS occurred in the late 1970s among menstruating women. It was shown to be related to the use of hyperabsorbant tampons by women who happened to be vaginally colonized by toxic shock syndrome toxin–(TSST)–positive strains of *S. aureus*. [Note: These tampons stimulated TSST expression, resulting in entry of the toxin into the circulation in the absence of true infection.] The incidence has decreased markedly since such tampons were removed from the market. Of the few cases of TSS that occur currently, approximately half are associated with ordinary *S. aureus* infections. Of the remainder, many result from a circulating enterotoxin rather than TSST. Figure 8.6 shows the desquamation (peeling or scaling of the skin) seen in TSS.

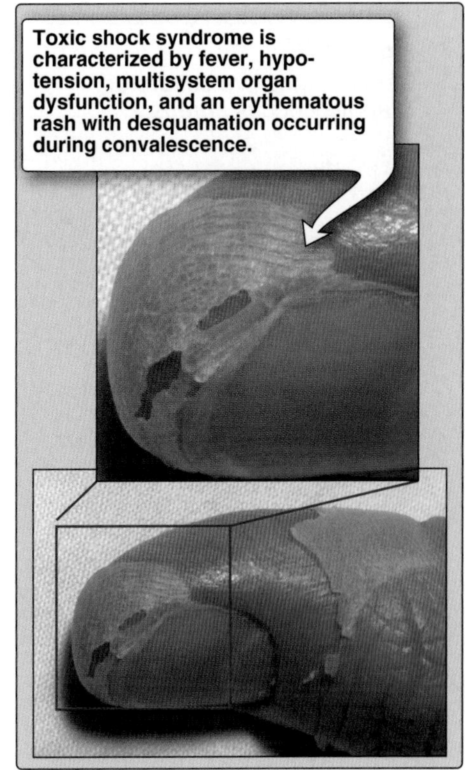

Toxic shock syndrome is characterized by fever, hypotension, multisystem organ dysfunction, and an erythematous rash with desquamation occurring during convalescence.

Figure 8.6
Desquamation of skin in toxic shock syndrome.

   b. **Staphylococcal gastroenteritis:** This is caused by ingestion of food contaminated with enterotoxin-producing *S. aureus*. Often contaminated by a food handler, these foods tend to be protein rich (for example, egg salad or cream pastry) or salty, like ham (*S. aureus* is salt tolerant), and improperly refrigerated. These heat-resistant toxins are able to withstand subsequent reheating. Symptoms, such as nausea, vomiting, and diarrhea, are acute following a short incubation period (less than 6 hours) and are triggered by local actions of the toxin on the GI tract rather than from infection. See p. 372 for a summary of foodborne illness. The short incubation period of staphylococcal food poisoning occurs because the toxin in the food has already been formed by the staphylococci before the food is ingested.

   c. **Scalded skin syndrome:** This involves the appearance of superficial bullae resulting from the action of an exfoliative toxin that attacks the intercellular adhesive of the stratum granulosum, causing marked epithelial desquamation (see Figure 8.12). The bullae may be infected or may result from toxin produced by organisms infecting a different site.

D. Laboratory identification

Identification of an isolate as a staphylococcus relies largely on microscopic and colony morphology and catalase positivity (Figure

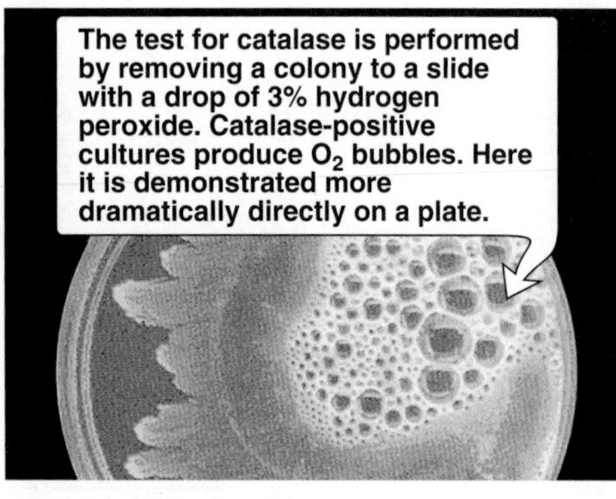

Figure 8.7
Catalase-positive culture of *Staphylococcus aureus*.

8.7). Bacteria stain strongly gram-positive, and are frequently seen in grapelike clusters (see Figure 8.2). *S. aureus* is distinguished from the coagulase-negative staphylococci primarily by coagulase positivity. In addition, *S. aureus* colonies tend to be yellow (hence "aureus," meaning golden) and hemolytic (see Figure 8.12), rather than gray and nonhemolytic like the coagulase-negative staphylococci. *S. aureus* is also distinguished from most coagulase-negative staphylococci by being mannitol-positive.

E. Immunity

S. aureus infections do not elicit strong or long-lasting immunity, as demonstrated by the continuing susceptibility of individuals to *S. aureus* infections throughout life.

F. Treatment

Serious *S. aureus* infections require aggressive treatment, including incision and drainage of localized lesions, as well as systemic antibiotics. Choice of antibiotics is complicated by the frequent presence of acquired antibiotic resistance determinants (see p. 64). Virtually all community and hospital-acquired *S. aureus* infections are now resistant to penicillin G due to penicillinase-encoding plasmids or transposons. This has required the replacement of the initial agent of choice, penicillin G, by β-lactamase-resistant penicillins, such as methicillin or oxacillin. However, increased use of methicillin and related antibiotics has resulted in *S. aureus* that is resistant to a number of β-lactam antibiotics, such as methicillin, oxacillin and amoxicillin (Figure 8.8). These strains are known as methicillin-resistant *S. aureus*.

1. **Hospital-acquired methicillin-resistant *S. aureus* (MRSA):** In recent decades, a high percentage (often in the range of 50 percent) of hospital *S. aureus* isolates has been found to be also resistant to methicillin or oxacillin. Antibiotic resistance is caused by chromosomal acquisition of the gene for a distinct penicillin-binding protein (PBP, see p. 57), PBP-2a. This protein codes for a new peptidoglycan transpeptidase with a low affinity for all currently available β-lactam antibiotics, and thus renders infections with MRSA unresponsive to β-lactam therapy. Compared with methicilllin-sensitive *S. aureus*, MRSA infections are associated with worse outcomes, including longer hospital and intensive care unit stays, longer durations of mechanical ventilation, and higher mortality rates. MRSA strains are also frequently resistant to many other antibiotics, some being sensitive only to glycopeptides such as vancomycin.

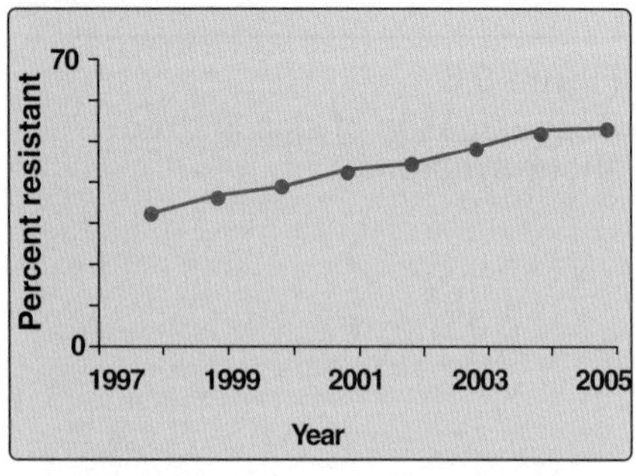

Figure 8.8
Trends in the prevalence of methicillin resistant strains of *Staphylococcus aureus*.

2. **Community-acquired MRSA (CA-MRSA):** Community acquired MRSA infections were documented in the mid-1990s, occurring in individuals who had no previous risk factors for MRSA infections, such as exposure to hospital. The most common clinical manifestations of CA-MRSA are skin and soft tissue infections such as abscesses or cellulitis (Figure 8.9). Less commonly, CA-MRSA can also cause severe diseases such as necrotizing pneumonia, osteomyelitis, and septicemia. Community-acquired MRSA has a

DRUG	HA-MRSA (Hospital strain)	CA-MRSA (Community strain)
Characteristics of patients	Patients are typically elderly, debilitated, and/or chronically ill.	Patients are typically young and healthy. Children students, athletes, and military service personnel are at risk.
Infection site	Bacteremia commonly occurs with no obvious infection site. Infection of surgical wounds, open ulcer, intravenous line, and urinary catheters often occur.	Infections often occur in skin and soft tissues, producing cellulitis and abscesses. Infections include necrotizing community pneumonia, septic shock, and bone and joint infections.
Transmission	Transmission occurs within health care settings. Only rarely is transmission among household contacts.	Transmission occurs in the community. May spread in families, sport teams, and other risk groups.
Medical history	Infections more likely in patients with a history of MRSA infections, recent surgery, admission to a hospital or nursing home. Antibiotic use, dialysis and permanent indwelling catheters are risk factors.	Patients show no significant medical history or health care contact.
Virulence of infecting strain	Spread of infection in the community is limited. PVL genes are usually absent.	Spread of infection in the community readily occurs. PVL genes are often present, predisposing to necrotising soft tissue or lung infections.
Antibiotic susceptibility	Multidrug antibiotic resistance often occurs, resulting in a limited choice of effective therapeutic agents.	CA-MRSA strains are often more virulent than HA-MRSA, but they tend to be susceptible to a broader array of antibiotics.

Figure 8.9
Comparison of hospital-acquired methicillin-resistant *Staphylococcus aureus* (HA-MRSA) with community-acquired methicillin-resistant *Staphylococcus aureus* (CA-MRSA). PVL = Panton-Valentine leukocidin.

number of characteristics that help distinguish it from hospital-associated MRSA. For example, CA-MRSA has a characteristic pattern of DNA fragments obtained upon enzymic cleavage and electrophoresis, and it produces specific toxins. CA-MRSA also exhibits a unique antibiotic resistance pattern, that is, CA-MRSA is sensitive to many antibiotics that do not show much activity against hospital-associated MRSA. These antibiotics include ciprofloxacin and clindamycin, with some CA-MRSA even sensitive to erythromycin, gentamicin, rifampin, tetracycline, and/or trimethoprim-sulfamethoxazole. Emerging antibiotic-resistant strains of *S. aureus* that infect otherwise healthy individuals (community-acquired infections) are often more virulent than the more common strains that originate in hospitals.

3. **Vancomycin resistance:** Vancomycin has been the agent of choice for empiric treatment of life-threatening MRSA *S. aureus* infections. Unfortunately, in 1997, several MRSAs were isolated that had also acquired low-level vancomycin resistance. The incidence of vancomycin resistance has increased steadily, prompting the use of alternative drugs such as quinupristin-dalfopristin, linezolid, and daptomycin. These agents have good *in vitro* activity against MRSA and most other clinically important gram-positive bacterial pathogens.

G. Prevention

There is no effective vaccine against *S. aureus*. Infection control procedures, such as barrier precautions and disinfection of hands and fomites, are important in the control of nosocomial *S. aureus* epidemics.

IV. COAGULASE-NEGATIVE STAPHYLOCOCCI

Of 12 coagulase-negative staphylococcal species that have been recovered as normal commensals of human skin and anterior nares, the most abundant and important is *S. epidermidis*. For this reason some clinical laboratories designate all coagulase-negative staphylococci as *S. epidermidis*, a practice that is not encouraged. The second most important coagulase-negative staphylococcus is *S. saprophyticus*, which has a special medical niche. Coagulase-negative staphylococcal species are important agents of hospital-acquired infections associated with the use of implanted prosthetic devices and catheters.

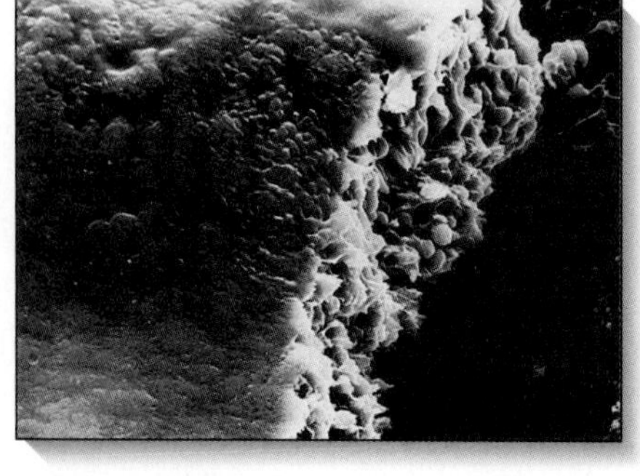

Figure 8.10
Staphylococcus epidermidis attached by its biofilm and growing on the surface of a cathether.

A. Staphylococcus epidermidis

S. epidermidis is present in large numbers as part of the normal flora of the skin (see p. 7). As such, it is frequently recovered from blood cultures, generally as a contaminant from skin. Despite its low virulence, it is a common cause of infection of implants such as heart valves and catheters (Figure 8.10). Acquired drug resistance by *S. epidermidis* is even more frequent than by *S. aureus*. Vancomycin sensitivity remains the rule, but vancomycin-resistant isolates have been reported. *S. epidermidis* produces an extracellular polysaccharide material called polysaccharide intercellular adhesin (sometimes called "slime"), that facilitates adherence to bioprosthetic material surfaces, such as intravenous catheters, and acts as a barrier to antimicrobial agents.

B. Staphylococcus saprophyticus

This organism is a frequent cause of cystitis in women, probably related to its occurrence as part of normal vaginal flora (see p. 10). It tends to be sensitive to most antibiotics, even penicillin G. *S. saprophyticus* can be distinguished from *S. epidermidis* and most other coagulase-negative staphylococci by its natural resistance to novobiocin (Figure 8.11). [Note: Urinary coagulase-negative staphylococcus is often presumed to be *S. saprophyticus*; but novobiocin resistance can be used for confirmation.]. Figure 8.12 presents a summary of diseases caused by staphylococci.

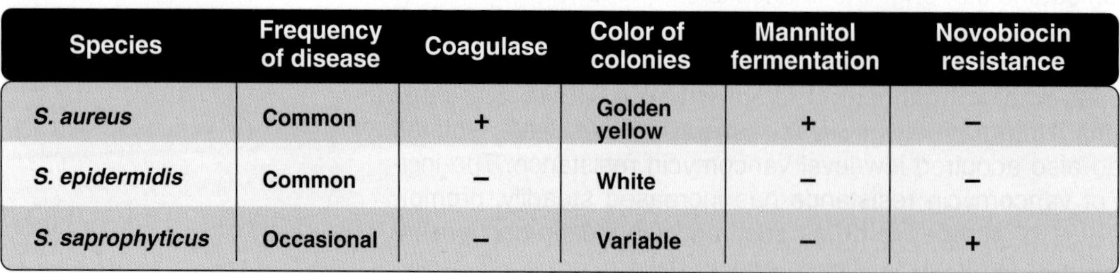

Species	Frequency of disease	Coagulase	Color of colonies	Mannitol fermentation	Novobiocin resistance
S. aureus	Common	+	Golden yellow	+	–
S. epidermidis	Common	–	White	–	–
S. saprophyticus	Occasional	–	Variable	–	+

Figure 8.11
Summary of various species of staphylococci.

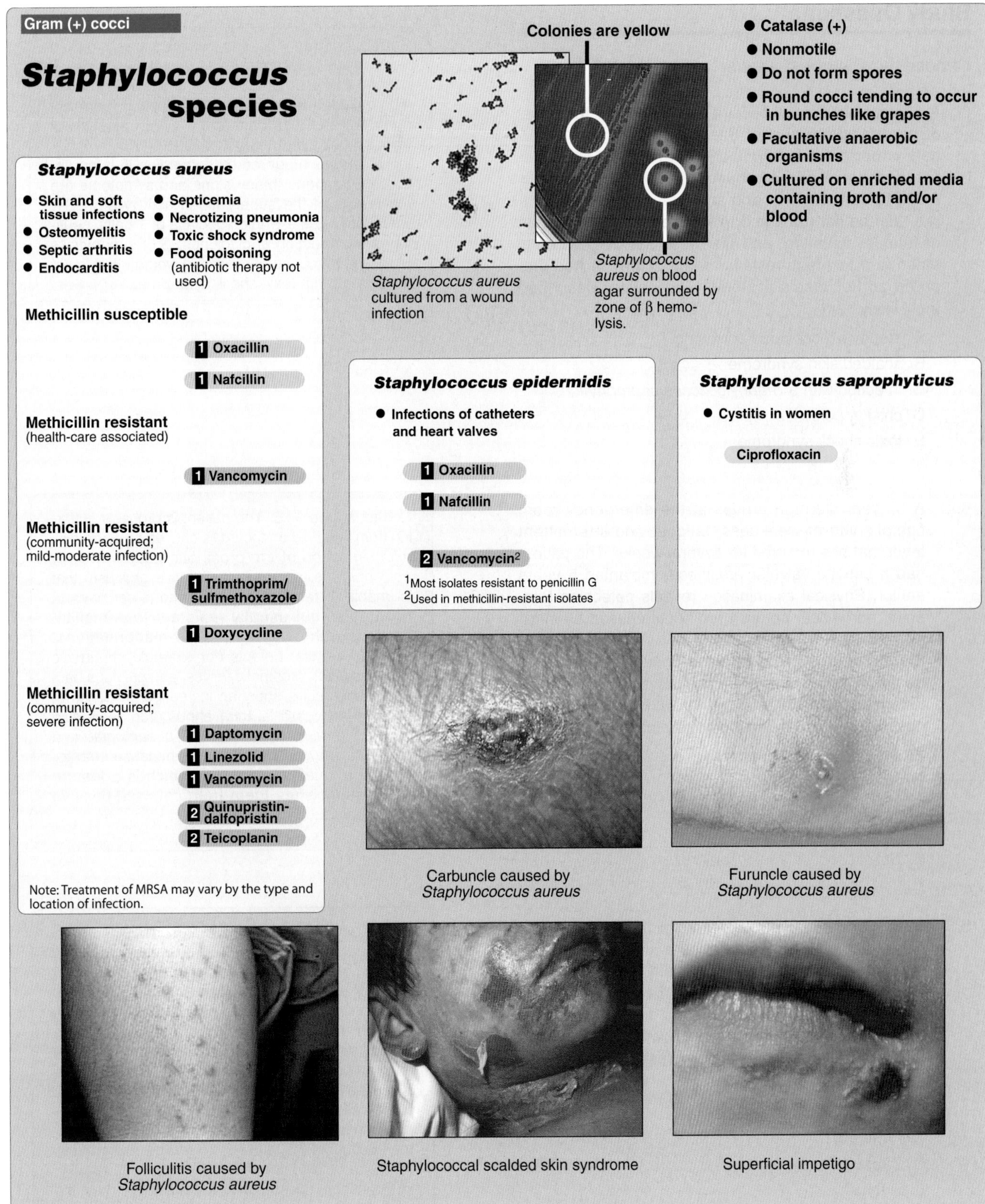

Figure 8.12
Summary of staphylococcal disease. 1 Indicates first-line drugs; 2 indicates alternative drugs.

Study Questions

Choose the ONE best answer

8.1 A 32-year-old woman became ill 4 days after the onset of her menstrual period. She presented in the emergency room with fever (104°F; normal = 98.6°F), elevated white blood cell count (16,000/mm^3; normal = 4,000 to 10,000/mm^3), and an erythematous, sunburn-like rash on her trunk and extremities. She complained of fatigue, vomiting, and diarrhea. She had recently eaten at a fast-food restaurant, but otherwise had prepared all her meals at home. The patient described most likely has:

A. staphylococcal food poisoning.
B. scalded skin syndrome.
C. infection with a *Staphylococcus saprophyticus.*
D. chickenpox.
E. toxic shock syndrome.

Correct answer = E. The patient shows signs of toxic shock syndrome. Toxic shock syndrome as defined in the outbreak of the late '70s and early '80s included an erythematous/peeling rash (not purpuric) and was caused by overproduction of toxic schock syndrome toxin (TSST)-1 by colonizing *S. aureus* triggered by something in hyperabsorbent tampons. Many signs and symptoms are the results of the superantigen activity of TSST, which activates a whole subclass of T cells, causing overproduction of cytokines. *S. saprophyticus* is a frequent cause of cystitis in women, but is not associated with toxic shock syndrome.

8.2 A 57-year-old man arrives at the emergency room complaining of weakness, fatigue, and intermittent fever that has recurred for several weeks. The patient had a cardiac valvular prosthesis implanted 5 years earlier. Physical examination reveals petechiae (pinpoint, nonraised, purplish red spots caused by intradermal hemorrhage) on the chest and stomach. Blood cultures grew catalase-positive, coagulase-negative, cocci. The gram-positive organisms failed to ferment mannitol, and their growth was inhibited by novobiocin. What is the most likely infectious agent?

A. *Staphylococcus aureus*
B. *Staphylococcus epidermidis*
C. *Staphylococcus saprophyticus*
D. *Streptococcus pneumoniae*
E. *Streptococcus agalactiae*

Correct answer = B. The patient is probably suffering from bacterial endocarditis caused by *S. epidermidis* infection of the prosthetic heart valve. *S. epidermidis* is a coagulase-negative organism that is unable to ferment mannitol and is sensitive to novobiocin but usually resistant to penicillin. Patients with congenital heart malformations, acquired valvular defects (for example, rheumatic heart disease), prosthetic valves, and previous bacterial endocarditis show an increased incidence of bacterial endocarditis. Intravenous drug users also have a high risk for infection. *S. pneumoniae* and *S. agalactiae* can be ruled out, because streptococci are catalase negative, which is a feature that distinguishes them from catalase-positive staphyococci.

8.3. An 18-month-old child was brought the pediatrician's office with what appeared to be a sunburn, although the parents denied that the child had been over exposed to the sun. The parents did recall seeing an area of redness and small blisters on the child's arm the night before. Which of the following virulence factors is critical to this disease manifestation?

A. Toxic shock syndrome toxin.
B. Panton-Valentine Leukocidin
C. Protein A
D. Capsule
E. Exfoliatin

Correct answer = E. Exfoliatin is a virulence factor, produced by some *Staphylococcus aureus* strains, cleaves desmosomes, resulting in loss of the outer layers of skin. This manifestation is also known as scalded skin syndrome. The toxic shock syndrome toxin is a superantigen produced by some *S. aureus* strains. This toxin causes systemic effects and has been associated with tampon use. Panton-Valentine Leukocidin is a hemolysin that lyses white blood cells and is produced by many community-acquired MRSA strains. Protein A is a virulence factor that allows *S. aureus* to evade an immune response by binding the Fc region of IgG, resulting in the inverse orientation of the antibody. Thus, the antibody cannot effectively opsonize the bacterium. The thin microcapsule of *S. aureus* is also associated with immune evasion.

Streptococci

9

I. OVERVIEW

Streptococci and staphylococci (see Chapter 8) constitute the main groups of medically important gram-positive cocci. Streptococci are gram-positive, nonmotile, and catalase negative. Clinically important genera include *Streptococcus* and *Enterococcus* (Figure 9.1). They are ovoid to spherical in shape and occur as pairs or chains (see Figure 9.16). Most are aerotolerant anaerobes because they grow fermentatively even in the presence of oxygen. Because of their complex nutritional requirements, blood enriched medium is generally used for their isolation. Diseases caused by this group of organisms include acute infections of the throat and skin caused by group A streptococci (*Streptococcus pyogenes*); female genital tract colonization, resulting in neonatal sepsis caused by group B streptococci (*Streptococcus agalactiae*); pneumonia, otitis media, and meningitis caused by *Streptococcus pneumoniae*; and endocarditis caused by the viridans group of streptococci.

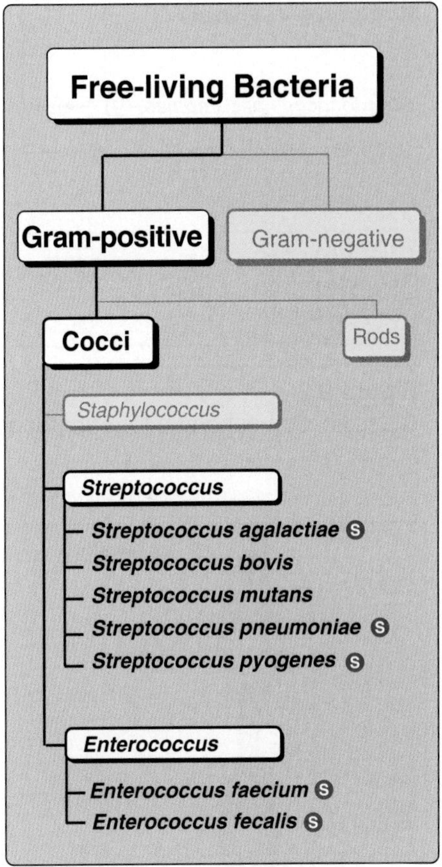

Figure 9.1
Classification of streptococci.
S See pp. 350–351 for summaries of these organisms.

II. CLASSIFICATION OF STREPTOCOCCI

Streptococci can be classified by several schemes, for example, by the hemolytic properties of the organisms, and according to the presence of specific surface antigens determined by immunologic assays.

A. Hemolytic properties on blood agar

α-Hemolytic streptococci cause a chemical change in the hemoglobin of red cells in blood agar, resulting in the appearance of a green pigment that forms a ring around the colony (see Figure 9.16). β-Hemolytic streptococci cause gross lysis of red blood cells, resulting in a clear ring around the colony (see Figure 9.16). γ-Hemolytic is a term applied to streptococci that cause no color change or lysis of red blood cells. The traditional division of streptococci based on the ability of the bacterial colony to hemolyze erythrocytes in the blood agar medium is still considered the first step in the classification of streptococci.

B. Serologic (Lancefield) groupings

Many species of streptococci have a polysaccharide in their cell walls known as C-substance, which is antigenic and easily extractable with dilute acid. The Lancefield scheme classifies primarily β-hemolytic streptococci into groups A through U on the basis of their C-sub-

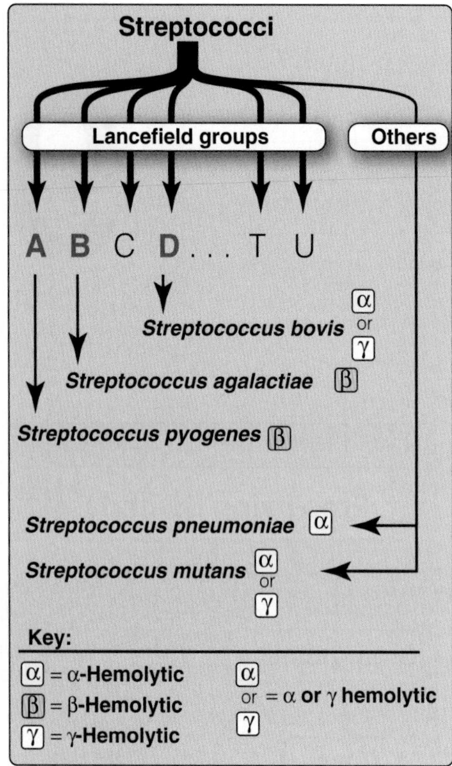

Figure 9.2
Classification schemes for streptococci.

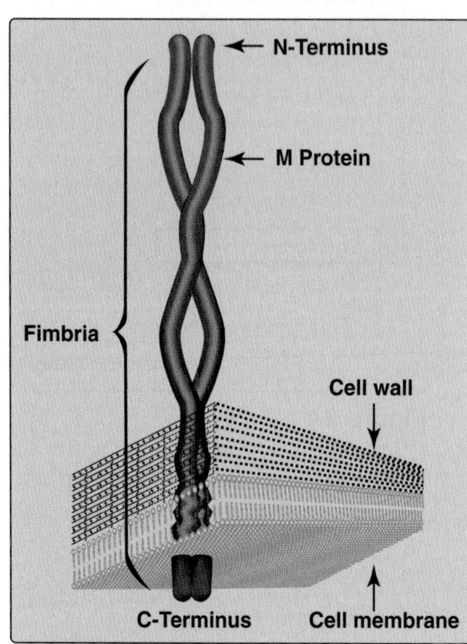

Figure 9.3
Schematic representation of the streptococcal M protein.

stance. The clinically most important groups of β-hemolytic streptococci are Types A and B (Figure 9.2). Commercial kits in which group-specific antisera are coupled to latex beads are now widely used for identification of β-hemolytic streptococci.

III. GROUP A β-HEMOLYTIC STREPTOCOCCI

S. pyogenes, the most clinically important member of this group of gram-positive cocci, is one of the most frequently encountered bacterial pathogens of humans worldwide. It can invade apparently intact skin or mucous membranes, causing some of the most rapidly progressive infections known. A low inoculum suffices for infection. Some strains of *S. pyogenes* cause postinfectious sequelae, including rheumatic fever and acute glomerulonephritis. Nasopharyngeal carriage is common especially in colder months and particularly among children. Unlike staphylococcal species, *S. pyogenes* does not survive well in the environment. Instead, its habitat is infected patients and also normal human carriers in whom the organism resides on skin and mucous membranes. *S. pyogenes* is usually spread person to person by skin contact and via the respiratory tract.

A. Structure and physiology

S. pyogenes cells usually form long chains when recovered from liquid culture (see Figure 9.16), but may appear as individual cocci, pairs, or clusters of cells in Gram stains of samples from infected tissue. Structural features involved in the pathology or identification of group A streptococci include:

1. **Capsule:** Hyaluronic acid, identical to that found in human connective tissue, forms the outermost layer of the cell. This capsule is not recognized as foreign by the body and, therefore, is nonimmunogenic. The capsule is also antiphagocytic.

2. **Cell wall:** The cell wall contains a number of clinically important components. Beginning with the outer layer of the cell wall, these components include the following (Figure 9.3):

   a. **M protein:** *S. pyogenes* is not infectious in the absence of M protein. M proteins extend from an anchor in the cell membrane, through the cell wall and then the capsule, with the N-terminal end of the protein exposed on the surface of the bacterium. M proteins are highly variable, especially the N-terminal regions, resulting in over 80 different antigenic types. Thus, individuals may have many *S. pyogenes* infections throughout their lives as they encounter new M protein types for which they have no antibodies. M proteins are antiphagocytic and they form a coat that interferes with complement binding.

   b. **Group A-specific C-substance:** This component is composed of rhamnose and N-acetylglucosamine. [Note: All group A streptococci, by definition, contain this antigen.]

   c. **Protein F (fibronectin-binding protein)** mediates attachment to fibronectin in the pharyngeal epithelium. M proteins and lipoteichoic acids also bind to fibronectin.

3. **Extracellular products:** Like *Staphylococcus aureus* (see p. 70), *S. pyogenes* secretes a wide range of exotoxins that often vary from one strain to another and that play roles in the pathogenesis of disease caused by these organisms (Figure 9.4).

B. Epidemiology

The only known reservoir for *S. pyogenes* in nature is the skin and mucous membranes of the human host. Respiratory droplets or skin contact spreads group A streptococcal infection from person to person, especially in crowded environments such as classrooms and children's play areas.

C. Pathogenesis

S. pyogenes cells, perhaps in an inhaled droplet, attach to the pharyngeal mucosa via actions of protein F, lipoteichoic acid, and M protein. The bacteria may simply replicate sufficiently to maintain themselves without causing injury in which case the patient is then considered colonized. Alternatively, bacteria may grow and secrete toxins, causing damage to surrounding cells, invading the mucosa, and eliciting an inflammatory response with attendant influx of white cells, fluid leakage, and pus formation. The patient then has streptococcal pharyngitis. Occasionally, there is sufficient spread that the bloodstream is significantly invaded, possibly resulting in septicemia and/or seeding of distant sites, where cellulitis (acute inflammation of subcutaneous tissue), fasciitis (inflammation of the tissue under the skin that covers a surface of underlying tissue), or myonecrosis (death of muscle cells) may develop rapidly or insidiously. However, direct inoculation of skin from another person's infection is probably more common as the pathogenesis of streptococcal skin and soft tissue infection.

D. Clinical significance

S. pyogenes is a major cause of cellulitis. Other more specific syndromes include:

1. **Acute pharyngitis or pharyngotonsilitis**: Pharyngitis is the most common type of *S. pyogenes* infection. *S. pyogenes* pharyngitis ("strep throat") is associated with severe, purulent inflammation of the posterior oropharynx and tonsillar areas (see Figure 9.16). [Note: If a sunburnlike rash develops on the neck, trunk, and extremities in response to the release of pyrogenic exotoxin to which the patient does not have antibodies, the syndrome is designated scarlet fever.] Many strep throats are mild, and many sore throats caused by viruses are severe. Hence, laboratory confirmation is important for accurate diagnosis and treatment of streptococcal pharyngitis, particularly for the prevention of subsequent acute rheumatic fever and rheumatic heart disease.

2. **Impetigo:** Although *S. aureus* is recovered from most contemporary cases of impetigo (see p. 72), *S. pyogenes* is the classic cause of this syndrome. The disease begins on any exposed surface (most commonly, the legs). Typically affecting children, it can cause severe and extensive lesions on the face and limbs (see Figure 9.16). Impetigo is treated with a topical agent such as mupirocin, or systemically with penicillin or a first-generation cephalosporin such

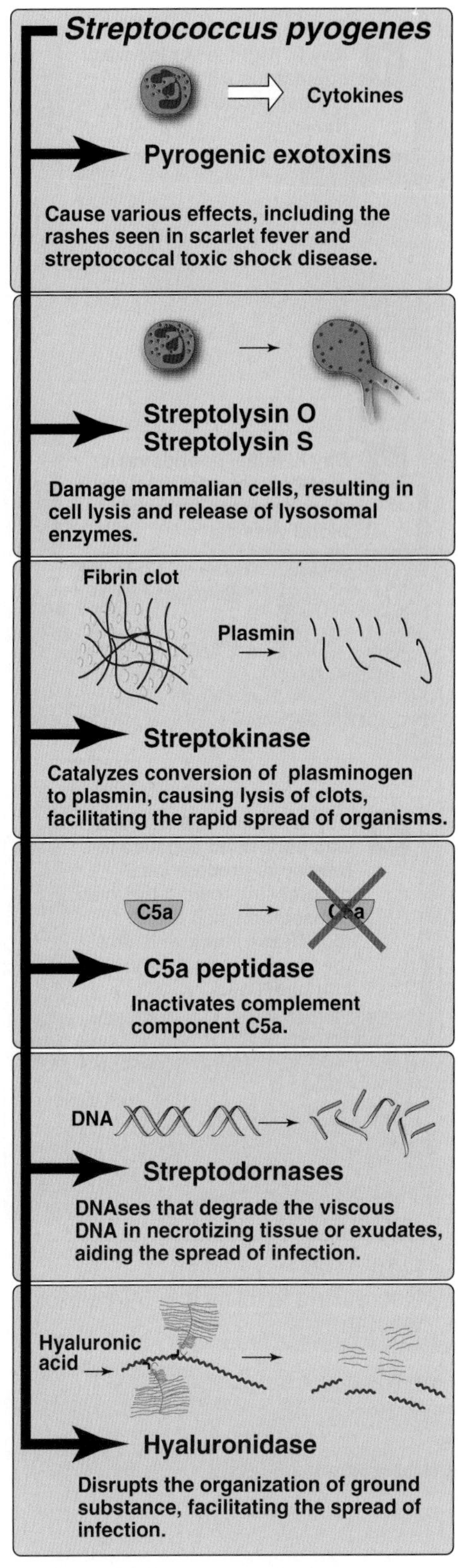

Streptococcus pyogenes
Cytokines
Pyrogenic exotoxins
Cause various effects, including the rashes seen in scarlet fever and streptococcal toxic shock disease.
Streptolysin O
Streptolysin S
Damage mammalian cells, resulting in cell lysis and release of lysosomal enzymes.
Fibrin clot
Plasmin
Streptokinase
Catalyzes conversion of plasminogen to plasmin, causing lysis of clots, facilitating the rapid spread of organisms.
C5a
C5a peptidase
Inactivates complement component C5a.
DNA
Streptodornases
DNAses that degrade the viscous DNA in necrotizing tissue or exudates, aiding the spread of infection.
Hyaluronic acid
Hyaluronidase
Disrupts the organization of ground substance, facilitating the spread of infection.

Figure 9.4
Cytolytic toxins and other exoenzymes produced by *Streptococcus pyogenes*.

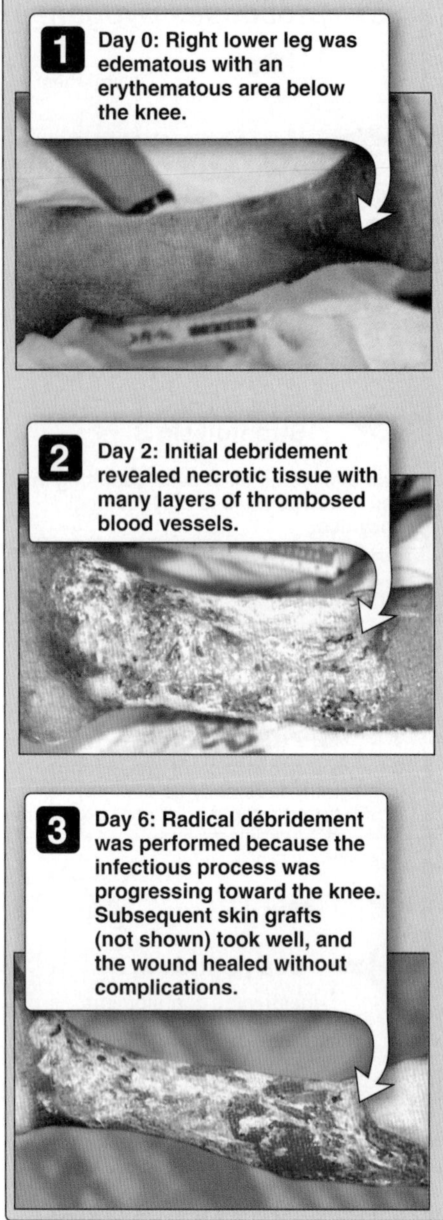

1
Day 0: Right lower leg was edematous with an erythematous area below the knee.
2
Day 2: Initial debridement revealed necrotic tissue with many layers of thrombosed blood vessels.
3
Day 6: Radical débridement was performed because the infectious process was progressing toward the knee. Subsequent skin grafts (not shown) took well, and the wound healed without complications.

Figure 9.5
Necrotizing fasciitis in a 59-year-old woman.

as cephalexin, which are effective against both *S. aureus* and *S. pyogenes*.

3. **Erysipelas:** Affecting all age groups, patients with erysipelas experience a fiery red, advancing erythema, especially on the face or lower limbs (see Figure 9.16).

4. **Puerperal sepsis:** This infection is initiated during, or following soon after, the delivery of a newborn. It is caused by exogenous transmission (for example, by nasal droplets from an infected carrier or from contaminated instruments) or endogenously, from the mother's vaginal flora. This is a disease of the uterine endometrium in which patients experience a purulent vaginal discharge and are systemically ill.

5. **Invasive group A streptococcal disease:** Common during the first half of the century, invasive group A streptococcal (GAS) disease became rare until its resurgence during the past decade. Patients may have a deep local invasion either without necrosis (cellulitis) or with it (necrotizing fasciitis/myositis) as shown in Figure 9.5. [Note: The latter disease led to the term "flesh-eating bacteria."] Invasive GAS disease often spreads rapidly, even in otherwise healthy individuals, leading to bacteremia and sepsis. Symptoms may include a toxic shock–like syndrome, fever, hypotension, multiorgan involvement, a sunburnlike rash, or a combination of these symptoms.

6. **Streptococcal toxic shock syndrome:** This syndrome is defined as isolation of group A β-hemolytic streptococci from blood or another normally sterile body site in the presence of shock and multiorgan failure. The syndrome is mediated by the production of streptococcal pyrogenic exotoxins that function as superantigens causing massive, nonspecific T-cell activation and cytokine release. Patients may initially present with flulike symptoms, followed shortly by necrotizing soft tissue infection, shock, acute respiratory distress syndrome, and renal failure. Treatment must be prompt and includes antistreptococcal antibiotics, usually consisting of high-dose penicillin G plus clindamycin.

7. **Post-streptococcal sequelae**

   a. **Acute rheumatic fever:** This autoimmune disease occurs 2 to 3 weeks after the initiation of pharyngitis. It is caused by cross-reactions between antigens of the heart and joint tissues, and the streptococcal antigen (especially the M protein epitopes). It is characterized by fever, rash, carditis, and arthritis. Central nervous system manifestions are also common including Sydenham's chorea, symptoms of which are uncontrolled movement and loss of fine motor control. Rheumatic fever is preventable if the patient is treated within the first 10 days following onset of acute pharyngitis.

   b. **Acute glomerulonephritis:** This rare, postinfectious sequela occurs as soon as 1 week after impetigo or pharyngitis ensues, due to a few nephritogenic strains of group A streptococci. Antigen–antibody complexes on the basement membrane of the glomerulus initiate the disease. There is no evidence that penicillin treatment of the streptococcal skin disease or pharyngitis (to eradicate the infection) can prevent acute glomerulonephritis.

E. Laboratory identification

Rapid latex antigen kits for direct detection of group A streptococci in patient samples are widely used. In a positive test, the latex particles clump together, whereas in a negative test, they stay separate, giving the suspension a milky appearance (Figure 9.6). These tests have high specificity but variable sensitivity compared with culture techniques. Specimens from patients with clinical signs of pharyngitis and a negative antigen detection test should undergo routine culturing for streptococcal identification. Depending on the form of the disease, specimens for laboratory analysis can be obtained from throat swabs, pus and lesion samples, sputum, blood, or spinal fluid. *S. pyogenes* forms characteristic small, opalescent colonies surrounded by a large zone of β hemolysis on sheep blood agar (see Figure 9.16). [Note: Hemolysis of the blood cells is caused by steptolysin S, which damages mammalian cells resulting in cell lysis.] This organism is highly sensitive to bacitracin, and diagnostic disks with a very low concentration of the antibiotic inhibit growth in culture. *S. pyogenes* is also catalase negative and optochin resistant. Group A C-substance can be identified by the precipitin reaction. Serologic tests detect a patient's antibody titer to streptolysin O (ASO test) after group A streptococcal infection. Anti-DNase B titers (ADB test) are particularly elevated following streptococcal infections of the skin.

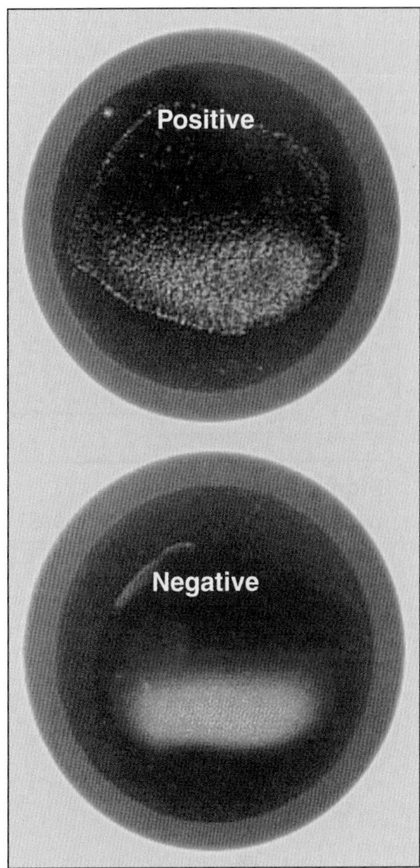

Figure 9.6
Latex agglutination for identification of group A β-hemolytic streptococci.

F. Treatment

Antibiotics are used for all group A streptococcal infections. *S. pyogenes* has not acquired resistance to penicillin G, which remains the antibiotic of choice for acute streptococcal disease. In a penicillin-allergic patient, a macrolide such as clarithromycin or azithromycin is the preferred drug (see Figure 9.16). Penicillin G plus clindamycin are used in treating necrotizing fasciitis and in streptococcal toxic shock syndrome. Clindamycin is added to penicillin to inhibit protein (i.e., toxin) synthesis so that a huge amount of toxin is not released abruptly from rapidly dying bacteria.

G. Prevention

Rheumatic fever is prevented by rapid eradication of the infecting organism. Prolonged prophylactic antibiotic therapy is indicated after an episode of rheumatic fever, because having had one episode of this autoimmune disease in the past is a major risk factor for subsequent episodes if the patient is again infected with *S. pyogenes.*

IV. GROUP B β-HEMOLYTIC STREPTOCOCCI

Group B streptococci, represented by the pathogen *S. agalactiae*, are gram-positive, catalase-negative organisms. *S. agalactiae* is found in the vaginocervical tract of female carriers, and the urethral mucous membranes of male carriers as well as in the gastrointestinal (GI) tract. *S. agalactiae* can be transmitted sexually among adults and from an infected mother to her infant at birth. Group B streptococci are a leading cause of meningitis and septicemia in neonates, with a high mortality rate. They are also an occasional cause of infections in postpartum women (endometritis) and individuals with impaired immune systems, in whom the organism may cause septicemia or pneumonia. Samples of blood, cervical swabs, sputum, or spinal fluid can be obtained for culture on blood agar. Latex agglutination tests can also demonstrate the presence of group B antigen in these samples. Group B streptococci are β hemolytic, with larger colonies and less hemolysis than group A. Most isolates remain sensitive to penicillin G and ampicillin, which are still the antibiotics of choice (see Figure 9.16). In life-threatening infections, an aminoglycoside can be added to the regimen. [Note: Pregnant carriers should be treated with ampicillin during labor if risk factors such as premature rupture of membranes or prolonged labor are present.] Intrapartum prophylaxis of group B streptococcal carriers and administration of antibiotics to their newborns reduce neonatal group B streptococcal sepsis by as much as 90 percent.

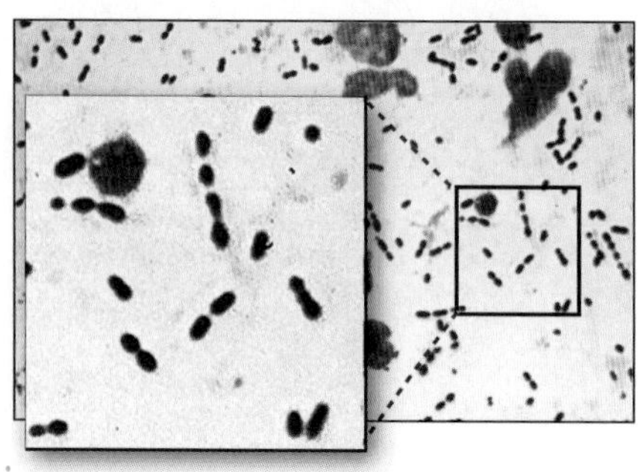

Figure 9.7
Streptococcus pneumoniae are gram-positive, nonmotile, encapsulated, lancet-shaped cocci.

V. STREPTOCOCCUS PNEUMONIAE (PNEUMOCOCCUS)

S. pneumoniae are gram-positive, nonmotile, encapsulated cocci (Figure 9.7). They are lancet shaped, and their tendency to occur in pairs accounts for their earlier designation as *Diplococcus pneumoniae*. *S. pneumoniae* is the most common cause of community-acquired pneumonia and adult bacterial meningitis and is an important cause of otitis media, sinusitis and mastoiditis. The risk of disease is highest among young children (Figure 9.8), older adults, smokers, and persons with certain chronic illnesses. Like other streptococci, *S. pneumoniae* is fastidious (has complex nutritional requirements) and routinely cultured on blood agar. It releases an α hemolysin that damages red cell membranes, causing colonies to be α hemolytic.

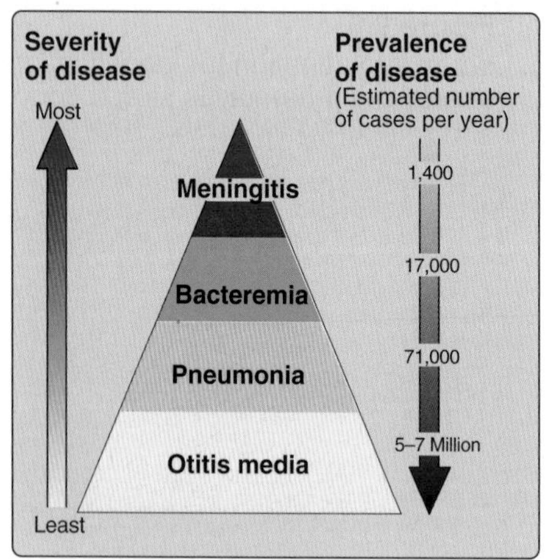

Figure 9.8
Comparison of severity and prevalence of some pneumococcal infections in children in the United States.

A. Epidemiology

S. pneumoniae is an obligate parasite of humans and can be found in the nasopharynx of many healthy individuals. This organism is extremely sensitive to environmental agents. Pneumococcal infections can be either endogenous or exogenous. For example, endogenous infection involves the spread of *S. pneumoniae* residing in the nasopharynx of a carrier who develops impaired resistance to the organism. Susceptibility to the infection may result from, for example, general debilitation such as that caused by malnutrition or alcoholism, respiratory damage following a prior viral infection, or from a depressed immune system. Patients with sickle cell disease or those who have had their spleens removed are particularly at risk for *S. pneumoniae* infection. Infection can also be exogenous, for example, by droplets from the nose of a carrier. Individuals such as those described above as susceptible to endogenous infection are also most likely to be infected by the exogenous route.

B. Pathogenesis

The bacterial capsule of *S. pneumoniae* is the most important virulence factor and is the basis for the classification of serotypes of this organism. The cell-associated enzymes pneumolysin and autolysin contribute to its pathogenicity (Figure 9.9).

1. **Capsule:** The *S. pneumoniae* polysaccharide capsule is both antiphagocytic and antigenic. Antiphagocytic properties of the capsule protect the bacteria from polymorphonuclear leukocyte attack, facilitating growth of the bacteria prior to the appearance of anticapsular antibodies. There are approximately 85 distinct capsular serotypes, some of which endow strains with greater virulence than others, as reflected by the fact that about 20 serotypes account for the vast majority of pneumococcal infections.

2. **Pili:** Pili enable the attachment of encapsulated pneumococci to the epithelial cells of the upper respiratory tract. Not all pneumococci are piliated, but those clinical isolates that express pili are more virulent. The genes required for regulation and assembly of the pilus are not present in all pneumococcal strains, but they can be horizontally transferred between strains on a pathogenicity "islet", which is small pathogenicity island. The chromosomal region responsible for production of the pneumococcal pilus is called the *rlrA* islet, named for the regulatory gene (*rlrA*) that is required for expression.

3. **Choline-binding protein A:** Choline binding protein A is a major adhesin allowing the pneumococcus to attach to carbohydrates on epithelial cells of the human nasopharynx.

4. **Autolysins:** Autolysins are enzymes that hydrolyze the components of a biological cell in which it is produced. LytA, B and C are peptidoglycan-hydrolyzing enzymes that are present in the bacterial cell wall and are normally inactive. However, these enzymes are readily activated (for example, by surface-active agents, β-lactam antibiotics, or stationary phase), resulting in cell lysis. Autolysin is thus responsible for the release of intracellular virulence factors (notably, pneumolysin).

5. **Pneumolysin:** Although retained within the cytosol of intact pneumococci, pneumolysin is thought to be an important virulence factor by virtue of its ability to attack mammalian cell membranes, causing lysis once it is released by autolysin from the interior of the bacterium. Pneumolysin binds to cholesterol and therefore interacts indiscriminately with all cell types. This toxin stimulates production of proinflammatory cytokines, inhibits the activity of polymorphonuclear leukocytes and activates complement.

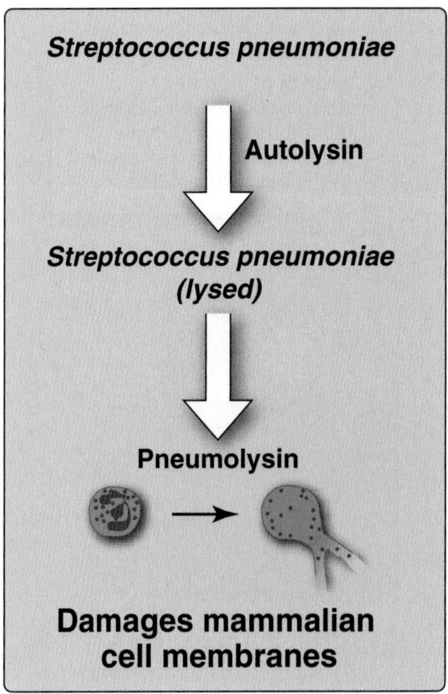

Figure 9.9
Cytolytic toxins produced by *Streptococcus pneumoniae.*

C. Clinical significance

1. **Acute bacterial pneumonia:** A leading cause of death, especially in older adults and those whose resistance is impaired, this disease is caused most frequently by *S. pneumoniae* (Figure 9.10). Pneumonia is frequently preceded by an upper or middle respiratory viral infection, which predisposes to *S. pneumoniae* infection

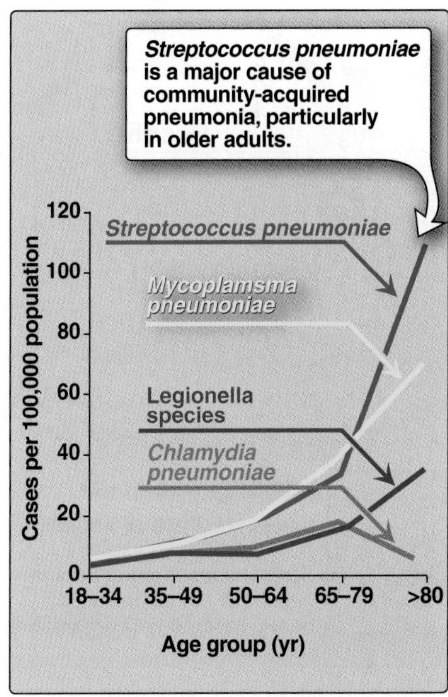

Figure 9.10
Age-specific rates of community-acquired pneumonia caused by specific pathogens.

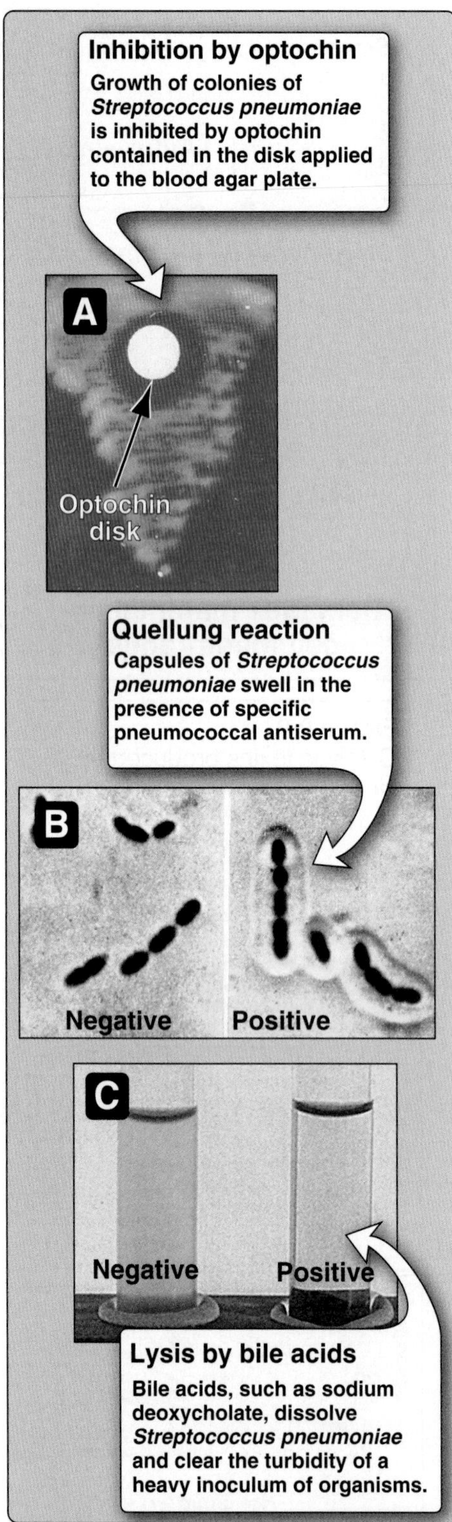

Inhibition by optochin
Growth of colonies of Streptococcus pneumoniae is inhibited by optochin contained in the disk applied to the blood agar plate.
A
Optochin disk
Quellung reaction
Capsules of Streptococcus pneumoniae swell in the presence of specific pneumococcal antiserum.
B
Negative
Positive
C
Negative
Positive
Lysis by bile acids
Bile acids, such as sodium deoxycholate, dissolve Streptococcus pneumoniae and clear the turbidity of a heavy inoculum of organisms.

Figure 9.11
Laboratory tests useful in the identification of *Streptococcus pneumoniae*.

of pulmonary parenchyma. Mechanisms by which virus infection predisposes an individual to streptococcal pneumonia include increased volume and viscosity of secretions that are more difficult to clear and secondary inhibition of the action of bronchial cilia by viral infection.

2. **Otitis media:** The most common bacterial infection of children, this disease (which is characterized by earache) is most frequently caused by pneumococcus, followed by *Haemophilus influenzae* and *Moraxella catarrhalis* (see p. 391). The traditional empiric treatment of pneumococcal otitis media with a β-lactam antibiotic (with or without a penicillinase-inhibitor) has been threatened by the spread of penicillin-resistant pneumococci.

3. **Bacteremia/sepsis:** In the absence of a focus of infection bacteremia/sepsis is commonly caused by pneumococcus, especially in individuals who are functionally or anatomically asplenic. This includes people with sickle cell disease who infarct their spleen and are functionally asplenic, although they still have a remnant of anatomical spleen.

4. **Meningitis:** *H. influenzae* was formerly the leading cause of bacterial meningitis in the United States. After a vaccine was developed against this organism, *S. pneumoniae* became the most common cause of adult bacterial meningitis (see p. 376). This disease has a high mortality rate, even when treated appropriately.

D. Laboratory identification

Specimens for laboratory evaluation can be obtained from a nasopharyngeal swab, blood, pus, sputum, or spinal fluid. α-Hemolytic colonies appear when *S. pneumoniae* is grown on blood agar overnight under aerobic conditions at 37°C. Lancet-shaped, gram-positive diplococci are observed on a Gram stain of the sample. Growth of these bacteria is inhibited by low concentrations of the surfactant optochin, and the cells are lysed by bile acids (Figure 9.11). Capsular swelling is observed when the pneumococci are treated with type-specific antisera (the Quellung reaction).

E. Treatment

S. pneumoniae isolates were highly sensitive to penicillin G, the initial agent of choice, until the late 1980s. Since then, the incidence of penicillin resistance has been increasing worldwide. The mechanism of this resistance is an alteration of one or more of the bacterium's penicillin-binding proteins (PBPs, see p. 57) rather than production of β-lactamase. Modified PBPs have a much-reduced affinity for penicillin G and for some, but not all, of the other β-lactams. Most resistant strains remain sensitive to third generation cephalosporins (such as cefotaxime or ceftriaxone), and all are still sensitive to vancomycin. These antibiotics are therefore the agents of choice for invasive infections by penicillin-resistant strains of *S. pneumoniae* (see Figure 9.16).

F. Prevention

There are two types of pneumococcal vaccine: pneumococcal polysaccharide vaccine (PPV) and pneumococcal conjugate vaccine (PCV13).

1. **Pneumococcal polysaccharide vaccine:** Introduced in the United States in 1983, PPV immunizes against 23 serotypes of *S. pneumoniae* and is indicated for the protection of high-risk individuals older than age 2 years. This vaccine protects against the pneumococcal strains responsible for 85 to 90 percent of infections, including prominent penicillin-resistant strains.

2. **Pneumococcal conjugate vaccine 13:** The polyvalent PCV 13, licensed in the United States in 2010, is effective in infants and toddlers (ages 6 weeks to 5 years). It is made up of 13 pneumococcal antigens conjugated to CRM197, a mutant nontoxic diphtheria toxin. Significant declines in the incidence of invasive pneumococcal disease occurred as a result of introduction of this and an earlier generation heptavalent conjugated vaccine (PCV 7). (Figure 9.12). In addition, the vaccines prevented greater numbers of invasive pneumococcal cases through indirect effects on pneumococcal transmission (that is, herd immunity) than through its direct effect of protecting vaccinated children. Young children do not elicit an immune response to oligosaccharide-only vaccines. However, if the oligosaccharide is conjugated to a protein, a protective immune response develops.

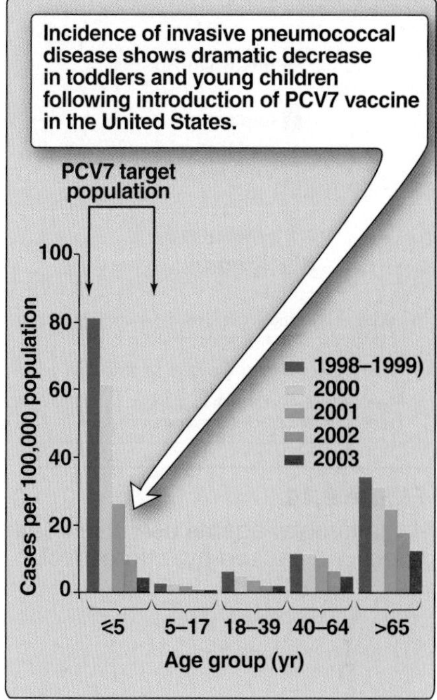

Figure 9.12
Incidence of vaccine-type invasive pneumococcal disease before and after the introduction of pneumococcal conjugate vaccine (PCV7), by age and year.

VI. ENTEROCOCCI

Enterococci contain a C-substance that reacts with group D antisera. Therefore, in the past, they were considered group D streptococci. Today, DNA analysis and other properties have placed them in their own genus, *Enterococcus*. The clinically most important species are *E. faecalis* and *E. faecium*. Enterococci can be α-, β-, or nonhemolytic. As a rule, enterococci are not very virulent, but they have become prominent as a cause of nosocomial infections as a result of their multiple antibiotic resistance. Figure 9.13 shows the microscopic appearance of *E. faecalis*.

A. Epidemiology

Enterococci are part of the normal fecal flora. However, they can also colonize oral mucous membranes and skin, especially in hospital settings. These organisms are highly resistant to environmental and chemical agents and can persist on fomites.

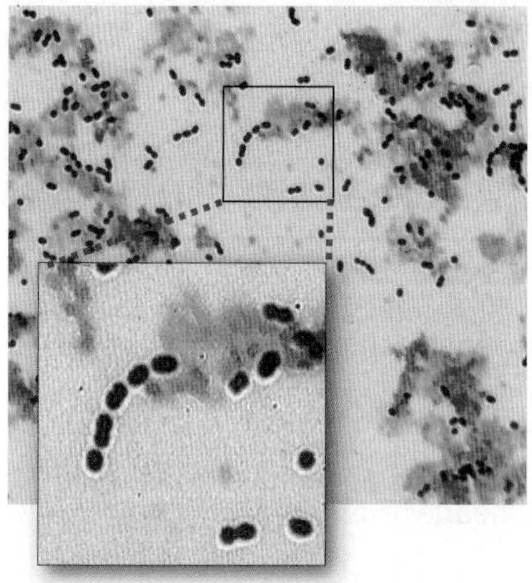

Figure 9.13
Enterococcus fecalis showing chain formation characteristic of *Streptococcus*.

B. Diseases

Enterococci seldom cause disease in normal, healthy individuals. However, under conditions in which host resistance is lowered or the integrity of the gastrointestinal or genitourinary tract has been

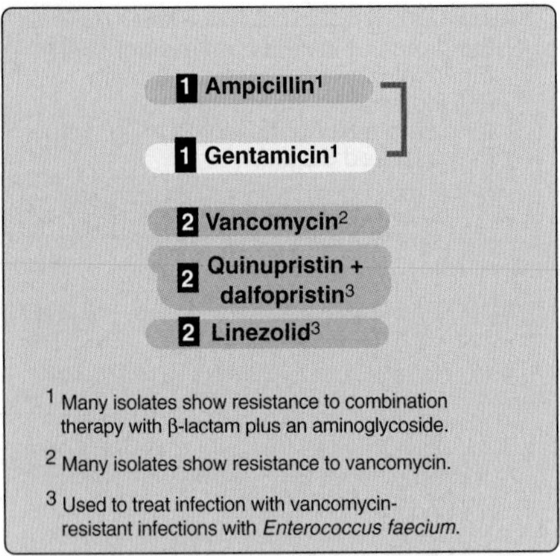

1 Ampicillin[1]
1 Gentamicin[1]
2 Vancomycin[2]
2 Quinupristin + dalfopristin[3]
2 Linezolid[3]
1 Many isolates show resistance to combination therapy with β-lactam plus an aminoglycoside.
2 Many isolates show resistance to vancomycin.
3 Used to treat infection with vancomycin-resistant infections with *Enterococcus faecium*.

Figure 9.14
Antimicrobial agents useful in treating infections caused by enterococci.

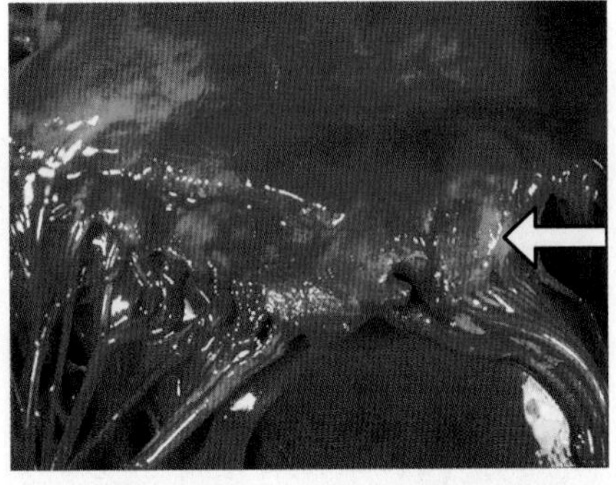

Figure 9.15
Streptococcal endocarditis showing vegetation of the mitral valve leaflet. [Note: Vegetation is a tissue outgrowth composed of fibrin, bacteria, and aggregated blood platelets adherent to a diseased heart valve.]

disrupted (for example, by instrumentation), enterococci can spread to normally sterile sites, causing urinary tract infections, bacteremia/sepsis, endocarditis, biliary tract infection, or intra-abdominal abscesses.

C. Laboratory identification

Enterococci are distinguished from the non–group D streptococci by their ability to survive in the presence of bile, and to hydrolyze the polysaccharide esculin, producing black colonies on esculin-containing plates. Unlike nonenterococcal group D streptococci, enterococci grow in 6.5 percent NaCl, and yield a positive pyrazin amidase (PYR) test. *E. faecalis* can be distinguished from *E. faecium* by their fermentation patterns, which are commonly evaluated in clinical laboratories

D. Treatment

Enterococci are naturally resistant to β-lactam antibiotics and aminoglycosides, but are sensitive to the synergistic action of a combination of these classes. In the past, the initial regimens of choice were penicillin +/– streptomycin or ampicillin +/– gentamicin (Figure 9.14). However, acquired resistance determinants in many current strains negate this synergy. In addition, isolates frequently have natural or acquired resistances to many other antibiotic classes, including glycopeptides such as vancomycin. Newer antibiotics, such as the combination of quinupristin and dalfopristin, are used to treat vancomycin-resistant infections. However, some enterococcal strains are resistant to all commercially available antibiotics. [Note: *E. faecium* is more likely to be vancomycin or multiply resistant than *E. faecalis*.]

E. Prevention

The rise of nosocomial infections by multiple drug–resistant enterococci is largely the result of selection due to high antibiotic usage in hospitals. Judicious use of antibiotics is an important factor in controlling the emergence of these infections.

VII. NONENTEROCOCCAL GROUP D STREPTOCOCCI

Streptococcus bovis is the most clinically important of the nonenterococcus group D streptococci. Part of normal fecal flora, they are either α– or nonhemolytic. *S. bovis* occasionally causes urinary tract infections and endocarditis, the latter especially in association with colon cancer. The organism is bile and esculin positive, but is PYR-negative, and does not grow in 6.5 percent salt (unlike the enterococci). It tends to be sensitive to penicillin and other antibiotics.

VIII. VIRIDANS STREPTOCOCCI

The viridans group of streptococci includes many gram-positive, catalase-negative, α– or γ–hemolytic species that constitute the main facultative oral flora. The viridans streptococci are relatively avirulent, but

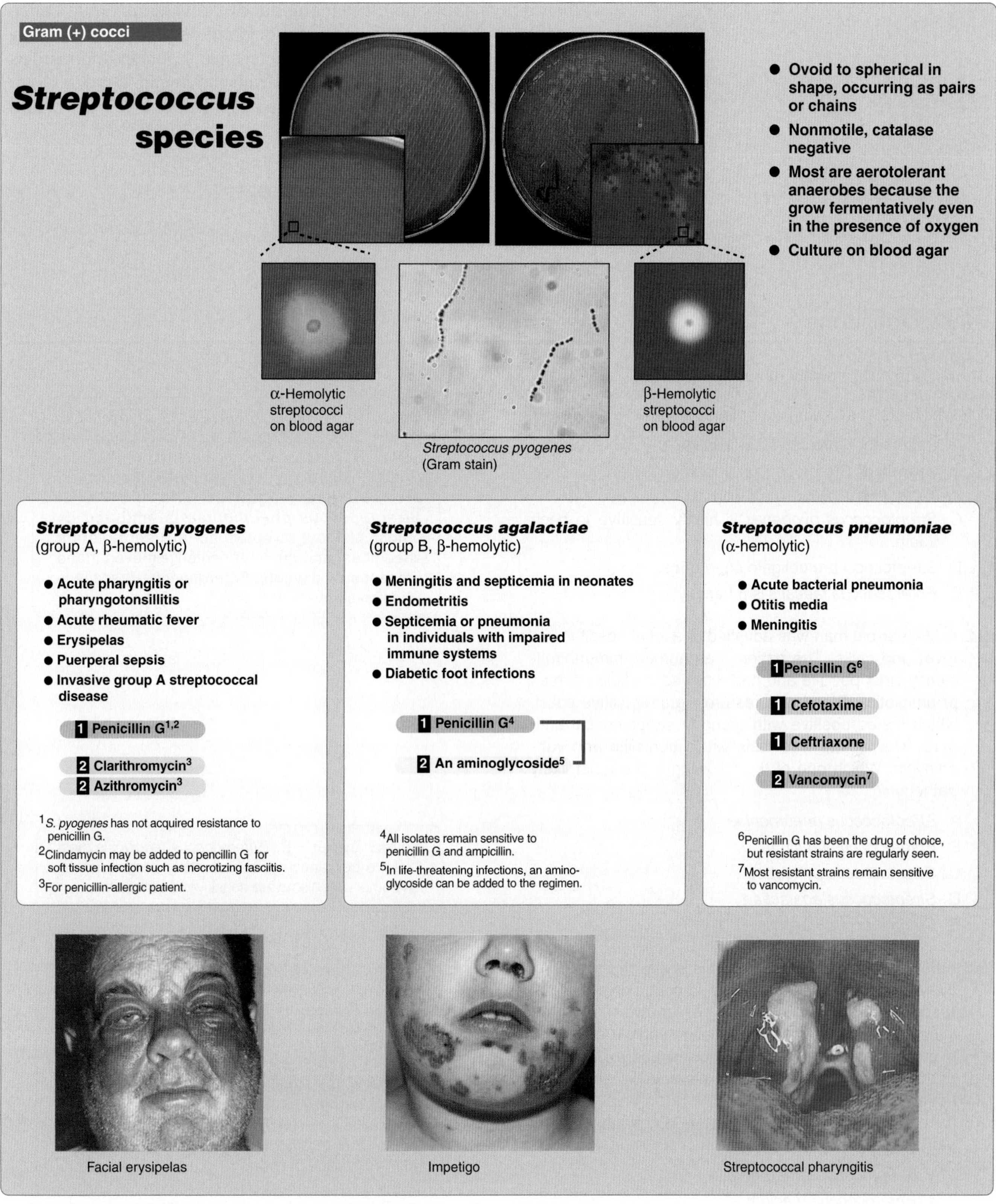

Gram (+) cocci
Streptococcus species
Ovoid to spherical in shape, occurring as pairs or chains
Nonmotile, catalase negative
Most are aerotolerant anaerobes because the grow fermentatively even in the presence of oxygen
Culture on blood agar
α-Hemolytic streptococci on blood agar
Streptococcus pyogenes (Gram stain)
β-Hemolytic streptococci on blood agar
Streptococcus pyogenes (group A, β-hemolytic)
Acute pharyngitis or pharyngotonsillitis
Acute rheumatic fever
Erysipelas
Puerperal sepsis
Invasive group A streptococcal disease
1 Penicillin G1,2
2 Clarithromycin3
2 Azithromycin3
1 S. pyogenes has not acquired resistance to penicillin G.
2 Clindamycin may be added to pencillin G for soft tissue infection such as necrotizing fasciitis.
3 For penicillin-allergic patient.
Streptococcus agalactiae (group B, β-hemolytic)
Meningitis and septicemia in neonates
Endometritis
Septicemia or pneumonia in individuals with impaired immune systems
Diabetic foot infections
1 Penicillin G4
2 An aminoglycoside5
4 All isolates remain sensitive to penicillin G and ampicillin.
5 In life-threatening infections, an aminoglycoside can be added to the regimen.
Streptococcus pneumoniae (α-hemolytic)
Acute bacterial pneumonia
Otitis media
Meningitis
1 Penicillin G6
1 Cefotaxime
1 Ceftriaxone
2 Vancomycin7
6 Penicillin G has been the drug of choice, but resistant strains are regularly seen.
7 Most resistant strains remain sensitive to vancomycin.
Facial erysipelas
Impetigo
Streptococcal pharyngitis

Figure 9.16
Summary of streptococcal disease. 1 Indicates first-line drugs; 2 indicates alternative drugs.

Streptococcus mutans and other members of the viridans group cause dental caries. In patients with abnormal or damaged heart valves, they can also infect these valves during a bacteremia, causing endocarditis (Figure 9.15). Therefore, at-risk patients with rheumatic, congenital, or sclerotic valvular disease should receive prophylactic penicillin before undergoing dental procedures.

Figure 9.16 summarizes streptococcal disease.

Study Questions

Choose the ONE correct answer

9.1 Which of the following statements is correct?

A. Streptococci are catalase positive.

B. Growth of *Streptococcus pneumoniae* is not sensitive to optochin.

C. *Streptococcus pyogenes* is highly sensitive to bacitracin.

D. Streptococci are obligate anaerobes.

E. *Enterococcus faecalis* is β-hemolytic.

Correct answer = C. *Streptococcus pyogenes* is highly sensitive to bacitracin, and diagnostic disks with a very low concentration of the antibiotic inhibit growth in culture. All streptococci are catalase negative. The growth of *Streptococcus pneumoniae* is inhibited by optochin. Most streptococci are aerotolerant anaerobes, and grow fermentatively even in the presence of oxygen. *Enterococcus faecalis* is γ hemolytic (no hemolysis).

9.2 A 55-year-old man was admitted to a local hospital with fever and chills. The patient was human immunodeficiency virus positive and had received multiple courses of antibiotics. Blood cultures grew gram-positive cocci, which tested positive with group D streptococcal antisera. The isolate was resistant to penicillin and vancomycin. Which one of the following is the most likely pathogen?

A. *Streptococcus pneumoniae*

B. *Enterococcus faecium*

C. *Streptococcus pyogenes*

D. *Streptococcus agalactiae*

E. *Streptococcus mutans*

Correct answer = B. *Enterococcus faecium* is most likely to be vancomycin or multiply drug-resistant. The other organisms are sensitive to vancomycin.

9.3 A 65-year-old male presents to his family physician with a rapid onset fever, chest pain and cough productive of rusty-yellow sputum. Chest X-ray shows focal lobar infiltrates. A Gram stain of a sputum sample contained many polymorphonuclear leukocytes and extracellular gram-positive diplococci. Capsule-specific antibodies bound to the diplococci resulted in a positive Quellung reaction. Which of the following is the most likely pathogen?

A. *Streptococcus pneumoniae*

B. *Enterococcus faecium*

C. *Streptococcus pyogenes*

D. *Streptococcus agalactiae*

E. *Enterococcus faecalis*

Correct answer = A. The most common cause of community acquired pneumonia in this age group is *Streptococcus pneumoniae*. The X-ray and microbiological findings are most consistent with a diagnosis of pneumococcal pneumonia. Following treatment, this patient should be advised to be vaccinated with the 23-valent pneumococcal vaccine. *Streptococcus pyogenes* does not typically present as pneumonia. *Streptococcus agalactiae* generally afflicts neonates. The enterococci (*Enterococcus faecium* and *Enterococcus faecalis*) do not exhibit the Quellung reaction and do not present as community acquired pneumonia.

Gram-positive Rods

10

I. OVERVIEW

The gram-positive rods discussed in this chapter (Figure 10.1) are not closely related, and they do not cause similar clinical conditions. The genus *Corynebacterium* includes *Corynebacterium diphtheriae*, the cause of the prototypic toxin-mediated disease diphtheria, as well as several usually harmless human commensals. *Bacillus* is a large genus of spore-forming bacteria, principally of soil origin. Anthrax is caused by *Bacillus anthracis. Listeria monocytogenes* causes various types of infection in populations such as newborns, pregnant women, and the immunocompromised.

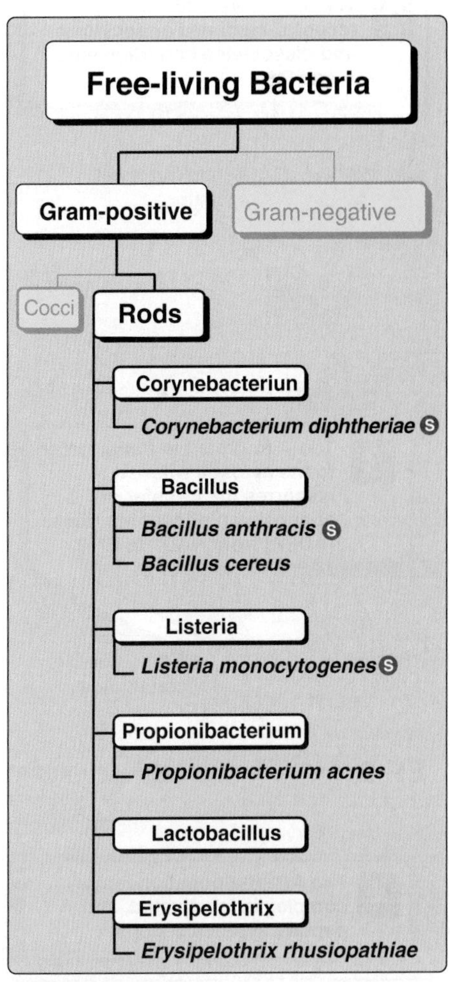

Figure 10.1
Classification of gram-positive rods.
See pp. 338, 332, and 343 for summaries of these organisms.

II. CORYNEBACTERIA

Corynebacteria are small, slender, pleomorphic, gram-positive rods of distinctive morphology that tend to stain unevenly. They are non-motile and unencapsulated, and they do not form spores. *Coryne-bacterium* is a large genus of diverse habitat. Most species are facultative anaerobes, and those associated with humans, including the pathogen *C. diphtheriae*, grow aerobically on standard laboratory media such as blood agar.

A. Corynebacterium diphtheriae

Diphtheria, caused by *C. diphtheriae*, is an acute respiratory or cutaneous disease and may be life threatening. The development of effective vaccination protocols and widespread immunization beginning in early childhood has made the disease rare in developed countries, and few present-day United States clinicians have seen a case of the disease. However, diphtheria is a serious disease throughout the world, particularly in those countries where the population has not been immunized.

1. **Epidemiology:** *C. diphtheriae* is found in the throat and nasopharynx of carriers and in patients with diphtheria. This disease is a local infection, usually of the throat, and the organism is primar-

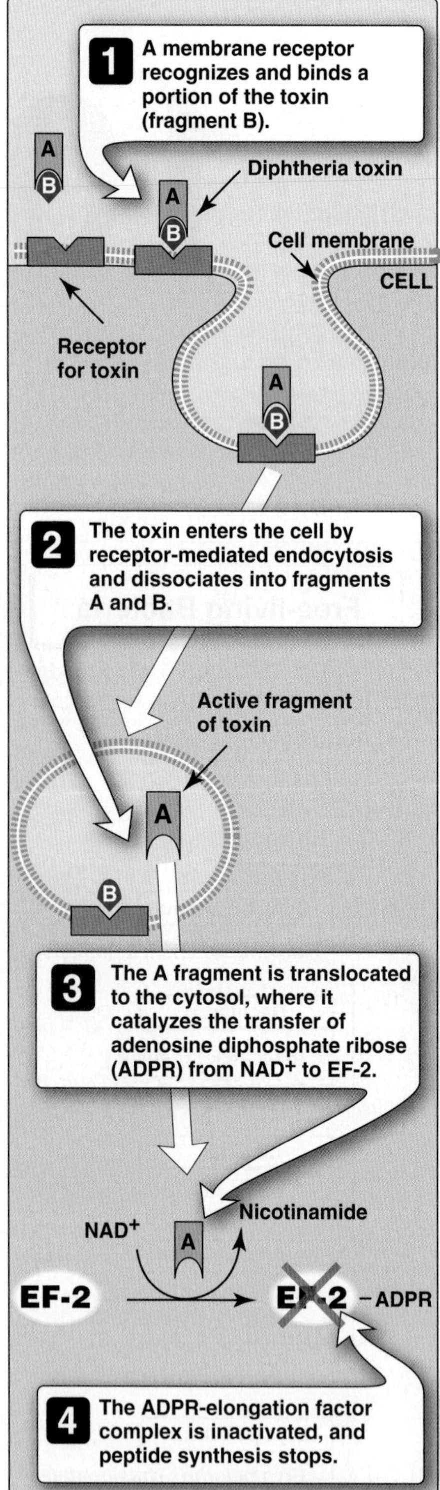
1
A membrane receptor recognizes and binds a portion of the toxin (fragment B).
A
B
Diphtheria toxin
Cell membrane
CELL
Receptor for toxin
2
The toxin enters the cell by receptor-mediated endocytosis and dissociates into fragments A and B.
Active fragment of toxin
3
The A fragment is translocated to the cytosol, where it catalyzes the transfer of adenosine diphosphate ribose (ADPR) from NAD+ to EF-2.
NAD+
Nicotinamide
EF-2
EF-2 –ADPR
4
The ADPR-elongation factor complex is inactivated, and peptide synthesis stops.

Figure 10.2
Action of diphtheria toxin. NAD^+ = nicotine adenine dinucleotide; EF-2 = eukaryotic polypeptide chain elongation factor.

ily spread by respiratory droplets, usually by convalescent or asymptomatic carriers. It is less frequently spread by direct contact with an infected individual or a contaminated fomite.

2. **Pathogenesis:** Diphtheria is caused by the local and systemic effects of a single exotoxin that inhibits eukaryotic protein synthesis. The toxin molecule is a heat-labile polypeptide that is composed of two fragments, A and B. Fragment B binds to susceptible cell membranes and mediates the delivery of fragment A to its target. Inside the cell, fragment A separates from fragment B and catalyzes a reaction between nicotine adenine dinucleotide (NAD^+) and the eukaryotic polypeptide chain elongation factor, EF-2[1] (Figure 10.2). The toxin is encoded on a β-corynephage and only those strains in which the phage is integrated into the *C. diphtheriae* chromosome produce toxin. Toxin gene expression is also regulated by environmental conditions. Low iron conditions induce toxin expression, whereas high iron conditions repress toxin production.

3. **Clinical significance:** Infection may result in one of two forms of clinical disease, respiratory or cutaneous, or in an asymptomatic carrier state.

   a. **Upper respiratory tract infection:** Diphtheria is a strictly localized infection, usually of the throat. The infection produces a distinctive thick, grayish, adherent exudate (pseudomembrane) that is composed of cell debris from the mucosa and inflammatory products (see Figure 10.5). It coats the throat and may extend into the nasal passages or downward in the respiratory tract, where the exudate sometimes obstructs the airways, even leading to suffocation. As the disease progresses, generalized symptoms occur caused by production and absorption of toxin (Figure 10.3). Although all human cells are sensitive to diphtheria toxin, the major clinical effects involve the heart and peripheral nerves. Cardiac conduction defects and myocarditis may lead to congestive heart failure and permanent heart damage. Neuritis of cranial nerves and paralysis of muscle groups, such as those that control movement of the palate or the eye, are seen late in the disease.

   b. **Cutaneous diphtheria:** A puncture wound or cut in the skin can result in introduction of *C. diphtheriae* into the subcutaneous tissue, leading to a chronic, nonhealing ulcer with a gray membrane. Rarely, exotoxin production leads to tissue degeneration and death.

4. **Immunity:** Diphtheria toxin is antigenic and stimulates the production of antibodies that neutralize the toxin's activity. [Note: Formalin treatment of the toxin produces a toxoid that retains the antigenic-

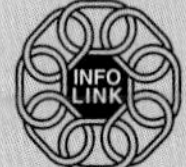
INFO LINK

[1]See Chapter 31 in ***Lippincott's Illustrated Reviews: Biochemistry*** for a discussion of polypeptide chain elongation.

ity but not the toxicity of the molecule. This is the material used for immunization against the disease (see p. 36).]

5. **Laboratory identification:** The presumptive diagnosis and decision to treat for diphtheria must be based on initial clinical observation. Diphtheria should be considered in patients who have resided in or traveled to an area in which diphtheria is prevalent, when they have pharyngitis, low-grade fever, and cervical adenopathy (swelling of the neck). Erythema of the pharynx progressing to adherent gray pseudomembranes increases suspicion of diphtheria. However, a definitive diagnosis requires isolation of the organism, which must then be tested for virulence using an immunologic precipitin reaction to demonstrate toxin production. *C. diphtheriae* can be isolated most easily from a selective medium, such as Tinsdale agar (see Figure 10.5), which contains potassium tellurite, an inhibitor of other respiratory flora, and on which the organism produces several distinctive black colonies with halos (see Figure 10.5). *C. diphtheriae* from clinical material or culture has a distinctive morphology when stained, for example, with methylene blue. This morphology includes characteristic bands and reddish (polychromatic) granules that are often seen in thin, sometimes club-shaped rods that appear in clumps, suggestive of Chinese characters or picket fences (see Figure 10.4). This presentation is often referred to as a "palisade arrangement" of cells. Initial decision to treat for diphtheria must be based on clinical observation. Culture and assay for toxin production are required for confirmation of the diagnosis.

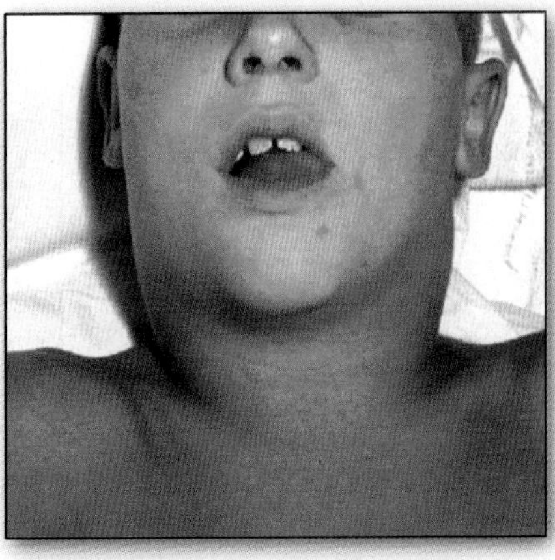

Figure 10.3
Diphtheria with marked swelling of the lymph nodes in the neck.

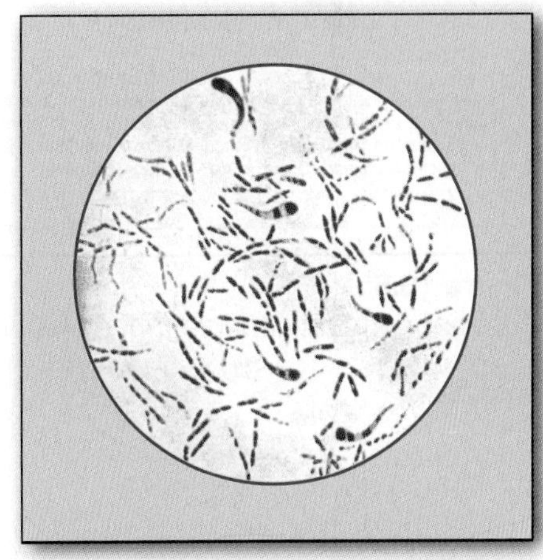

Figure 10.4
Corynebacterium diphtheriae.

6. **Treatment:** Treatment of diphtheria requires prompt neutralization of toxin, followed by eradication of the organism. A single dose of horse serum antitoxin inactivates any circulating toxin, although it does not affect toxin already bound to a cell-surface receptor. [Note: Serum sickness caused by a reaction to the horse protein may cause complications in approximately 10 percent of patients.] *C. diphtheriae* is sensitive to several antibiotics, and passive immunization with preformed diphtheria toxin antibodies is a mandatory part of treatment of diphtheria. Because diphtheria is highly contagious, suspected diphtheria patients must be isolated. Antibiotic treatment, such as erythromycin or penicillin (Figure 10.5), slows the spread of infection and, by killing the organism, prevents further toxin production. Supportive care directed especially at respiratory and cardiac complications is an essential part of the management of patients with diphtheria.

7. **Prevention:** The cornerstone of diphtheria prevention is immunization with toxoid, usually administered in the DTaP triple vaccine, together with tetanus toxoid and pertussis antigens (see p. 38). The initial series of injections should be started in infancy. Booster injections of diphtheria toxoid (with tetanus toxoid) should be given at approximately 10-year intervals throughout life. The control of an epidemic outbreak of diphtheria involves rigorous immunization and a search for healthy carriers among patient contacts.

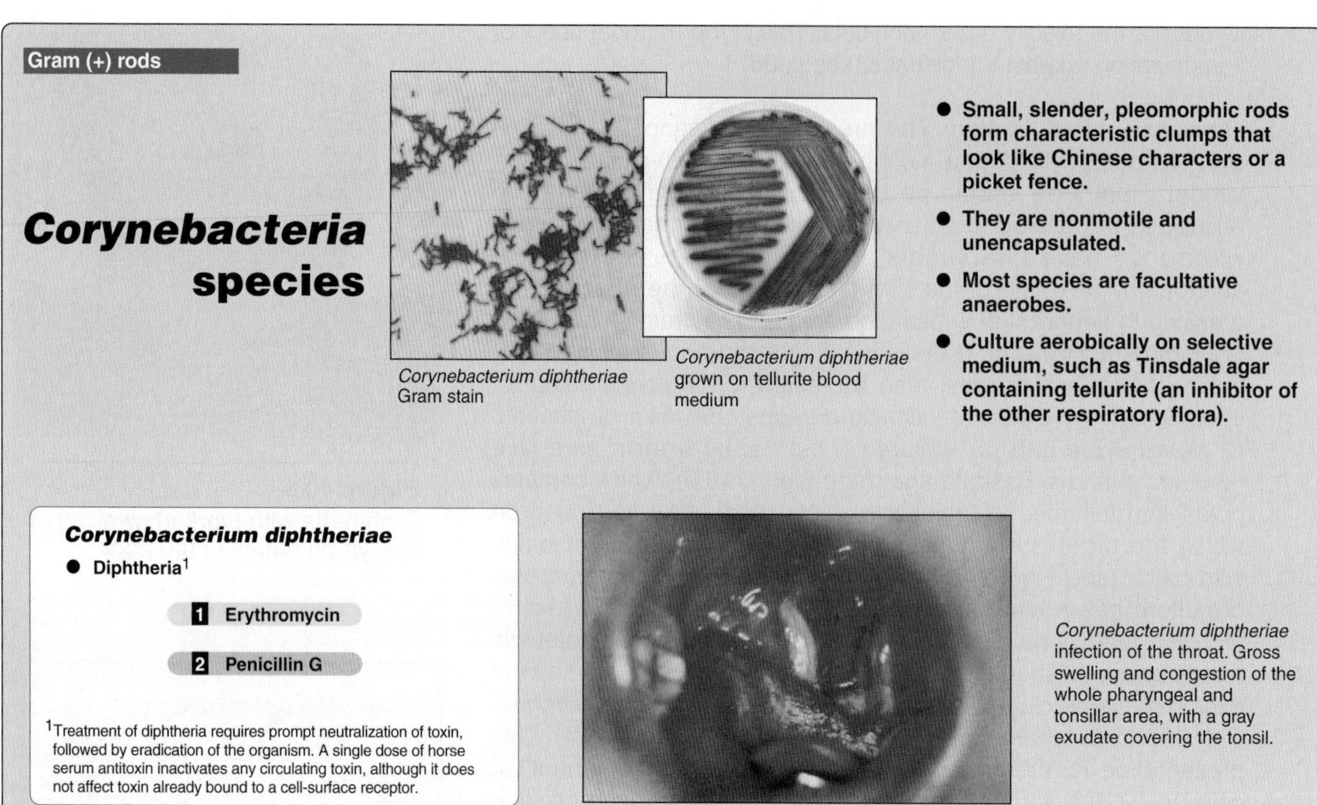

Figure 10.5
Summary of *Corynebacterium diphtheriae* disease. 1 Indicates first-line drugs; 2 indicates alternative drugs.

B. Diphtheroids

Several other corynebacterium species that morphologically resemble the type species, *C. diphtheriae*, are common commensals of the nose, throat, nasopharynx, skin, urogenital tract, and conjunctiva. They are therefore called diphtheroids and are generally unable to produce exotoxin, but a few cause disease in rare circumstances such as in immunosuppressed individuals.

III. BACILLUS SPECIES

Species of the genus *Bacillus* are gram-positive, form endospores, and are either strict aerobes or aerotolerant anaerobes (that is, they can grow in the presence of oxygen, but do not require it). Most of the 70 or so species of *Bacillus* are found in soil and water and are usually encountered in the medical laboratory as airborne contaminants. *B. anthracis*, the cause of the disease anthrax, is clinically the most important member of this genus.

A. Bacillus anthracis

Anthrax is a rare disease in the United States. For example, from 1984 to 1997, only three case of cutaneous anthrax were reported.

However, in 2001, 20 new cases occurred—11 cutaneous and 11 inhalation anthrax. These infections resulted from probable exposure to *B. anthracis* powder sent through the mail.

1. **Epidemiology:** Anthrax is an enzootic disease of worldwide occurrence. [Note: The term enzootic disease applies to a population of animals (equivalent to endemic disease in a human population, that is, its occurrence changes little over time). This is as compared to an epizootic disease, which attacks a large number of animals at the same time (similar to a human epidemic).] Anthrax affects principally domestic herbivores (for example, sheep, goats, and horses) and is transmitted to humans by contact with infected animal products or contaminated dust (Figure 10.6). Infection is usually initiated by the subcutaneous inoculation of spores through incidental skin abrasions. Less frequently, the inhalation of spore-laden dust causes a pulmonary form of anthrax. [Note: Sometimes an occupational hazard, this form of pneumonia is known as "woolsorter's disease."] *B. anthracis* spores may remain viable for many years in contaminated pastures and in bones, wool, hair, hides, and other animal materials. These spores, like those of clostridia (see p. 53), are highly resistant to physical and chemical agents. In the United States, a veterinary vaccine in widespread use makes domestic animal sources of the disease quite rare. Contaminated agricultural imports may account for the few cases seen and lead occasionally to the quarantine of goods from endemic areas. *B. anthracis* is a potential bioterrorism agent because it can be easily grown in large quantities. Moreover, the spores are resistant to destruction and can be formulated into an aerosol for wide dissemination. Physicians must be prepared to recognized anthrax even though it is rarely seen in the United States.

2. **Pathogenesis:** *B. anthracis* produces a unique capsule that is comprised of poly-D-glutamic acid and is antiphagocytic. Elaboration of this capsule is essential for full virulence. The organism also produces two plasmid-coded exotoxins: edema toxin and lethal toxin. Both toxins are AB type toxins with activity and binding domains. The binding subunit shared by both toxins is called protective antigen (so named because of its use in producing protective anthrax vaccines). This domain mediates cell entry of both toxins. The activity subunits are called edema factor and lethal factor. Edema factor is a calmodulin-dependent adenylyl cyclase, which causes elevation of intracellular cAMP, resulting in the severe edema usually seen in *B. anthracis* infections. Lethal factor is responsible for tissue necrosis. Lethal factor complexed with protective antigen is known as lethal toxin, whereas edema factor complexed with protective antigen is known as edema toxin.

3. **Clinical significance**

   a. **Cutaneous anthrax:** About 95 percent of human cases of anthrax are cutaneous. Upon introduction of organisms or spores that germinate, a papule develops. It rapidly evolves into a painless, black, severely swollen "malignant pustule,"

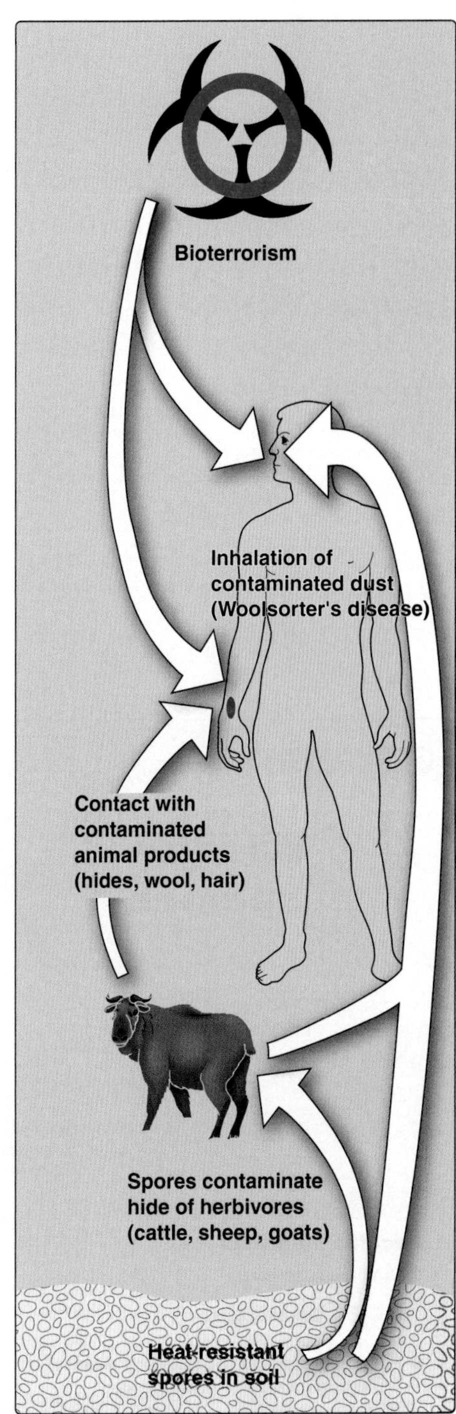

Figure 10.6
Anthrax in animal and human hosts.

which eventually crusts over. The organisms may invade regional lymph nodes and then the general circulation, leading to fatal septicemia. Although some cases remain localized and heal, the overall mortality in untreated cutaneous anthrax is about 20 percent.

b. **Pulmonary anthrax** (**woolsorter's disease**)**:** Caused by inhalation of spores, the pulmonary form is characterized by progressive hemorrhagic lymphadenitis (inflammation of the lymph nodes), hemorrhagic mediastinitis (inflammation of the mediastinum) and has a mortality rate approaching 100 percent if left untreated.

4. **Laboratory identification:** *B. anthracis* is easily recovered from clinical materials, where it is often present in massive numbers. Microscopically, the organisms appear as blunt-ended bacilli that occur singly; in pairs; or frequently in long chains (Figure 10.7). They do not sporulate often in clinical samples but do so in culture. The spores are oval and centrally located. On blood agar, the colonies are large, grayish, and nonhemolytic, with an irregular border. Unlike many bacillus species, *B. anthracis* is nonmotile

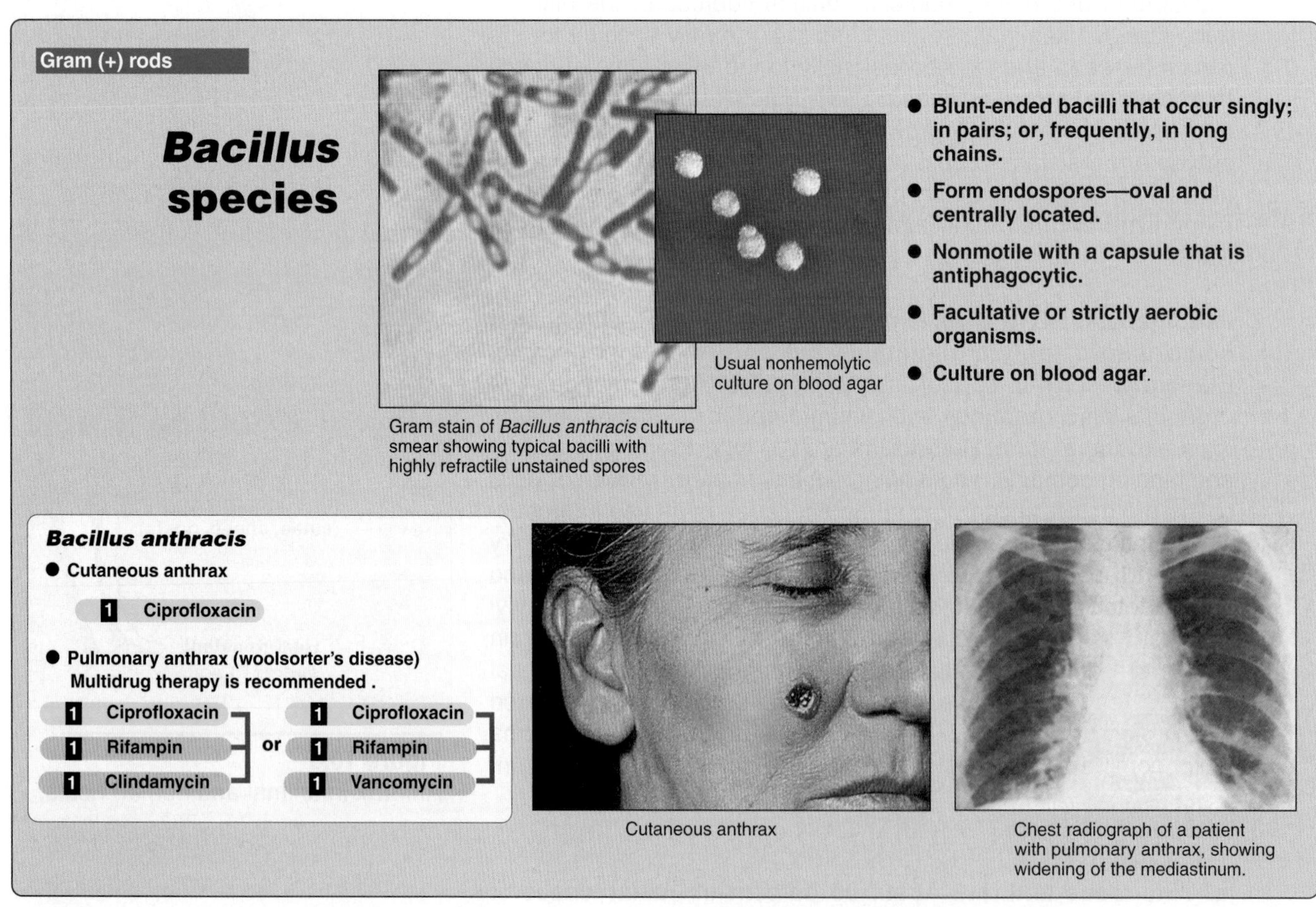

Figure 10.7
Summary of anthrax disease. 1 Indicates first-line drugs.

and is encapsulated *in vivo*. A direct immunofluorescence assay aids in identification of the organism.

5. **Treatment:** *B. anthracis* is sensitive to a variety of antibiotics. Cutaneous anthrax responds to ciprofloxacin (see Figure 10.7). Penicillin is not recommended because of inducible β-lactamase in *B. anthracis*. Multidrug therapy (for example, ciprofloxacin plus rifampin plus vancomycin) is recommended for inhalation anthrax. Aggressive therapy is indicated for inhalation anthrax both because of the severity of the disease and the fact that the disease is often not diagnosed until late in the course of the illness.

6. **Prevention:** A cell-free vaccine is available for workers in high-risk occupations (see p. 37). Postexposure prophylaxis with ciprofloxacin or doxycycline is recommended. [Note: Because of the resistance of endospores to chemical disinfectants, autoclaving is the most reliable means of decontamination.]

B. Other bacillus species

Uncommonly, other species of bacillus are implicated in opportunistic lesions, particularly following trauma or the placement of artificial devices and catheters. A commonly identified species is *Bacillus cereus*. Strains of this species produce a tissue-destructive exotoxin. *B. cereus* also causes food poisoning by means of enterotoxins with either emetic or diarrheal effects.

IV. LISTERIA

Listeria species are slender, short, gram-positive rods (see Figure 10.9). They do not form spores. Sometimes they occur as diplobacilli or in short chains, and they are avid intracellular parasites that may be seen within the cytoplasm of host cells in tissue samples. *Listeria* species are catalase-positive, and display a distinctive tumbling motility by light microscopy in liquid medium, which is most active after growth at 25°C. These characteristics distinguish it from *Streptococcus* (catalase negative) or *Corynebacterium* (nonmotile) species, both of which may be confused morphologically with *Listeria*. *Listeria* species grow on a variety of enriched media.

A. Epidemiology

Listeria monocytogenes is the only species that infects humans, although the *Listeria* species are widespread among animals in nature. *Listeria* infections, which may occur as sporadic cases or in small epidemics, are usually foodborne. For example, studies have shown that 2 to 3 percent of processed dairy products (including ice cream and cheese), 20 to 30 percent of ground meats, and a majority of retail poultry samples are contaminated with *L. monocytogenes*. [Note: Because *L. monocytogenes* is capable of growth at 4°C, refrigeration does not reliably suppress its growth in food.] One to 15 percent of healthy humans are asymptomatic intestinal carri-

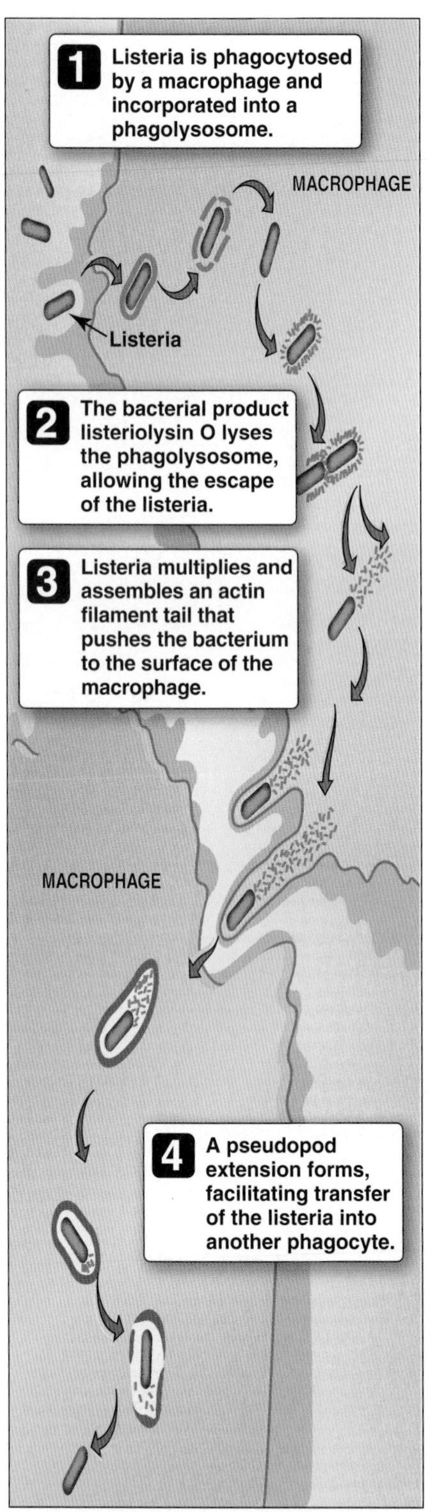

1 Listeria is phagocytosed by a macrophage and incorporated into a phagolysosome.
MACROPHAGE
Listeria
2 The bacterial product listeriolysin O lyses the phagolysosome, allowing the escape of the listeria.
3 Listeria multiplies and assembles an actin filament tail that pushes the bacterium to the surface of the macrophage.
MACROPHAGE
4 A pseudopod extension forms, facilitating transfer of the listeria into another phagocyte.

Figure 10.8
Life cycle of *Listeria monocytogenes* in host macrophages.

ers of the organism. *Listeria* infections are most common in pregnant women, fetuses and newborns, and in immunocompromised individuals, such as older adults and patients receiving corticosteroids. In the United States, some 2,000 cases are reported each year, with 450 deaths and 100 stillbirths. Blood cultures are indicated in pregnant febrile women when no alternate pathology (for example, urinary tract infection) is readily detected.

B. Pathogenesis

L. monocytogenes is an intracellular parasite that has been used extensively to study phagocytosis and immune activation of macrophages. The organism attaches to and enters a variety of mammalian cells, apparently by normal phagocytosis. Once internalized, it escapes from the phagocytic vacuole by elaborating a membrane-damaging toxin called listeriolysin O. [Note: Mutants lacking a functional listeriolysin O are avirulent.] *L. monocytogenes* grows in the cytosol and stimulates changes in cell function that facilitate its direct passage from cell to cell. The organisms induce a reorganization of cellular actin such that short filaments and actin-binding proteins adhere to the bacteria, creating a cometlike "tail." This complex appears to propel the organisms through the cell to pseudopods in contact with adjacent cells. Bacterium-produced membrane-degrading phospholipases then mediate the passage of the organism directly to a neighboring cell, allowing avoidance of the extracellular milieu, including cells of the immune system (Figure 10.8).

C. Clinical significance

Septicemia and meningitis are the most commonly reported forms of *L. monocytogenes* infection (listeriosis). A variety of focal lesions are less frequently seen such as granulomatous skin lesions. Pregnant women, usually in the third trimester, may have a milder "flulike" illness. In this as well as in asymptomatic vaginal colonization, the organism can be transmitted to the fetus and result in spontaneous abortion. Alternatively, the organism can also be transmitted to a newborn following birth, resulting in neonatal meningitis. (*L. monocytogenes* is a relatively common cause of newborn meningitis). Immunocompromised individuals, especially those with defects in cellular immunity, are susceptible to serious generalized infections.

D. Laboratory identification

The organism can be isolated from blood, cerebrospinal fluid, and other clinical specimens by standard bacteriologic procedures. On blood agar, *L. monocytogenes* produces a small colony surrounded by a narrow zone of β hemolysis (Figure 10.9). *Listeria* species can be distinguished from various streptococci by morphology, motility, and the production of catalase.

E. Treatment and prevention

A variety of antibiotics have been successfully used to treat *L. monocytogenes* infections, including ampicillin and trimetho-

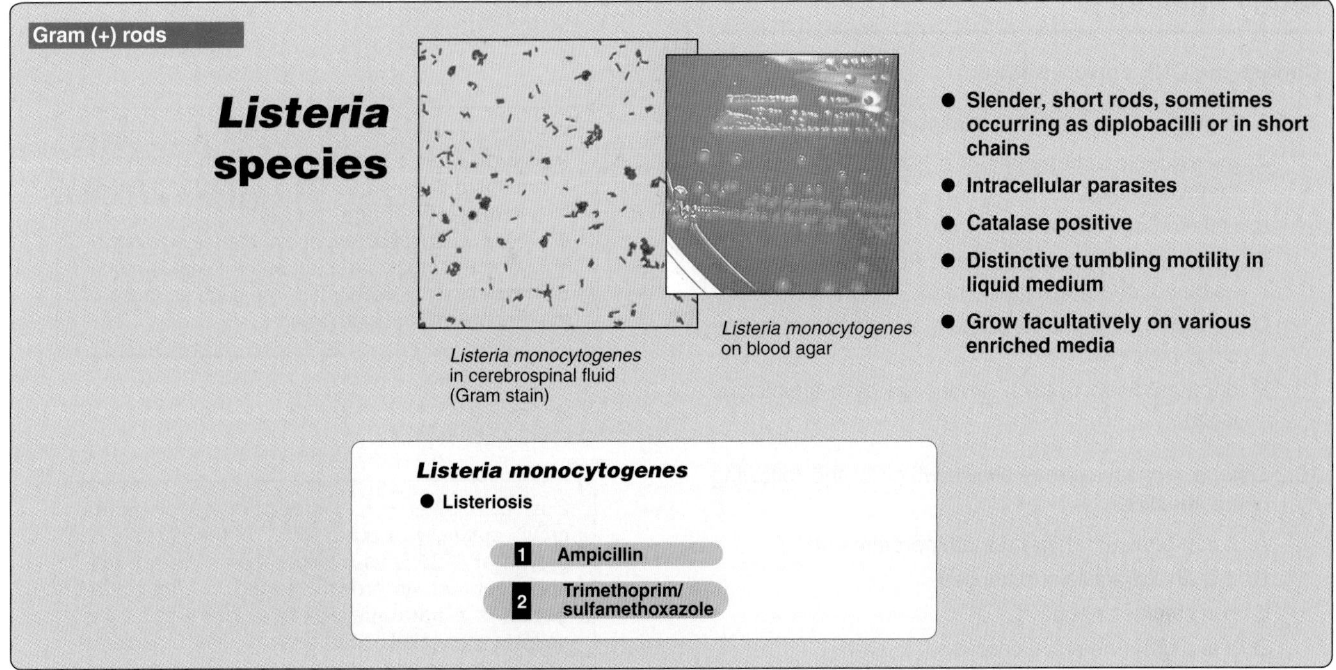

Figure 10.9
Summary of *Listeria* species. 1 Indicates first-line drugs; 2 indicates alternative drugs.

prim/sulfamethoxazole (see Figure 10.9). Prevention of *L. monocytogenes* infections can be accomplished by proper food preparation and handling, as well as removal of contaminated products from the food supply.

V. OTHER NON-SPORE-FORMING, GRAM-POSITIVE RODS

Propionibacterium is a genus of anaerobic or microaerophilic rods of diphtheroidlike morphology. They are common inhabitants of normal skin, and, in rare instances, have been reported as causes of endocarditis and infections of plastic implants. *P. acnes*, often a strict anaerobe, has been implicated as a contributing cause of acne. Various species of *Lactobacillus* are part of the commensal flora of human mucous membranes. They produce large quantities of lactic acid during fermentation and have been thought to assist in maintaining the acid pH of normal mucous epithelia. Acid production by oral lactobacilli may play a role in the progression of dental caries, especially in dentine. *Erysipelothrix rhusiopathiae* is a filamentous, gram-positive rod that causes disease in animals and, rarely, a skin infection called erysipeloid in people who commonly handle animal products (for example, butchers, veterinarians, and fishermen).

Study questions

Choose the ONE correct answer

10.1 A diagnosis of diphtheria is confirmed by:

A. microscopic appearance of organisms stained with methylene blue.
B. isolation of a typical colony on Tinsdale agar.
C. isolation of typical organisms from materials such as blood, showing invasiveness.
D. detection of β phage plaques in cultures of suspicious isolates.
E. demonstration of toxin production by a suspicious isolate.

Correct answer = E. Observation of diphtheria toxin production is required to prove the diagnosis. Items A and B are presumptive indicators. β Phage is a temperate phage, and lytic activity is not observed. *Cornyebacterium diphtheriae* is noninvasive, and the organism (but not the toxin) is recovered only from surface infections such as those of the oropharynx and skin lesions.

10.2 *Listeria monocytogenes* shows which of the following characteristics?

A. It can grow at refrigerator temperatures (4°C).
B. It is an extracellular pathogen.
C. It is catalase negative.
D. It is a gram-negative coccus.
E. It is strictly a human pathogen.

Correct answer = A. *Listeria. monocytogenes* grows optimally at 30 to 37°C, but is capable of growth at 4°C. Thus, refrigeration does not reliably suppress its growth in food. *L. monocytogenes* is a catalase-positive, gram-positive, obligate intracellular pathogen. These organisms are found in cattle, other warmblooded animals, and fish, where they can cause disease.

10.3 A 26-year-old woman, 8 months pregnant, visits her obstetrician complaining of fever, myalagia and backache of recent onset. Three weeks earlier, the patient had been a weekend guest at a rural farmhouse, where all the food was reported to be "unprocessed" and "natural." A culture of the patient's blood shows gram-positive rods that are catalase positive and display a distinctive tumbling motility in liquid medium. What is the most likely source of the woman's infection?

A. Well-done roast beef
B. Fresh, raw cow's milk
C. Home-baked bread
D. Homemade applesauce
E. Baked apple pie

Correct answer = B. The woman is most likely experiencing listerosis. *Listeriae* are common in the gastrointestinal tract and milk of cattle, but are normally killed by pasteurization. Unpasteurized milk was presumably consumed at the farm.

10.4 A 45-year-old cattle rancher presents to his physician with a wound on his forearm that resembles a large scab. Samples collected from the wound were cultured and examined. The bacteria recovered were Gram positive, nonmotile rods with square ends. The cultured bacteria formed irregularly shaped, nonhemolytic colonies on blood agar plates and individual cells from the plates had a centrally located spore. What is the most likely cause of this infection?

A. *Listeria monocytogenes*
B. *Staphylococcus aureus*
C. *Legionella pneumophila*
D. *Corynebacterium diphtheriae*
E. *Bacillus anthracis*

Correct answer = E. This cattle rancher is suffering from cutaneous anthrax, which is an occupational hazard. The scab like wound is called an eschar and results from localized edema and tissue destruction caused by the two toxins produced by *Bacillus anthracis*. The microbiological characteristics of the organism are consistent with a diagnosis of *B. anthracis* infection. The other microorganisms do not have the chacteristics described.

Neisseriae

11

I. OVERVIEW

The genus *Neisseria* consists of gram-negative, aerobic cocci. Two *Neisseria* species are pathogenic for humans—*Neisseria gonorrhoeae* (commonly called gonococcus), the causal agent of gonorrhea and *Neisseria meningitidis* (commonly called meningococcus), a frequent cause of meningitis. Gonococci and meningococci are nonmotile diplococci that cannot be distinguished from each other under the microscope. However, they can be differentiated in the laboratory by sugar-use patterns, and the sites of their primary infections. Both bacteria are classified as pyogenic cocci because infections by these organisms are also characterized by the production of purulent (puslike) material comprised largely of white blood cells. Neisseriae and organisms that are easily confused with them are discussed in this chapter (Figure 11.1.)

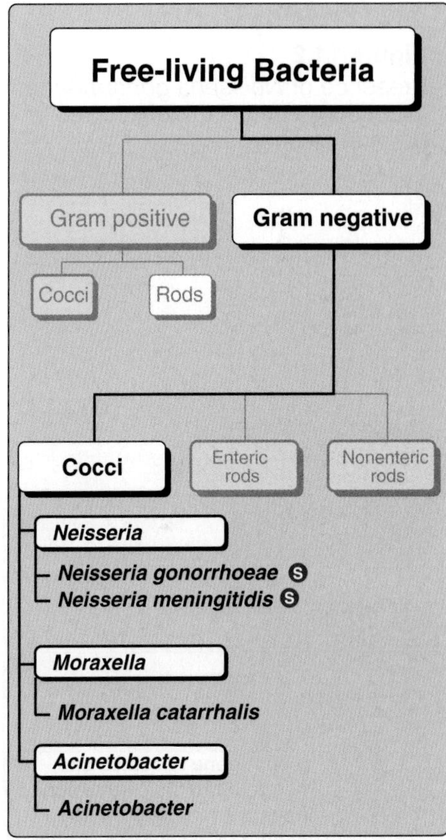

Figure 11.1
Classification of *Neisseria* and related organisms. See pp. 345–346 for summaries of these organisms.

II. NEISSERIA GONORRHOEAE

Gonorrhea is one of the most frequently reported infectious diseases in the United States. The causal agent, *N. gonorrhoeae*, a gram-negative diplococcus, is frequently observed within the polymorphonuclear leukocytes of clinical samples obtained from infected patients (Figure 11.2). *N. gonorrhoeae* is usually transmitted during sexual contact or, more rarely, during the passage of a baby through an infected birth canal. It does not survive long outside the human body because it is highly sensitive to dehydration.

A. Structure

Gonococci are unencapsulated (unlike meningococci, see p. 105), piliated, and nonmotile, and they resemble a pair of kidney beans.

1. **Pili:** These hairlike surface appendages are made of helical aggregates of repeating peptide subunits called pilin. Pili enhance attachment of the organism to host epithelial and mucosal cell surfaces. They are, therefore, important virulence factors. Pili are also antigenic. At least twenty gonococcal genes code for pilin, most of which are not expressed at any given time because they lack promoters (that is, they are "silent"). By shuffling and recombining chromosomal regions of these genes, a single strain of *N. gonorrhoeae* can, at different times, synthesize ("express") multiple pilins that have different amino acid sequences. This process, known as antigenic variation by gene conversion, allows the

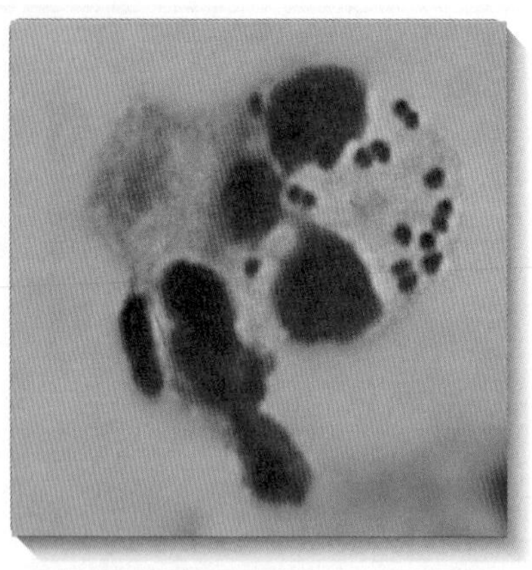

Figure 11.2
Presence of *Neisseria gonorrhoeae* in polymorphonuclear leukocytes in urethral discharge.

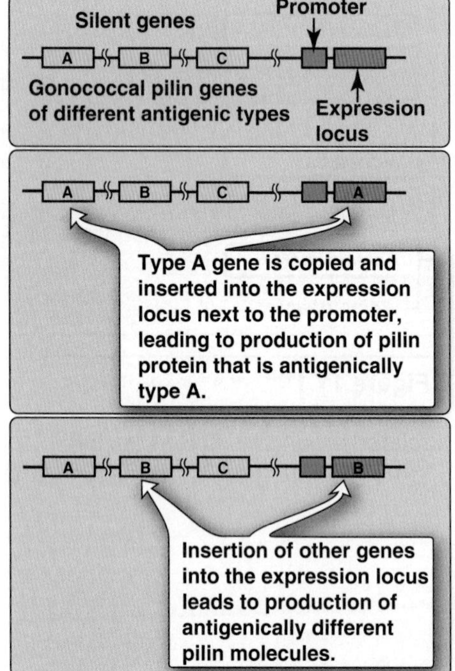

Figure 11.3
Antigenic variation in the gonococcus.

organism to produce antigenically different pilin molecules at high frequency (Figure 11.3).

2. **Lipooligosaccharide:** Gonococcal lipooligosaccharides (LOS) have shorter, more highly branched, nonrepeat O-antigenic side chains than do lipopolysaccharides found in other gram-negative bacteria (see p. 13). The bactericidal antibodies in normal human serum are IgM molecules directed against LOS antigens. The gonococcus is also capable of high-frequency variation of the LOS antigens presented on the cell surface. Variation occurs as a consequence of phase variation of one of several genes involved in the biosynthesis of LOS. If the biosynthetic gene is in the off phase, terminal saccharide moieties cannot be added, resulting in presentation of an antigenically distinct LOS molecule.

3. **Porin proteins:** The gonococcus expresses a single porin type, known as PorB. Different strains express either PorB1A or PorB1B; however, the porin proteins are not subject to a high frequency phase or antigenic variation like other outer membrane antigens.

4. **Opacity proteins:** Opacity (Opa) proteins (formerly called PII proteins) are so named due to their tendency to impart an opaque quality to gonococcal colonies. The gonococcus has the capacity to express up to 11 different Opa proteins, but generally only one or a few are expressed simultaneously. Opa proteins are subject to phase variation by virtue of the presence of numerous polymeric repeats (CTCTT) in the coding regions. If an Opa protein is expressed, an increase or decrease in the number of repeats shifts the protein out of the reading frame, resulting in phase variation to the off phase. Different Opa proteins bind to distinct receptors on host cells. Therefore shifting expression from one Opa protein to another results in changes in host cell tropism.

B. Pathogenesis

Pili and Opa proteins facilitate adhesion of the gonococcus to epithelial cells of the urethra, rectum, cervix, pharynx, and conjunctiva, thereby making colonization possible. In addition, both gonococci and meningococci produce an IgA protease that cleaves IgA_1, helping the pathogen to evade immunoglobulins of this subclass. The gonococcus requires iron for growth and survival *in vivo*. The pathogen acquires this necessary nutrient by expression of specific transport systems that remove and internalize the iron from human iron binding proteins including transferrin, lactoferrin and hemoglobin. To establish infection in human males, the gonococcus must express proteins that facilitate iron acquisition from either transferrin or lactoferrin.

C. Clinical significance

Gonococci most often colonize the mucous membrane of the genitourinary tract or rectum. There, the organisms may cause a localized infection with the production of pus or may lead to tissue invasion, chronic inflammation, and fibrosis. A higher proportion of females than males are generally asymptomatic, and these individuals act as the reservoir for maintaining and transmitting gonococcal infections. [Note: More than one sexually transmitted disease (STD) may be acquired at the same time, such as, gonorrhea in combination with syphilis (*Treponema pallidum* infection), *Chlamydia*, human immunodeficiency virus, or hepatitis B virus. Patients with gonorrhea may, therefore, need treatment for more than one pathogen.]

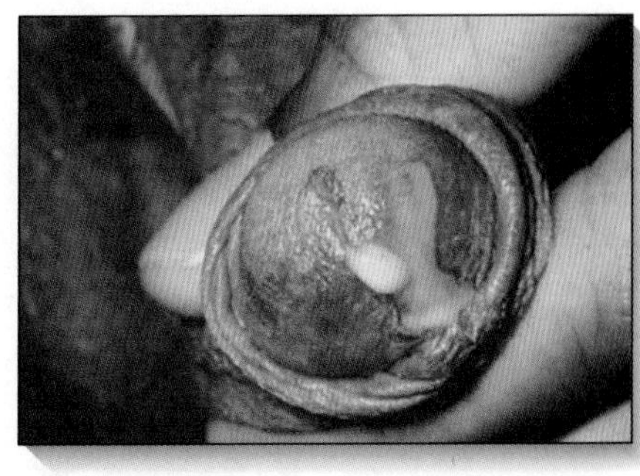

Figure 11.4
Urethral discarge of gonorrhea.

1. **Genitourinary tract infections:** Symptoms of gonococcal infection are more acute and easier to diagnose in males. The patient typically presents with a yellow, purulent urethral discharge and painful urination (Figure 11.4). In females, infection occurs in the endocervix and extends to the urethra and vagina. A greenish-yellow cervical discharge is most common, often accompanied by intermenstrual bleeding. The disease may progress to the uterus, causing salpingitis (inflammation of the fallopian tubes), pelvic inflammatory disease (PID), and fibrosis. Infertility occurs in approximately 20 percent of women with gonococcal salpingitis, as a result of tubal scarring. *N. gonorrhoeae* is a common cause of pelvic inflammatory disease in females.

2. **Rectal infections:** Prevalent in men who have sex with men, rectal infections are characterized by constipation, painful defecation, and purulent discharge.

3. **Pharyngitis:** Pharyngitis is contracted by oral-genital contact. Infected individuals may show a purulent pharyngeal exudate, and the condition may mimic a mild viral or a streptococcal sore throat (see p. 81).

4. **Ophthalmia neonatorum**: This infection of the conjunctival sac is acquired by newborns during passage through the birth canals of infected mothers (Figure 11.5). If untreated, acute conjunctivitis may lead to blindness. Treatment is systemic ceftriaxone IM or IV in a single dose. Infants born to mothers who are known to have a birth canal infected with gonococcus or are at high risk of having this are also given a systemic dose of ceftriaxone prophylactically, even in the absence of clinically evident ophthalmia. Topical erythromycin ointment is only used for routine prophylaxis in circumstances of relatively low risk.

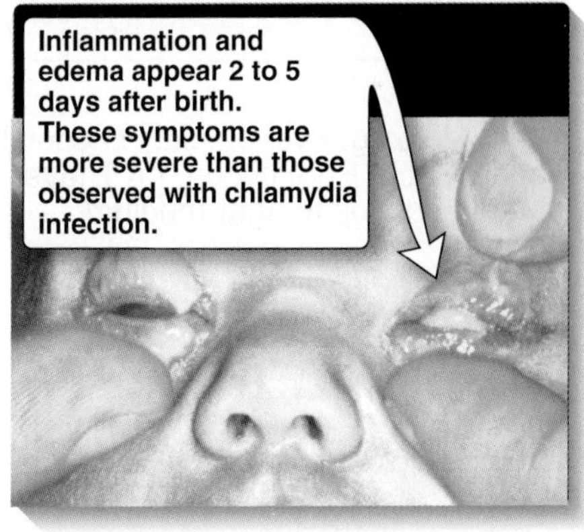

Figure 11.5
Gonococcal ophthalmia neonatorum.

5. **Disseminated infection:** Most strains of gonococci have a limited ability to multiply in the bloodstream. Therefore, bacteremia with gonococci is rare. In contrast, meningococci multiply rapidly in blood (see p. 105). However, some strains of *N. gonorrhoeae* do invade the bloodstream and may result in a disseminated infection in which the organism can cause fever; a painful, purulent arthritis; and small, single, scattered pustules on the skin, whose base becomes erythematous (red) due to dilation or congestion of capillaries. Necrosis may develop. [Note: Gonococcal infection is the most common cause of septic arthritis in sexually active adults.] Disseminated infections are seen in both men and women but are more common in women, particularly during pregnancy and menses. All patients treated for disseminated infection should also receive a 7-day course of doxycycline to eliminate potentially concurrent infection with *Chlamydia*. Gonorrhea is most common in adolescents and young adults (Figure 11.6). (A summary of organisms causing the most common STDs is presented in Figure 33.2.)

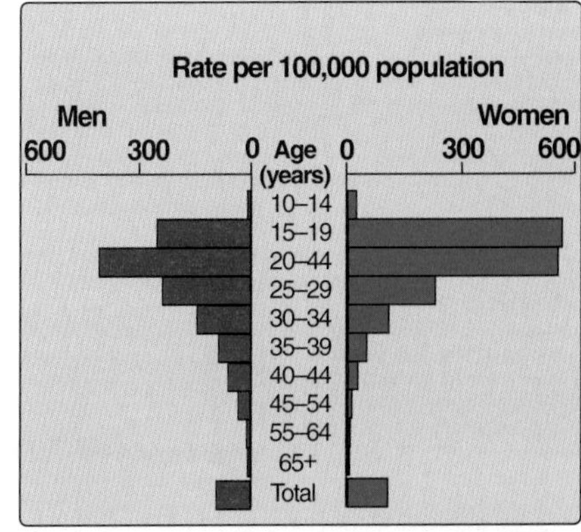

Figure 11.6
Incidence of gonorrhea in the United States (2009) according to age and sex.

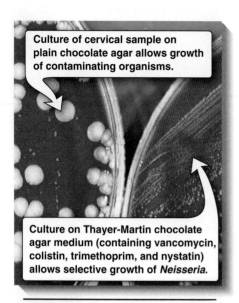

Figure 11.7
Left: Mixed growth on plain chocolate agar. Right: Pure culture on Thayer-Martin chocolate agar medium.

D. Laboratory identification

In the male, the finding of numerous neutrophils containing gram-negative diplococci in a smear of urethral exudate permits a provisional diagnosis of gonococcal infection and indicates that the individual should be treated. In contrast, a positive culture is needed to diagnose gonococcal infection in the female as well as at sites other than the urethra in the male. If disseminated gonococcal infection is suspected, appropriate cultures should be set up as indicated, for example, of skin lesions, joint fluid, and blood.

1. **Growth conditions for culture:** *N. gonorrhoeae* grows best under aerobic conditions, and most strains require enhanced CO_2. *N. gonorrhoeae* utilizes glucose as a carbon and energy source but not maltose, lactose, or sucrose. [Note: *N. meningitidis* utilizes both glucose and maltose (see p. 107).] All members of the genus are oxidase-positive. [Note: The oxidase test (see p. 24) is used to identify *Neisseriae*, but does not distinguish between gonococci, meningococci, and nonpathogenic *Neisseriae*.]

2. **Selective media:** Gonococci, like pneumococci, are very sensitive to heating or drying. Cultures must be plated promptly or, if this is not possible, transport media must be used to extend the viability of the organism to be cultured. Thayer-Martin medium (chocolate agar supplemented with several antibiotics that suppress the growth of nonpathogenic *Neisseriae* and other normal and abnormal flora) is typically used to isolate gonococci (Figure 11.7). The use of this medium is important for cultures that are typically obtained from sites such as the genitourinary tract or rectum, where there is normally an abundance of flora. On nonselective media, the normal flora overgrows the gonococci. Culture of *N. gonorrhoeae* on Thayer-Martin agar remains the "gold standard" for diagnosis.

E. Treatment and prevention

More than 20 percent of current isolates of *N. gonorrhoeae* are resistant to penicillin, tetracycline, cefoxitin, and/or spectinomycin. Penicillin-resistant organisms are called PPNG—penicillinase-producing *N. gonorrhoeae*. These strains contain plasmids that carry the gene for β-lactamase of the TEM type (encoded in a transposable element), such as is seen in *Escherichia coli* and *Haemophilus influenzae*. The frequency of PPNG in the United States is now sufficiently high that penicillin is no longer recommended for treatment of gonorrhea. However, most organisms still respond to treatment with third-generation cephalosporins; for example, a single intramuscular dose of ceftriaxone is the recommended therapy for uncomplicated gonococcal infections of the urethra, endocervix, or rectum. Intramuscular spectinomycin is indicated in patients who are allergic to cephalosporins. Many patients with gonorrhea have coexisting chlamydial infections. Therefore, doxycycline, a tetracycline effective against *Chlamydia*, is often included as part of the treatment regimen for gonorrhea. Prevention of gonorrhea involves evaluation and management of sexual contacts of the patient, generally using a dose of an effective antibiotic prophylactically in an exposed individual even in the absence of symptoms. The use of barrier methods is also a preventive measure against gonorrhea as is the case for all sexually transmitted infections. No vaccine is available for gonorrhea.

III. NEISSERIA MENINGITIDIS

N. meningitidis is one of the most frequent causes of meningitis. Infection with *N. meningitidis* can also take the form of a fulminant meningococcemia, with intravascular coagulation, circulatory collapse, and potentially fatal shock, but without meningitis. In each case, symptoms can occur with extremely rapid onset and great intensity. Outbreaks of meningitis, most common in winter and early spring, are favored by close contact between individuals, such as occurs in schools, institutions, and military barracks. Severe epidemics also occur periodically in developing nations, such as in sub-Saharan Africa and Latin America. *N. meningitidis* tends to strike young, previously well individuals and can progress over a matter of hours to death.

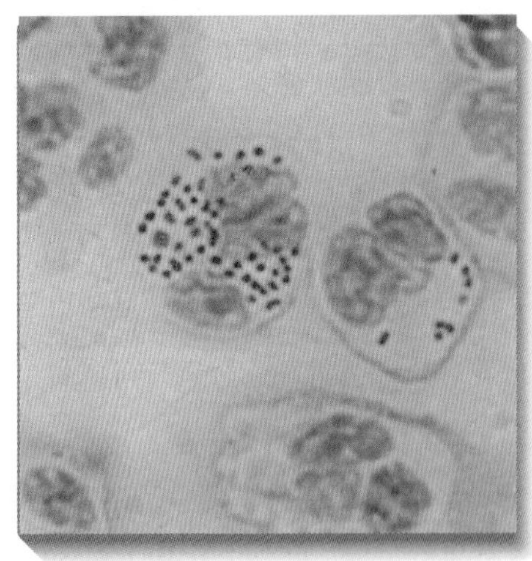

Figure 11.8
Smear of purulent cerebrospinal fluid showing *Neisseria meningitidis*.

A. Structure

Like *N. gonorrhoeae*, *N. meningitidis* is a nonmotile, gram-negative diplococcus, shaped like a kidney bean, which always appears in pairs (Figure 11.8). It is also piliated and the pili allow attachment of the organism to the nasopharyngeal mucosa where it is harbored both in carriers and in those with meningococcal disease. When meningococcus is isolated from blood or spinal fluid, it is invariably encapsulated. The meningococcal polysaccharide capsule is antiphagocytic and, therefore, the most important virulence factor. [Note: Antibodies to the capsule carbohydrate are bactericidal.]

1. **Serogroups:** The polysaccharide capsule is antigenically diverse, which allows the identification of at least 13 capsular polysaccharide types, called serogroups (Figure 11.9). Most infections are caused by serogroups A, B, C, W-135, and Y, although approximately 90 percent of cases of meningococcal disease are caused by serogroups A, B, and C. Serogroup A is usually responsible for massive epidemics in developing countries. In the United States, *N. meningitidis* serogroup B is the predominant cause of disease and mortality, followed by group C. Organisms that do not have a capsule are called unencapsulated.

EPIDEMIOLOGIC CLASSIFICATION	ANTIGENIC DETERMINANT
Serogroups (>13)	Polysaccharide capsule
Serotypes (>20)	Outer membrane proteins

Figure 11.9
Antigenic determinants of *Neisseria meningitidis*.

2. **Serotypes:** A second classification system called serotyping (serotypes 1, 2,...20) is also a serologic classification (see Figure 11.9) that is based on the properties of the outer membrane proteins (see p. 102). The meningococcus expresses PorA- and PorB-type porins. There is no predicable relationship between serogroups and serotypes.

B. Epidemiology

Transmission occurs through inhalation of respiratory droplets from a carrier or a patient in the early stages of the disease. In addition to contact with a carrier, risk factors for disease include recent viral or mycoplasma upper respiratory tract infection, active or passive smoking, and complement deficiency. In susceptible persons, pathogenic strains may invade the bloodstream and cause systemic

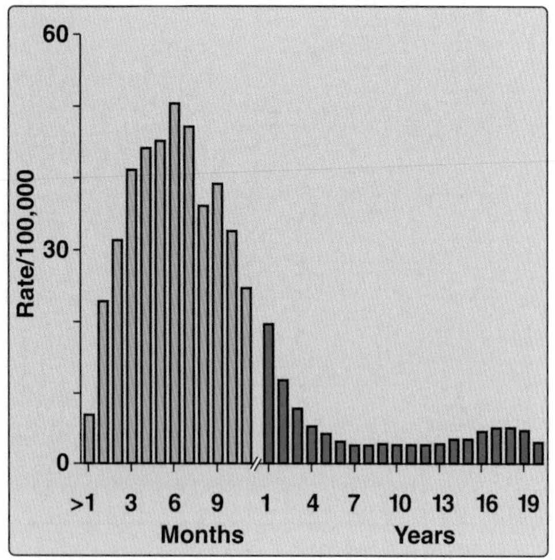

Figure 11.10
Incidence of meningococcal infection according to age.

illness after an incubation period of 2 to 10 days. The incidence of meningococcal disease in the United States is highest among infants younger than age 1 year (Figure 11.10). An incidence peak among adolescents and young adults led the Centers for Disease Control to recently recommend vaccination of this at-risk group. Humans are the only natural host.

C. Pathogenesis

Antiphagocytic properties of the meningococcal capsule aid in the maintenance of infection. LOS, released during autolysis and in outer membrane vesicles, is responsible for the toxic effects found in disseminated meningococcal disease. As noted on p. 102, gonococci and meningococci make an IgA protease that cleaves IgA_1 and, thus, helps the pathogens to evade immunoglobulins of this subclass. [Note: Nonpathogenic *Neisseriae* do not make this protease.]

D. Clinical significance

N. meningitidis initially colonizes the nasopharynx, resulting in a largely asymptomatic meningococcal pharyngitis. In young children and other susceptible individuals, the organism can cause disseminated disease by spreading through the blood, leading to meningitis and/or fulminating septicemia. *N. meningitidis* is currently a leading cause of meningitis.

1. **Meningitis:** The epithelial lining of the nasopharynx normally serves as a barrier to bacteria. Therefore, most persons colonized by *N. meningitidis* remain well. As a rare event, meningococci penetrate this barrier and enter the bloodstream where they rapidly multiply (meningococcemia). In patients with fulminant septicemia, meningococci can be detected in peripheral blood smears—an unusual occurrence. If the disease is not severe, the patient may have only a fever and other nonspecific symptoms. However, the organism can seed from the blood to other sites, for example, by crossing the blood-brain barrier and infecting the meninges. There they multiply and induce an acute inflammatory response, accompanied by an influx of polymorphonuclear leukocytes, resulting in a purulent meningitis. Joint symptoms and a petechial and/or purpuric rash are also commonly observed in meningococcal infections (Figure 11.11). Within several hours the initial fever and malaise can evolve into severe headache, a rigid neck, vomiting, and sensitivity to bright lights—symptoms characteristic of meningitis. Coma can occur within a few hours. A summary of the major organisms causing meningitis is shown in Figure 33.5, p. 376. The gold standard for diagnosis of systemic meningococcal infection is the isolation of *N. meningitidis* from a usually sterile body fluid, such as blood or cerebrospinal fluid (CSF). In performing a Gram stain on CSF, the clinical sample is centrifuged to concentrate the organisms, because 10^5 to 10^6 bacteria per ml are required for this test.

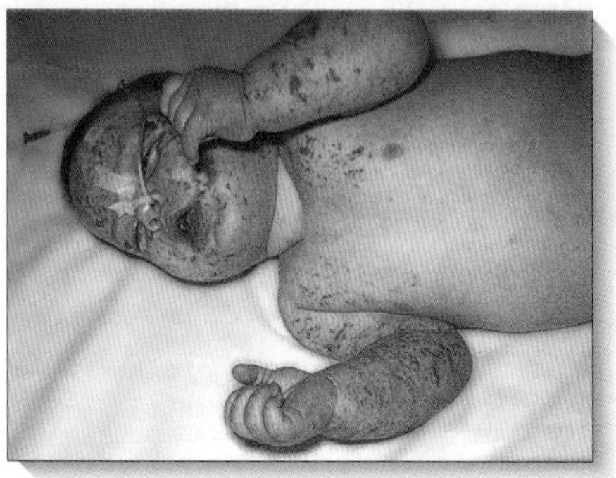

Figure 11.11
Petechial and/or purpuric rash and neck extension characteristic of meningococcal meningitis.

2. **Septicemia:** Meningococci can cause a life-threatening septicemia in an apparently healthy individual in less than 12 hours. Up to 30 percent of patients with meningitis progress to fulminant sep-

ticemia. In this condition, the clinical presentation is one of severe septicemia and shock, for which the bacterial endotoxin (LOS) is largely responsible. Acute, fulminant meningococcal septicemia is seen mainly in very young children (the Waterhouse-Friderichsen syndrome). It is characterized by large, purple, blotchy skin hemorrhages, vomiting and diarrhea, circulatory collapse, adrenal necrosis, and death within 10 to 12 hours.

E. Laboratory identification

Under the light microscope, *N. meningitidis* obtained from CSF and skin lesion aspirates appear as gram-negative diplococci, often in association with polymorphonuclear leukocytes (see Figure 11.8). Carriers can be detected by culturing swabs from the nasopharyngeal region.

1. **Culture conditions:** Meningococci are cultured on chocolate agar with increased CO_2. The sample must be plated promptly or, if this is not possible, transport medium must be used to extend the viability of the organism to be cultured. Unlike gonococci, meningococci are usually cultured from CSF or blood, which are normally sterile; therefore a selective medium is not required, and plain chocolate agar is sufficient. [Note: Thayer-Martin medium (see p. 104) is required for samples obtained from a skin lesion or nasopharyngeal swab, to eliminate contaminating organisms.]

2. **Additional tests:** All *Neisseria* species are oxidase-positive. To differentiate between species, sugar utilization tests are used (Figure 11.12). *N. meningitidis* utilizes both glucose and maltose, whereas *N. gonorrhoeae* uses only glucose (see Figure 11.12). In bacterial meningitis, the CSF shows increased pressure, elevated protein, decreased glucose (partly resulting from its consumption as a bacterial nutrient), and many neutrophils. The presence of an infecting organism or of antigenic capsular substance confirms the diagnosis. Figure 11.13 compares the characteristics of *N. gonorrhoeae* and *N. meningitidis.*

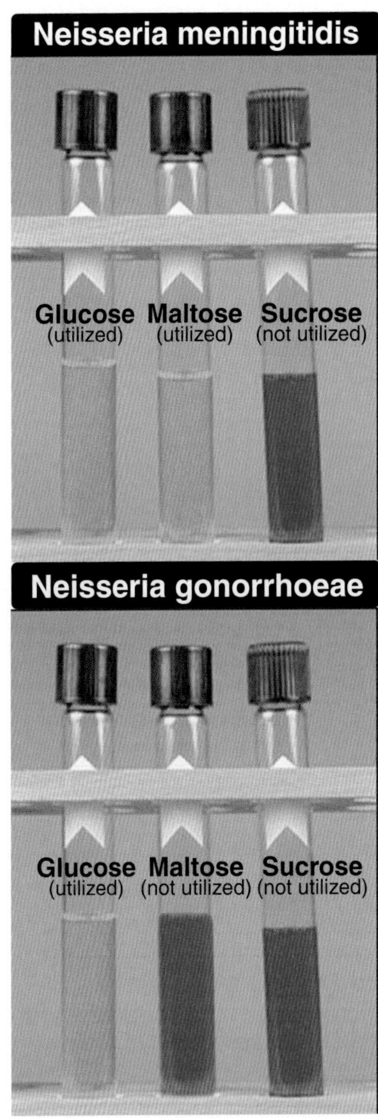

Figure 11.12
Neisseria meningitidis produces acid from oxidation of glucose and maltose, but not from sucrose. The acid turns the pH indicator phenol red from red to yellow.

F. Treatment and prevention

Bacterial meningitis is a medical emergency. Accordingly, antibiotic treatment cannot await a definitive bacteriologic diagnosis. High fever, headache, and a rash typical of meningococcal infection are treated immediately in an effort to prevent progression to fulminant septicemia which has a high mortality rate. Blood cultures should be drawn and antibiotic therapy should not be delayed while waiting for

	GLUCOSE UTILIZATION	MALTOSE UTILIZATION	PLASMIDS	VACCINE AVAILABLE	POLY-SACCHARIDE CAPSULE	β-LACTAMASE PRODUCTION	OXIDASE
Neisseria gonorrhoeae	+	–	Common	–	–	Common	+
Neisseria meningitidis	+	+	Rare	Serogroups A, C, W-135, Y	+	None	+

Figure 11.13
Differential bacteriologic features of *Neisseria gonorrhoeae* and *Neisseria meningitidis.*

lumbar puncture to be performed. Pretreatment with antibiotics can substantially diminish the probability of a positive CSF culture but the diagnosis can often still be established from the pretreatment blood cultures; and organisms may continue to be visible on Gram stain of the CSF. Meningitis can be effectively treated with penicillin G or ampicillin (both of which can pass the inflamed blood-brain barrier) in large intravenous doses. When the etiology of the infection is unclear, cefotaxime or ceftriaxone is recommended. Prompt treatment reduces mortality to about 10 percent. Because of the intense inflammatory reaction that accompanies bacterial meningitis, many authorities recommend a dose of the corticosteroid dexamethasone shortly prior to, or together with, the first dose of antibiotic.

1. **Diagnosis:** Gram stains on CSF can be performed immediately, and latex agglutination tests with serogroup-specific anticapsular antibody can be used to obtain rapid presumptive identification of serogroup-specific meningococci in CSF.

SEROGROUP CLASSIFICATION	COMMENT
A	Usually responsible for massive epidemics in developing countries.
B	Does not elicit an effective immune response.
B, C	Responsible for most endemic meningitis in the United States.
A, C, W-135,Y	Effective capsular vaccine is available.

Figure 11.14
Characteristics of the common serogroups of *Neisseria meningitidis*.

2. **Vaccines:** A conjugate meningococcal vaccine (MCV4) was approved in the United States in 2005 for use in adolescents and adults ages 11 to 55 years, and has replaced the unconjugated polysaccharide vaccine. MCV4 is a tetravalent vaccine that contains capsular polysaccharides from serogroups A, C, W-135, and Y conjugated to diphtheria toxoid. The conjugated vaccines elicit a T cell-dependent memory response that increases the effectiveness of the vaccine, resulting in an improved primary response to the vaccine and a strong response on subsequent exposure to the pathogen. The serogroup B polysaccharide capsule is a self-antigen and therefore does not elicit an effective immune response. Figure 11.14 summarizes vaccines and serogroups.

3. **Prophylaxis:** Prophylactic rifampin is given to family members because of the inevitability of their close contact and thus exposure. Other drugs used for prophylaxis include oral ciprofloxacin and intramuscular ceftriaxone. Figure 11.15 summarizes the diseases caused by *Neisseria* species.

IV. MORAXELLA

Members of the genus *Moraxella* are nonmotile, gram-negative coccobacilli that are generally found in pairs. *Moraxella* are aerobic, oxidase-positive, fastidious organisms that do not ferment carbohydrates. The most important pathogen in the genus is *Moraxella* (formerly, *Branhamella*) *catarrhalis*. This organism can cause infections of the respiratory system, middle ear, eye, CNS, and joints.

V. ACINETOBACTER

Members of the genus *Acinetobacter* are nonmotile coccobacilli that are frequently confused with *Neisseriae* in gram-stained samples. Generally encapsulated, oxidase-negative, and obligately aerobic, they do not ferment carbohydrates. *Acinetobacter baumanii* is an important nosocomial (hospital-acquired) pathogen.

Gram (–) cocci

Neisseria species

Neisseria gonorrhoea in clumps within polymorphonuclear leukocytes in urethral exudate.

Neisseria meningitidis in cerebrospinal fluid of patient with meningitis.

- "Kidney bean"–shaped diplococci
- Pili important in attachment to mucosa
- Oxidase positive
- Aerobic
- Nonmotile
- Pyogenic

Neisseria gonorrhoeae

Neisseria gonorrhoeae infection of human epithelial cells. A bacteria microcolony is seen attaching to the host cell via surface appendages called Type IV pili (cobwed-like structures), which induce the formation of host cell microvilli. (Photos courtesy of Dustin L. Higashi, Al Agellon, and Magdalene So).

- Maltose not utilized for energy
- Grown on Thayer-Martin medium
- No polysaccharide capsule

- Ophthalmia neonatorum
  - 1 Ceftriaxone[1]
  - 1 Erythromycin[2]
  - 1 Silver nitrate[2]

[1]Systemic [2]Topical for routine prophylaxis in circumstances of relatively low risk

- Uncomplicated gonorrhea
  - 1 Ceftriaxone[1]
  - 1 Doxycycline[2]

[1]A single 1-gram dose of azithromycin is used in persons with cephalosporin allergy.

[2]A tetracycline is added when *Chlamydia* is a suspected co-pathogen.

Neisseria meningitidis

- Meningitis
- Meningococcemia
- Waterhouse-Friderichsen syndrome
  - 1 Penicillin G[1]
  - 2 Cefotaxime
  - 2 Ceftriaxone

[1]Resistant strains have emerged, and sensitivity testing should be performed.

Note: Rifampin can be used prophylactically to treat family members or other close contacts of an infected individual

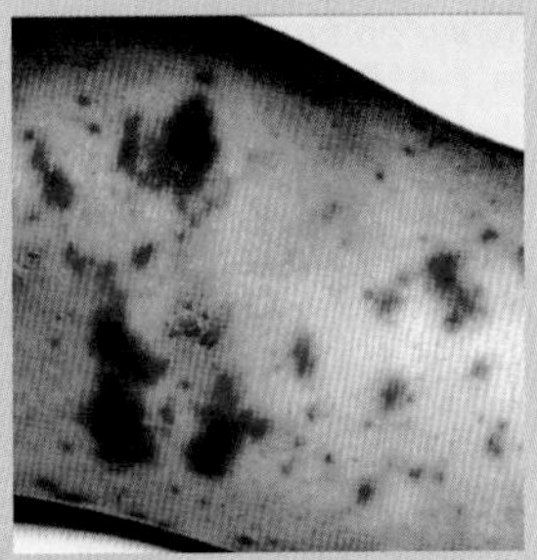

Purpuric rash characteristic of meningococcemia.

- Maltose utilized for energy
- Grown on chocolate agar
- Most common cause of meningitidis in persons between ages 2 and 18 years.
- Polysaccharide capsule
- Vaccine for serogroups Y, W-135, C, and A

Figure 11.15

Summary of *Neisseria* diseases. 1 Indicates first-line drugs; 2 indicates alternative drugs.

Study Questions

Choose the ONE best answer

11.1 A 20-year-old, sexually-active female presents at her family physician's office with fever, painful arthritis of the right knee, and several small pustules on her extremities. Material from the pustules and joint fluid were collected for culture on modified Thayer-Martin medium. Which of the following results are consistent with a diagnosis of gonococcal infection?

A. Growth of small colonies consisting of gram-negative diplococci. Bacteria grown on plates are catalase and oxidase positive.
B. Growth of small colonies consisting of gram-positive cocci. Bacteria growth on plates are catalase and oxidase positive.
C. Growth of small colonies consisting of gram-negative diplococci. Bacteria growth on plates are catalase and oxidase negative.
D. Growth of large mucoid colonies consisting of gram-negative bacilli. Bacteria growth on plates are catalase and oxidase negative.
E. Growth of gram-negative diplococci within polymorphonuclear leukocytes. Bacteria can utilize glucose and maltose as a carbon sources.

Correct answer = A. Gonococcal infection is the most common cause of septic arthritis in sexually active adults. *Neisseria gonorrhoeae* can be cultured from the joint fluid and pustular material, following dissemination from the genital tract to the skin and joints. Gonococci grow on modified Thayer-Martin medium to form small colonies that are oxidase positive and catalase positive. *N. gonorrhoeae* following Gram stain appears as a gram-negative diplococcus. Although *N. gonorrhoeae* is often found within polymorphonuclear leukocytes when clinical specimens are stained directly, these human cells would not be present after culturing on Modified Thayer-Martin medium.

11.2 Which of the following neisserial virulence factors is subject to high-frequency antigenic variation by a mechanism involving recombination between silent and expressed chromosomal loci?

A. Lipooligosaccharide
B. Capsule
C. Porin
D. Pilin
E. Opacity proteins

Correct answer = D. Althoough the synthesis of lipooligosaccharide (LOS) is phase variable, the mechanism does not involve recombination between silent and expressed genes. LOS varies by a mechanism known as slipped-strand mispairing, which results in changes in the number of single nucleotide repeats within the LOS biosynthetic genes. If the biosynthetic gene has the appropriate number of repeats, the gene is in frame, which results in enzymatic modification of the LOS structure. Capsule and porin are not subject to high frequency variation. Opacity proteins (Opa) vary by a mechanism similar to that described for LOS. Slipped-strand mispairing results in changes in the number of CTCTT repeats within the *opa* structural gene. Some Opa proteins are synthesized because the number of repeats results in the proteins being in frame. Other Opa proteins are not expressed because the number of repeats within the gene results in the protein being out of frame.

11.3 Which of the following neisserial virulence factors is part of the tetravalent vaccine that protects against some but not all serogroups of *Neisseria meningitidis*?

A. Lipooligosaccharide
B. Capsule
C. Porin
D. Pilin
E. Opacity proteins

Correct answer = B. *N. meningitidis* has a polysaccharide capsule that is an important surface-exposed virulence factor. The chemical composition of the capsule defines the serogroup of the meningococcal strain. There are 13 known serogroups. The meningococcal vaccine contains 4 of the 13 different capsule types, making it a tetravalent vaccine. Note that serogroup B capsule is a self-antigen and is therefore not part of the vaccine. Serogroup B *N. meningitidis* is endemic in industrialized countries but the vaccine is not protective against this serogroup.

Gastrointestinal Gram-negative Rods

12

I. OVERVIEW

All of the organisms covered in this chapter are routinely found in the gastrointestinal (GI) tract of humans or other animals. Many also have alternative habitats in soil or water. All are relatively hardy but are sensitive to drying, and all grow in the presence or absence of oxygen, being facultative anaerobes. They contain lipopolysaccharide (LPS), which is both antigenic and an important virulence factor (endotoxin). These gram-negative rods belong to diverse taxonomic groups. These facultative organisms constitute only a fraction of the total microbial flora of the GI tract as most bowel organisms are either gram-positive or gram-negative anaerobes. Different enteric gram-negative rods cause diseases within the GI tract, outside the GI tract, or in both locations. For example, diseases caused by members of the genera *Escherichia*, *Salmonella*, *Yersinia*, and *Campylobacter* can be both GI and extraintestinal; those caused by members of the genera *Shigella*, *Helicobacter*, and *Vibrio* are primarily GI; and those caused by members of the genera *Enterobacter*, *Klebsiella*, *Serratia*, and *Proteus* are primarily extraintestinal. Fecal contamination is commonly important in the transmission of those organisms that cause GI diseases. Gram-negative rods discussed in this chapter are listed in Figure 12.1.

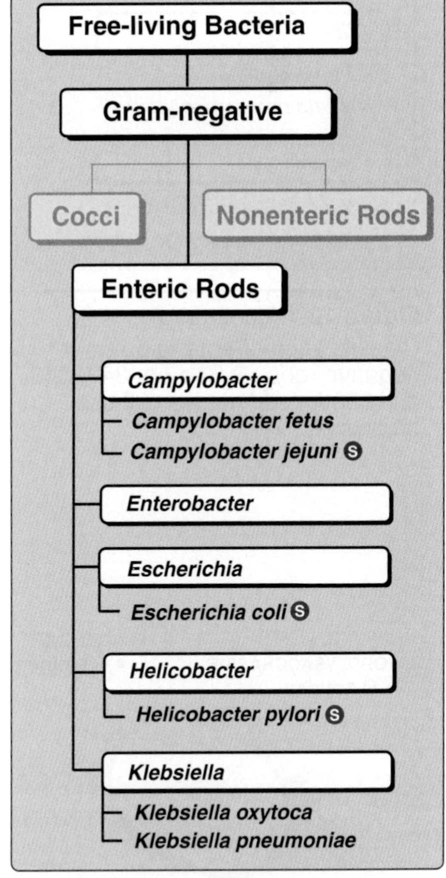

Figure 12.1
Classification of enteric gram-negative rods (figure continues on the next page). Ⓢ See pp. 335, 339, and 341 for summaries of these organisms.

II. ESCHERICHIA COLI

Escherichia coli is part of the normal flora of the colon in humans and other animals but can be pathogenic both within and outside of the GI tract. [Note: The differences in the degree of virulence of various *E. coli* strains is correlated with the acquisition of plasmids, integrated prophages, and pathogenicity islands.] *E. coli* has fimbriae or pili that are important for adherence to host mucosal surfaces, and different strains of the organism may be motile or nonmotile. Most strains can ferment lactose (that is, they are Lac^+) in contrast to the major intestinal pathogens, *Salmonella* (see p. 115) and *Shigella* (see p. 119), which cannot ferment lactose (that is, they are Lac^-). *E. coli* produces both acid and gas during fermentation of carbohydrates.

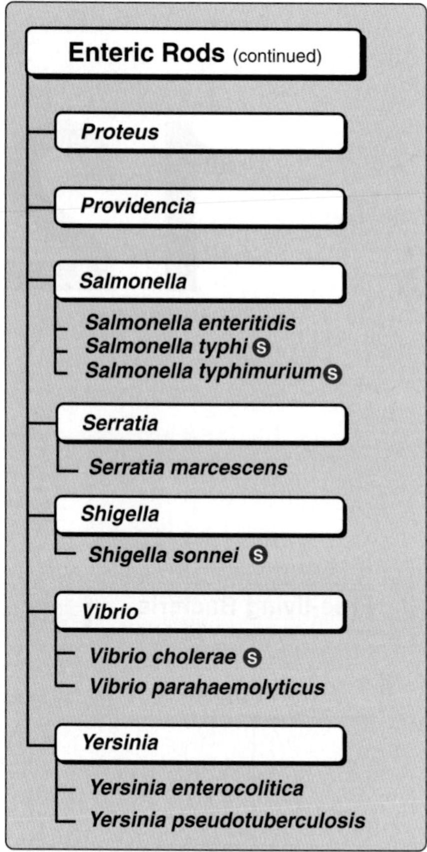

Figure 12.1 (continued)
Classification of enteric gram-negative rods. Ⓢ See pp. 347, 348, and 353 for summaries of these organisms.

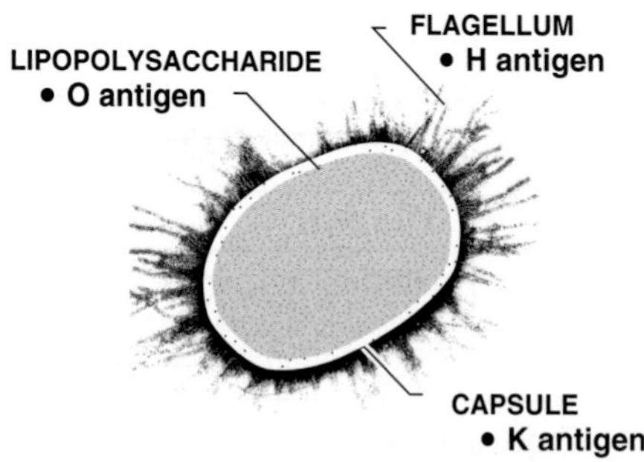

Figure 12.2
Electron micrograph of *Escherichia coli* showing virulence factors.

A. Structure and physiology

E. coli shares many properties with the other Enterobacteriaceae. They are all facultative anaerobes (see p. 22), they all ferment glucose, and they all can generate energy by aerobic or anaerobic respiration (using nitrate, nitrite, or fumarate as terminal electron acceptors). They all lack cytochrome c oxidase (that is, they are oxidase negative). Typing strains is based on differences in three structural antigens: O, H, and K (Figure 12.2). The O antigens (somatic or cell wall antigens) are found on the polysaccharide portion of the LPS. These antigens are heat stable and may be shared among different Enterobacteriaceae genera. O antigens are commonly used to serologically type many of the enteric gram-negative rods. The H antigens are associated with flagella, and, therefore, only flagellated (motile) Enterobacteriaceae such as *E. coli* have H antigen. The K antigens are located within the polysaccharide capsules. Among *E. coli* species, there are many serologically distinct O, H, and K antigens, and specific serotypes are associated with particular diseases. For example, a serotype of *E. coli* possessing O157 and H7 (designated O157:H7) causes a severe form of hemorrhagic colitis (see p. 113).

B. Clinical significance: intestinal disease

Transmission of intestinal disease is commonly by the fecal–oral route, with contaminated food and water serving as vehicles for transmission. At least five types of intestinal infections that differ in pathogenic mechanisms have been identified (Figure 12.3): enterotoxigenic (ETEC), enteropathogenic (EPEC), enterohemorrhagic (EHEC), enteroinvasive (EIEC), and enteroaggregative (EAEC). *E. coli* all are basically the same organism, differing only by the acquisition of specific pathogenic traits. EHEC *E. coli* infection should be suspected in all patients with acute bloody diarrhea, particularly if associated with abdominal tenderness and absence of fever.

1. **Enterotoxigenic *E. coli*:** ETEC are a common cause of traveler's diarrhea. Transmission occurs through food and water contaminated with human waste or by person-to-person contact. ETEC colonize the small intestine (pili facilitate the binding of the organism to the intestinal mucosa). In a process mediated by enterotoxins (see p. 51), ETEC cause prolonged hypersecretion of chloride ions and water by the intestinal mucosal cells, while inhibiting the reabsorption of sodium. The gut becomes full of fluid, resulting in significant watery diarrhea that continues over a period of several days. Enterotoxins include a heat-stable toxin (ST) that works by causing an elevation in cellular cyclic guanosine monophosphate (cGMP) levels, whereas a heat-labile toxin (LT) causes elevated cyclic adenosine monophosphate (cAMP) (Figure 12.4). [Note: LT is essentially identical to cholera toxin (see p. 121).]

2. **Enteropathogenic *E. coli*:** EPEC are an important cause of diarrhea in infants, especially in locations with poor sanitation. The newborn becomes infected perinatally. The EPEC attach to mucosal cells in the small intestine by use of bundle-forming pili

STRAIN *Escherichia coli*	ABBREVIATION	SYNDROME	THERAPY[1]
Enterotoxigenic *E. coli*	ETEC	Watery diarrhea	Antibiotics may be useful.[2]
Enteropathogenic *E. coli*	EPEC	Watery diarrhea of long duration, mostly in infants, often in developing countries	Antibiotics may be useful.[2]
Enterohemorrhagic *E. coli*	EHEC	Bloody diarrhea; Hemorrhagic colitis and hemolytic uremic syndrome (HUS)	Avoid antibiotics because of the possible risk of potentiating HUS.
Enteroinvasive *E. coli*	EIEC	Bloody diarrhea	Rehydrate and correct electrolyte abnormalities.
Enteroaggregative *E. coli*	EAEC	Persistent watery diarrhea in children and patients infected with HIV	Rehydrate and correct electrolyte abnormalities.

Figure 12.3
Characteristics of intestinal infections caused by *Eschericia coli.* Fluoroquinolones are commonly used in adults for traveler's diarrhea but are not recommended for children. [1]Rehydration and correction of electrolyte abnormalities are essential for all diarrheal illnesses. [2]Rifaximin is approved for the treatment of diarrhea caused by noninvasive strains of *E. coli* in patients age12 years and older. Rifaximin is a nonabsorable, gastrointestinal-selective, oral antibiotic.

(BfpA). Characteristic lesions in the small intestine called attaching and effacing lesions (A/E), in addition to destruction of the microvilli, are caused by injection of effector proteins into the host cell by way of a type III secretion system (T3SS). EPEC cells are presented at the apex of pedestals elicited by dramatic cytoskeletal rearrangements, induced by the T3SS effectors. EPEC are not invasive and, thus, do not cause bloody diarrhea. Toxins are not elaborated by EPEC strains. Watery diarrhea results, which, on rare occasions, may become chronic.

3. **Enterohemorrhagic E. coli:** EHEC bind to cells in the large intestine via BfpA and, similar to EPEC, produce A/E lesions. However, in addition, EHEC produce one of two exotoxins (Shiga-like toxins 1 or 2), resulting in a severe form of copious, bloody diarrhea (hemorrhagic colitis) in the absence of mucosal invasion or inflammation. Serotype O157:H7 is the most common strain of *E. coli* that produce Shiga-like toxins. This strain is also associated with outbreaks of a potentially life-threatening, acute renal failure (hemolytic uremic syndrome, or HUS) characterized by fever, acute renal failure, microangiopathic hemolytic anemia and thrombocytopenia in children younger than ages 5 to 10 years. The primary reservoir of EHEC is cattle. Therefore, the possibility of infection can be greatly decreased by thoroughly cooking ground beef and pasteurizing milk.

4. **Enteroinvasive E. coli:** EIEC cause a dysentery-like syndrome with fever and bloody stools. Plasmid-encoded virulence factors are nearly identical to those of *Shigella* species. These virulence factors allow the invasion of epithelial cells (Ipa) and intercellular spread by use of actin-based motility. In addition, EIEC strains produce a hemolysin (HlyA).

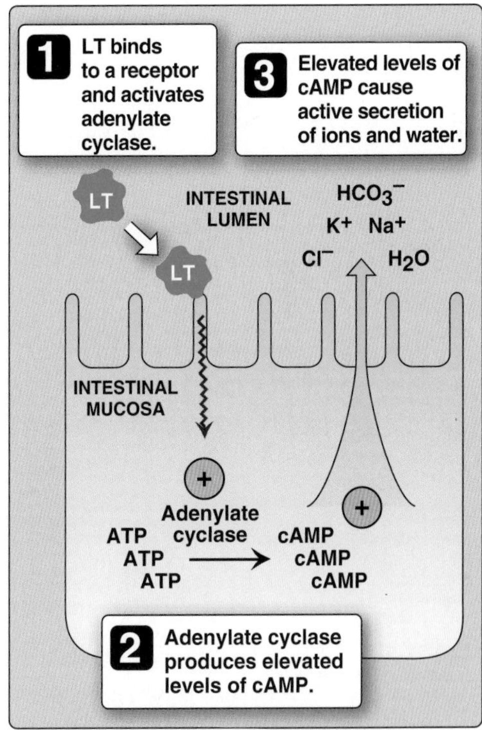

Figure 12.4
The action of *Escherichia coli* LT (heat-labile toxin). [Note: ST (heat-stable toxin) activates guanylate cyclase, causing production of cyclic guanosine monophosphate (cGMP) that also causes secretion.]

5. **Enteroaggregative E. coli:** EAEC also cause traveler's diarrhea and persistent diarrhea in young children. Adherence to the small intestine is mediated by aggregative adherence fimbriae. The adherent rods resemble stacked bricks and result in shortening of microvilli. EAEC strains produce a heat-stable toxin that is plasmid encoded. An outbreak of *E. coli* infections in Germany in 2011, resulting in many cases of HUS and several deaths, was caused by a hybrid strain. The causative agent was an EAEC strain that had acquired the phage-encoded gene to produce Shiga-like toxin 2. The resulting strain was capable of tight adherence to the small intestine in addition to toxin production, which resulted in HUS.

C. Clinical significance: extraintestinal disease

The source of infection for extraintestinal disease is frequently the patient's own flora, in which the individual's own *E. coli* is nonpathogenic in the intestine. However, it causes disease in that individual when the organism is found, for example, in the bladder or bloodstream (normally sterile sites).

1. **Urinary tract infection:** *E. coli* is the most common cause of urinary tract infection (UTI), including cystitis and pyelonephritis. Women are particularly at risk for infection. Uncomplicated cystitis (the most commonly encountered UTI) is caused by uropathogenic strains of *E. coli*, characterized by P fimbriae (an adherence factor) and, commonly, hemolysin, colicin V, and resistance to the bactericidal activity of serum complement. Complicated UTI (pyelonephritis) may occur in settings of obstructed urinary flow, which may be caused by nonuropathogenic strains.

2. **Neonatal meningitis:** *E. coli* is a major cause of this disease occurring within the first month of life. The K1 capsular antigen, which is chemically identical to the polysaccharide capsule of group B *Neisseria meningitidis*, is particularly associated with such infections.

3. **Nosocomial (hospital-acquired) infections:** These include sepsis/bacteremia, endotoxic shock, and pneumonia.

D. Laboratory identification

1. **Intestinal disease:** Because *E. coli* is normally part of the intestinal flora, detection in stool cultures of disease-causing strains is generally difficult. EIEC strains often do not ferment lactose and may be detected on media such as MacConkey agar (see p. 23). EHEC, unlike most other strains of *E. coli*, ferment sorbitol slowly, if at all, and may be detected on MacConkey sorbitol agar. Current molecular techniques, such as polymerase chain reaction, may be employed to identify *E. coli* strains producing Shiga-like toxins.

2. **Extraintestinal disease:** Isolation of *E. coli* from normally sterile body sites (for example, the bladder or cerebrospinal fluid) is diagnostically significant. Specimens may be cultured on MacConkey

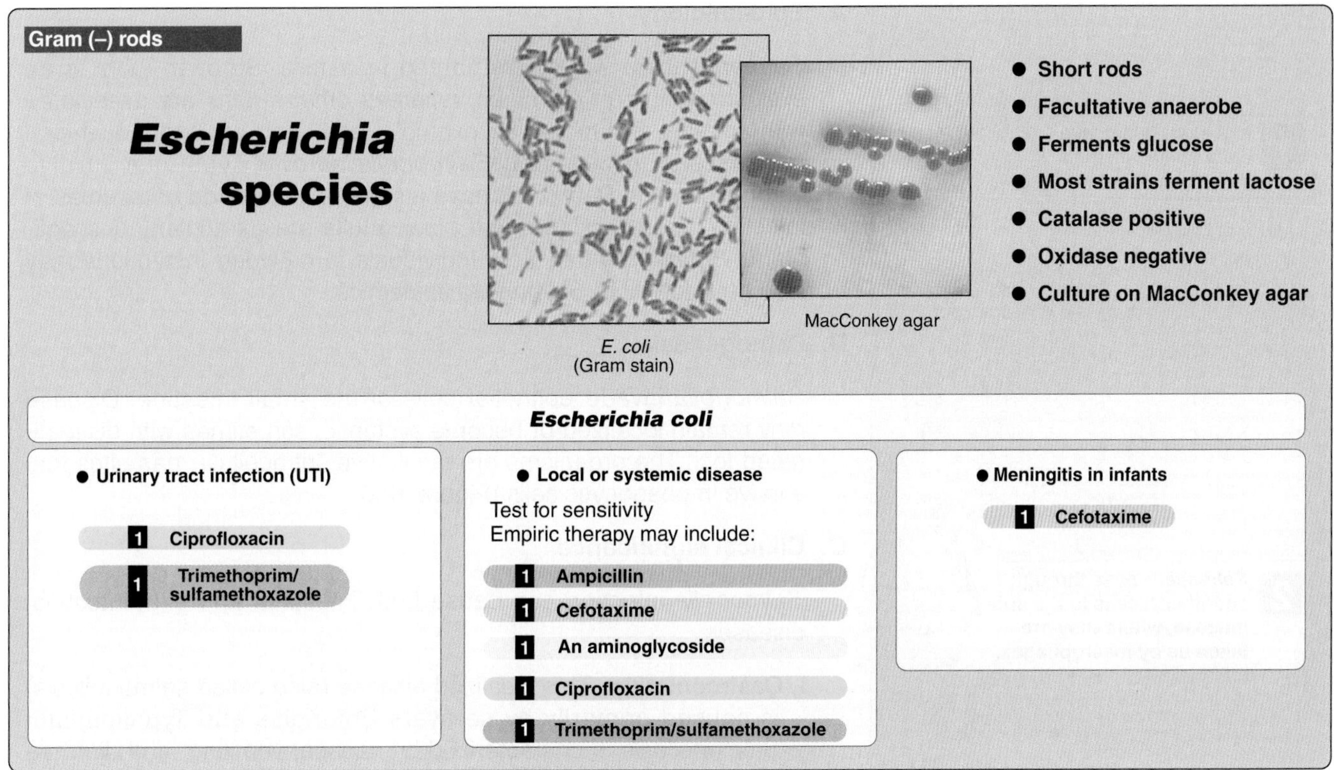

Figure 12.5
Summary of *Escherichia* species. 1 Indicates first-line drugs.

agar. Strains of *E. coli* can be further characterized on the basis of serologic tests.

E. Prevention and treatment

Intestinal disease can best be prevented by care in selection, preparation, and consumption of food and water. Maintenance of fluid and electrolyte balance is of primary importance in treatment. Antibiotics may shorten duration of symptoms, but resistance is nevertheless widespread. Extraintestinal diseases require antibiotic treatment (Figure 12.5). Antibiotic sensitivity testing of isolates is necessary to determine the appropriate choice of drugs.

III. SALMONELLA

Members of the genus *Salmonella* can cause a variety of diseases, including gastroenteritis and enteric (typhoid) fever. Although *Salmonella* classification has undergone numerous revisions, currently, all strains affecting humans are grouped in a single species, *Salmonella enteritidis*, which has approximately 2,500 different serotypes, or serovars, including the clinically significant serotypes Typhimurium and Typhi. Most strains of *Salmonella* are Lac$^-$ and produce acid and gas during fermentation of glucose. They also produce H_2S from sulfur-containing amino acids.

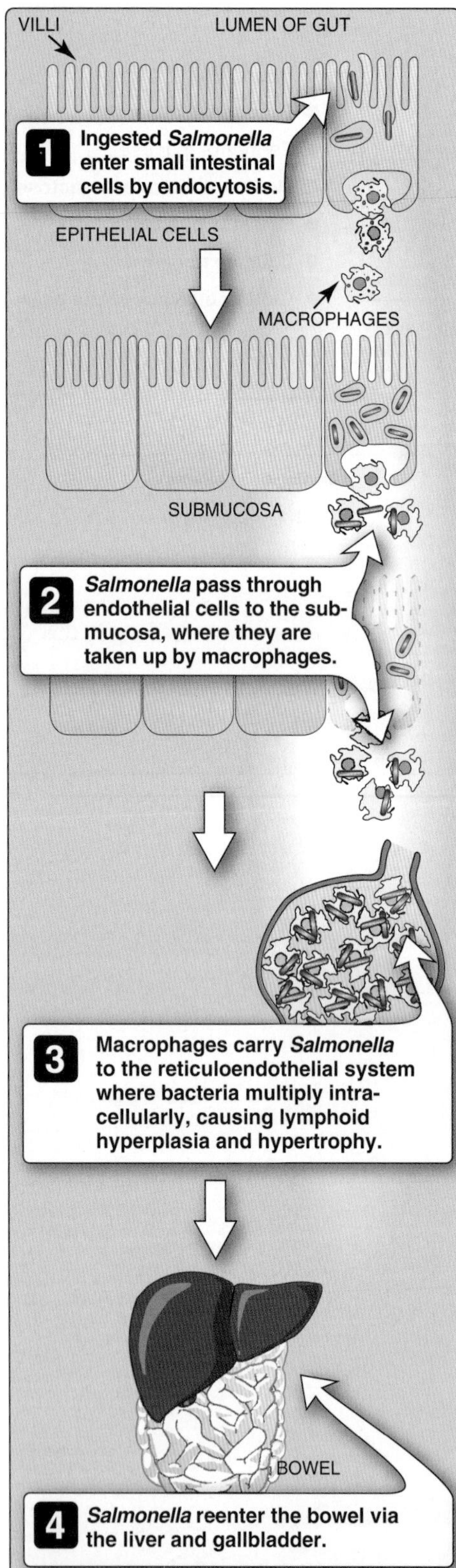

Figure 12.6
Mechanism of *Salmonella* infection causing enteric fever.

A. Epidemiology

Salmonella are widely distributed in nature. Serovar Typhi is an exclusively human pathogen, whereas other strains are associated with animals and foods (for example, eggs and poultry). Fecal–oral transmission occurs and *Salmonella* serovar Typhi may involve chronic carriers. Pet turtles have also been implicated as sources of infection. Young children and older adults are particularly susceptible to *Salmonella* infection. Individuals in crowded institutions may also be involved in *Salmonella* epidemics.

B. Pathogenesis

Salmonella invade epithelial cells of the small intestine. Disease may remain localized or become systemic, sometimes with disseminated foci. The organisms are facultative, intracellular parasites that survive in phagocytic cells (Figure 12.6).

C. Clinical significance

Salmonella infection can cause both intestinal and extraintestinal diseases.

1. **Gastroenteritis:** This localized disease (also called salmonellosis) is caused primarily by serovars Enteriditis and Typhimurium. Salmonellosis is characterized by nausea, vomiting, and diarrhea (usually nonbloody), which develop generally within 48 hours of ingesting contaminated food or water. Fever and abdominal cramping are common. In uncompromised patients, disease is generally self-limiting (48 to 72 hours), although convalescent carriage of organisms may persist for a month or more. More than 95 percent of cases of *Salmonella* infection are foodborne, and salmonellosis accounts for approximately 30 percent of deaths resulting from foodborne illnesses in the United States.

2. **Enteric or typhoid fever:** This is a severe, life-threatening systemic illness, characterized by fever and, frequently, abdominal symptoms. It is caused primarily by serovar Typhi. Nonspecific symptoms may include chills, sweats, headache, anorexia, weakness, sore throat, cough, myalgia, and either diarrhea or constipation. About 30 percent of patients have a faint and evanescent (transient) maculopapular rash on the trunk (rose spots). The incubation period varies from 5 to 21 days. Untreated, mortality is approximately 15 percent. Among survivors, the symptoms generally resolve in 3 to 4 weeks. Timely and appropriate antibiotic therapy reduces mortality to less than 1 percent and speeds resolution of fever. Complications can include intestinal hemorrhage and/or perforation and, rarely, focal infections and endocarditis. A small percentage of patients become chronic carriers. [Note: Infected gallbladders are the main source of chronic carriage.] Typhoid fever remains a global health problem. In the United States, however, typhoid fever has become less prevalent and is now primarily a disease of travelers and immigrants.

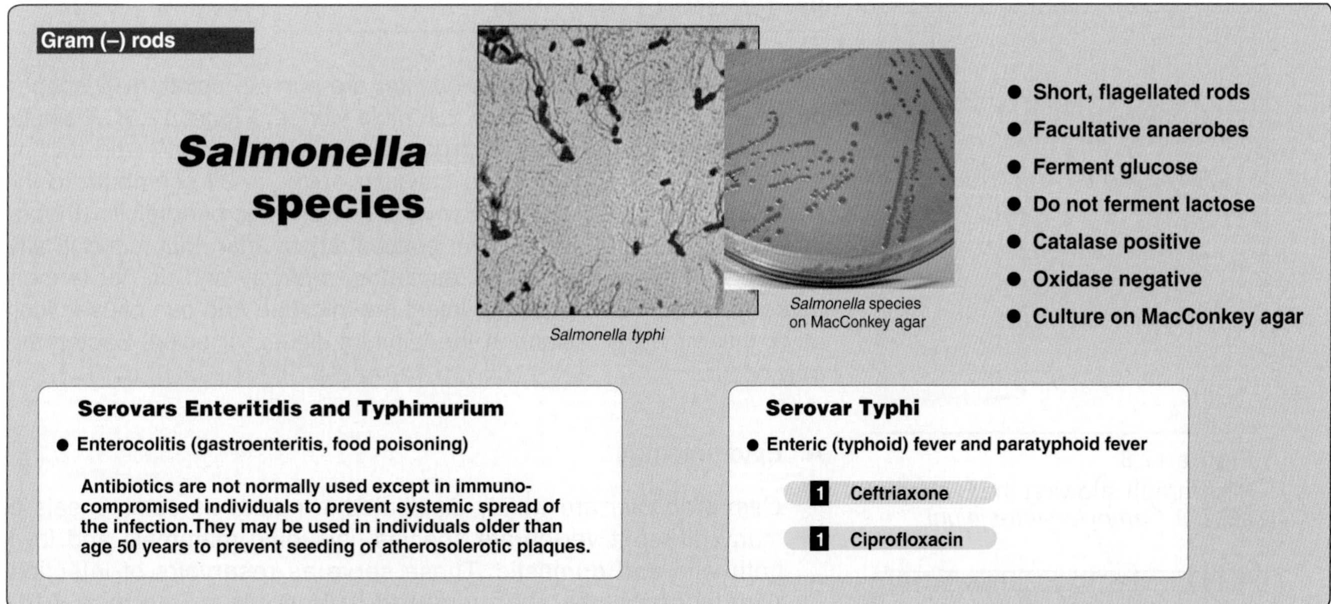

Figure 12.7
Summary of *Salmonella* disease. 1 Indicates first-line drugs.

3. **Other sites of Salmonella infection:** Sustained bacteremia is often associated with vascular *Salmonella* infections that occur when bacteria seed atherosclerotic plaques. *Salmonella* can also cause abdominal infections (often of the hepatobiliary tract and spleen); osteomyelitis; septic arthritis; and, rarely, infections of other tissues or organs. Chronic carriage of non-typhoidal serovars may develop, although this is rare.

D. Laboratory identification

In patients with diarrhea, *Salmonella* can typically be isolated from stools on MacConkey agar or selective media (Figure 12.7). For patients with enteric fever, appropriate specimens include blood, bone marrow, urine, stool, and tissue from typical rose spots (if they are present).

E. Treatment and prevention

For gastroenteritis in uncompromised hosts, antibiotic therapy is often not needed and may prolong the convalescent carrier state. For enteric fever, appropriate antibiotics include β-lactams and fluoroquinolones (see Figure 12.7). Prevention of *Salmonella* infection is accomplished by proper sewage disposal, correct handling of food, and good personal hygiene. Two different vaccines are available to prevent typhoid fever: One vaccine is delivered orally and consists of live attenuated *Salmonella* serovar Typhi. The other vaccine consists of the Vi capsular polysaccharide and is delivered parenterally. Vaccination is recommended for people who travel from developed countries to endemic areas including Asia, Africa, and Latin America.

IV. CAMPYLOBACTER

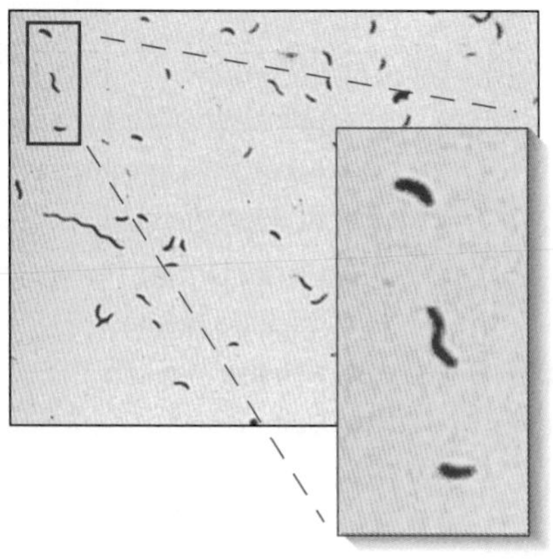

Figure 12.8
Micrograph showing the S-shaped cells of *Campylobacter jejuni.*

Members of the genus *Campylobacter* are curved, spiral, or S-shaped organisms that microscopically resemble vibrios (Figure 12.8). A single, polar flagellum provides the organism with its characteristic darting motility. Somatic, flagellar, and capsular antigens all contribute to the numerous serotypes. Most *Campylobacter* are microaerophilic (that is, they require oxygen but at lower concentrations than that found in air). Members of this genus use a respiratory pathway and do not ferment carbohydrates. *Campylobacter* infect the intestine and can cause ulcerative, inflammatory lesions in the jejunum, ileum, or colon. Bacteremia may occur.

A. Epidemiology

Campylobacter are widely distributed in nature as commensals of many different vertebrate species, including mammals and fowl, both wild and domestic. These serve as reservoirs of infection. *Campylobacter* are transmitted to humans primarily via the fecal–oral route through direct contact, exposure to contaminated meat (especially poultry), or contaminated water supplies.

B. Pathogenesis and clinical significance

Campylobacter may cause both intestinal and extraintestinal disease. The characteristics of some common forms of bacterial foodborne illness are shown in Figure 12.9. [Note: Food infection should be distinguished from food poisoning. Food infections (like *Campylobacter*) have longer incubation periods and require colonization by the bacterium. Food poisonings have shorter incubation periods and only require ingestion of the toxin.] *C. jejuni* typically causes an acute enteritis in otherwise healthy individuals following a 1- to 7-day incubation. The disease lasts days to several weeks and, generally, is self-limiting. Symptoms may be both systemic (fever, headache, myalgia) and intestinal (abdominal cramping and diarrhea, which may or may not be bloody). *Campylobacter jejuni* is a cause of both traveler's diarrhea and pseudoappendicitis (symptoms simulating appendicitis without inflammation of the appendix). Bacteremia (often transient) may occur, most often in infants and older adults. Sustained bacteremia usually reflects host compromise. Complications include septic abortion, reactive arthritis, and Guillain-Barré syndrome. Important virulence factors include a cytotoxin that may be involved in inflammatory colitis and an enterotoxin (related to cholera toxin) that results in increased adenylyl cyclase activity and, therefore, electrolyte and fluid imbalance. *Campylobacter* is currently one of the leading causes of foodborne disease in the United States.

Bacteria that may cause food poisoning due to preformed toxins

Bacillus cereus
Clostridium botulinum
Clostridium perfringens
Staphylococcus aureus

Because the toxins are ingested preformed and no microbial growth within the host is required, symptoms occur rapidly, usually within 2–12 hour

Bacteria that may cause foodborne illness after food is ingested

Campylobacter jejuni
Escherichia coli
***Salmonella* species**
Listeria monocytogenes
***Shigella* species**
Vibrio cholerae

Because microbial growth within the host is required, symptoms occur more slowly, usually after at least 24 hours.

Figure 12.9
Characteristics of common forms of bacterial foodborne illness.

C. Laboratory identification

Campylobacter can be isolated from feces using special selective media and microaerophilic conditions. Because of their small size, these organisms are not retained by bacteriologic filters that hold back most other bacteria. Thus, filtration of the fecal suspension may enhance recovery rate. Presumptive diagnosis can be made on

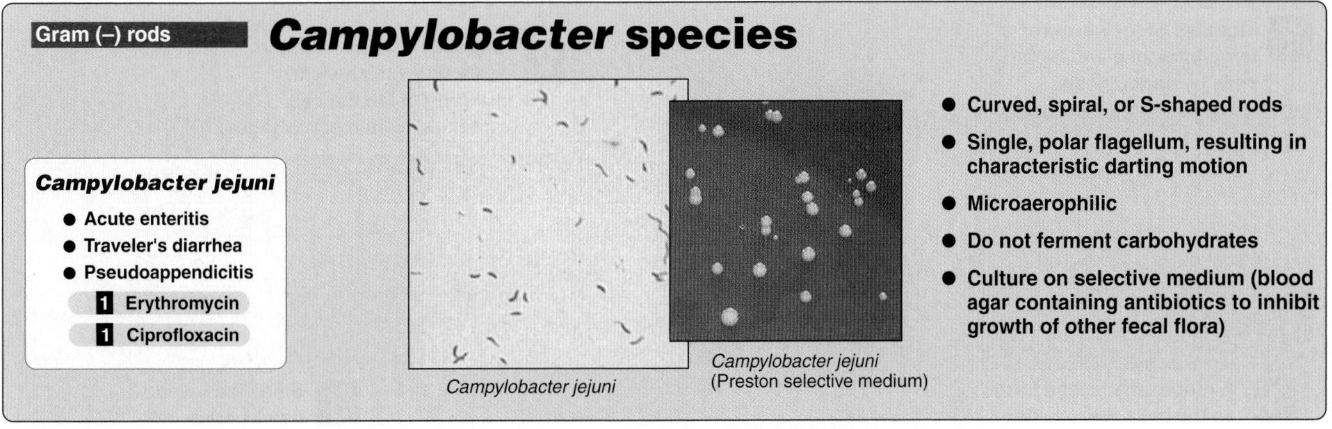

Figure 12.10
Summary of *Campylobacter* disease. 1 Indicates first-line drugs.

the basis of finding curved organisms with rapid, darting motility in a wet mount of feces.

D. Treatment and prevention

Diarrhea should be treated symptomatically with fluid and electrolyte replacement. For patients with more severe symptoms (for example, high fever, bloody diarrhea, worsening illness, or illness of more than 1 week's duration), antibiotics should be administered. For *C. jejuni*, ciprofloxacin is the drug of choice, but other antibiotics are also effective (Figure 12.10). For *Campylobacter fetus*, ampicillin or third-generation cephalosporins are effective. Thorough cooking of potentially contaminated foods (for example, poultry) and pasteurization of milk and milk products are essential to prevention of campylobacteriosis. Also, surfaces used to prepare raw meat or poultry should be disinfected before using them for uncooked food such as salads.

V. SHIGELLA

Shigella species cause shigellosis (bacillary dysentery), a human intestinal disease that occurs most commonly among young children. Shigellae are nonmotile, unencapsulated, and Lac$^-$. Most strains do not produce gas in a mixed-acid fermentation of glucose.

A. Epidemiology

Shigella are typically spread from person to person, with contaminated stools serving as a major source of organisms. Humans are the only natural host for *Shigella* species. Flies and contaminated food or water can also transmit the disease. Shigellosis has a low infectious dose: Approximately 10–100 viable organisms are sufficient to cause disease. Therefore, secondary cases within a household are common, particularly under conditions of crowding or poor sanitation. The 40 serotypes of *Shigella* are organized into four groups (A, B, C, and D) based on the serologic relatedness of their polysaccharide O antigens. Group D (*Shigella sonnei*) is the

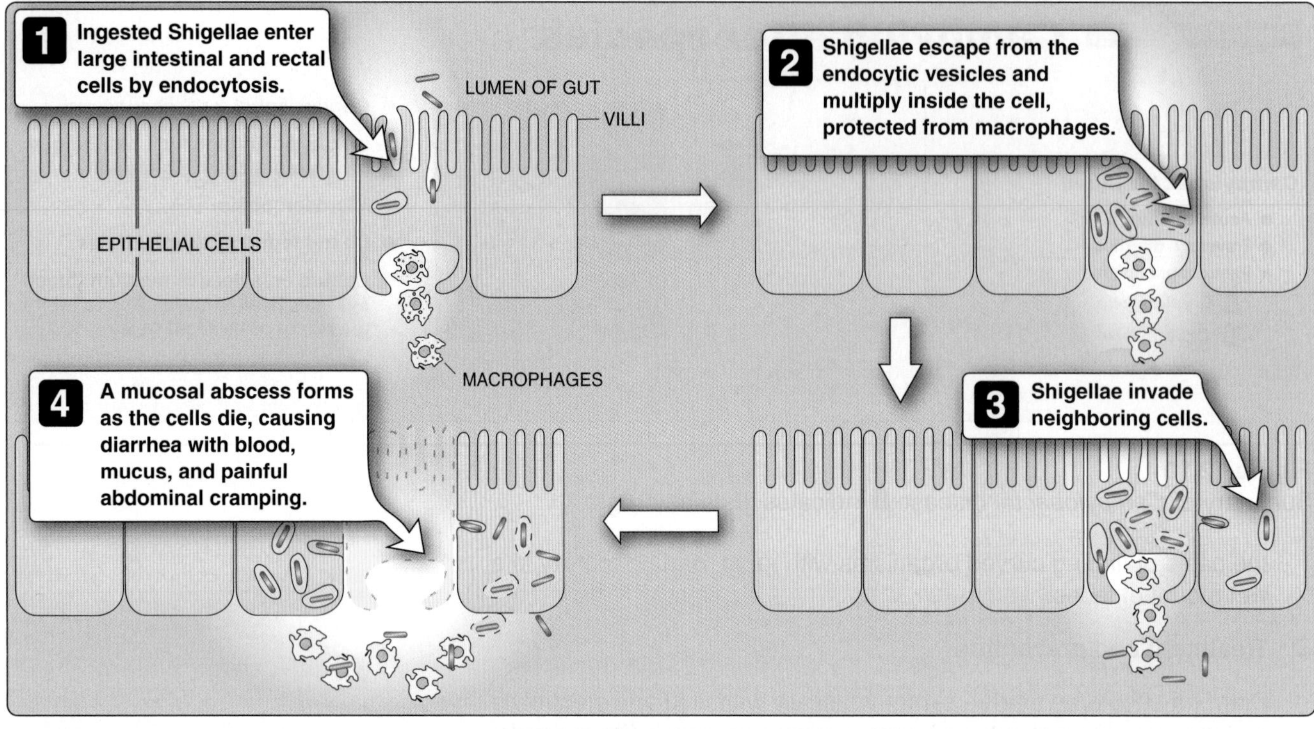

Figure 12.11
Mechanism of *Shigella* infection causing diarrhea.

serogroup found most commonly in the United States. *Shigella flexneri* is the second most common species isolated in the United States and has been associated with outbreaks among sexually active men who have sex with men. *Shigella dysenteriae* causes the most serious infections, including HUS similar to that caused by EHEC. *S. dysenteriae* type 1 produces Shiga toxin, which is structurally and genetically very similar to Shiga-like toxins 1 and 2 produced by *E. coli* virotypes. All Shiga and Shiga-like toxins are capable of resulting in HUS in susceptible individuals.

B. Pathogenesis and clinical significance

Shigellae invade and destroy the mucosa of the large intestine. Infection rarely penetrates to deeper layers of the intestine and does not lead to bacteremia (Figure 12.11). The Shigellae invade the colonic epithelium by expression of plasmid-encoded virulence genes that encode a type III secretion system. Injection of effector proteins results in bacterial engulfment. The same plasmid encodes proteins that allow the Shigellae to polymerize actin at one pole, thereby propelling the bacterium though the cytoplasm and into adjacent cells. This virulence plasmid is also possessed by EIEC. An exotoxin (Shiga toxin) with enterotoxic and cytotoxic properties has been isolated from *S. dysenteriae* type 1, and its toxicity results in the development of hemorrhagic colitis and HUS. Shigellae cause classic bacillary dysentery, characterized by diarrhea with blood, mucus ("currant jelly" stools), and painful abdominal cramping. The disease is generally most severe in the very young; older adults; and among malnourished individuals, in whom shigellosis may lead to

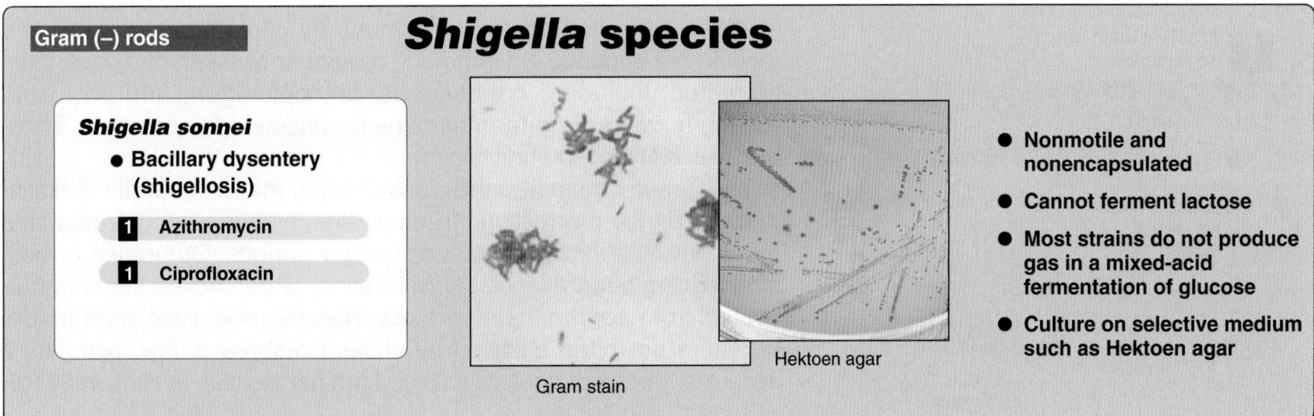

Gram (-) rods
Shigella species
Shigella sonnei
• Bacillary dysentery (shigellosis)
1 Azithromycin
1 Ciprofloxacin
Gram stain
Hektoen agar
• Nonmotile and nonencapsulated
• Cannot ferment lactose
• Most strains do not produce gas in a mixed-acid fermentation of glucose
• Culture on selective medium such as Hektoen agar

Figure 12.12
Summary of *Shigella* disease. **1** Indicates first-line drugs.

severe dehydration and, sometimes, death. Among uncompromised populations, untreated dysentery commonly resolves in a week but may persist longer.

C. Laboratory identification

During acute illness, organisms can be cultured from stools using differential, selective Hektoen agar or other media specific for intestinal pathogens.

D. Treatment and prevention

Antibiotics (for example, ciprofloxacin or azithromycin) can reduce the duration of illness and the period of shedding organisms but usage is controversial because of widespread antibiotic resistance (Figure 12.12). Protection of the water and food supply and personal hygiene are crucial for preventing *Shigella* infections. Candidate vaccines in advanced development stages include a conjugate vaccine composed of O-antigen polysaccharides from Shigellae and a live attenuated vaccine.

VI. VIBRIO

Members of the genus *Vibrio* are short, curved, rod-shaped organisms. Vibrios are closely related to the family Enterobacteriaceae. They are rapidly motile by means of a single polar flagellum. [Note: This contrasts with the peritrichous flagella (distributed all over the surface) of the motile Enterobacteriaceae.] O and H antigens are both present, but only O antigens are useful in distinguishing strains of vibrios that cause epidemics. Vibrios are facultative anaerobes. The growth of many *Vibrio* strains either requires or is stimulated by NaCl. Pathogenic vibrios include: 1) *Vibrio cholerae*, serogroup O1 strains that are associated with epidemic cholera; 2) non-O1 *V. cholerae* and related strains that cause sporadic cases of choleralike and other illnesses; and 3) *Vibrio parahaemolyticus* and other halophilic vibrios, which cause gastroenteritis and extraintestinal infections.

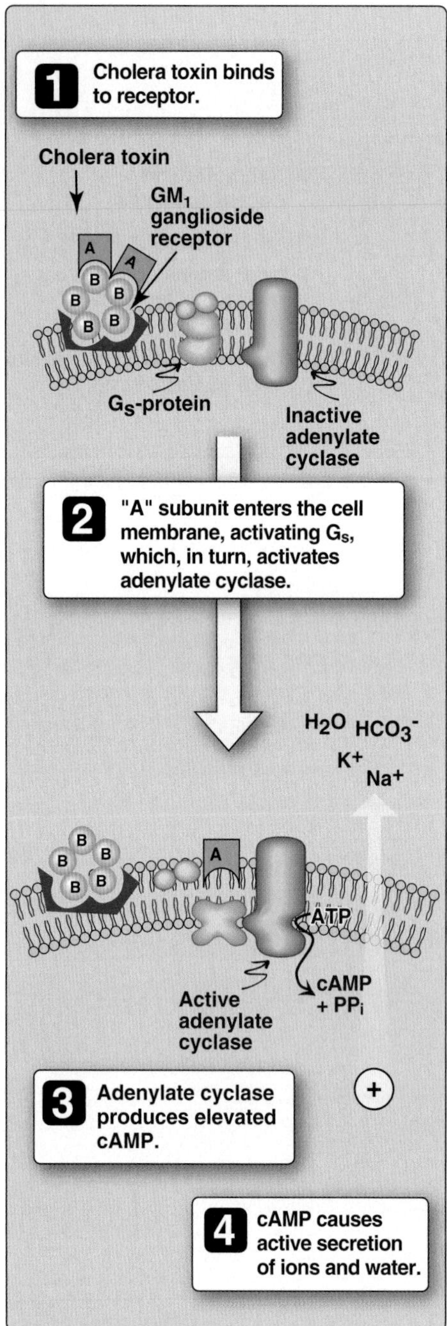

Figure 12.13
Action of cholera toxin. cAMP = cyclic adenosine monophosphate, PP_i = pyrophosphate.

A. Epidemiology

V. cholerae is transmitted to humans by contaminated water and food. In the acquatic environment, a number of reservoirs have been identified, including crustaceans, phytoplankton, and protozoa. Among humans, long-term carriage is considered uncommon. There are two biotypes (subdivisions) of the species *V. cholerae*: classic and El Tor. In contrast to the classic strain, the El Tor strain is distinguished by the production of hemolysins, higher carriage rates, and the ability to survive in water for longer periods. Outbreaks of both strains have been associated with raw or undercooked seafood harvested from contaminated waters. Natural (and even man-made) disasters are often followed by cholera outbreaks. For example, a severe outbreak of cholera followed the earthquake in Haiti in 2010.

B. Pathogenesis

Following ingestion, *V. cholerae* infects the small intestine. Adhesion factor(s) are important for colonization and virulence. Achlorhydria and/or treatments that lessen gastric acidity, greatly reduce the infectious dose. The organism is noninvasive but adheres to the epithelium by expression of pili called Tcp, or toxin-coregulated pili. These pili are coordinately expressed along with cholera toxin, which is an enterotoxin that initiates an outpouring of fluid (Figure 12.13). Cholera toxin is a multimeric protein composed of an A and a B subunit. The B subunit (consisting of five identical monomers) binds to the GM_1 ganglioside receptor of cells lining the intestine. The A subunit has two components: The A2 subunit tethers the A1 subunit to the B pentamer, and the A1 subunit is an adenosine diphosphate (ADP)-ribosyl transferase that ADP-ribosylates the membrane-bound G_s protein.[1] Modified G_s protein activates adenylyl cyclase, which produces elevated levels of intracellular cAMP. This, in turn, causes an outflowing of ions and water to the lumen of the intestine.

C. Clinical significance

Full-blown cholera is characterized by massive loss of fluid and electrolytes from the body. After an incubation period ranging from hours to a few days, profuse watery diarrhea ("rice-water" stools) begins. Untreated, death from severe dehydration causing hypovolemic shock may occur in hours to days, and the death rate may exceed 50 percent. Appropriate treatment reduces the death rate to less than 1 percent. [Note: Non-O1 *V. cholerae* and other nonhalophilic vibrios cause sporadic cases of cholera indistinguishable from that caused by *V. cholerae*, serotype O1. They also cause milder illness, comparable to that caused by enterotoxigenic *E. coli*.] Patients with suspected cholera need to be treated prior to laboratory confirmation, because death by dehydration can occur within hours.

D. Laboratory identification

V. cholerae grows on standard media such as blood and MacConkey agars. Thiosulfate-citrate-bile salts–sucrose medium can enhance isolation. The organism is oxidase positive, but further bio-

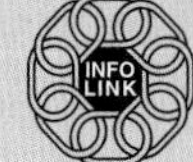

[1]See Chapter 8 in ***Lippincott's Illustrated Reviews: Biochemistry*** for a discussion of the mechanism of action of G_s proteins.

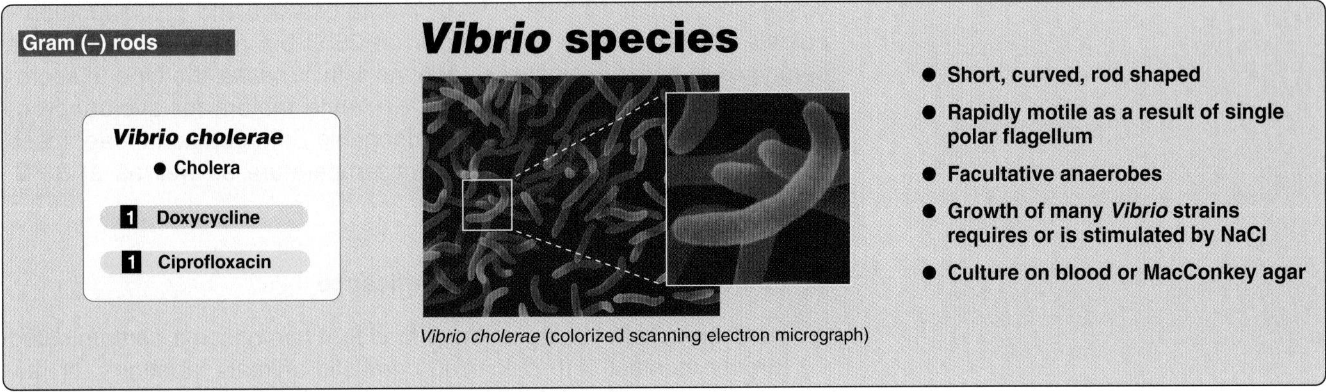

Gram (–) rods
Vibrio species
Vibrio cholerae
● Cholera
1 Doxycycline
1 Ciprofloxacin
● Short, curved, rod shaped
● Rapidly motile as a result of single polar flagellum
● Facultative anaerobes
● Growth of many Vibrio strains requires or is stimulated by NaCl
● Culture on blood or MacConkey agar

Vibrio cholerae (colorized scanning electron micrograph)

Figure 12.14
Summary of *Vibrio* disease. 1 Indicates first-line drugs.

chemical testing is necessary for specific identification of *V. cholerae*.

E. Treatment and prevention

Replacement of fluids and electrolytes is crucial in preventing shock and does not require bacteriologic diagnosis. Antibiotics (doxycycline is the drug of choice) can shorten the duration of diarrhea and excretion of the organism (Figure 12.14). Prevention relies primarily on public health measures that reduce fecal contamination of water supplies and food. Adequate cooking of foods can minimize transmission. Vaccines that are only modestly protective are available in many other countries but not in the United States.

F. Vibrio parahaemolyticus and other halophilic, noncholera vibrios

These organisms are characterized by a requirement for higher-than-usual concentrations of NaCl and their ability to grow in 10 percent NaCl. They are common in coastal seawaters. *Vibrio parahaemolyticus* is associated with outbreaks of GI illness that result from ingestion of contaminated and inadequately cooked seafood, especially shellfish and crustaceans. The disease is self-limiting, and antibiotics do not alter the course of infection. Neither human carriers nor other mammalian reservoirs have been identified. Other halophilic, noncholera vibrios are associated with soft tissue infections and septicemia resulting either from contact of wounds with contaminated seawater or from ingestion of contaminated seafood. For soft tissue infections, prompt administration of antibiotics, such as tetracycline, fluoroquinolones or cefotaxime, is important, and surgical drainage/debridement may be required. Bacteremia is associated with high mortality, especially when caused by *Vibrio vulnificus*.

VII. YERSINIA

The genus *Yersinia* includes three species of medical importance: *Yersinia enterocolitica* and *Yersinia pseudotuberculosis*, both potential pathogens of the GI tract that are discussed in this chapter, and *Yersinia pestis*, the etiologic agent of bubonic plague, which is discussed in Chapter 13 (see p. 143). *Y. enterocolitica* and *Y. pseudotuberculosis* are both motile when grown at 25°C but not at 37°C. Multiple serotypes of both species exist, and, as with *Y. pestis*, the type III secretion system and Yop proteins are virulence factors for avoidance of phagocytosis. In contrast to most pathogenic Enterobacteriaceae, these strains of *Yersinia* grow well at room temperature as well as at 37°C. Most strains are Lac^-.

A. Pathogenesis and clinical significance

Infection occurs via ingestion of food that has become contaminated through contact with colonized domestic animals, abattoirs, or raw meat (especially pork). *Y. enterocolitica* is a relatively uncommon cause of enterocolitis in the United States, and *Y. pseudotuberculosis* is even rarer. Infection results in ulcerative lesions in the terminal ileum, necrotic lesions in Peyer patches, and enlargement of mesenteric lymph nodes. Enterocolitis caused by *Yersinia* is characterized by fever, abdominal pain, and diarrhea. When accompanied by right lower quadrant tenderness and leukocytosis, the symptoms are clinically indistinguishable from appendicitis. Symptoms commonly resolve in 1 to 3 weeks. Sequelae may include reactive polyarthritis and erythema nodosum. Other, less common clinical presentations include exudative pharyngitis and, in compromised patients, septicemia.

B. Laboratory identification

Yersinia can be cultured from appropriate specimens on MacConkey or cefsulodin-irgasan-novobiocin (CIN, a medium selective for *Yersinia*) agars. Identification is based on biochemical screening. In the absence of a positive culture, serologic tests for anti-Yersinia antibodies may assist in diagnosis.

C. Treatment and prevention

Reducing infections and outbreaks rests on measures to limit potential contamination of meat, ensuring its proper handling and preparation. Antibiotic therapy (for example, with ciprofloxacin or trimethoprim-sulfamethoxazole) is essential for systemic disease

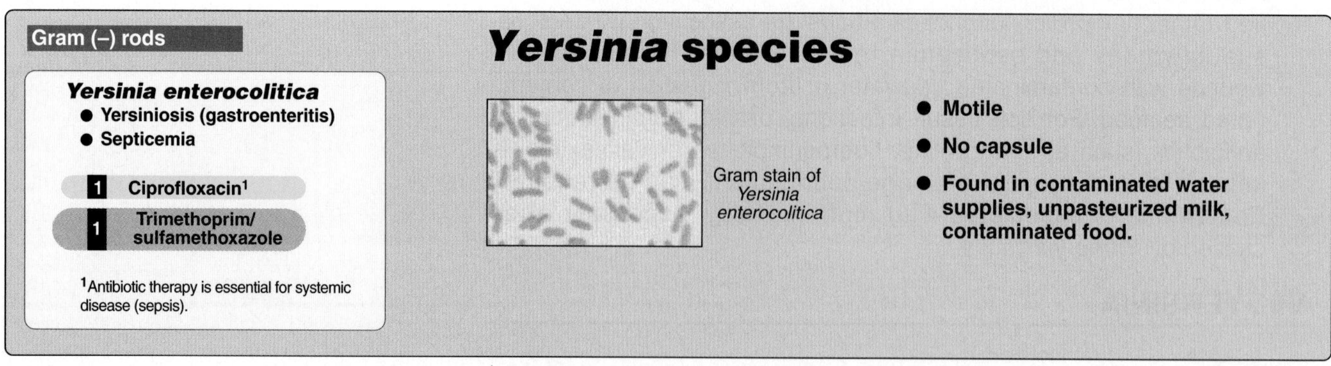

Figure 12.15
Summary of *Yersinia enterocolitica* disease. ■ Indicates first-line drugs.

(sepsis), but is of questionable value for self-limited diseases such as enterocolitis (Figure 12.15).

VIII. HELICOBACTER

Members of the genus *Helicobacter* are curved or spiral organisms (Figure 12.16). They have a rapid, corkscrew motility resulting from multiple polar flagella. *Helicobacter pylori*, the species of human significance, is microaerophilic, and produces urease. It causes acute gastritis and duodenal and gastric ulcers. *H. pylori* (and several other *Helicobacter* species) are unusual in their ability to colonize the stomach, where low pH normally protects against bacterial infection. *H. pylori* infections are relatively common and worldwide in distribution.

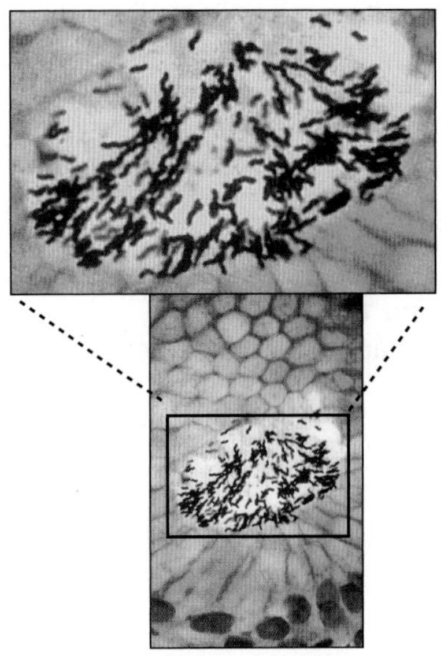

Figure 12.16
Helicobacter pylori in a gastric pit.

A. Pathogenesis

Transmission of *H. pylori* is thought to be from person to person, because the organism has not been isolated from food or water. Untreated, infections tend to be chronic, even lifelong. *H. pylori* colonizes gastric mucosal (epithelial) cells in the stomach and metaplastic gastric epithelium in the duodenum or esophagus but does not colonize the rest of the intestinal epithelium. The organism survives in the mucus layer that coats the epithelium and causes chronic inflammation of the mucosa (Figure 12.17). Although the organism is noninvasive, it recruits and activates inflammatory cells. Urease released by *H. pylori* produces ammonia ions that neutralize stomach acid in the vicinity of the organism, favoring bacterial multiplication. Ammonia may also both cause injury and potentiate the effects of a cytotoxin produced by *H. pylori*.

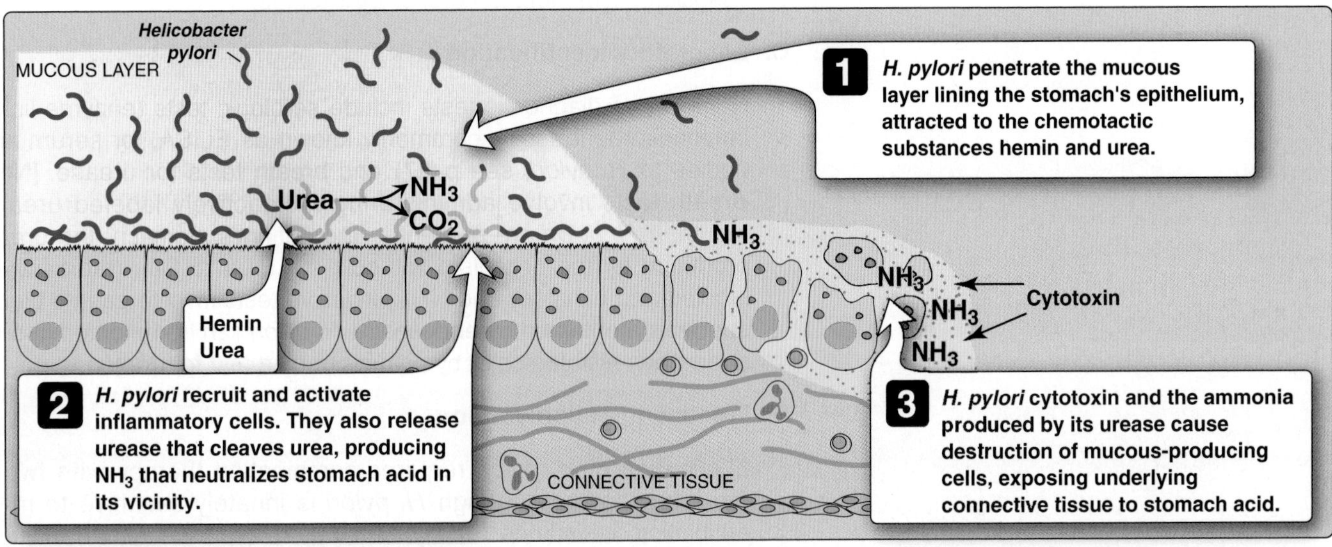

Figure 12.17
Helicobacter pylori infection, resulting in ulceration of the stomach.

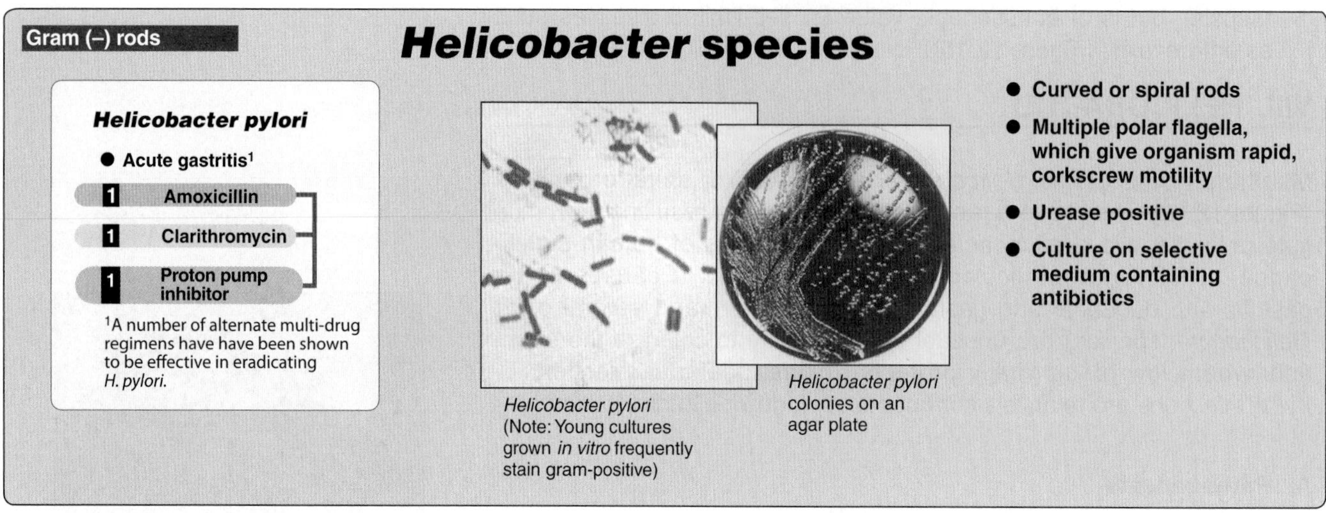

Figure 12.18
Summary of *Helicobacter* disease. **1** Indicates first-line drugs.

B. Clinical significance

Initial infection with *H. pylori* causes acute gastritis, sometimes with diarrhea that lasts about 1 week. The infection usually becomes chronic, with diffuse, superficial gastritis that may be associated with epigastric discomfort. Both duodenal ulcers and gastric ulcers are closely correlated with infection by *H. pylori*. [Note: *H. pylori* infection is found in more than 95 percent of duodenal ulcer patients and in nearly all patients with gastric ulcers who do not use aspirin or other nonsteroidal anti-inflammatory drugs, both risk factors for gastric ulcers.] *H. pylori* infection appears to be a risk factor for development of gastric carcinoma and gastric B-cell lymphoma (mucosa-associated lymphoid tumors, or MALTomas).

C. Laboratory identification

Noninvasive diagnostic tests include serologic tests (enzyme-linked immunosorbent assay, commonly known as ELISA, for serum antibodies to *H. pylori*, see p. 27) and breath tests for urease. [Note: Breath tests involve administering radioactively labeled urea by mouth. If *H. pylori* are present in the patient's stomach, the urease produced by the organism will split the urea to CO_2 (radioactively labeled and exhaled) and NH_3.] Invasive tests involve gastric biopsy specimens obtained by endoscopy. *H. pylori* can be detected in such specimens histologically, by culture, or by a test for urease.

D. Treatment and prevention

Elimination of *H. pylori* requires combination therapy with two or more antibiotics. Although *H. pylori* is innately sensitive to many antibiotics, resistance readily develops. A typical regimen includes amoxicillin plus clarithromycin plus a proton pump inhibitor such as omeprazole (Figure 12.18).

IX. OTHER ENTEROBACTERIACEAE

Other genera of Enterobacteriaceae, such as *Klebsiella*, *Enterobacter*, *Proteus*, and *Serratia*, which can be found as normal inhabitants of the large intestine, include organisms that are primarily opportunistic and often nosocomial pathogens. Widespread antibiotic resistance among these organisms necessitates sensitivity testing to determine the appropriate antibiotic treatment.

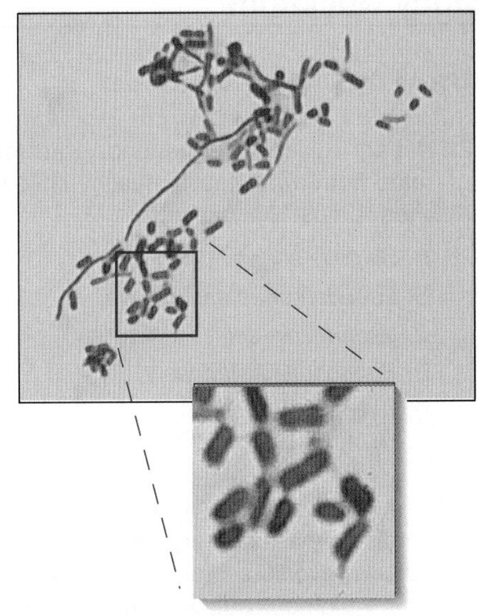

Figure 12.19
Micrograph showing rod-shaped *Klebsiella pneumoniae* cells.

A. Enterobacter

Enterobacter species are motile and Lac$^+$. They rarely cause primary disease in humans but frequently colonize hospitalized patients, especially in association with antibiotic treatment, indwelling catheters, and invasive procedures. These organisms may infect burns, wounds, and the respiratory (causing pneumonia) and urinary tracts.

B. Klebsiella

Klebsiellae are large, nonmotile bacilli that possess a luxurious capsule (Figure 12.19). They are Lac$^+$. *Klebsiella pneumoniae* and *Klebsiella oxytoca* cause necrotizing lobar pneumonia in individuals compromised by alcoholism, diabetes, or chronic obstructive pulmonary disease. *K. pneumoniae* also causes UTI and bacteremia, particularly in hospitalized patients. The organism formerly known as *Calymmatobacterium granulomatis* has been reclassified as *Klebsiella granulomatis*, based upon genome sequence analysis. *K. granulomatis* causes donovanosis, or granuloma inguinale, which is a sexually transmitted infection that is rare in the United States but endemic in Africa, India, South America, and Australia. The disease presents, after a prolonged incubation period, as subcutaneous nodules that break down, revealing one or more painless granulomatous lesions. The gram-negative rods can be identified within mononuclear cells by staining the material collected from the border of lesions.

C. Serratia

Serratia are motile and ferment lactose slowly, if at all. The species of *Serratia* that most frequently causes human infection is *Serratia marcescens*. *Serratia* can cause extraintestinal infections such as those of the lower respiratory and urinary tracts, especially among hospitalized patients.

D. Proteus, Providencia, and Morganella

Members of these genera are agents of urinary tract and other extraintestinal infections. *Proteus* species are relatively common causes of uncomplicated as well as nosocomial UTI. Other extraintestinal infections, such as wound infections, pneumonias, and septicemias, are associated with compromised patients. *Proteus* organisms produce urease, which catalyzes the hydrolysis of urea to ammonia. The resulting alkaline environment promotes the precipitation of struvite stones containing insoluble phosphates of magnesium and phosphate.

Study Questions

Choose the ONE correct answer

12.1 A Lac$^+$, glucose-fermenting, gram-negative rod isolated from a previously healthy child with bloody diarrhea is most likely to be:

A. *Shigella sonnei.*
B. *Pseudomonas aeruginosa.*
C. *Escherichia coli.*
D. *Salmonella enterica.*
E. *Helicobacter pylori.*

Correct answer = C. *Escherichia coli* is Lac$^+$, and enteroinvasive strains characteristically cause a dysentery-like syndrome. *Shigella* characteristically causes bloody diarrhea (dysentery) but is Lac$^-$. *Pseudomonas aeruginosa* characteristically causes infections in compromised hosts and is Lac$^-$. *Salmonella* is also Lac$^-$. *Helicobacter pylori* causes gastritis.

12.2 A male older adult, hospitalized and recovering from cardiac bypass surgery, develops pneumonia. Sputum culture reveals a gram-negative rod that produces a green pigment but does not ferment carbohydrates. The most likely organism is:

A. *Klebsiella pneumoniae.*
B. *Serratia* species.
C. *Proteus* species.
D. *Enterobacter* species.
E. *Pseudomonas aeruginosa.*

Correct answer = E. All five organisms are opportunists capable of causing pneumonia in compromised patients. However, the first four are members of the family Enterobacteriaceae and, by definition, can ferment carbohydrates. In addition, none of these organisms are known to produce a green pigment, although *Serratia* may produce a red pigment. *Pseudomonas aeruginosa* is an obligate aerobe that uses respiratory pathways exclusively. Production of green pyocyanin pigment regularly occurs.

12.3 An older, alcoholic male develops severe, necrotizing lobar pneumonia. The organism is Lac$^+$ and produces a luxuriant capsule. The most likely agent is:

A. *Klebsiella pneumoniae.*
B. *Serratia* species.
C. *Yersinia pseudotuberculosis.*
D. *Pseudomonas aeruginosa.*
E. *Campylobacter fetus.*

Correct answer = A. The combination of necrotizing pneumonia and an alcoholic patient suggests *Klebsiella pneumoniae*, and the laboratory data (Lac$^+$ and a luxuriant capsule) are consistent. Although *Serratia* can cause pneumonia in compromised patients, necrosis is not a characteristic feature. Moreover, the organism ferments lactose slowly, if at all, and does not have a luxuriant capsule. *Yersinia pseudotuberculosis* is Lac$^-$ and rarely causes pneumonia. *Pseudomonas aeruginosa* can cause pneumonia in compromised patients but does not ferment lactose. *Campylobacter fetus* typically causes bacteremia and disseminated infections.

12.4 A young man returned from a backpacking trip in Mexico suffering from a high fever, pain in the abdomen, and watery diarrhea. The emergency room doctor noted a faint rash on the patient's abdomen and chest. A blood specimen was collected and plated on MacConkey agar, incubated at 37°C in ambient air. Lac$^-$ colonies grew on the plates. The cultured organism was a gram-negative rod that did not produce Shiga or Shiga-like toxins. The most likely etiological agent for this man's disease is:

A. Enterohemorrhagic *Escherichia coli*
B. *Shigella* dysenteriae
C. *Salmonella typhi*
D. *Helicobacter pylori*
E. *Campylobacter jejuni*

Correct answer = C. This person is suffering from typhoid fever, caused by *Salmonella enterica* serovar *typhi.* Both enterohemorrhagic *Escherichia coli* and *Shigella dysenteriae* produce Shiga or Shiga-like toxins, which were not detected in this case. Both *Helicobacter pylori* and *Campylobacter jejuni* are curved organisms, which is not consistent with the cell morphology of the organism causing this infection. Moreover, neither *H. pylori* nor *C. jejuni* can be cultured on typical primary plating media such as MacConkey agar.

Other Gram-negative Rods

13

I. OVERVIEW

Although not part of a closely related family, the organisms covered in this chapter do share two significant features of structure and physiology. First, they all have a gram-negative cell envelope and, therefore, contain lipopolysaccharide (LPS), which is a virulence factor. Second, they grow in the presence of oxygen and, therefore, cause infections at sites where oxygen tension is high (for example, in the lungs, and other vital tissues). It is helpful to consider these organisms as follows: 1) those that are primarily or exclusively pathogens of the human respiratory tract (*Haemophilus*, *Bordetella* and *Legionella*), 2) *Pseudomonas,* an organism that can infect a wide variety of tissues and whose virulence is potentiated by certain immune compromise, and 3) those that are primarily pathogens of animals (that is, zoonotic organisms, such as *Brucella, Francisella,* and *Pasteurella,* for which humans are accidental hosts). Although *Yersinia pestis* is a member of the family Enterobacteriaceae (covered in Chapter 12), it is included in this chapter because it is a nongastrointestinal, gram-negative rod. *Bartonella*, another unusual gram-negative rod that is responsible for trench fever and cat scratch disease, is also described here. The organisms covered in this chapter are listed in Figure 13.1.

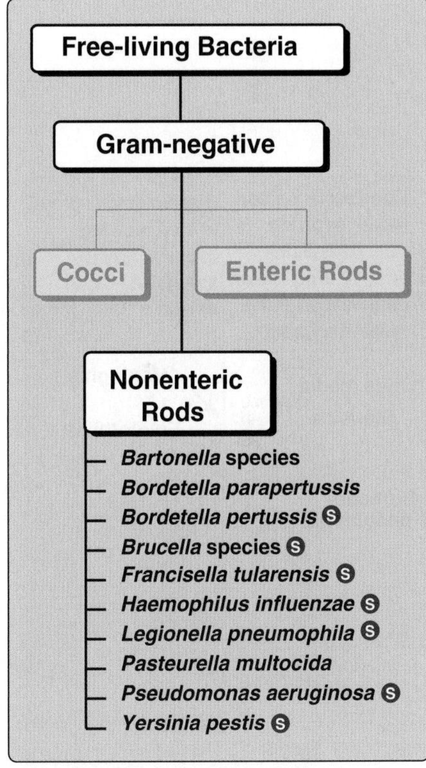

Figure 13.1
Classification of other gram-negative rods. See pp. 333, 334, 340, 342, 346, and 353 for summaries of these organisms.

II. HAEMOPHILUS

Cells of *Haemophilus influenzae*—the major human pathogen of this genus—are pleomorphic, ranging from coccobacilli to long, slender filaments. *H. influenzae* may produce a capsule (six capsular types have been distinguished) or may be unencapsulated (Figure 13.2). The capsule is an important virulence factor. Serious, invasive *H. influenzae* disease is associated particularly with capsular type b (Hib), which is composed of polyribose phosphate. Hib is especially important as a pathogen of young children, although it can cause disease in individuals of all age groups. Nontypeable (unencapsulated) strains may also cause serious disease and are a significant cause of pneumonia among older adults and individuals with chronic lung disease.

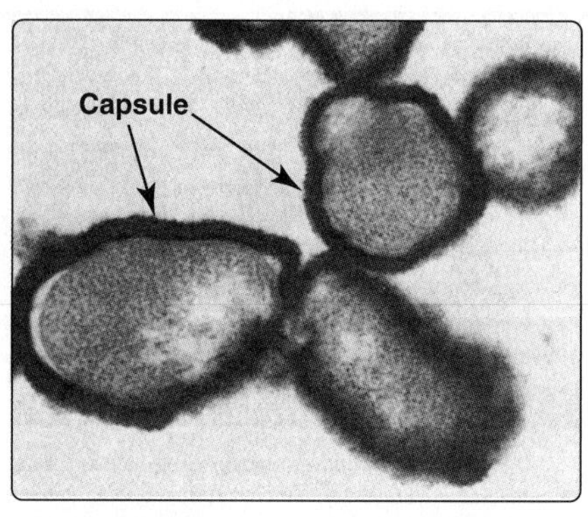

Figure 13.2
Haemophilus influenzae (electron micrograph) showing thick capsules.

A. Epidemiology

H. influenzae is a normal component of the upper respiratory tract flora in humans and may also colonize the conjunctiva and genital tract. Humans are the only natural hosts, and colonization begins shortly after birth, with unencapsulated strains and Hib being carried most frequently. *H. influenzae* illnesses are usually sporadic in occurrence.

B. Pathogenesis

H. influenzae is transmitted by respiratory droplets. Immunoglobulin A (IgA) protease produced by the organism degrades secretory IgA, facilitating colonization of the upper respiratory tract mucosa. From this site, *H. influenzae* can enter the bloodstream and disseminate to distant sites. Diseases caused by *H. influenzae*, therefore, fall into two categories (Figure 13.3). First, disorders such as otitis media, sinusitis, epiglottitis, and bronchopneumonia result from contiguous spread of the organism from its site of colonization in the respiratory tract. Second, disorders such as meningitis, septic arthritis, and cellulitis result from invasion of the bloodstream, followed by localization of *H. influenzae* in these and other areas of the body.

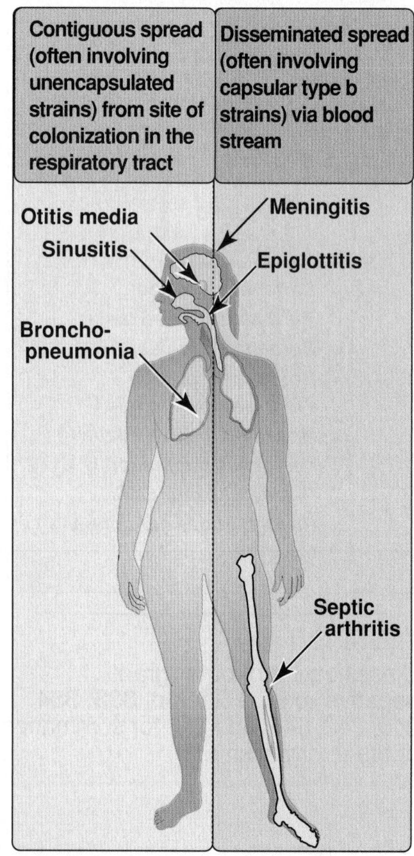

Figure 13.3
Infections caused by *Haemophilus influenzae.*

C. Clinical significance

H. influenzae has been a leading cause of bacterial meningitis, primarily in infants and very young children, frequently in conjunction with an episode of otitis media. A vaccine against *H. influenzae* type b, administered to infants, has dramatically decreased the frequency of such infections (Figure 13.4). Clinically, *H. influenzae* meningitis is indistinguishable from other purulent meningitides and may be gradual in onset or fulminant (sudden onset with great severity). Mortality from meningitis is high in untreated patients, but appropriate therapy reduces mortality to about 5 percent. Survivors may be left with permanent neurologic sequelae, especially deafness.

D. Laboratory identification

A definitive diagnosis generally requires identification of the organism (for example, by culture on chocolate agar). *H. influenzae* is fastidious and requires supplementation with hemin, factor X, and nicotinamide adenine dinucleotide (NAD^+), factor V. *H. influenzae* can be cultured on chocolate agar (lysed blood cells provide these growth factors) but cannot be grown on blood or MacConkey agar. Isolation from normally sterile sites and fluids, such as blood, cerebrospinal fluid (CSF), and synovial fluid, is significant, whereas isolation from pharyngeal cultures is inconclusive. Rapid diagnosis is crucial because of the potentially fulminant course of type b infections. In cases of meningitis, Gram staining of CSF commonly reveals pleomorphic, gram-negative coccobacilli (Figure 13.5). Type b capsule may be identified directly in CSF, either by the capsular swelling (quellung) reaction (see p. 26) or by immunofluorescent staining (see p. 28). Capsular antigen may be detected in CSF or other body fluids using immunologic tests, such as latex agglutination, countercurrent immunoelectrophoresis, ELISA, and radioimmunoassay.

E. Treatment

When invasive *H. influenzae* is suspected, a suitable antibiotic (for example, a third-generation cephalosporin, such as ceftriaxone or cefotaxime) should be started as soon as appropriate specimens have been taken for culture (see Figure 13.5). Antibiotic sensitivity testing is necessary because of emergence of strains resistant to antibiotics commonly used to treat *H. influenzae* (for example, strains with β-lactamase-mediated ampicillin resistance). Sinusitis, otitis media, and other upper respiratory tract infections are treated with trimethoprim-sulfamethoxazole or ampicillin plus clavulanate.

F. Prevention

Active immunization against Hib is effective in preventing invasive disease and also reduces respiratory carriage of Hib (see Figure 13.4). The current vaccine, generally given to children younger than age 2 years, consists of Hib polyribose phosphate (PRP) capsular carbohydrate conjugated to a carrier protein (see p. 35). Rifampin is given prophylactically to individuals in close contact with a patient infected with *H. influenzae*—particularly those patients with invasive disease (for example, *H. influenzae* meningitis).

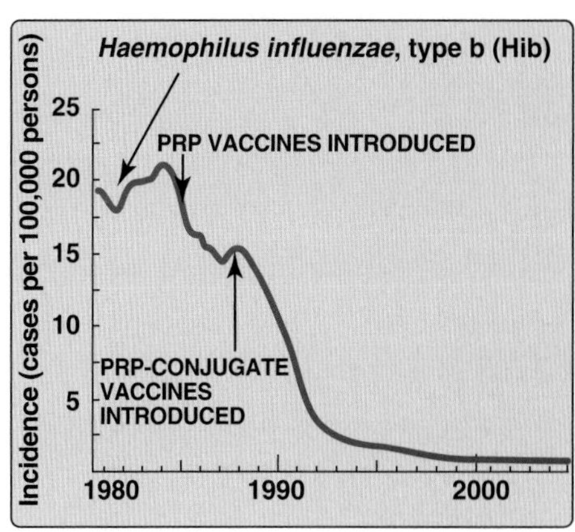

Figure 13.4
Incidence of *Haemophilus influenzae* type b meningitis in a pediatric population in the United States. PRP = polyribose phosphate.

Gram (–) rods

***Haemophilus* species**

Gram stain of *Haemophilus influenzae*

Haemophilus influenzae on chocolate agar

- **Pleomorphic in shape, ranging from small coccobacilli to long slender filaments**
- **Obligate parasites, requiring hemin and NAD+ for growth**
- **Culture on chocolate agar containing hemin and NAD+**

Haemophilus influenzae

- **Otitis media**
- **Sinusitis**
- **Pneumonia**
- **Bacterial meningitis**
- **Epiglottitis**
- **Septic arthritis**

1 Ampicillin/clavulanate[1]

1 Cefotaxime[2]

1 Ceftriaxone[2]

2 Trimethoprim-sulfamethoxazole[3]

[1]Non-life-threatening illness
[2]Meningitis, epiglottitis, and other life-threatening illness
[3]Respiratory infections and otitis; not meningitis

Gross specimen from patient with bacterial meningitis, showing copious purulent exudate covering base of brain

Figure 13.5
Summary of *Haemophilus* disease. **1** Indicates first-line drugs; **2** indicates alternative drugs. NAD = nicotinamide adenine dinucleotide.

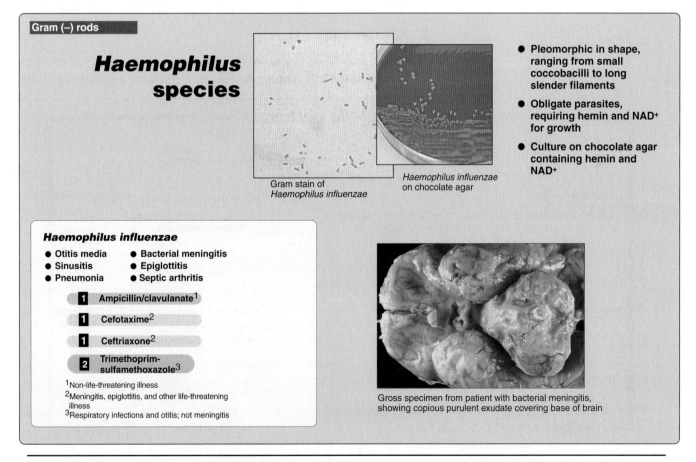

III. BORDETELLA

Bordetella pertussis and *Bordetella parapertussis* are the human pathogens of this genus. The former causes the disease pertussis (also known as whooping cough), and the latter causes a mild pertussis-like illness. Whooping cough is a highly contagious disease and a significant cause of morbidity and mortality worldwide (51 million cases and 600,000 deaths each year). Members of the genus *Bordetella* are aerobic. They are small, encapsulated coccobacilli that grow singly or in pairs. They can be serotyped on the basis of cell-surface molecules including adhesins and fimbriae.

A. Epidemiology

The major mode of transmission of *Bordetella* is via droplets spread by coughing, but the organism survives only briefly outside the human respiratory tract. The incidence of whooping cough among different age groups can vary substantially, depending on whether active immunization of young children is widespread in the community. In the absence of an immunization program, disease is most common among young children (ages 1 to 5 years). Adolescent and adult household members, whose pertussis immunity has disappeared, are an important reservoir of pertussis for young children.

B. Pathogenesis

B. pertussis binds to ciliated epithelium in the upper respiratory tract (see Figure 13.9). There, the bacteria produce a variety of toxins

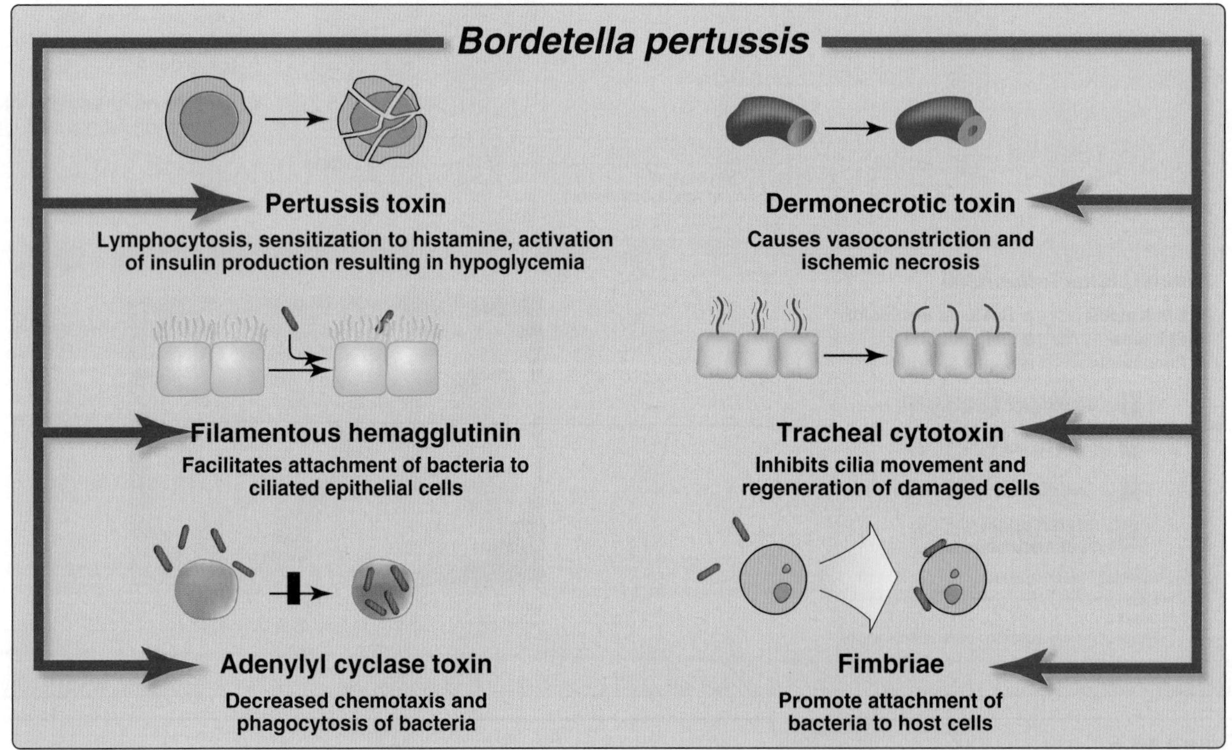

Figure 13.6
Toxins and virulence factors produced by *Bordetella pertussis*.

and other virulence factors that interfere with ciliary activity, eventually causing death of these cells (Figure 13.6).

C. Clinical significance

The incubation period for pertussis generally ranges from 1 to 3 weeks (Figure 13.7). The disease can be divided into two phases: catarrhal and paroxysmal.

1. **Catarrhal phase:** This phase begins with relatively nonspecific symptoms, such as rhinorrhea, mild conjunctival infection (hyperemia, or bloodshot conjunctivae), malaise, and/or mild fever, and then progresses to include a dry, nonproductive cough. Patients in this phase of disease are highly contagious.

2. **Paroxysmal phase:** With worsening of the cough, the paroxysmal phase begins. The term "whooping cough" derives from the paroxysms of coughing followed by a "whoop" as the patient inspires rapidly. Large amounts of mucus may be produced. Paroxysms may cause cyanosis and/or end with vomiting. [Note: Whooping may not occur in all patients.] Pertussis typically causes leukocytosis that can be quite striking as the total white blood cell count sometimes exceeds 50,000 cells/μL (normal range = 4,500–11,000 white blood cells/μL), with a striking predominance of lymphocytes. Following the paroxysmal phase, convalescence requires at least an additional 3 to 4 weeks. During this period, secondary complications, such as infections (for example, otitis media and pneumonia) and central nervous system (CNS) dysfunction (for example, encephalopathy or seizures), may occur. Disease is generally most severe in infants.

D. Laboratory identification

Presumptive diagnosis may be made on clinical grounds once the paroxysmal phase of classic pertussis begins. Pertussis may be suspected in an individual who has onset of catarrhal symptoms within 1 to 3 weeks of exposure to a diagnosed case of pertussis. Culture of *B. pertussis* on Bordet-Gengou or Regan-Lowe media (selective and enrichment media) from the nasopharynx of a symptomatic patient supports the diagnosis. The organism produces pin-

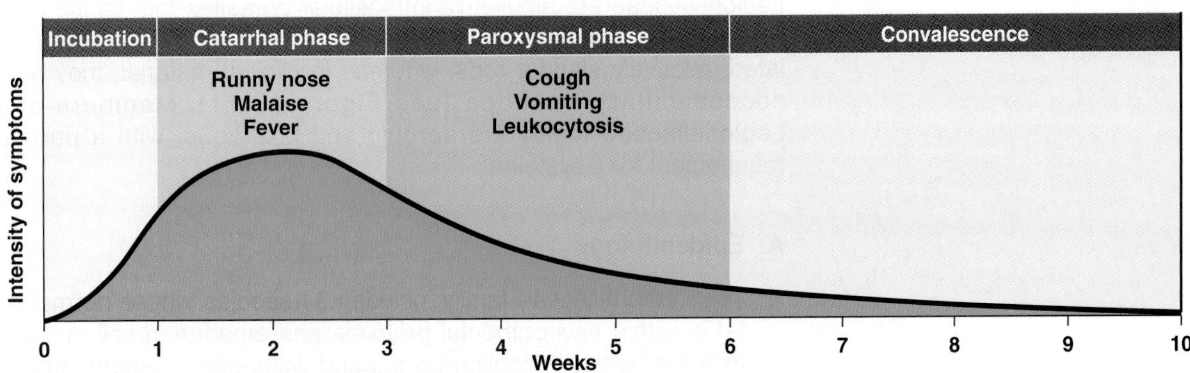

Figure 13.7
Clinical presentation of *Bordetella pertussis* disease.

point colonies in 3 to 6 days on selective agar medium (for example, one that contains blood and charcoal), which serves to absorb and/or neutralize inhibitory substances and is supplemented with antibiotics to inhibit growth of normal flora. More rapid diagnosis may be accomplished using a direct fluorescent antibody test to detect *B. pertussis* in smears of nasopharyngeal specimens. Serologic tests for antibodies to *B. pertussis* are primarily useful for epidemiologic surveys.

E. Treatment

Erythromycin is the drug of choice for infections with *B. pertussis*, both as chemotherapy (where it reduces both the duration and severity of disease) and as chemoprophylaxis for household contacts (see Figure 13.9). For erythromycin treatment failures, trimethoprim-sulfamethoxazole is an alternative choice. Patients are most contagious during the catarrhal stage and during the first 2 weeks after onset of coughing. Treatment of the infected individuals during this period limits the spread of infection among household contacts.

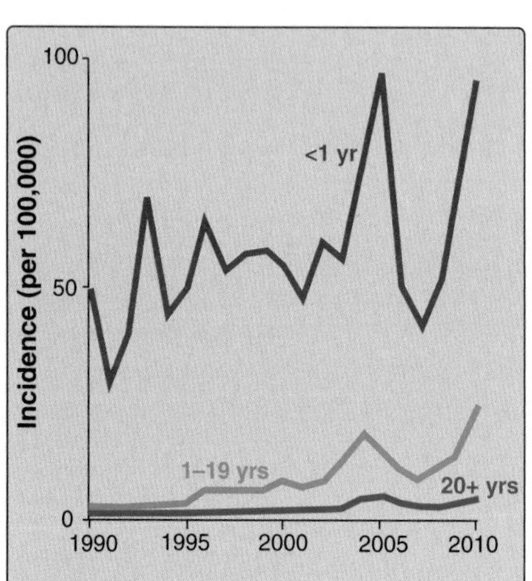

Figure 13.8
Incidence of pertussis by age group, United States.

F. Prevention

Pertussis vaccine is available and has had a significant effect on lowering the incidence of whooping cough. It contains proteins purified from *B. pertussis* and is formulated in combination with diphtheria and tetanus toxoids (see p. 38). To protect infants who are at greatest risk of life-threatening *B. pertussis* disease (Figure 13.8), immunization is generally initiated when the infant is 2 months old. Widespread use of pertussis vaccine was followed by a dramatic decrease in reported pertussis in the United States for decades, until the middle of the first decade of the 21st century. However, because neither disease- nor vaccine-induced immunity is durable, there has been a resurgence, with reported cases in 2010 the highest since the 1950's. A new vaccine, licensed for adolescents and adults, and vaccination of women even during the last trimester of pregnancy, may help to reduce reported pertussis in the United States.

IV. LEGIONELLA

Legionellaceae are facultative intracellular parasites that cause primarily respiratory tract infections. In nature, *Legionella* cells are unencapsulated, relatively slender rods, whereas in clinical material, they appear coccobacillary in shape (see Figure 13.11). Members of the Legionellaceae family are aerobic and fastidious, with a particular requirement for L-cysteine.

A. Epidemiology

The Legionellaceae family includes 34 species whose normal habitat is within environmental protozoa and amebae in soil and water, including water in cooling towers and distribution systems. About 85 to 90 percent of human disease is caused by a single species,

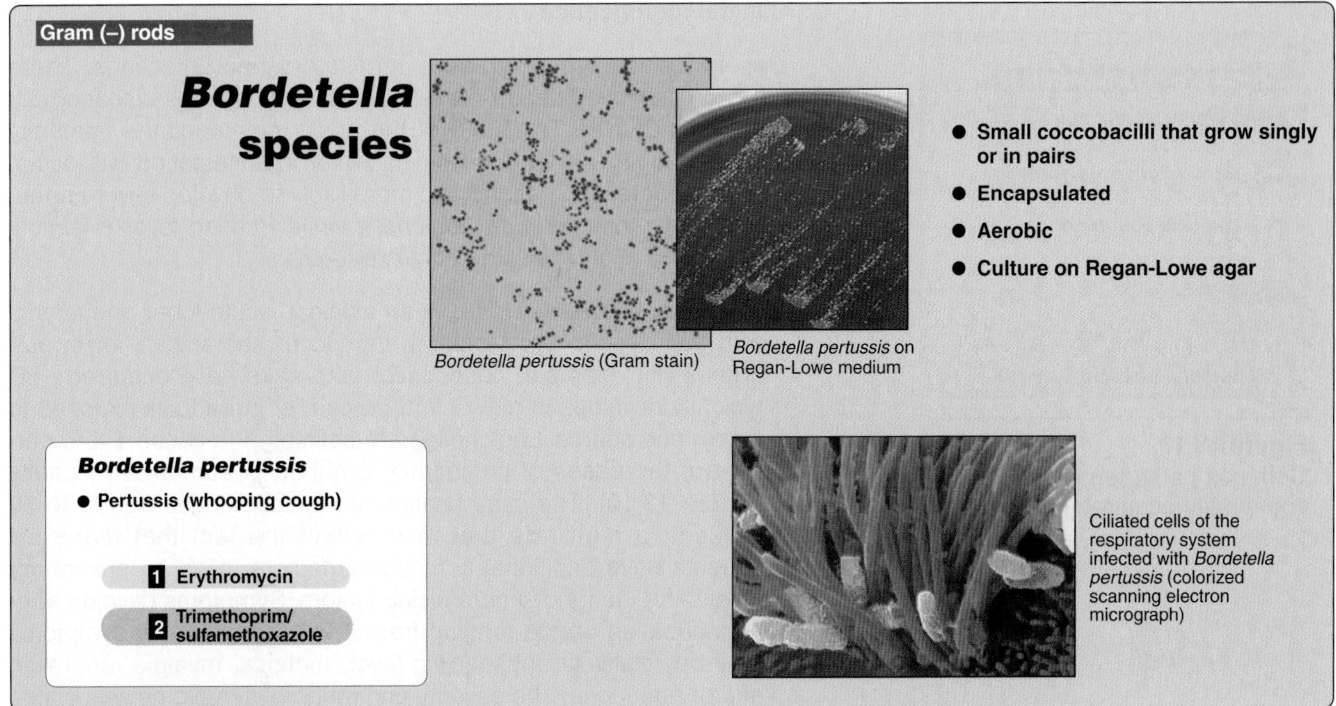

Gram (–) rods
Bordetella species
Small coccobacilli that grow singly or in pairs
Encapsulated
Aerobic
Culture on Regan-Lowe agar
Bordetella pertussis (Gram stain)
Bordetella pertussis on Regan-Lowe medium
Bordetella pertussis
Pertussis (whooping cough)
1 Erythromycin
2 Trimethoprim/ sulfamethoxazole
Ciliated cells of the respiratory system infected with Bordetella pertussis (colorized scanning electron micrograph)

Figure 13.9
Summary of *Bordetella* disease. 1 Indicates first-line drugs; 2 indicates alternative drugs.

Legionella pneumophila. Most infections result from inhalation of aerosolized organisms within amebas or within environmental biofilm but, occasionally, may follow other exposures (for example, swimming in contaminated water). Both sporadic cases and localized outbreaks may occur. One famous outbreak occurred in 1976 during a convention of American Legion members (hence the name, *Legionella*). Cases of legionellosis in the United States nearly tripled from 2000 to 2009. The organism is chlorine tolerant and, thus, survives water treatment procedures. There is no person-to-person spread of the disease. Growth within the environmental ameba induces the expression of key virulence factors that make the *Legionellae* more fit for infection of human macrophages.

B. Pathogenesis

The organism gains entry to the upper respiratory tract by aspiration of water containing the organism or by inhalation of a contaminated aerosol. Failure to clear the organisms permits them to reach the lungs. Alveolar macrophages in the lung bed normally constitute an important line of defense for clearing invading organisms. Although the macrophages do phagocytose *L. pneumophila*, the resulting phagosome fails to fuse with a lysosome. Instead, the organisms multiply within the protected environment of the phagosome until the cell ruptures, releasing a new crop of bacteria.

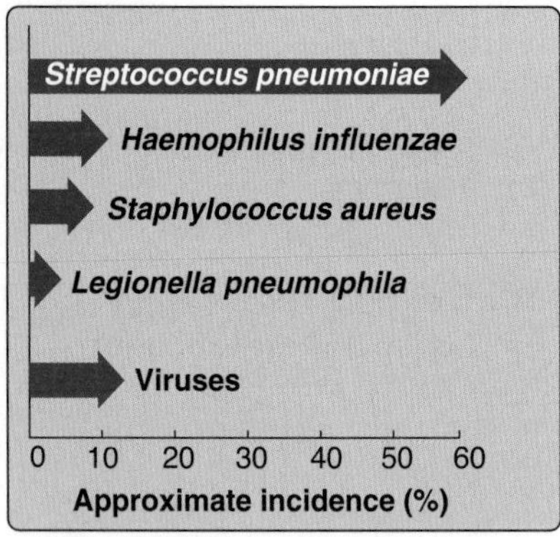

Figure 13.10
Common pathogens causing community-acquired pneumonia.

C. Clinical significance

Legionellaceae primarily cause respiratory tract infections. There are two distinctly different presentations: Legionnaires disease (LD) and Pontiac fever. The state of the host's cell-mediated immunity plays a critical role in determining which manifestation will occur. Immunosuppressed patients are more likely to develop severe pneumonia when infected with *Legionella* while Pontiac fever is almost always seen in otherwise healthy individuals.

1. **Legionnaires disease:** This is an atypical, acute lobar pneumonia with multisystem symptoms. It may occur sporadically or in outbreaks (for example, nosocomial outbreaks have occurred). LD typically develops in only 1 to 5 percent of individuals exposed to a common source. Legionellae are estimated to cause 1 to 5 percent of the cases of community-acquired pneumonias in adults (Figure 13.10). The case fatality rate for LD ranges from 5 to 30 percent, a high rate that may reflect the fact that many LD patients have additional contributing factors, such as pulmonary disease or immunocompromising factors. Symptoms develop after an incubation period ranging from 2 to 10 days. Early symptoms may be relatively nonspecific: fever, malaise, myalgia, anorexia, and/or headache. The severity and range of symptoms associated with LD vary substantially. A cough that is only slightly productive then occurs, sometimes with respiratory compromise. Diarrhea (watery rather than bloody stools) occurs in 25 to 50 percent of cases. Nausea, vomiting, and neurologic symptoms may also occur. Risk factors associated with a presentation of LD include advanced age, smoking or chronic lung disease, immune suppression due to cancer or its treatment, kidney disease, and diabetes.

2. **Pontiac fever:** This is an influenza-like illness that characteristically infects otherwise healthy individuals. The attack rate among those exposed to a common source is typically 90 percent or more. Recovery is usually complete within 1 week. No specific therapy is required.

D. Laboratory identification

LD cannot be diagnosed unambiguously on the basis of clinical presentation or radiologic appearance of lungs. Although the organism can be Gram stained, the Gimenez stain is more useful for visualization. The definitive method of diagnosis involves the culturing of *Legionella* from respiratory secretions, using buffered (pH 6.9) charcoal yeast extract (Figure 13.11) enriched with L-cysteine, iron, and α-ketoglutarate. Visible colonies form in 3 to 5 days. A urinary antigen test using an enzyme immunoassay is available and has several advantages over culture. For example, the test positivity can persist for days even during administration of antibiotic therapy, making it useful in patients who receive empiric anti-Legionella therapy. Further, the results of the urinary antigen test can be available within hours, whereas culture results require 3 to 5 days. However, it is important to note that the urinary tract antigen test only detects

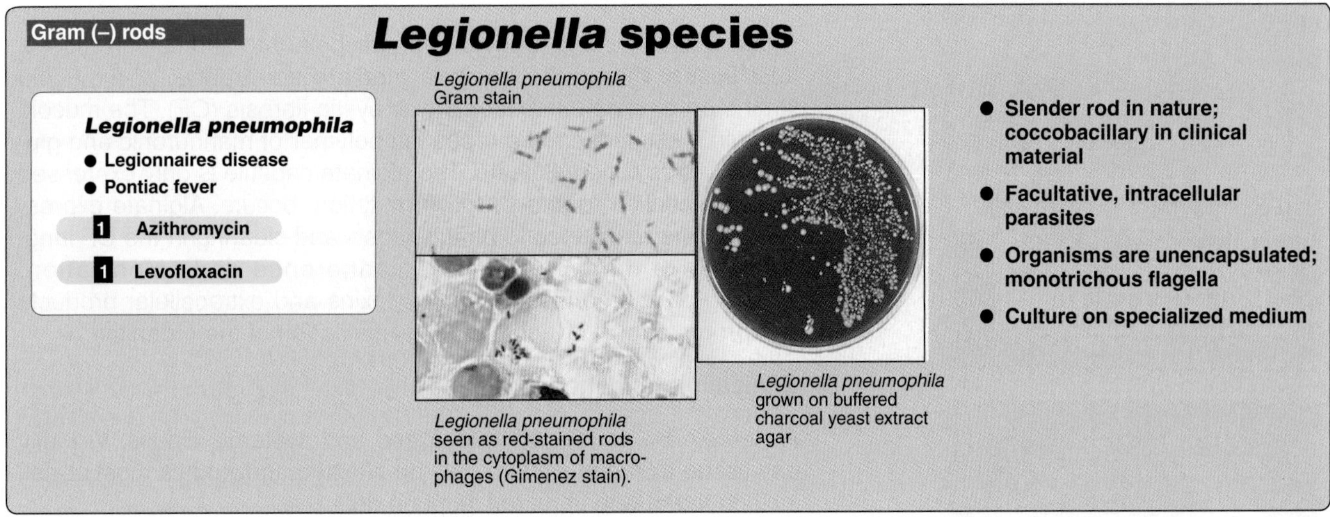

Gram (–) rods
Legionella species
Legionella pneumophila
• Legionnaires disease
• Pontiac fever
1 Azithromycin
1 Levofloxacin
Legionella pneumophila
Gram stain
Legionella pneumophila
seen as red-stained rods
in the cytoplasm of macro-
phages (Gimenez stain).
Legionella pneumophila
grown on buffered
charcoal yeast extract
agar
• Slender rod in nature; coccobacillary in clinical material
• Facultative, intracellular parasites
• Organisms are unencapsulated; monotrichous flagella
• Culture on specialized medium

Figure 13.11
Summary of *Legionella* disease. 1 Indicates first-line drugs.

infection with serogroup A *L. pneumophila*. Therefore, a negative antigen test does not rule out infection with all Legionellae. When LD is suspected, both a urinary antigen test and *Legionella* culture of a respiratory specimen should be ordered.

E. Treatment

Macrolides, such as erythromycin or azithromycin, are the drugs of choice for LD. Fluoroquinolones are also effective (see Figure 13.11). Pontiac fever is usually treated symptomatically, without antibiotics.

V. PSEUDOMONAS

Pseudomonas aeruginosa, the primary human pathogen in the genus *Pseudomonas*, is widely distributed in nature. It is found in soil, water, plants, and animals. Although it may colonize healthy humans without causing disease, it is also a significant opportunistic pathogen and a major cause of nosocomial (hospital-acquired) infections. *P. aeruginosa* is regularly a cause of nosocomial pneumonia, nosocomial urinary tract infections, surgical site infections, infections of severe burns, and infections of patients undergoing either chemotherapy for neoplastic disease or antibiotic therapy. *P. aeruginosa* is motile (it has polar flagella) and aerobic or facultative. *P. aeruginosa* does not ferment carbohydrates but can utilize alternate electron acceptors, such as nitrate, in anaerobic respiration. Nutritional requirements are minimal, and the organism can grow on a wide variety of organic substrates. In fact, *P. aeruginosa* can even grow in laboratory water baths, hot tubs, intravenous (IV) tubing, and other water-containing vessels. This explains why the organism is responsible for so many nosocomial infections.

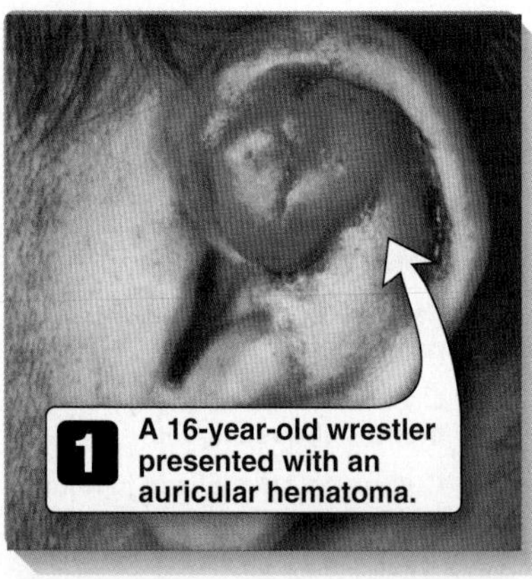

1
A 16-year-old wrestler presented with an auricular hematoma.

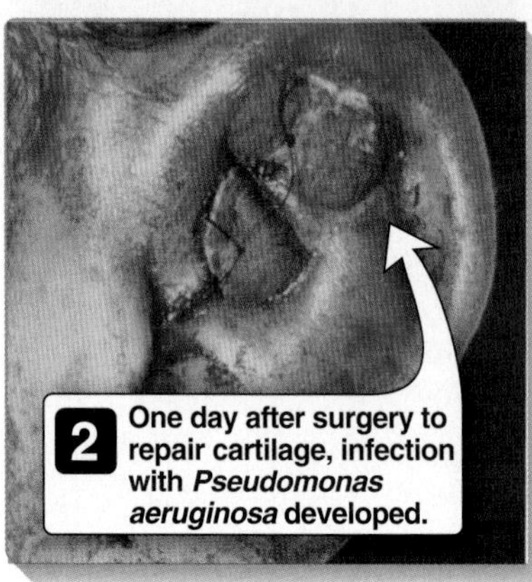

2
One day after surgery to repair cartilage, infection with *Pseudomonas aeruginosa* developed.

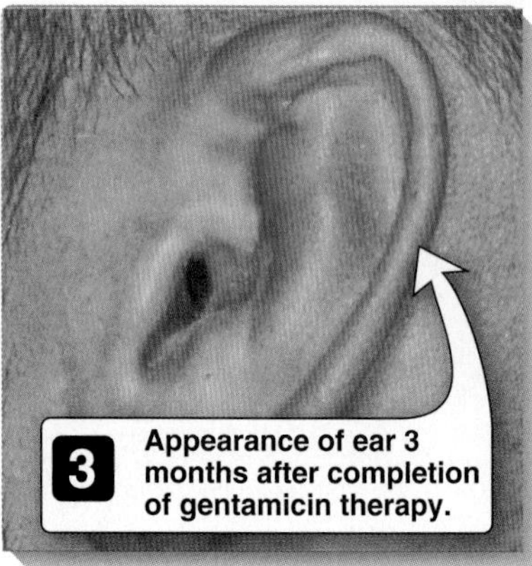

3
Appearance of ear 3 months after completion of gentamicin therapy.

Figure 13.12
Pseudomonas infection of the pinna of the ear.

A. Pathogenesis

P. aeruginosa disease begins with attachment to and colonization of host tissue. Pili on the bacteria mediate adherence, and mucoid strains predominate in patients with cystic fibrosis (CF). The mucoid capsule is composed of a repeating polymer of mannuronic and glucuronic acids called alginate. The alginate capsule is only expressed after a so-called "patho-adaptive mutation" occurs. Alginate expression confers resistance to phagocytosis and clearing in the CF lung. Host tissue damage facilitates adherence and colonization. *P. aeruginosa* produces numerous toxins and extracellular products that promote local invasion and dissemination of the organism.

B. Clinical significance

P. aeruginosa causes both localized and systemic illness. Virtually any tissue or organ system may be affected. Individuals most at risk include those with impaired immune defenses.

1. **Localized infections:** These may occur in the eye (causing keratitis and endophthalmitis following trauma), ear (causing external otitis, or swimmer's ear, and invasive and necrotizing otitis externa, particularly in older adult diabetic patients or trauma patients), skin (causing wound infection, as shown in Figure 13.12, and pustular rashes occurring in epidemics associated with use of contaminated whirlpools, hot tubs, and swimming pools), urinary tract (particularly in hospitalized patients who have been subjected to catheterization, instrumentation, surgery, or renal transplantation), respiratory tract (causing pneumonia in individuals with chronic lung disease, congestive heart failure, or cystic fibrosis, particularly in patients who have been intubated or are on ventilators for longer than than a few days), gastrointestinal tract (causing infections ranging from relatively mild diarrheal illness in children to severe, necrotizing enterocolitis in infants and neutropenic cancer patients), and the CNS (causing meningitis and brain abscesses, particularly in association with trauma, surgery, or tumors of the head or neck). Localized infections have the potential to lead to disseminated infection. [Note: The organism has a propensity to invade blood vessel walls.]

2. **Systemic infections:** Infections reflecting systemic spread of the organism include bacteremia (most common in patients whose immune systems have been compromised), secondary pneumonia, bone and joint infections (in IV drug users and patients with urinary tract or pelvic infections), endocarditis (in IV drug users and patients with prosthetic heart valves), CNS (mainly when the meninges are breached), and skin/soft tissue infections. *P. aeruginosa* is feared because it can cause severe hospital-acquired infections, especially in immunocompromised hosts. It is often antibiotic resistant due to expression of a number of efflux pumps, complicating the choice of therapy.

C. Laboratory identification

P. aeruginosa can be isolated by plating on a variety of media, both nonselective (for example, blood agar) and moderately selective (for

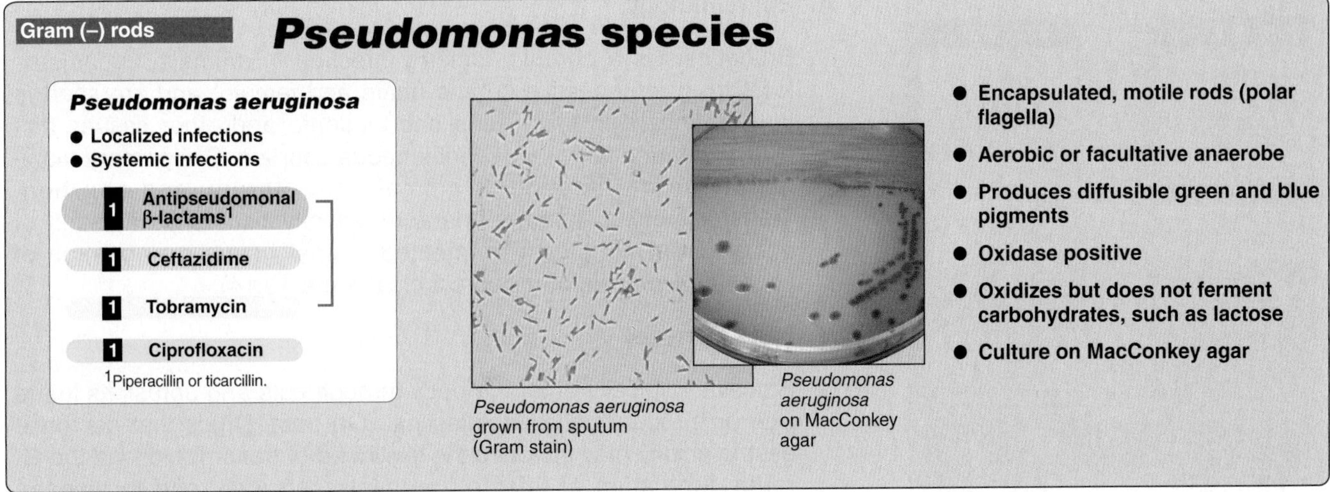

Gram (–) rods
Pseudomonas species
Pseudomonas aeruginosa
● Localized infections
● Systemic infections
1 Antipseudomonal β-lactams¹
1 Ceftazidime
1 Tobramycin
1 Ciprofloxacin
¹Piperacillin or ticarcillin.
Pseudomonas aeruginosa grown from sputum (Gram stain)
Pseudomonas aeruginosa on MacConkey agar
● Encapsulated, motile rods (polar flagella)
● Aerobic or facultative anaerobe
● Produces diffusible green and blue pigments
● Oxidase positive
● Oxidizes but does not ferment carbohydrates, such as lactose
● Culture on MacConkey agar

Figure 13.13
Summary of *Pseudomonas* disease. **1** Indicates first-line drugs.

example, MacConkey agar as shown in Figure 13.13). Identification is based on the results of a battery of biochemical and other diagnostic tests. Serologic typing is used in the investigation of clusters of cases, which may stem from exposure to a common source. [Note: A clue to its presence is a characteristic fruity odor, both in the laboratory and at the bedside.] *P. aeruginosa* typically produces a blue-green pigment called pyocyanin and is oxidase positive.

D. Treatment and Prevention

Specific therapy varies with the clinical presentation and the antibiotic sensitivity pattern of the isolate. It is difficult to find antibiotics effective against *P. aeruginosa* because of its rapid development of resistance mutations and its own innate mechanisms of antibiotic resistance. *Pseudomonas* infections typically occur in patients with impaired defenses. Therefore, aggressive antimicrobial therapy (often a combination of two bactericidal antibiotics, such as an aminoglycoside, an antipseudomonal β-lactam, or a quinolone) is generally required (see Figure 13.13).

VI. BRUCELLA

Members of the genus *Brucella* are primarily pathogens of animals (domestic and feral). Thus, brucellosis (undulant fever) is a zoonosis (a disease of animals that may be transmitted to humans under natural conditions). Different species of *Brucella* are each associated with particular animal species: *Brucella abortus* (cattle), *Brucella melitensis* (goats and sheep), *Brucella suis* (swine), *Brucella canis* (dogs), and *Brucella ovis* (sheep). All but *B. ovis* are known to cause disease in humans. The brucellae are aerobic, facultatively intracellular parasites that can survive and multiply within host phagocytes. Cells of the genus *Brucella* are unencapsulated, small coccobacilli arranged singly or in pairs (see Figure 13.15). LPS is the major virulence factor as well as the major cell wall antigen.

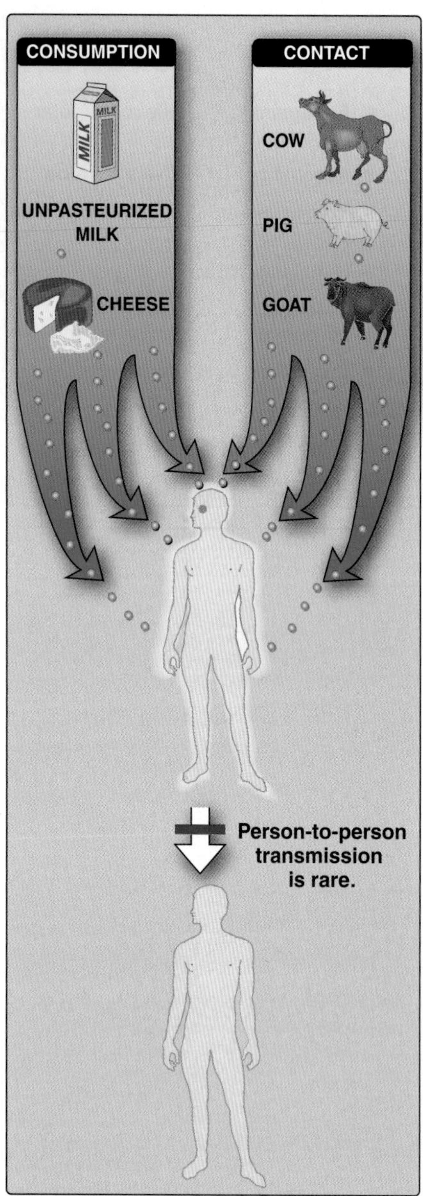

Figure 13.14
Transmission of *Brucella.*

A. Epidemiology

Brucellosis is a chronic, lifelong infection in animals. Organisms localize in reproductive organs (male and female) and are shed in large numbers in milk, urine, the placenta and other tissues discharged during delivery or spontaneous abortion. The primary manifestations of infection in animals are sterility and abortion. Transmission to humans characteristically occurs as a result of either direct contact with infected animal tissue or ingestion of unpasteurized milk or milk products (Figure 13.14).

B. Pathogenesis

Brucellae typically enter the body through cuts and abrasions in the skin or through the gastrointestinal (GI) tract. Drugs that decrease gastric acidity may increase the likelihood of transmission via the GI route. Inhalation of infected aerosols can also lead to disease among abattoir workers. Once the organisms gain entry, they are transported via the lymphatic system to the regional lymph nodes, where they multiply. The organisms are then carried by the blood to organs that are involved in the reticuloendothelial system, including the liver, spleen, kidneys, bone marrow, and other lymph nodes.

C. Clinical significance

The incubation period for *Brucella* infections ranges from 5 days to several months but typically lasts several weeks. Symptoms are nonspecific and flulike (malaise, fever, sweats, anorexia, GI symptoms, headache, and back pains) and may also include depression. Symptom onset may be abrupt or insidious. Objective clinical findings are often few and mild, in contrast to the patient's subjective evaluation. Untreated, patients may develop an undulating pattern of fever (temperatures repeatedly rise then fall, hence the name "undulant fever," the traditional name for brucellosis). Subclinical infections occur. Manifestations of brucellosis may involve any of a variety of organ systems, including the GI tract and the skeletal, neurologic, cardiovascular, and pulmonary systems. In industrialized countries, brucellosis is largely an occupational disease, occurring in ranchers, dairy farmers, abattoir workers, and veterinarians.

D. Laboratory identification

Because the nonspecific symptoms may not point to a diagnosis of brucellosis, a detailed history is often crucial, including the patient's occupation, exposure to animals, travel to countries where brucella infection is prevalent, and ingestion of potentially contaminated foods. The organism can be cultured from blood and other body fluids or from tissue specimens. Multiple blood specimens should be cultured. For plated materials, colonies may appear in 4 to 5 days, whereas longer times are required for blood cultures, and these are routinely examined for up to 1 month before being declared negative.

E. Treatment

Combination therapy involving doxycycline and rifampin is generally recommended for brucellosis (Figure 13.15). Prolonged treatment

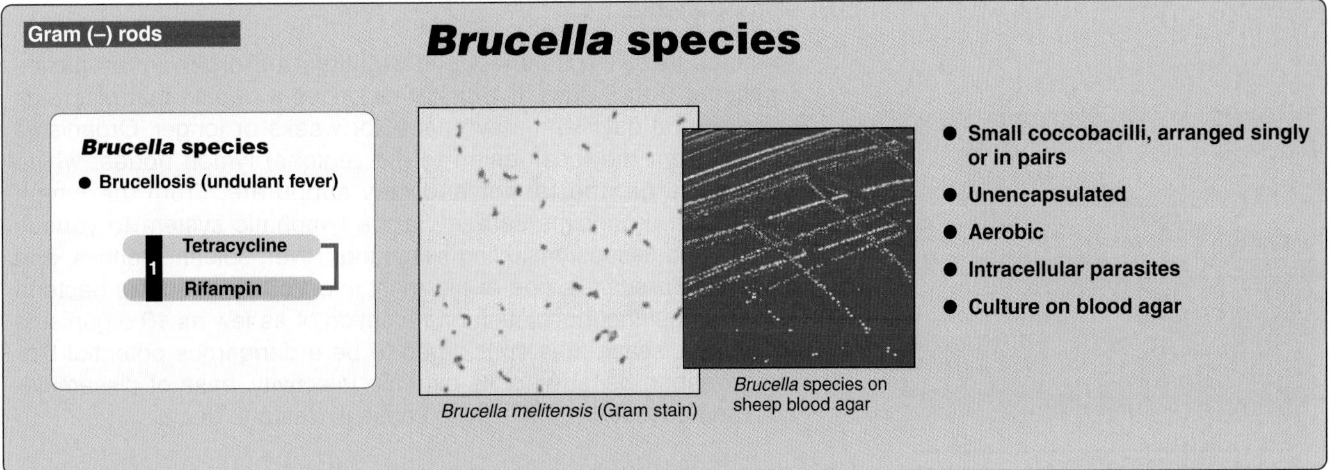

Figure 13.15
Summary of *Brucella* disease. **1** Indicates first-line drugs.

(for example, 6 weeks) is generally necessary to prevent relapse and reduce the incidence of complications.

VII. FRANCISELLA TULARENSIS

Francisella tularensis is primarily a pathogen of animals. Thus, tularemia (also known as rabbit fever and deerfly fever) is a zoonosis. The cells are small, pleomorphic coccobacilli that possess a polysaccharide capsule, which, although nontoxic, is a virulence factor (Figure 13.16). Members of the genus *Francisella* are facultative intracellular parasites that can survive and multiply within host macrophages as well as in other types of cells. The organisms are facultative anaerobes.

A. Epidemiology

The host range of *F. tularensis* is broad and includes wild mammals and birds. A number of biting or blood-sucking arthropods (for example, ticks, lice, and mites) can serve as vectors. Infection of humans occurs as a result of contact with infected animal tissues or the bite of an infected arthropod. Within particular geographic regions, specific vertebrates and invertebrate vectors are associated with transmission. For example, in the United States, the major (but not exclusive) endemic tularemic area encompasses Arkansas, Missouri, and Oklahoma. Incidence is most common in the summer months, a fact that reflects the arthropod transmission of the disease. During the winter months, a smaller peak incidence occurs, which reflects exposure of hunters to infected animal carcasses. Infection is also more common in males, because they have a greater exposure risk. Tularemia is an occupational risk for veterinarians, hunters, and trappers (see Figure 13.18), domestic livestock workers, and meat handlers. Recreational activities that increase exposure to ticks and biting flies also increase the risk of acquiring tularemia. There is no person-to-person transmission.

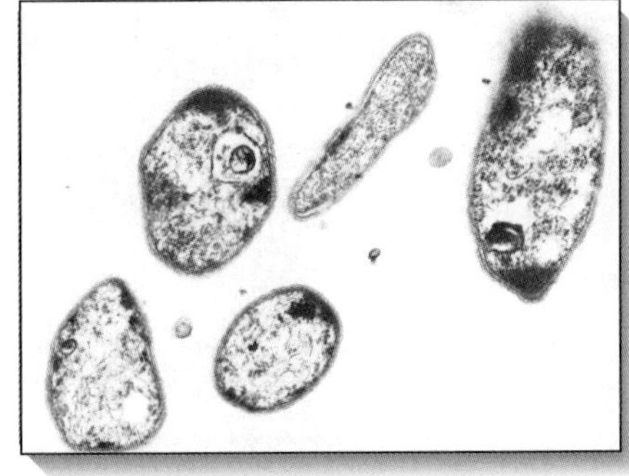

Figure 13.16
Electron micrograph showing the pleomorphic cells of *Francisella tularenis*.

B. Pathogenesis

In cases involving cutaneous inoculation, the organism multiplies locally for 3 to 5 days. It typically produces a papule that ulcerates after several days and may persist for weeks or longer. Organisms spread from the local lesion to the regional lymph nodes, which become large and tender and may suppurate. From the lymph nodes, the organisms spread via the lymphatic system to various organs and tissues, including skin, lungs, liver, spleen, kidneys, and CNS. *F. tularensis* is one of the most infectious pathogenic bacteria known, requiring inoculation or inhalation of as few as 10 organisms to cause disease. It is considered to be a dangerous potential biologic weapon because of its extreme infectivity, ease of dissemination, and substantial capacity to cause illness and death.

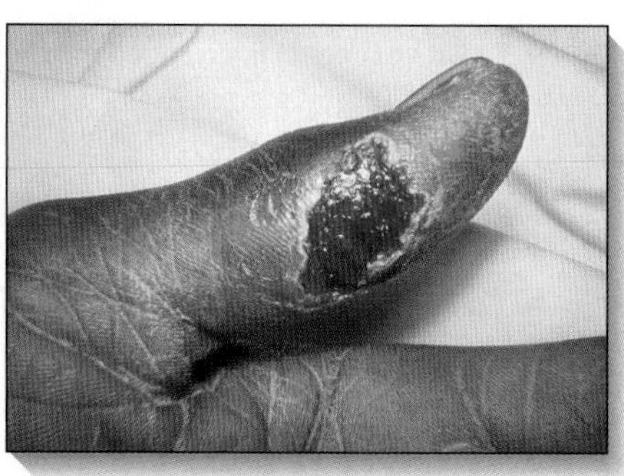

Figure 13.17
Thumb with skin ulcer of tularemia.

C. Clinical significance

Tularemia varies in severity from mild to fulminant and fatal. Clinical presentation, infectious dose, and length of the incubation period depend on the virulence of the organism, portal of entry, and host immunity. Onset of symptoms is usually abrupt. The most common symptoms are flulike (chills, fever, headache, malaise, anorexia, and fatigue), although respiratory and GI symptoms may also occur.

1. **Ulceroglandular tularemia:** The most common presentation of tularemia is ulceroglandular (Figure 13.17). Ulcers may result from contact with contaminated animal products (typically on the hands and/or forearms) or from insect bites (commonly on the trunk and/or lower extremities). Multiple lesions may occur. The location of affected lymph nodes also reflects the type of exposure. Lymphadenopathy is characteristic.

2. **Other forms of tularemia:** Tularemia characterized by lymphadenopathy without evidence of ulceration is known as glandular tularemia. In these cases, the ulcer may have been minimal or may have even healed prior to medical attention. In oculoglandular tularemia, the organism gains entry through the conjunctiva, which becomes inflamed. In pharyngeal tularemia, the organism gains entry through the pharynx and causes a severe sore throat. In pneumonic tularemia, the prominent feature of initial presentation is pulmonary. The pneumonia may be primary, a result of inhalation of infectious aerosols, or secondary, a result of hematogenous dissemination of the organisms from a primary site elsewhere in the body to the lungs. Systemic illness without lymphadenopathy or ulcerations is called typhoidal tularemia.

D. Laboratory identification

Clinical presentation and history consistent with possible exposure is of primary importance in diagnosis. Results of routine laboratory tests are not specific to tularemia. The organism may be cultured from ulcer scrapings, lymph node biopsies, gastric washings, and sputum but rarely from blood. *F. tularensis* is nutritionally fastidious and requires a sulfhydryl source such as cysteine. The organism is highly infectious, and laboratories must take special precautions when culturing specimens to avoid laboratory transmission. For this reason, the laboratory should be notified when there is suspicion of tularemia.

E. Treatment

The drug of choice for treatment of the forms of tularemia discussed above is streptomycin or gentamicin plus a tetracycline (Figure 13.18).

VIII. YERSINIA PESTIS

The genus *Yersinia* is a member of the family Enterobacteriaceae, which is presented in Chapter 12. The most clinically notorious member of this genus is *Yersinia pestis*, which causes plague, rather than enteric disease and, therefore, is being discussed separately from the rest of the family. In common with other Yersiniae, *Y. pestis* is a small rod that stains bipolarly (see Figure 13.21). *Y. pestis* produces a variety of plasmid-encoded virulence factors that are immunosuppressive or

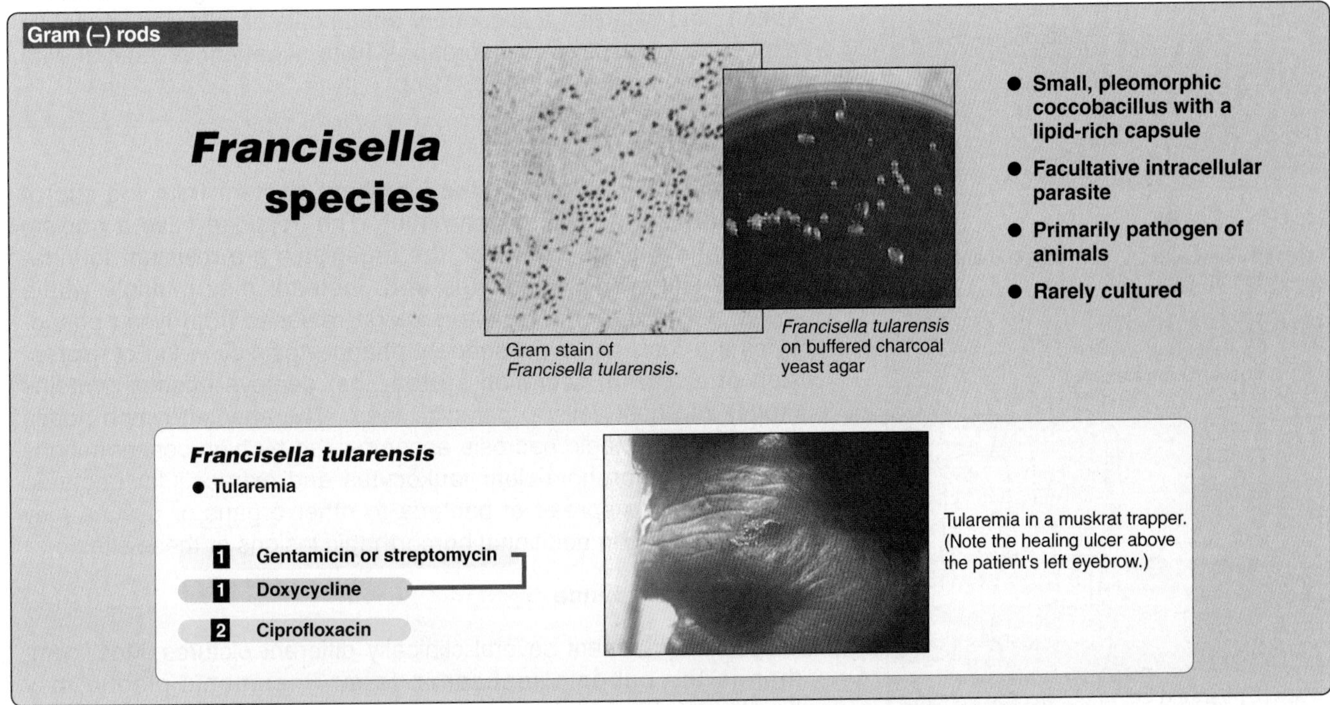

Gram (–) rods
Francisella species
Gram stain of Francisella tularensis.
Francisella tularensis on buffered charcoal yeast agar
Small, pleomorphic coccobacillus with a lipid-rich capsule
Facultative intracellular parasite
Primarily pathogen of animals
Rarely cultured
Francisella tularensis
Tularemia
1 Gentamicin or streptomycin
1 Doxycycline
2 Ciprofloxacin
Tularemia in a muskrat trapper. (Note the healing ulcer above the patient's left eyebrow.)

Figure 13.18
Summary of *Francisella* species. 1 Indicates first-line drugs; 2 indicates alternative drugs.

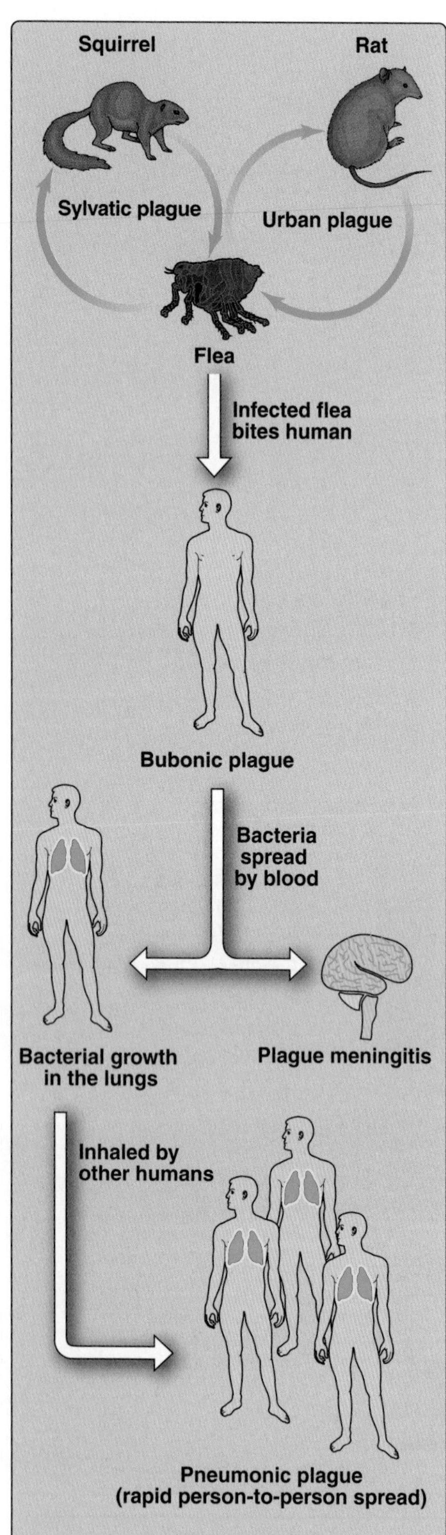

Figure 13.19
Epidemiology and pathology of plague.

antiphagocytic. These virulence factors include the Yop proteins, which are secreted by a type III secretion system; the Pla protease, which is a plasminogen activator that prevents blood clotting; and a proteinacious capsule (F1 antigen), which is antiphagocytic.

A. Epidemiology

Plague is predominantly a zoonosis with worldwide distribution. In the United States, the Southwest has been a primary focus of *Y. pestis* infection, although the distribution of human cases has been expanding into the Northwest and south-central states. The organism can infect a variety of mammals. For example, rats are common reservoirs in urban areas of some countries (urban plague). However, in the United States, plague is predominantly found in the wild, where prairie dogs and ground squirrels are the most important reservoirs (sylvatic plague). Household pets, particularly cats allowed to roam in plague-enzootic areas, may also become infected. Wild carnivores that ingest infected rodents can also be a source of transmission to humans who hunt or come into contact with these animals. Plague is characteristically transmitted by fleas, which serve to maintain the infection within the animal reservoir. Humans are generally accidental and dead-end hosts. Plague can also be transmitted by ingestion of contaminated animal tissue or via the respiratory route (pneumonic plague). [Note: The latter occurs either when organisms reach the lung via the bloodstream and establish a secondary pneumonia or following inhalation exposure to respiratory secretions from a patient or animal with plague pneumonia (Figure 13.19).]

B. Pathogenesis

Organisms are carried by the lymphatic system from the site of inoculation to regional lymph nodes. The Yersinae have a tropism for lymphoid tissue. However, the organisms are resistant to intracellular killing by phagocytes and, instead, may multiply within these cells. Furthermore, the bacteria released from lysed phagocytes are resistant to subsequent phagocytosis by virtue of expression of a type III secretion system that deploys effector proteins (Yops) into host cells to paralyze them. The affected lymph nodes display hemorrhagic necrosis accompanied by high concentrations of both polymorphonuclear leukocytes and extracellular bacteria. Hematogenous spread of bacteria to other organs or tissues may occur, resulting in additional hemorrhagic lesions at these sites.

C. Clinical significance

Plague may present several clinically different pictures. Most common is the bubonic/septicemic form. Pneumonic plague may develop as a result of spread to the lungs during septicemic plague or may be spread person-to-person via the respiratory route. Less common presentations include plague meningitis (typically a secondary focus resulting from hematogenous spread of the organisms), cutaneous plague, and pharyngitis (the latter two generally acquired by handling or ingesting contaminated animal tissue).

1. **Bubonic (septicemic) plague:** The infectious cycle begins when a flea ingests a blood meal from an animal that is infected and bacteremic. *Y. pestis* produces a biofilm that blocks the flea's midgut. This blockage prevents the flea from digesting the blood meal so it is consequently starved and voraciously feeds searching for a productive meal. *Y. pestis* multiplies in this environment. When the flea next attempts to feed, it regurgitates these bacteria from its foregut into the new animal's skin. The incubation period (from flea bite to development of symptoms) is generally 2 to 8 days. Onset of nonspecific symptoms, such as high fever, chills, headache, myalgia, and weakness that proceeds to prostration, is characteristically sudden. Within a short time, a characteristic, painful bubo develops (Figure 13.20). Buboes (pronounced swellings comprised of one or more infected nodes and surrounding edema that led to the term "bubonic plague") are typically located in the groin but may also occur in axillae or on the neck. As the disease proceeds, blood pressure generally drops, potentially leading to septic shock and death. Mortality of untreated bubonic plague generally exceeds 50 percent, with untreated and highly contagious pneumonic plague being invariably fatal unless promptly treated. Other manifestations associated with bubonic plague include pustules or vesicles containing leukocytes and *Y. pestis*. Purpura and necrosis of extremities may occur during systemic disease. [Note: Ingestion of contaminated meat or exposure to airborne bacilli can result in primary lesions in the pharynx. These produce a severe tonsillitis and cervical buboes.] Septicemic plague is a variation in which the patient is overwhelmed by massive bacteremia before the characteristic buboes develop.

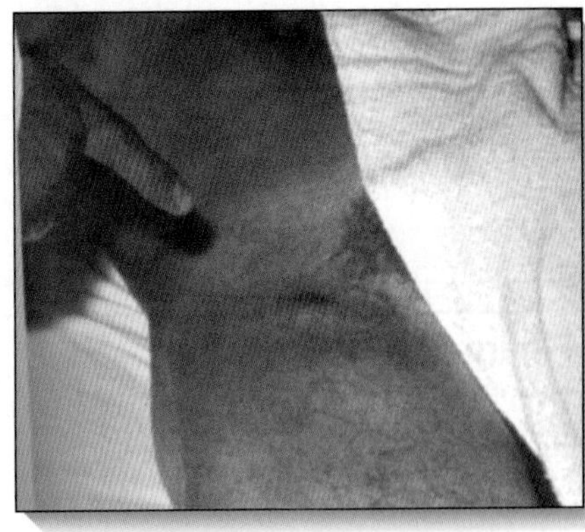

Figure 13.20
Bubo characteristic of infections due to *Yersinia pestis*.

2. **Pneumonic plague:** If plague bacilli reach the lungs, they cause hemorrhagic pneumonia that, if untreated, is rapidly fatal. It is also highly contagious person to person. The organisms can cause pneumonic plague directly if inhaled.

3. **Plague meningitis:** This results from hematogenous dissemination of organisms to the meninges. It may occur following inadequately treated bubonic plague or, like septicemic plague, may occur without, or prior to, development of a bubo. Organisms can be demonstrated in the CSF.

D. Laboratory identification

Diagnosis of *Y. pestis* infection may be made presumptively on the basis of clinical presentation. Laboratory identification can be initiated by a gram-stained smear, and culture of an aspirate from a bubo (or from CSF or sputum in the case of meningitis or pneumonic presentations). Blood cultures should be sent to the laboratory. The organism grows on both MacConkey and blood agar media, although colonies grow somewhat more slowly than those of other Enterobacteriaceae.

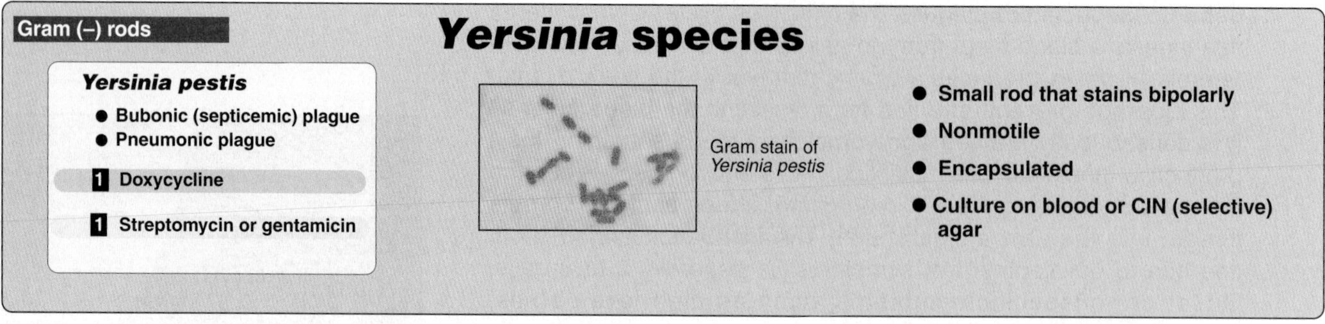

Figure 13.21
Summary of *Yersinia pestis* disease. 1 Indicates first-line drugs. CIN = cefsulodin-Irgasan-novobiocin.

E. Treatment and prevention

Streptomycin is the drug of choice, but gentamicin and doxycycline are acceptable alternatives (Figure 13.21). For plague meningitis, chloramphenicol offers good penetration into the CSF. Because of the potential for overwhelming septicemia, rapid institution of antibiotic therapy is crucial. Supportive therapy is essential for patients with signs of shock. A formalin-killed vaccine is available for those at high risk of acquiring plague. For individuals in enzootic areas, efforts to minimize exposure to rodents and fleas are important. Sick or dead rodents should never be touched with bare hands because infected fleas will seek attachment to a warm, living animal.

IX. BARTONELLA

Members of the genus *Bartonella* (formerly, *Rochalimaea*), facultative, intracellular parasites, can be cultivated on special media in the laboratory. Two species have been implicated in human diseases.

A. Bartonella quintana

Bartonella quintana causes trench fever, an often mild, relapsing fever with a maculopapular rash. The organism has a reservoir in humans, and its vector is the human body louse. The disease is, therefore, associated with humans living in poor sanitary conditions. Specific diagnosis can be aided by culture of clinical materials and serologic tests. Broad-spectrum antibiotics are effective in the treatment of the disease (Figure 13.22).

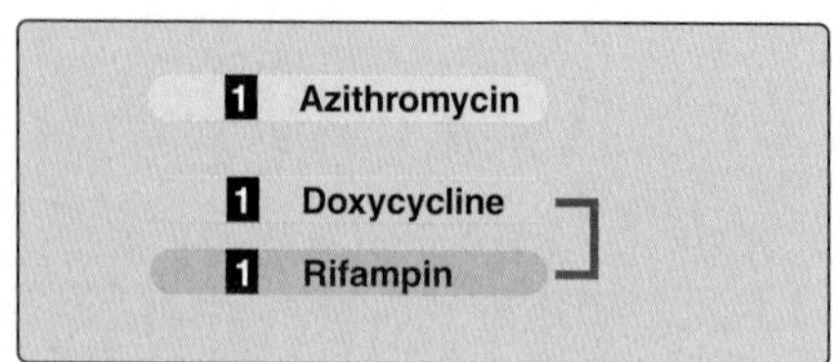

Figure 13.22
Antimicrobial agents useful in therapy of infections caused by *Bartonella* species.
1 Indicates first-line drugs.

B. Bartonella henselae

Bartonella henselae was recently shown to be associated with most cases of cat scratch disease, a syndrome that has been familiar to physicians for decades, but whose etiology had been elusive. The illness is characterized by small abscesses at the site of a cat (less commonly, other pets) scratch or bite. This is followed by fever and localized lymphadenopathy. *B. henselae* is also responsible for several other types of infections such as bacillary angiomatosis (a disease of small blood vessels of the skin and visceral organs) seen primarily in immunocompromised patients such as those with AIDS. *B. henselae* infections are successfully treated with rifampin in combination with doxycycline (see Figure 13.22).

X. PASTEURELLA

Members of the genus *Pasteurella* primarily colonize mammals and birds, both domestic and feral. Therefore, *Pasteurella* infections are considered zoonoses. The major human pathogen in this genus is *Pasteurella multocida*, which can cause either disease or asymptomatic infections. Pasteurellae are coccobacilli or rods that often exhibit bipolar staining, and some strains are encapsulated (Figure 13.23). Virulence factors include the organism's capsule and endotoxin. Pasteurellae are aerobes or facultative anaerobes.

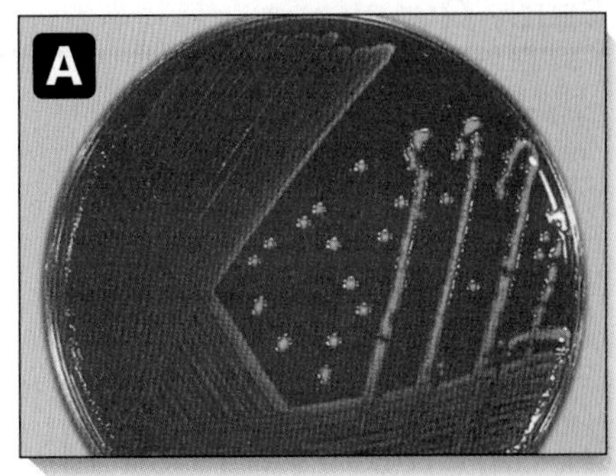

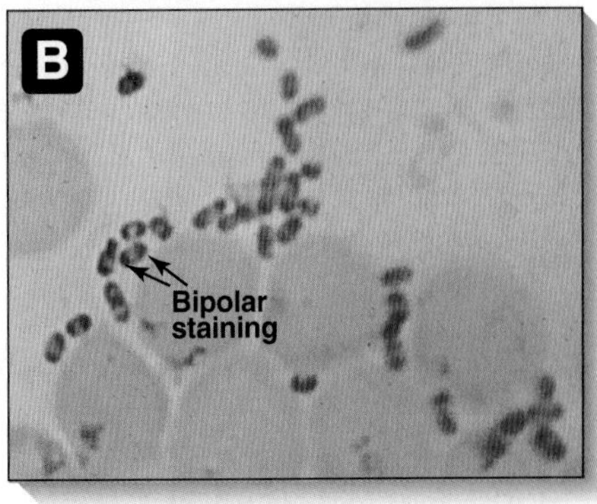

Figure 13.23
Pasteurella multocida. A. Culture on blood agar showing small, translucent nonhemolytic colonies. B. Blood smear, Wright stain. (Note bipolar staining.)

A. Epidemiology

The majority of *Pasteurella* infections in humans are soft tissue infections that follow an animal bite or cat scratch. A smaller fraction of human *Pasteurella* infections occur either following a non-bite animal exposure or in the absence of any known animal exposure. The source of Pasteurellae in the latter infections is suspected to be nasopharyngeal colonization of the patient.

B. Clinical significance

P. multocida infection should be suspected in cases of acute, painful cellulitis that develop within 24 hours of an animal bite or cat scratch. Soft tissue infections are characterized by the rapid onset of acute local inflammation within hours of the bite or scratch. Lesions often begin to drain within 1 to 2 days. Manifestations of *P. multocida* infection include cellulitis, lymphangitis; lymphadenitis, fever, and local complications, such as osteomyelitis and arthritis, which can result in extended disability.

C. Laboratory identification

Laboratory diagnosis (essential in non–bite/scratch-associated cases) can be accomplished by culturing the organism on blood agar and performing appropriate biochemical tests.

D. Treatment

For soft tissue infections, wounds should be cleansed, irrigated, and debrided. Deep-seated infections require surgical drainage and prolonged antibiotic treatment. Penicillin is the drug of choice (Figure 13.24). Fatal infections are uncommon and usually reflect underlying host compromise.

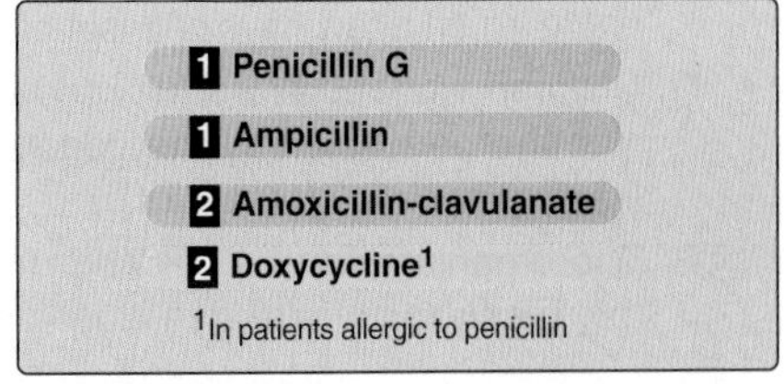

1 Penicillin G
1 Ampicillin
2 Amoxicillin-clavulanate
2 Doxycycline[1]
[1] In patients allergic to penicillin

Figure 13.24
Antimicrobial agents useful in therapy of infections caused by *Pasteurella multocida*. 1 Indicates first-line drugs; 2 indicates alternative drugs.

Study Questions

Choose the ONE correct answer

13.1 Which of the following is true of *Haemophilus influenzae*?

A. Invasive infections are most commonly associated with encapsulated strains.
B. Most invasive infections occur in infants during the neonatal period.
C. Most human infections are acquired from domestic pets.
D. The organism can be readily cultured on sheep blood agar in an environment of elevated CO_2.
E. Older adults are rarely at risk for infection with this organism because they typically have a high level of immunity.

Correct answer = A. The capsule is antiphagocytic, and facilitates hematogenous dissemination of *Haemophilus influenzae.* Although *H. influenzae* is an important pathogen of infants and young children, passive transfer of maternal immunoglobulin G may afford neonates protection. Immunity begins to wane in older adults, increasing the risk of infection for this population. Humans are the only natural host for *H. influenzae. H. influenzae* requires both hemin, X factor, and nicotinamide adenine dinucleotide (NAD), V factor, which are not available in sheep blood agar. Heating the blood lyses the erythrocytes, releasing both X and V factors, and simultaneously inactivating an NAD-inactivating enzyme present in blood. Media made with such heated blood is termed "chocolate agar." The organism does prefer elevated CO_2.

13.2 For which of the following organisms is there no known animal reservoir?

A. *Francisella tularensis*
B. *Pasteurella multocida*
C. *Bordetella pertussis*
D. *Brucella melitensis*
E. *Yersinia pestis*

Correct answer = C. *Francisella tularensis* has a broad host range, including wild and domestic mammals, birds, and house pets. *Pasteurella multocida* primarily colonizes mammals and birds, both domestic and feral. *Brucella melitensis* primarily infects sheep and goats. *Yersinia pestis* infects a variety of mammals.

13.3 Which of the following statements about *Bordetella pertussis* infection is true?

A. Infection causes a leukocytosis characterized primarily by a marked elevation in polymorphonuclear leukocytes.
B. Isolation of the organism from clinical specimens is greatest during the early stages of illness.
C. Clinical diagnosis of whooping cough can usually be made within a few days of onset of initial symptoms.
D. Children who receive a full series of immunizations with the pertussis vaccine generally develop solid, lifelong immunity to pertussis.
E. The organism can be cultured on standard laboratory media such as sheep blood agar.

Correct answer = B. *Bordetella pertussis* typically causes a lymphocytic leukocytosis. Initial symptoms of *Bordetella* infection are relatively nonspecific (rhinorrhea, etc.). The characteristic paroxysmal coughing begins somewhat later. Maintenance of solid immunity depends on repeated exposure to the organism, either through natural causes or by administration of booster shots. Growth of *Bordetella* requires a medium containing a substance such as charcoal to absorb or neutralize inhibitory substances and also antibiotics that inhibit the growth of normal flora.

13.4 Which of the following is transmitted to humans via an arthropod vector?

A. *Pseudomonas aeruginosa*
B. *Legionella pneumophila*
C. *Yersinia pestis*
D. *Brucella abortus*
E. *Pasteurella multocida*

Correct answer = C. *Yersinia pestis* can be transmitted to humans via the bite of an infected flea. The organism can also be transmitted person to person via the respiratory route if the lungs of the source patient or animal are infected. *Brucella abortus* infection is acquired via skin abrasions or ingestion. *Pseudomonas aeruginosa* is transmitted via direct inoculation into the respiratory tract, urinary tract, or into wounds in the hospital setting. *Legionella pneumophila* is acquired by inhalation of environmental ameba containing the bacteria. Free-living *L. pneumophila,* after multiplying in protozoa within water systems, can also be inhaled, resulting in Legionnaire disease or Pontiac fever. *Pasteurella multocida* is most commonly transmitted to humans via the bite of an infected animal.

Clostridia and Other Anaerobic Rods

14

I. OVERVIEW

The organisms discussed in this chapter are all obligate anaerobes. These microorganisms obtain energy exclusively by fermentation, and the presence of oxygen is inhibitory to their growth. Their sensitivity to oxygen limits the conditions under which these organisms can colonize the human body or cause disease. The obligate anaerobic genus, *Clostridium*, consists of gram-positive, spore-forming rods that are associated with soft tissue and skin infections (for example, cellulitis and fasciitis), and antibiotic-associated colitis and diarrhea. These organisms also synthesize some of the most potent exotoxins known. For example, the toxins of specific clostridial species cause botulism, tetanus, gas gangrene, and pseudomembranous colitis. A number of anaerobic, gram-negative rods, such as *Bacteroides* and related genera, are frequently involved in visceral and other abscesses, although these are generally polymicrobic (mixed) infections in which some facultative bacteria are also involved. The organisms discussed in this chapter are listed in Figure 14.1.

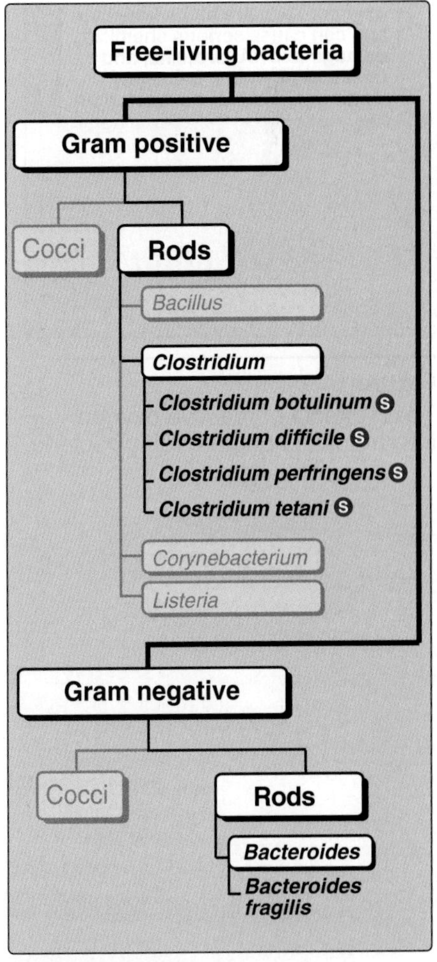

Figure 14.1
Classification of organisms in this chapter. Ⓢ See pp. 336–337 for summaries of these organisms.

II. CLOSTRIDIA

Clostridia are the anaerobic gram-positive rods of greatest clinical importance. Other clinically important gram-positive rods are aerobic. Clinically significant species of *Clostridium* include *Clostridium perfringens*, which causes histotoxic (tissue destructive) infections (myonecrosis) and food poisoning; *Clostridium difficile*, which causes pseudomembranous colitis associated with antibiotic use; *Clostridium tetani*, which causes tetanus ("lockjaw"); and *Clostridium botulinum*, which causes botulism.

A. General features of clostridia

Clostridia are large, gram-positive, blunt-ended rods. They form endospores, and the position of the developing spore within the vegetative cell is useful in identifying the species (see Figure 14.10). Most species are motile.

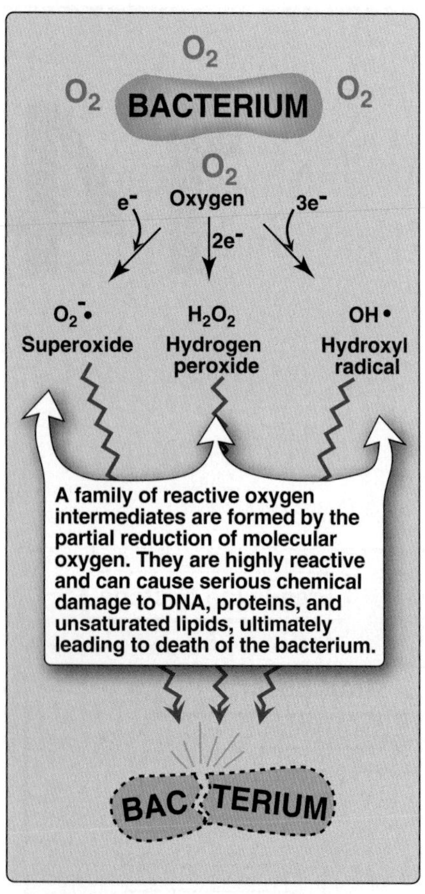

Figure 14.2
Toxic effects of reactive oxygen intermediates on anaerobic bacteria.

1. **Physiology:** *Clostridia* cannot use free oxygen as the terminal electron acceptor in energy production as do aerobic organisms (see p. 22). Instead, they use a variety of small organic molecules, such as pyruvate, as the final electron acceptors in the generation of energy. In the vegetative state, *Clostridia* are also variably inhibited or damaged by O_2 (Figure 14.2). [Note: The reasons for this damage are not entirely clear. One explanation is that some *Clostridia* lack enzymes such as peroxidases, catalase, or superoxide dismutase. These enzymes allow aerobes to detoxify reactive oxygen species including peroxides and hydroxyl radicals. Without the capacity to produce these detoxifying enzymes, *Clostridia* are damaged or growth-inhibited under aerobic conditions.] *Clostridia* grow on enriched media in the presence of a reducing agent, such as cysteine or thioglycollate (to maintain a low oxidation-reduction potential) or in an O_2-free, gaseous atmosphere provided by an air-evacuated glove box, sealed jar, or other device.

2. **Epidemiology:** *Clostridia*, part of the intestinal flora in humans and other mammals, are found in soil, sewage, and aquatic settings, particularly those with high organic content. A number of clostridial species produce destructive and invasive infections when introduced into tissues (for example, by a break in the skin resulting from surgery or trauma). Their presence in infectious processes is opportunistic and often is due to the patient's normal flora. Endospore formation facilitates their persistence in the environment. Spores are resistant to chemical disinfectants and may withstand ultraviolet irradiation or boiling temperatures for some time, although not standard autoclaving conditions (121°C for 15 minutes at increased pressure).

B. Clostridium perfringens

C. perfringens is a large, nonmotile, gram-positive, encapsulated bacillus. It is ubiquitous in nature, with its vegetative form as part of the normal flora of the vagina and gastrointestinal (GI) tract. Its spores are found in soil. [Note: Spores are rarely seen in the body or following *in vitro* cultivation.] When introduced into tissue, however, *C. perfringens* can cause anaerobic cellulitis and myonecrosis (gas gangrene). Some strains of *C. perfringens* also cause a common form of food poisoning.

1. **Pathogenesis:** *C. perfringens* secretes a variety of exotoxins, enterotoxins, and hydrolytic enzymes that facilitate the disease process (Figure 14.3).

   a. **Exotoxins:** *C. perfringens* elaborates at least 12 exotoxins, designated by Greek letters. The most important of these, and the one that seems to be required for virulence in tissue, is α toxin. α Toxin is a lecithinase (phospholipase C) that degrades lecithin in mammalian cell membranes, causing lysis of endothelial cells as well as erythrocytes, leukocytes, and platelets. Other *C. perfringens* exotoxins have hemolytic or other cytotoxic and necrotic effects, either locally or when dispersed in the bloodstream. Perfringolysin O, or theta (θ) toxin, is a cholesterol-dependent hemolysin and an important virulence factor. *C. perfringens* strains are grouped A through E on the basis of their spectrum of exotoxins. Type A strains, which produce both α toxin and enterotoxin, are responsible for most human clostridial infections.

b. **Enterotoxin:** *C. perfringens* enterotoxin, a small, heat-labile protein, acts in the lower portion of the small intestine. The molecule binds to receptors on the epithelial cell surface and alters the cell membrane, disrupting ion transport (primarily in the ileum) and leading to loss of fluid and intracellular proteins. Interestingly, enterotoxin-producing strains are unusually heat resistant, the spores remaining viable for longer than an hour at 100°C, enhancing their threat as foodborne pathogens.

c. **Degradative enzymes:** *C. perfringens* is a metabolically vigorous organism that produces a variety of hydrolytic enzymes, including proteases, DNases, hyaluronidase, and collagenases, which liquefy tissue and promote the spread of infection. The resulting degradation products serve as fermentation substrates for the rapid metabolism of *C. perfringens*. This organism has one of the fastest doubling times recorded, at less than 10 minutes.

2. **Clinical significance:** The disease processes initiated by *C. perfringens* result from a combination of infection and the production of exotoxins and/or enterotoxins and degradative enzymes.

a. **Myonecrosis (gas gangrene):** Clostridial spores are introduced into tissue, for example, by contamination with infected soil, or by endogenous transfer from the intestinal tract. Severe and open wounds, such as compound fractures and other ischemia-producing injuries (for example, crush injuries), are a prime predisposing condition. α Toxin and other exotoxins are secreted, and extensive cell death ensues. Production of enzymes that break down extracellular matrix facilitates the spread of infection. Fermentation of tissue carbohydrates, lipids, and amino acids yields gas, and an accumulation of gas bubbles in the subcutaneous spaces produces a crinkling sensation on palpation (crepitation), hence, the name "gas gangrene" (Figure 14.4). [Note: The rapidly accumulating gas itself is a virulence factor because it dissects along tissue planes. By enlarging these potential spaces, the clostridia progress much more rapidly due to the decreased resistance they create with gas.] The majority of infections resulting in necrosis of muscle are due to *Clostridium* species (gas gangrene) and group A streptococci. The exudates are copious and foul smelling. As the disease progresses, increased capillary permeability allows exotoxins to be carried from damaged tissue to other organs, resulting in systemic effects, such as shock, renal failure, and intravascular hemolysis. Untreated clostridial myonecrosis is uniformly fatal within days of the initiation of gangrene.

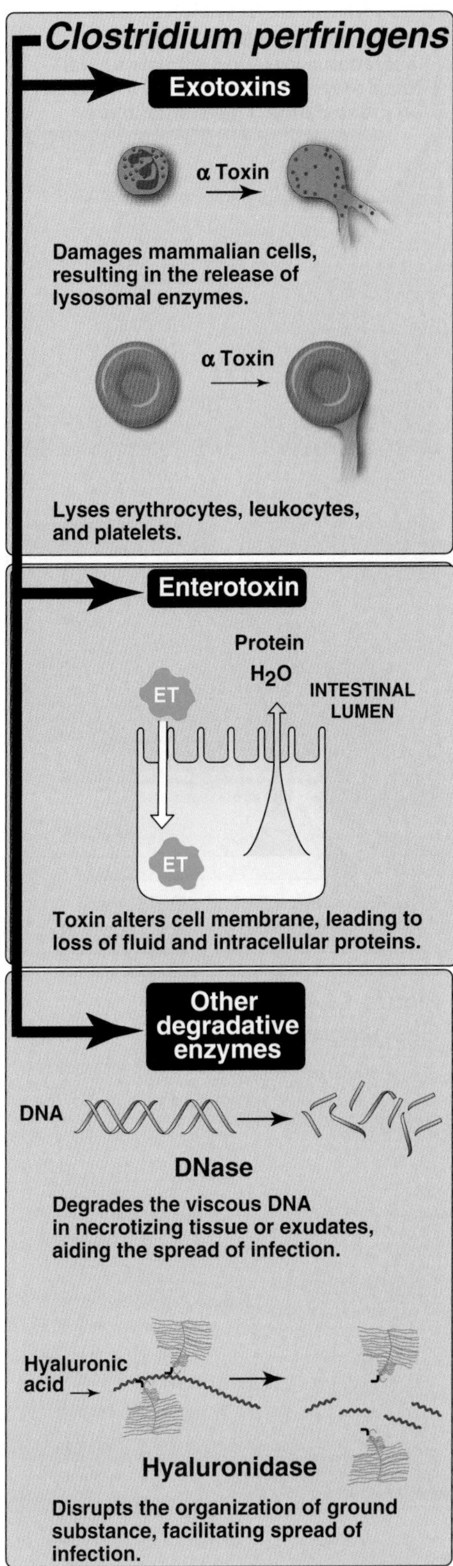

Figure 14.3
Toxins and degradative enzymes produced by *Clostridium perfringens*. ET = enterotoxin.

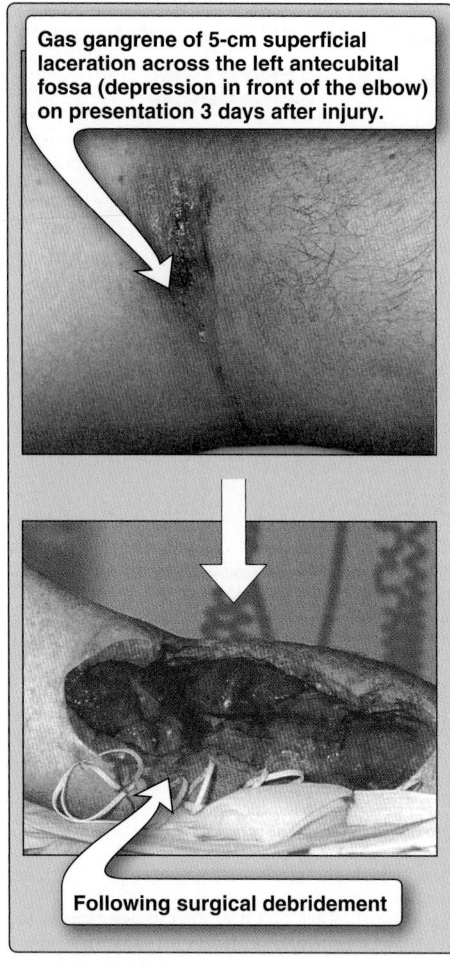

Gas gangrene of 5-cm superficial laceration across the left antecubital fossa (depression in front of the elbow) on presentation 3 days after injury.
Following surgical debridement

Figure 14.4
Gas gangrene of arm.

b. Anaerobic cellulitis: This is a clostridial infection of connective tissue in which the spread of bacterial growth along fascial planes (fasciitis) does not involve invasion of muscle tissue. Necrotizing processes play a more limited role, but surgical intervention is generally unsuccessful (unless it is carried out very promptly and aggressively) because of the rapid spread of infection and compromise of blood supply due to swelling beneath tight fascia.

c. Foodborne infection: *C. perfringens* is a common cause of foodborne infection in the United States. Typically, the onset of nausea, abdominal cramps, and diarrhea occurs 8 to 18 hours after eating contaminated food. Fever is absent and vomiting rare. The attack is usually self-limited, with recovery within 1 to 2 days. The occurrence of clinical symptoms requires a large inoculum of 10^8 organisms or greater. Therefore, a typical episode of clostridial enterotoxin food poisoning involves cooking that fails to inactivate spores, followed by holding the food for several hours under conditions that allow bacterial germination and several cycles of growth. Vegetative cells are consumed in the contaminated product, and *C. perfringens* then reproduces following ingestion (food infection) and produces toxin *in vivo*. Meats, meat products, and gravy are the most commonly implicated foods in *C. perfringens* foodborne illness.

d. Necrotic enteritis: Outbreaks of a necrotizing bowel disease with high mortality (greater than 50 percent) caused by *C. perfringens* have been sporadically reported.

e. Clostridial endometritis: This condition is a grave complication of incomplete abortion or the use of inadequately sterilized instruments. Gangrenous infection of uterine tissue is followed by illness due to toxins and bacteremia.

3. Laboratory identification: Diagnosis of clostridial myonecrosis or cellulitis rests largely on clinical presentation. The presence of clostridia in clinical materials may be adventitious (that is, an accidental contamination). With Gram stain, however, specimens from diseased tissue usually show vegetative clostridial forms (large, gram-positive rods), accompanied by other bacteria and cellular debris. When cultured anaerobically on blood agar, *C. perfringens* grows rapidly, producing colonies with a unique double zone of hemolysis due to production of α toxin (partial hemolysis) and perfringolysin O (complete hemolysis) as shown in Figure 14.5. In food infection, the organism can be sought in suspected food and the patient's feces. Gram stain and other laboratory findings greatly help planning of antibiotic therapy in patients with clinical manifestations of gas gangrene.

4. Treatment and prevention: The key to both prevention and treatment of gas gangrene is immediate and thorough removal of foreign material and devitalized tissue and exposure of the wound to O_2. Hyperbaric oxygen chambers increase the tissue O_2 tension in the affected part and inhibit the pathologic process. If debridement is unable to control the progression of the gangrene, amputation, when anatomically possible, is mandatory in gangrene. Supplementary to this is the administration of antibiotics in high doses. *C. perfringens* is sensitive to penicillin and several common inhibitors of prokaryotic protein synthesis (see Figure 14.10). Because clostridial infections usually involve a mixture of species, the use of broad-spectrum antibiotics is appropriate.

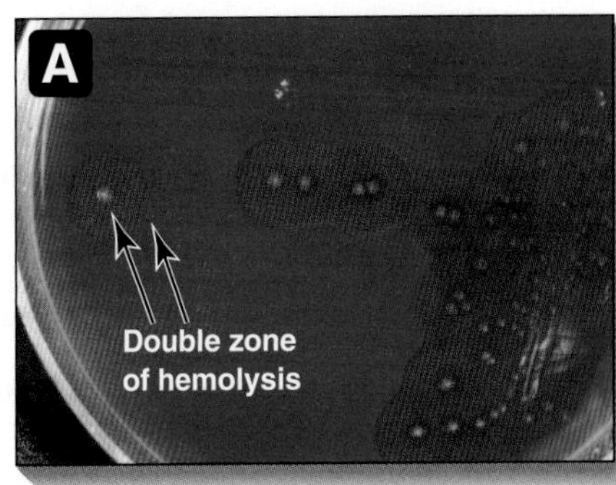

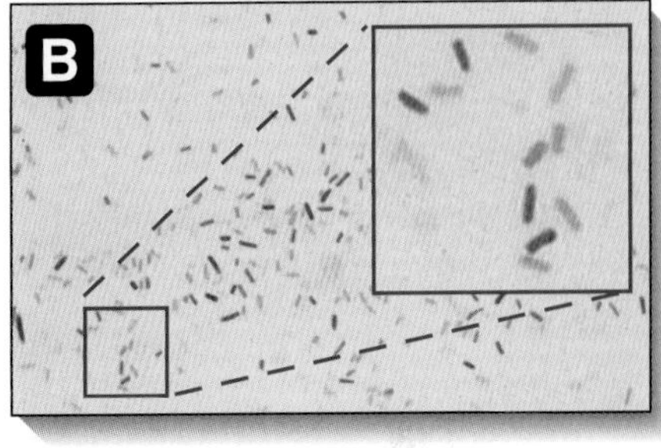

Figure 14.5
Clostridium perfringens. A. Colonies on blood agar showing double zone of hemolysis. B. Photomicrograph of Gram stain.

C. Clostridium botulinum

C. botulinum causes botulism, which occurs in several clinical forms. Botulism is caused by the action of a neurotoxin that is one of the most potent poisons known and causes a flaccid paralysis. Contact with the organism itself is not required, and the the disease can be solely due to ingestion of toxin-contaminated food.

1. **Epidemiology:** *C. botulinum* is found worldwide in soil and aquatic sediments, and the spores frequently contaminate vegetables and meat or fish. Under appropriate conditions, including a strictly anaerobic environment at neutral or alkaline pH, the organism germinates, and toxin is produced during vegetative growth. Because the toxin is often elaborated in food, outbreaks frequently occur in families or other eating groups.

2. **Pathogenesis:** There are several types of botulinum toxin, designated A through G, but human disease is almost always caused by types A, B, or E. The botulinum and tetanus toxins constitute a homologous set of proteins whose neurotoxicity arises from proteolytic cleavage of specific synaptic vesicle peptides, causing subsequent failure of neurotransmission. In contrast to tetanus toxin, which causes constant contraction (spasms, see p. 154), botulinum toxins affect peripheral cholinergic synapses by blocking the neuromuscular junction and inhibiting release of the neurotransmitter acetylcholine, preventing contraction and causing flaccid paralysis (Figure 14.6). Both botulinum and tetanus toxins are AB-type toxins comprised of an activity domain (A) and a binding domain (B).

3. **Clinical significance:**

   a. **Classic botulism:** Food poisoning in which a patient first begins to experience difficulties in focusing vision, swallowing, and other cranial nerve functions, 12 to 36 hours after ingesting toxin-containing food but not necessarily viable organisms is classic botulism. There is no fever or sign of sepsis. A progressive paralysis of striated muscle groups develops, and mortality rate is about 15 percent, with the patient usually succumbing to respiratory paralysis. Recovery, which involves regeneration of the damaged nerves, is protracted, lasting several weeks.

   b. **Infant botulism:** The most common form of botulism in the United States today is infant botulism, or a cause of floppy

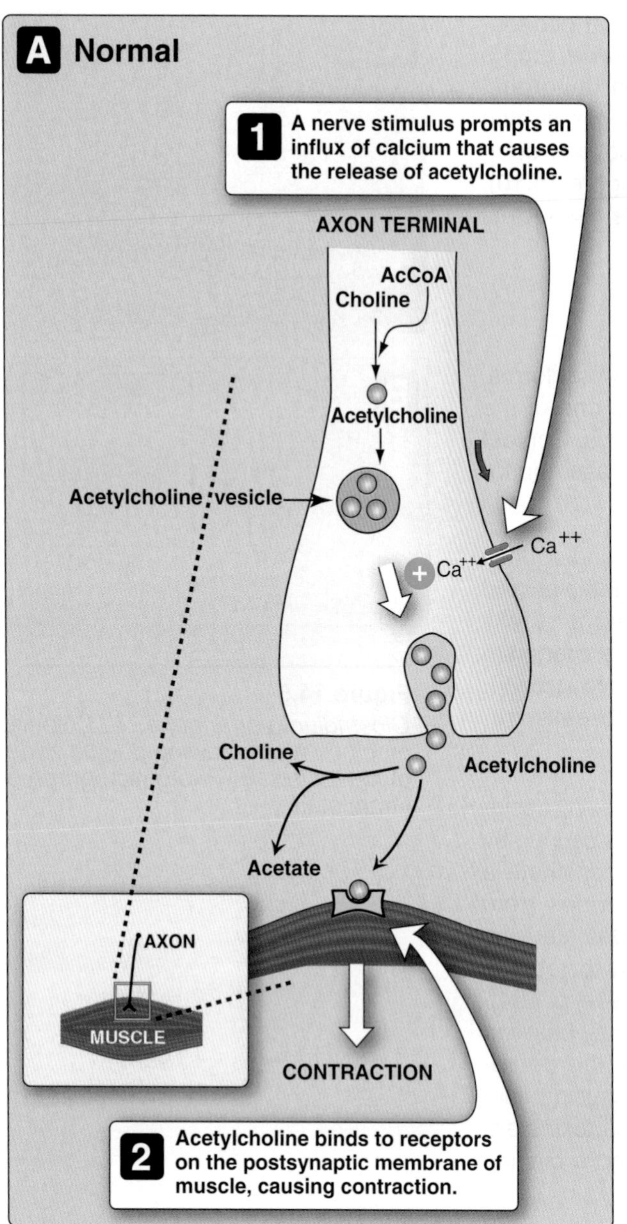

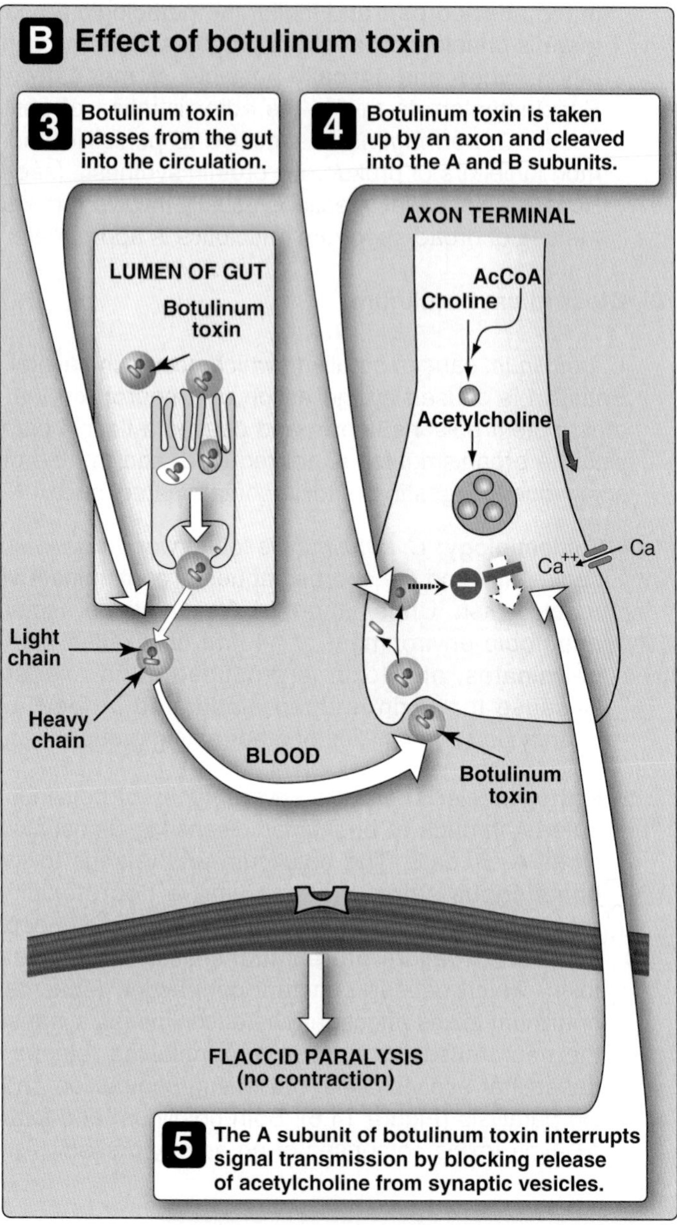

Figure 14.6
Mechanism of botulinum toxin. AcCoA = acetyl CoA.

baby syndrome (see Figure 14.10). An infant has yet to develop mature colonic microbial flora. Therefore, without competition, *C. botulinum* can colonize the large bowel of infants and produce toxin. The botulinum toxin is produced *in vivo* and slowly absorbed. Constipation, feeding problems, lethargy, and poor muscle tone are common early signs. Supplementation of infant foods (cereals or formula) with raw honey, which is contaminated with *C. botulinum* spores, may transmit the organism. The condition is possibly a cause of sudden infant death syndrome, but recovery is the usual outcome, following symptomatic treatment that may be prolonged.

c. **Wound botulism:** A rare form of botulism occurs when a wound becomes contaminated with the organism, and toxin is absorbed from that site. The molecular pathogenesis of this infection is similar to that of tetanus.

4. **Laboratory identification:** The organism can be cultured and identified by standard anaerobic methods (see p. 22). Toxin is also identifiable in serum, stool, and food.

5. **Treatment and prevention:** Antitoxin, which neutralizes unbound botulinum toxin, should be administered as soon as possible in suspected botulinal intoxication. A trivalent (A, B, E) horse antiserum is available from the Centers for Disease Control. Supportive measures, including mechanical ventilation, may be required. In wound and infant botulism, the infection can be treated with penicillin or other antibiotics to which the organism is sensitive. The toxin is inactivated at boiling temperatures, although killing of botulinal spores requires moist heat under pressure (autoclaving). [Note: Even the most severe cases of botulism do not result in immunity.]

D. Clostridium tetani

The introduction of *C. tetani* spores into even small wounds via contaminated soil is probably a common occurrence. But a combination of the extreme O_2 sensitivity of vegetative *C. tetani* and widespread immunization against its exotoxin, make the resulting disease, tetanus, rare in developed countries. In the United States, the disease is seen most often in older individuals who have not received their immunization boosters regularly and whose immunity has, therefore, waned. Growth of *C. tetani* is completely local, but it produces a powerful neurotoxin that is transported to the central nervous system, where it causes spastic paralysis.

1. **Epidemiology:** *C. tetani* spores are common in barnyard, garden, and other soils. The most typical focus of infection in tetanus is a puncture wound caused, for example, by a splinter. Introduced foreign bodies or small areas of cell killing create a nidus of devitalized material in which tetanus spores can germinate and grow. Special circumstances may also lead to tetanus, for example, after severe burns, surgery or ischemia. Illicit drugs can contain spores that are introduced by injection.

2. **Pathogenesis:** Tetanus toxin, called tetanospasmin, is an extremely potent toxin. It is transported from an infected locus by retrograde neuronal flow or blood. A plasmid-coded exotoxin of a single antigenic type, it is produced as a single polypeptide that is cleaved to generate the mature toxin of two chains held together by a disulfide bond. The heavy fragment (B, or binding subunit) mediates binding to neurons and cell penetration of the light fragment (A, or activity subunit). The A subunit blocks neurotransmitter release at inhibitory synapses, thereby causing severe, prolonged muscle spasms (Figure 14.7). The A fragment has

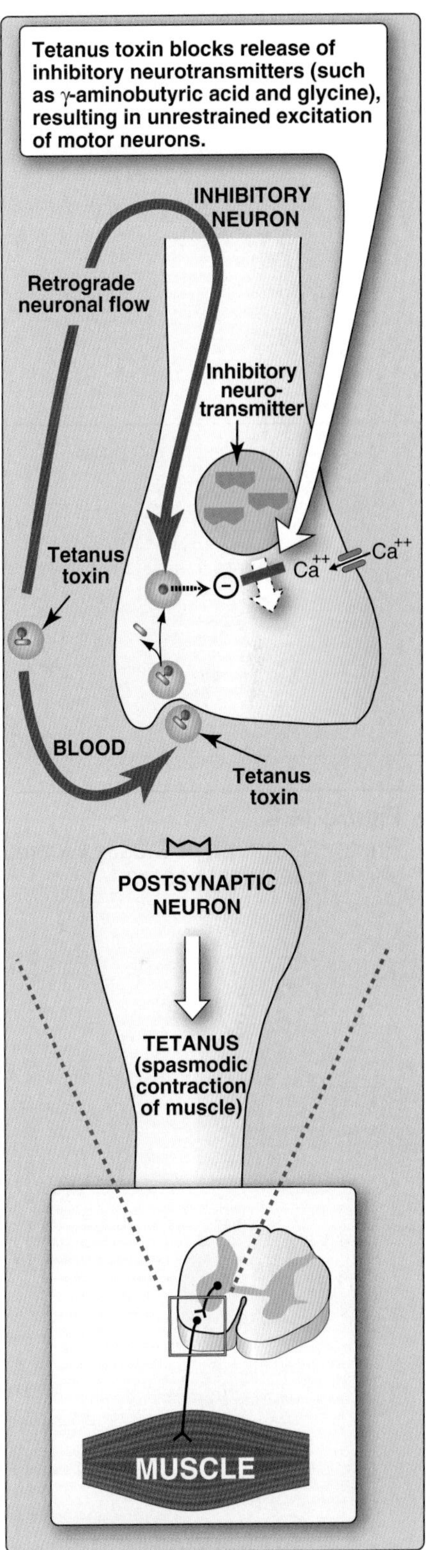

Figure 14.7
Mechanism of tetanus toxin.

been shown to be a protease, cleaving a small synaptic vesicle protein (synaptobrevin) and abolishing the flow of inhibitory neurotransmitters, including glycine and γ-aminobutyric acid.

3. **Clinical significance:** Tetanus has an incubation period varying from 4 days to several weeks. A shorter period is usually associated with more severe disease and wounds closer to the brain. Tetanus presents as a spastic paralysis, in which muscle spasms often first involve the site of infection. In the early stages of the disease, the jaw muscles are affected, so that the mouth cannot open (trismus, or "lockjaw"). Gradually, other voluntary muscles become involved (see Figure 14.10), and any external stimulus (for example, noise or bright light) precipitates a painful spasm and, sometimes, convulsions. Death, which occurs in 50 to 60 percent of cases, is usually the result of paralysis of chest muscles leading to respiratory failure.

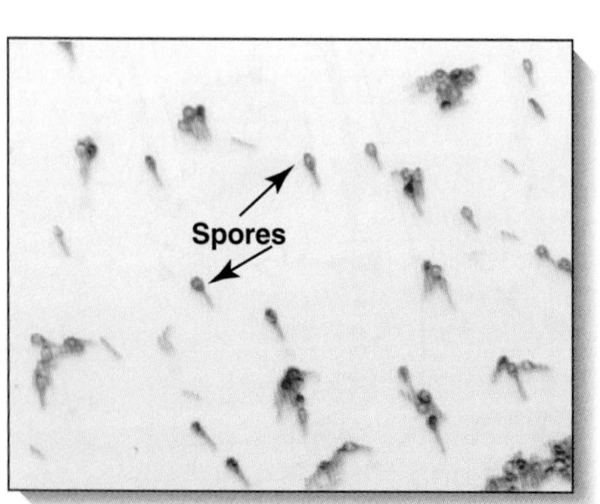

Figure 14.8
Photomicrograph of *Clostridium tetani* showing terminal spores.

4. **Laboratory identification:** Because treatment must be initiated immediately, the diagnosis of tetanus is based largely on clinical findings. The focus of infection is often a trivial wound that may be difficult to locate. *C. tetani* has a characteristic morphology, with a long, slender rod and round, terminal spore (racket-shaped bacillus) as shown in Figure 14.8, and characteristic swarming growth on anaerobic blood agar.

5. **Treatment:** Prompt administration of antitoxin to neutralize any toxin not yet bound to neurons is the first order of treatment. Treatment with human hyperimmune globulin (tetanus immune globulin) is preferred, but, in countries where it is not available, horse antitoxin is used. The organism is sensitive to penicillin, and this drug can be used to eradicate the infection, together with debridement of necrotic tissue at the entry wound. Therapy includes treatment with sedatives and muscle relaxants to minimize spasms and attention to maintenance of ventilation.

6. **Prevention:** Active immunization with tetanus toxoid (formalin-inactivated toxin) prevents tetanus. It is usually administered to children as a triple vaccine with diphtheria toxoid and pertussis antigens (DTaP). Recent studies have confirmed that circulating antibody levels gradually decline and that many older individuals lose protection. Therefore, booster immunizations with a preparation of diphtheria and tetanus toxoids given every 10 years throughout life are recommended. Tetanus immunoglobulin can be used to give immediate passive immunity to injury victims with no history of immunization. Active immunization should also be started. Antitoxin and toxoid, administered in different areas of the body, can be given simultaneously.

E. Clostridium difficile

Diarrhea, a common complication of antimicrobial drug treatment, can range from loose stools to life-threatening pseudomembranous colitis (PMC) as shown in Figure 14.10. *C. difficile* is estimated to be responsible for at least one fourth of antibiotic-associated diarrheas

(AADs) in hospitalized patients and almost all cases of PMC. After its introduction to a site, the environment (that is, dust, bedding, toilets, etc.) becomes persistently contaminated with spores, and new residents are easily colonized. They are then at higher risk for developing the adverse intestinal effect of antibiotic treatments.

1. **Pathogenesis:** *C. difficile* is a minor component of the normal flora of the large intestine. When antimicrobial treatment suppresses more predominant species in this community, *C. difficile* proliferates. Pathogenic strains produce two toxic polypeptides, designated toxins A and B. Toxin A is an enterotoxin that causes excessive fluid secretion, but also stimulates an inflammatory response, and has some cytopathic effect in tissue culture. Toxin B is a cytotoxin. In tissue culture, it disrupts protein synthesis and causes disorganization of the cytoskeleton. Both toxins A and B are glucosyltransferases that glucosylate and inactivate Rho-family guanosine triphosphate–binding proteins.

2. **Clinical significance:** Virtually all antimicrobial drugs have been reported as predisposing to clostridial AAD and colitis (Figure 14.9). The three drugs most commonly implicated are clindamycin, ampicillin, and the cephalosporins. The severity of disease varies widely from mild diarrhea through varying degrees of inflammation of the large intestine to a fulminant PMC. The pseudomembranous exudate, composed of mucus, fibrin, inflammatory cells, and cell debris overlying an ulcerated epithelium, is best demonstrated by endoscopy. PMC often begins some time after cessation of drug treatment or may recur after what should be adequate therapy. This is a consequence of the stability and persistence of the spores formed by *C. difficile*.

3. **Laboratory identification:** *C. difficile* can be cultured from stools and identified by routine anaerobic procedures, but the more rapid and useful tests are directed at demonstrating toxin production in stool extracts. Enzyme immunoassays (ELISA, see p. 27) for exotoxins A and B have replaced earlier immunologic or tissue culture cytotoxicity assays. Polymerase chain reaction–based detection strategies are also widely available.

4. **Treatment:** Discontinuance of the predisposing drug and fluid replacement usually lead to resolution of the symptoms. Relapses, however, are common. Oral administration of metronidazole or vancomycin is usually added (Figure 14.10). Reconstitution of the host's normal colonic flora may aid in the recovery.

Frequently associated

- Ampicillin
- Amoxicillin
- Cephalosporins
- Clindamycin

Occassionally associated

- Penicillins other than ampicillin
- Sulfonamides
- Erythromycin
- Trimethoprim
- Quinolones

Rarely or never associated

- Parenteral aminoglycoside
- Tetracyclines
- Chloramphenicol
- Metronidazole
- Vancomycin

Figure 14.9
The potential of antimicrobial drugs to induce *Clostridium difficile* diarrhea and colitis.

III. ANAEROBIC GRAM-NEGATIVE RODS

Anaerobic gram-negative rods are normally the most common organisms in the oral cavity (particularly the gingiva), female genital tract, and lower GI tract, where they outnumber *Escherichia coli* 1,000:1. They are, therefore, frequently recovered from infections in various parts of the body (for example, gram-negative anaerobic rods are recovered in about 10 percent of bacteremias). Gram-negative rods generally

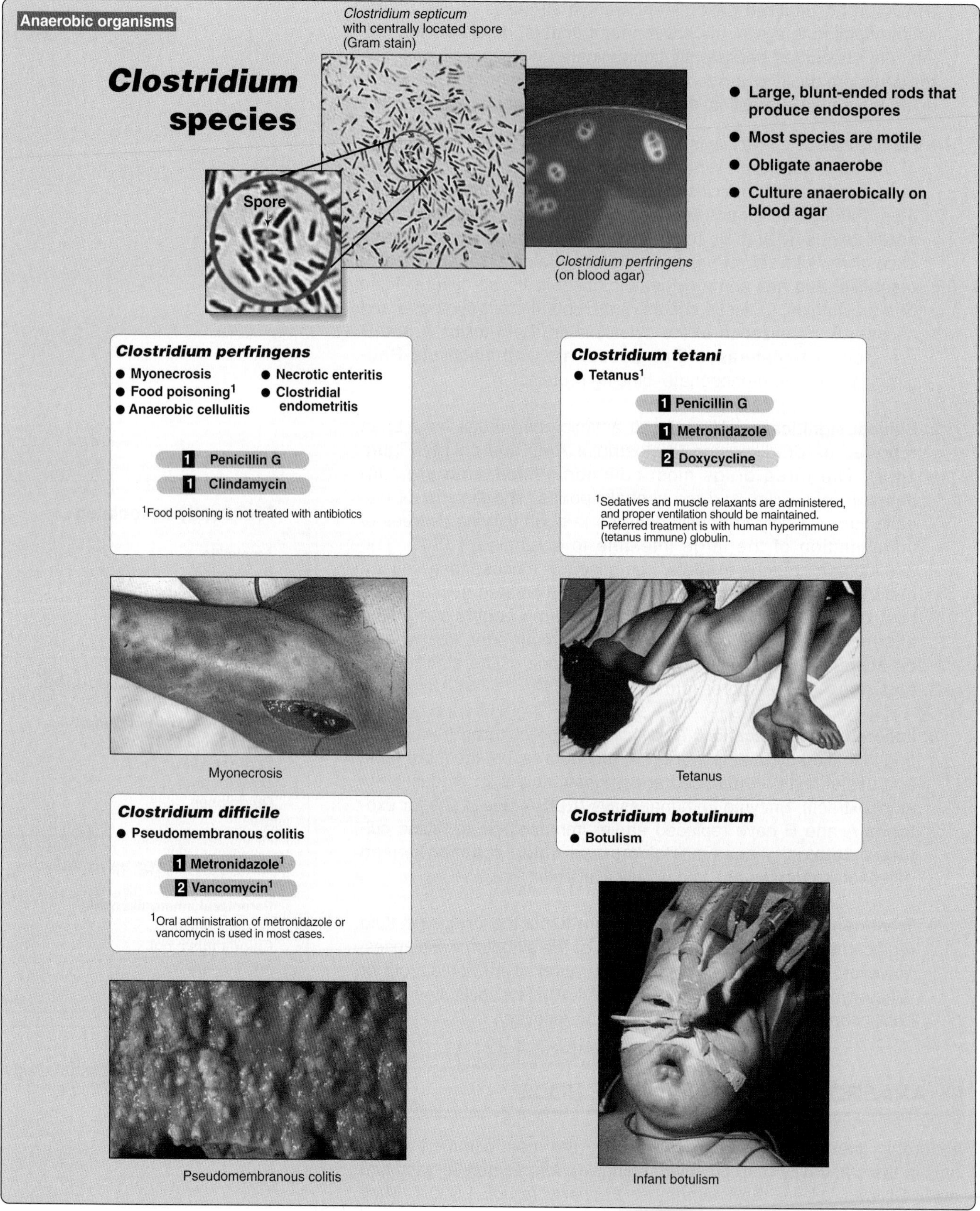

Figure 14.10
Summary of *Clostridium* species. 1 Indicates first-line drugs; 2 indicates alternative drugs.

constitute the majority of organisms associated with anaerobic abscesses. Organisms in this group may breach the host epithelial barrier and establish infection in any body tissue. This usually occurs because of trauma, an incident such as a ruptured appendix, or because of compromised immune status. A localized abscess is the most common lesion, and the infectious process often involves two or more species of organisms. For example, various facultative organisms help lower the pO_2, thus providing the anaerobic environment required by the coinfecting gram-negative rods (Figure 14.11).

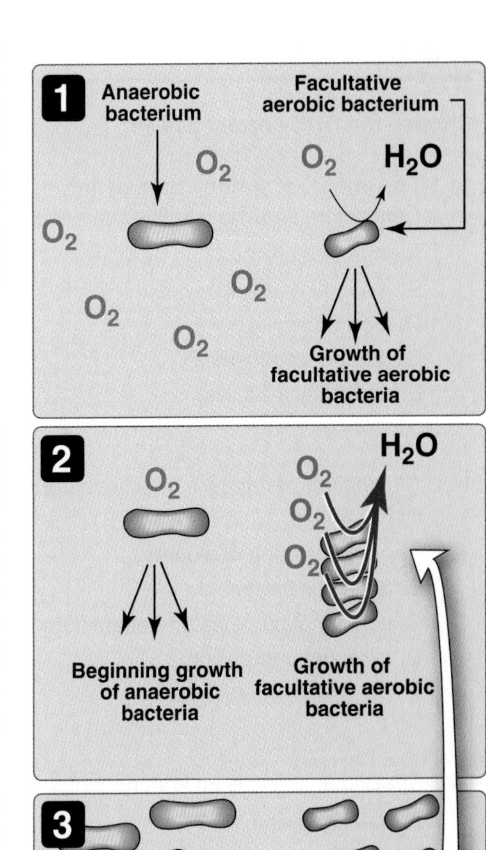

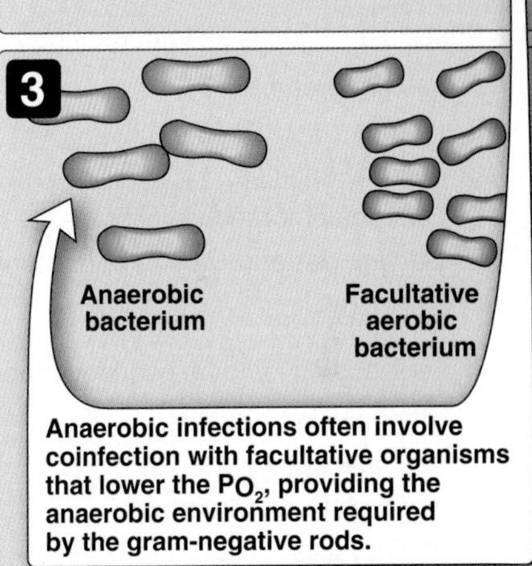

Figure 14.11
Anaerobic organisms growth is facilitated by facultative aerobic bacteria.

A. Bacteroides

Members of the genus *Bacteroides* are the predominant anaerobes found in the human colon. They are part of the normal flora and only cause disease when they gain access to tissues or the blood during bowel penetration (for example, during surgery or trauma). They are, however, the most common cause of serious infections by anaerobic organisms. *Bacteroides* are slender rods or coccobacilli. Their polysaccharide capsule is an important virulence factor, conveying resistance to phagocytosis. Purified capsule alone is sufficient to induce abscess formation in laboratory animals, indicating that this polysaccharide is key to the pathology seen with *Bacteroides* infections.

1. **Epidemiology:** *Bacteroides* are transmitted from the colon to the blood or peritoneum following abdominal trauma. Therefore, the source of infection is endogenous (it is not transmitted from person to person).

2. **Pathology and clinical significance:** The major disease-causing *Bacteroides* species is *Bacteroides fragilis*. When released from the colon into the blood, *B. fragilis* multiplies rapidly, causing bacteremia. If it is introduced into the abdominal cavity, *B. fragilis* causes peritonitis, and/or abdominal abscesses.

3. **Laboratory identification:** Exudates from mixed anaerobic lesions are often copious and noticeably foul smelling. A Gram stain of such exudates shows numerous faint, slender, gram-negative rods, usually in mixed flora. The organisms are easily obscured by debris and polymorphonuclear leukocytes. *B. fragilis* can be cultured on blood agar under anaerobic conditions. Gas chromatography can be used to identify the characteristic short-chain fatty acids produced by the organism, and biochemical tests can determine its sugar fermentation pattern.

4. **Treatment and prevention:** Drug resistance is common among the *Bacteroides*. Metronidazole is the antibiotic of choice for *B. fragilis* infections. Alternative choices include ampicillin-sulbactam, imipenem-cilastatin, ticarcillin-clavulanate, cefoxitin, or clindamycin. Aminoglycosides are, of course, ineffective against anaerobes (see p. 42). Surgical drainage of any abscess is essential to ensure penetration of drugs. To prevent *Bacteroides* contamination of a surgical wound, a perioperative antibiotic, such as cefoxitin, can be administered.

Study Questions

Choose the ONE correct answer

14.1 The most common form of infection caused by *Clostridium botulinum* in this country is:

A. infant botulism.
B. wound infection.
C. food poisoning.
D. primary septicemia.
E. anaerobic cellulitis.

Correct answer = A. Currently, the most common form of botulism in the United States occurs in infants. Malignant food poisoning (C) was the first-described form of infection and is probably the best known. A wound focus is rare (B). *Clostridium botulinum* is noninvasive and causes neither septicemia (D) nor cellulitis (E).

14.2 *Clostridium perfringens* infections are commonly associated with:

A. contamination of wounds.
B. antibiotic treatment.
C. consumption of water contaminated with sewage.
D. immunosuppression.
E. preexisting lung disease.

Correct answer = A. Contamination of wounds is the most common route of infection by this organism. However, the symptoms of gastroenteritis associated with some strains of *Clostridium perfringens* are usually caused by contamination of food.

14.3 Specific antitoxin is an important part of treatment in:

A. gas gangrene.
B. tetanus.
C. necrotic enteritis.
D. pseudomembranous colitis.
E. *Bacteroides* and *Prevotella* infections.

Correct answer = B. Tetanus antitoxin is an essential reagent in wound prophylaxis and the treatment of clinical disease. It neutralizes only that toxin that has not bound the neuronal receptors. In the case of gas gangrene (A), numerous clinical studies have shown no advantage in the use of antitoxin preparations, and, presumably, the same would be true for necrotic enteritis and pseudomembranous colitis (C and D). Possible toxins among the gram-negative anaerobes are poorly described, and no therapeutic antisera are available (E).

14.4 A predisposing factor in pseudomembranous colitis is:

A. clindamycin treatment.
B. neonatal age.
C. diet high in dairy products.
D. cholecystitis.
E. older age (older than age 60 years).

Correct answer = A. Antibiotic treatment is often complicated by gastrointestinal disturbances, including pseudomembranous colitis. Certain drugs, including clindamycin, are more likely to cause this complication.

14.5 A 67-year-old man, who is an avid gardener, presents at an emergency department. He is suffering from spastic paralysis, which began in his right hand and now extends to his jaw muscles. The causative agent of this infection produces a virulence factor with which of the following activities?

A. Overstimulation of T cells with resulting massive release of cytokines
B. Blockage of the release of the neurotransmitter acetylcholine from synaptic vesicles
C. Adenosine diphosphate–ribosylation of EF-2, resulting in inhibition of protein synthesis
D. Blockage of the release of the inhibitory neurotransmitter glycine
E. Glucosylation of Rho-family GTPases

Correct answer = D. This man is suffering from tetanus, caused by the exotoxin produced by *Clostridium tetani*. This is a ubiquitous organism found widely in the soil. Although most people are immunized against tetanus, immunity is not lifelong and requires periodic booster immunizations. Tetanospasmin produced by *C. tetani* prevents the release of inhibitory neurotransmitters by cleaving synaptobrevins in synaptic vesicles. The effect of this toxin is a systemic, spastic paralysis that can result in death if not aggressively treated with antitoxin.

Spirochetes

15

I. OVERVIEW

Spirochetes are long, slender, motile, flexible, undulating, gram-negative bacilli that have a characteristic corkscrew or helical shape. Depending on the species, they can be microaerophilic, aerobic, or anaerobic. Some species can be grown in laboratory culture (either cell free culture or tissue culture), whereas others cannot. Some species are free living, and some are part of the normal flora of humans and animals. Spirochetes that are important human pathogens are confined to three genera (Figure 15.1): *Treponema* (*Treponema pallidum* causes syphilis), *Borrelia* (*Borrelia burgdorferi* causes Lyme disease and *Borrelia recurrentis* and *Borrelia hermsii* cause relapsing fever), and *Leptospira* (*Leptospira interrogans* causes leptospirosis).

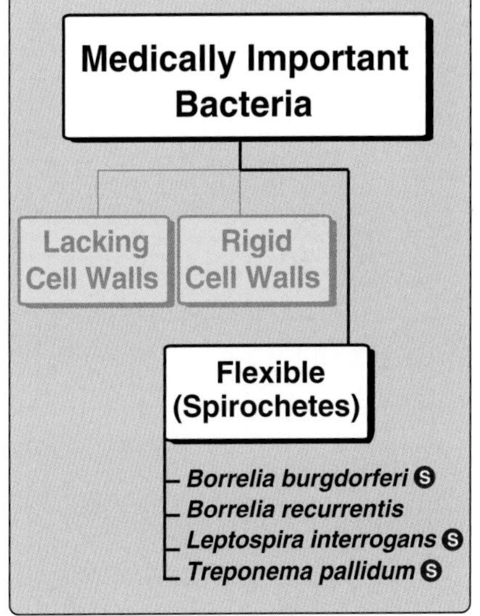

Figure 15.1
Classification of spirochetes.
S See pp. 334, 342, and 352 for summaries of these organisms.

II. STRUCTURAL FEATURES OF SPIROCHETES

Spirochetes have a unique structure that is responsible for motility. As illustrated in Figure 15.2, the spirochete cell has a central protoplasmic cylinder bounded by a plasma membrane and a typical gram-negative cell wall. Unlike in other bacilli, this cylinder is enveloped by an outer membrane composed of glycolipids and lipoproteins[1]. Between the peptidoglycan and the outer sheath are located multiple periplasmic flagella that do not protrude from the cell but are oriented axially. Bundles of these endoflagella (axial filaments) span the entire length of the cell and are anchored at both ends. Although the mechanics are not totally clear, it is likely that these axial periplasmic flagella rotate like the external flagella of other motile bacteria, propelling the cell in a corkscrew-like manner. Spirochetes can move through highly viscous solutions with little impediment, and it is theorized that this kind of motion is responsible for the ability of spirochete pathogens to penetrate and invade host tissue, just as a corkscrew penetrates cork.

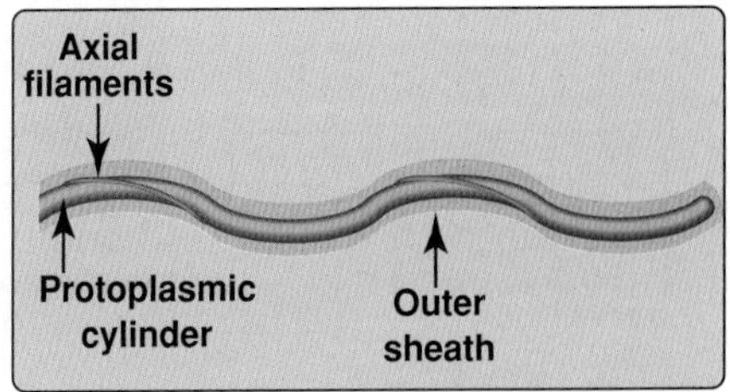

Figure 15.2
Spirochete morphology.

III. TREPONEMA PALLIDUM

Syphilis is primarily a sexually transmitted infection caused by the spirochete *T. pallidum*. Starting with a small lesion (chancre), several progressive stages of the disease can span a period of 30 years or more, often ending in syphilitic dementia or cardiovascular damage. The

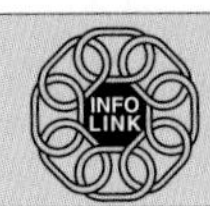

[1]See Chapters 17 and 18 in ***Lippincott's Illustrated Reviews: Biochemistry*** for a discussion of glycolipids and lipoproteins.

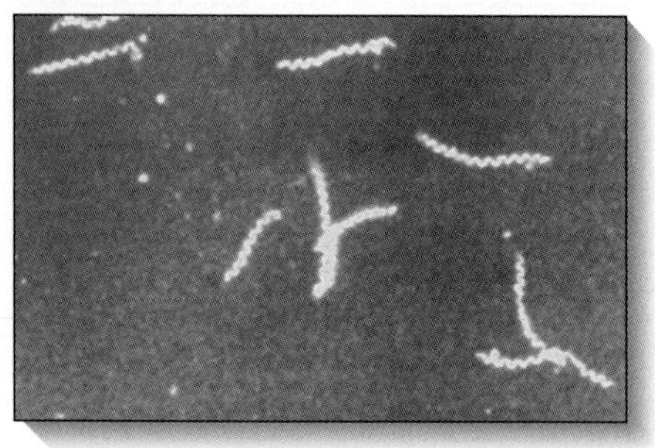

Figure 15.3
Dark-field microscopy of *Treponema pallidum.*

causative organism of syphilis is extremely fastidious and fragile. It cannot be cultured in cell-free systems and is sensitive to disinfectants, heat, and drying. *T. pallidum* is so thin that it cannot be observed by conventional light microscopy but requires immunofluorescent or dark-field techniques (Figure 15.3). The outer surface of the spirochete is sparse in proteins, and the organism is only weakly antigenic. *T. pallidum* secretes hyaluronidase, an enzyme that disrupts ground substance and probably facilitates dissemination of the organism. Unlike typical gram-negative bacteria, most spirochetes, including *T. pallidum*, do not have lipopolysaccharide (LPS), or endotoxin, in the outer leaflet of the outer membrane. Genome sequence analysis identified genes with similarity to those encoding typical cytolysins or hemolysins, but the genes for secretion of these substances are absent. Antigenic variation of surface proteins plays an important role in immune evasion.

A. Pathogenesis

Transmission of *T. pallidum* is almost always by sexual contact or transplacentally (congenital syphilis). This is understandable because the organism is so sensitive to environmental factors that survival outside of the host for more than a few minutes is highly unlikely. The organism enters the body through a break in the skin or by penetrating mucous membranes such as those of the genitalia.

B. Clinical significance

1. **Syphilis:** Syphilis occurs in three stages (Figure 15.4). The first symptom of primary syphilis is a hard, painless genital or oral ulcer (chancre) that develops at the site of inoculation. The average period between infection and the appearance of the chancre is about 3 weeks but varies with the number of infecting organ-

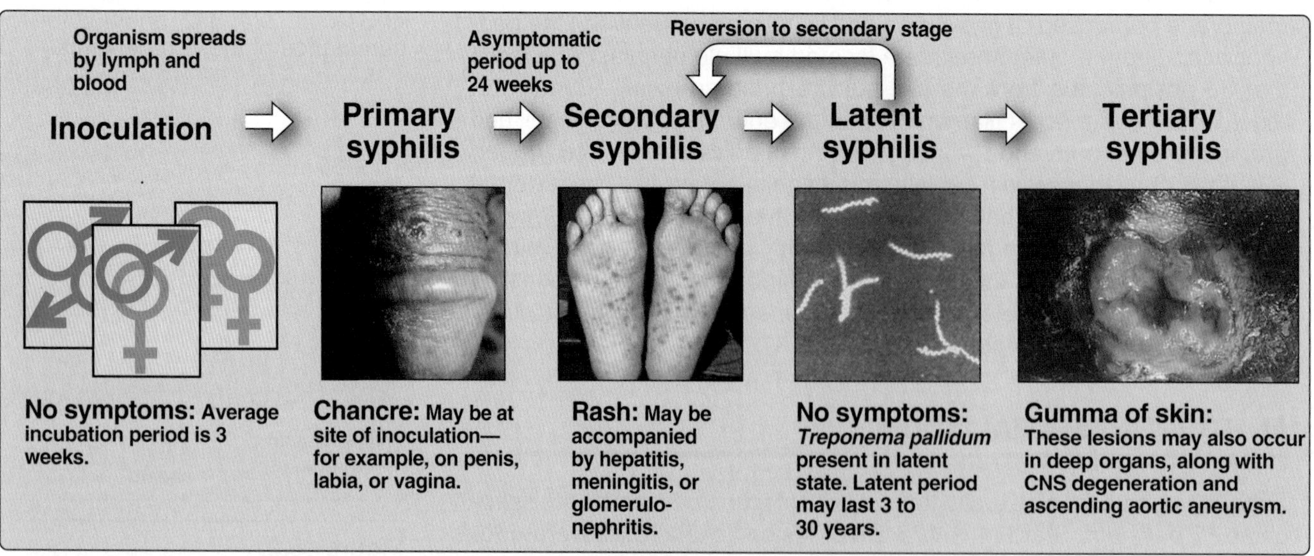

Figure 15.4
Clinical stages of untreated syphilis. CNS = central nervous systems.

isms. This primary lesion heals spontaneously, but the organism continues to spread throughout the body via the lymph and blood. An asymptomatic period ensues, lasting as long as 24 weeks, followed by the secondary stage. This stage is characterized by the appearance of a red, maculopapular rash on almost any part of the body, including the palms of the hands and soles of the feet. Also present are pale, moist, flat papules seen primarily in the anogenital region (where they are called condylomata lata), armpits, and mouth. Both primary and secondary lesions teem with *T. pallidum* and are extremely infectious. The secondary stage may be accompanied by multiorgan involvement, causing hepatitis, meningitis, nephritis, or chorioretinitis. Upon healing of the secondary lesions, the disease enters a latent period that can last for many years. In approximately 40 percent of infected individuals, the disease progresses to a tertiary stage, characterized by degeneration of the nervous system; cardiovascular lesions, such as ascending aortic aneurysms; and granulomatous lesions (gummas) in the liver, skin, and bones.

2. **Congenital syphilis:** *T. pallidum* can be transmitted through the placenta to a fetus after the first 10 to 15 weeks of pregnancy. Infection can cause fetal or infant death or spontaneous abortion. Infected infants who live develop a condition similar to secondary syphilis, including a variety of central nervous system (CNS) and structural abnormalities. Treatment of the pregnant mother with appropriate antibiotics prevents congenital syphilis.

3. **Other treponemal infections:** Three geographically localized treponemal diseases closely mimic syphilis. They include bejel (found in hot, arid areas of Africa, Southeast Asia, and the Middle East), yaws (found in humid, tropical countries and shown in Figure 15.5), and pinta (found in South and Central America, Mexico, and the Phillipines). Unlike syphilis, direct skin contact, crowded living conditions, and poor hygiene contribute to the spread of these diseases. Sexual contact is not usually the mode of transmission, and congenital infections occur rarely if at all. All three diseases are curable with penicillin.

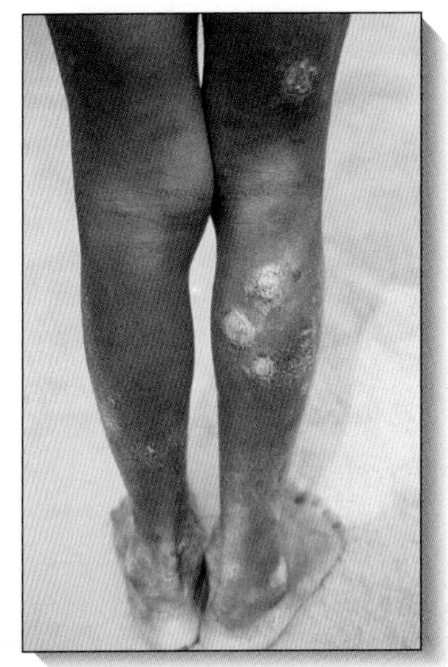

Figure 15.5
Yaws: early stage.

C. Laboratory identification

Although treponemal spirochetes from primary and secondary lesions can be detected microscopically using immunofluorescent stain or dark-field illumination (see Figure 15.3), syphilis is usually diagnosed serologically. Infection with *T. pallidum* elicits two kinds of antibodies: 1) antitreponemal antibodies that are specific to the treponemal surface proteins and 2) nontreponemal antibodies (reagin), that are directed against normal phospholipid components of mammalian membranes, such as cardiolipin[2]. Serologic tests using both kinds of antibodies are available. Antitreponemal antibody tests are more specific than reagin-based tests but remain positive during and after successful treatment and, are, therefore, not useful

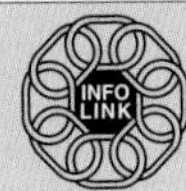

[2]See Chapter 17 in ***Lippincott's Illustrated Reviews: Biochemistry*** for a discussion of the structure of cardiolipin.

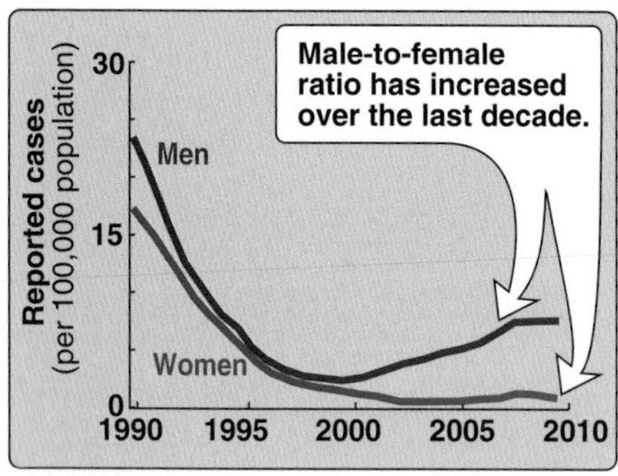

Figure 15.6
Incidence of primary and secondary syphilis.

for monitoring therapy. Cardiolipin-based tests are less specific and liable to give more false positives. [Note: Nonspecific tests are, therefore, confirmed by a specific test (usually fluorescent treponemal antibody).] They are, nevertheless, useful in screening and for monitoring therapy because tests for reagin usually become negative about 1 year after successful treatment.

D. Treatment and prevention

One single treatment with penicillin is curative for primary and secondary syphilis, and no antibiotic resistance has been reported. In cases of patient sensitivity to penicillin, alternate therapy with erythromycin or tetracyclines may also be effective (see Figure 15.7). In spite of an inexpensive and highly effective cure, there are still over 10,000 new cases of syphilis in the United States each year (Figure 15.6). There is no vaccine against *T. pallidum*, and prevention depends on safe sexual practices. More than one sexually transmitted disease (STD) can be passed on at the same time. Therefore, when any STD has been diagnosed, the possibility of the infected individual also having syphilis should be considered. For example, concomitant HIV infection makes treatment of syphilis more difficult, sometimes requiring longer courses of therapy and definitely requiring longer and more intensive follow-up.

IV. BORRELIA BURGDORFERI

Members of the genus *Borrelia* are relatively large spirochetes which, like *Treponema*, have endoflagella that make them highly motile (see Figure 15.12). *Borrelia* species are unusual among bacteria in that they have linear rather than circular plasmid and chromosomal DNA. Like *T. pallidum*, *Borrelia* do not produce endotoxin or exotoxins.

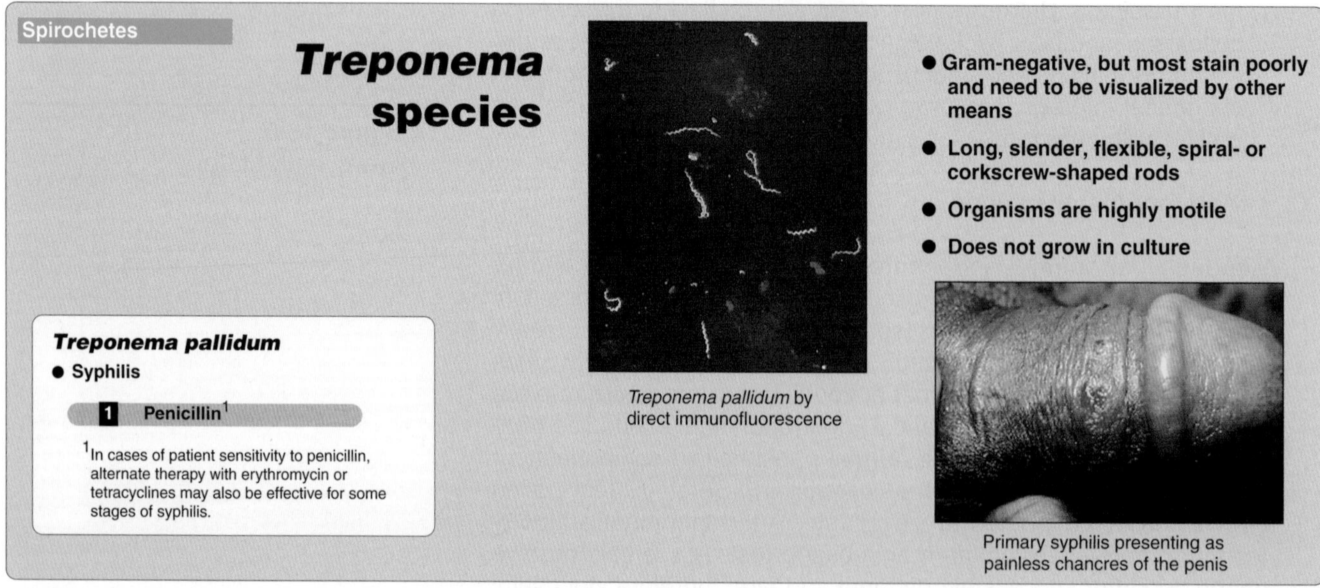

Figure 15.7
Summary of *Treponema* species. **1** Indicates first-line drugs.

A. Pathogenesis

Lyme disease is caused by the spirochete *B. burgdorferi*, which is transmitted by the bite of a small tick of the genus *Ixodes* (Figure 15.8). [Note: The tick must be attached for at least 24 hours before there is transmission of bacteria. This blood meal results in a heavily engorged tick.] Mice and other small rodents serve as primary reservoirs for the spirochete, but deer and other mammals serve as hosts for the ticks. Lyme disease is currently the most common arthropod-transmitted disease in the United States, averaging at least 20,000 cases per year. Lyme disease in Europe and Asia can be caused by other *Borrelia* species, including *Borrelia garinii* and *Borrelia afzelii*, which are associated with different late-stage symptoms.

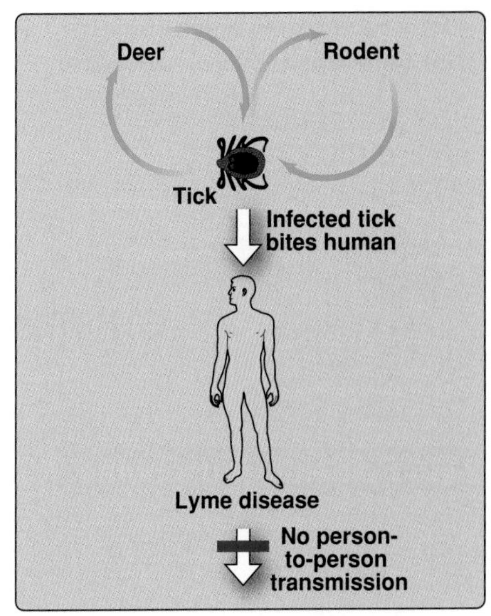

Figure 15.8
Transmission of Lyme disease.

B. Clinical significance

The first stage of Lyme disease begins 3 to 32 days after a tick bite, when a characteristic red, circular lesion with a clear center (erythema migrans) appears at the site of the bite (Figure 15.9). Flulike symptoms often accompany the erythema. The organism spreads via the lymph or blood to musculoskeletal sites, skin, CNS, heart, and other tissues and organs. Weeks to months after the onset, the second stage of the disease begins, with symptoms such as arthritis, arthralgia, cardiac complications, and neurologic complications such as meningitis. Months to years later, the third stage begins with the appearance of chronic arthritis, progressive CNS disease, chronic skin manifestations, and cardiac dysfunction. Lyme disease is rarely fatal but can result in a poor quality of life if untreated. Although caused by different spirochetes, the general similarities in the progression of Lyme disease and syphilis are striking.

C. Laboratory identification

Unlike *T. pallidum*, *B. burgdorferi* can be cultured, but the procedure is difficult and takes 6 to 8 weeks. Serologic tests have been used to

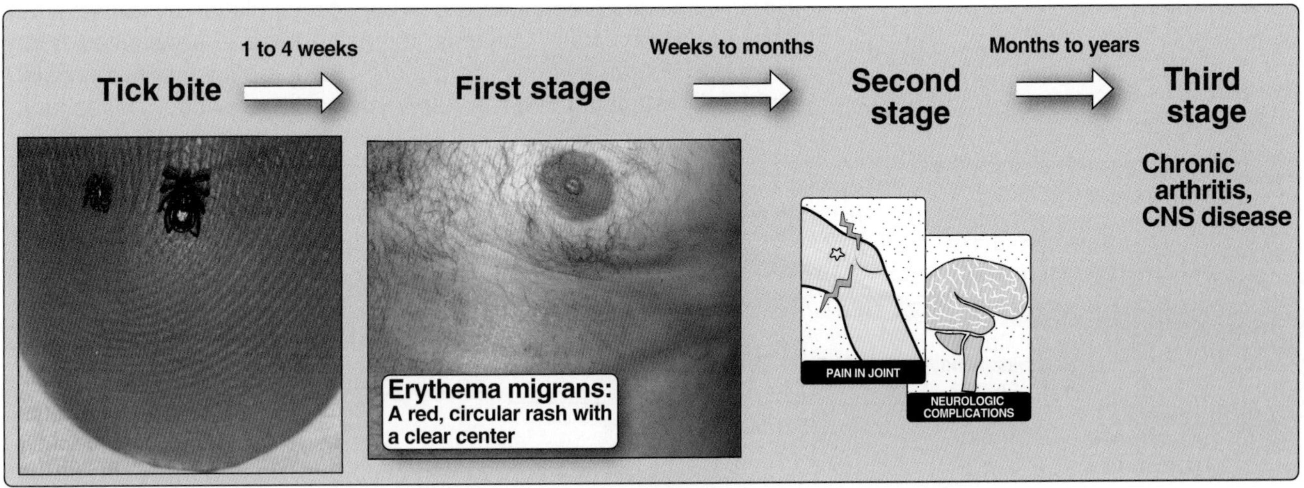

Figure 15.9
Clinical stages of untreated Lyme disease. CNS = central nervous system.

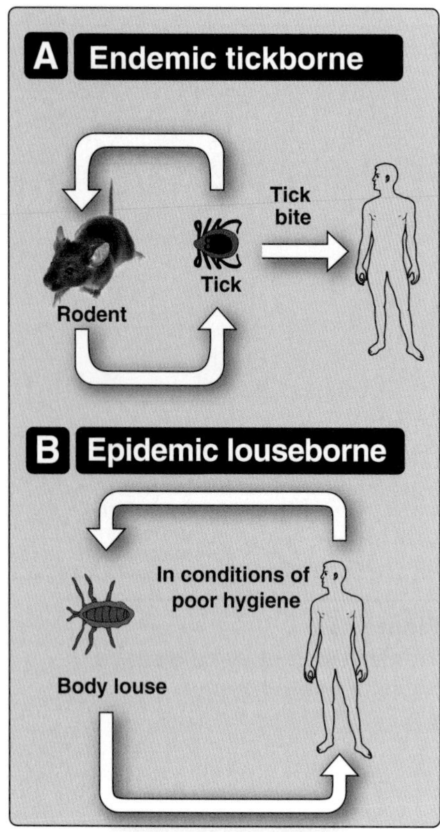

Figure 15.10
Endemic versus epidemic relapsing fever by *Borrelia recurrentis.*

diagnose Lyme disease, but the number of false positives can outnumber the true positives. Such tests should be used only as confirmation of a strong clinical suspicion. A two-stage testing process that involves an enzyme-linked immunosorbent assay (or, ELISA) followed by Western blot is recommended for the most definitive confirmatory serologic diagnosis.

D. Treatment and prevention

Doxycycline is the most recommended treatment for the early stages of the disease (see Figure 15.12). If arthritic symptoms have already appeared, longer courses of antibiotics (ceftriaxone) are used. Prevention of infection also includes use of insect repellents and wearing clothing that sufficiently protects the body from tick bites.

V. RELAPSING FEVER SPIROCHETES

Epidemic relapsing fever is caused by *B. recurrentis* whereas endemic relapsing fever can be caused by a variety of *Borrelia* species, including *B. hermsii*, *Borrelia turicatae,* and *Borrelia parkeri*. Relapsing fever is characterized by several cycles of apparent recovery, each followed by a relapse. A most striking property of the relapsing fever spirochetes is their ability to change surface protein antigens. This ability accounts for the relapsing nature of the disease because, with each relapse, a new antigenic variant arises.

A. Pathogenesis

Distinctions can be made between endemic and epidemic relapsing fever. Endemic relapsing fever can be caused by a variety of *Borrelia* species, occurs in most areas of the world, and is transmitted by soft-bodied ticks. Endemic relapsing fever is a zoonosis, because it is transmitted from small mammal reservoirs to humans by vectors. The tick vectors also serve as reservoirs because the *Borrelia* species are maintained in the tick population by transovarial passage. By contrast, epidemic relapsing fever is transmitted from human to human by body lice (Figure 15.10), so it is not a zoonosis. Epidemic relapsing fever is associated with crowded, unsanitary,

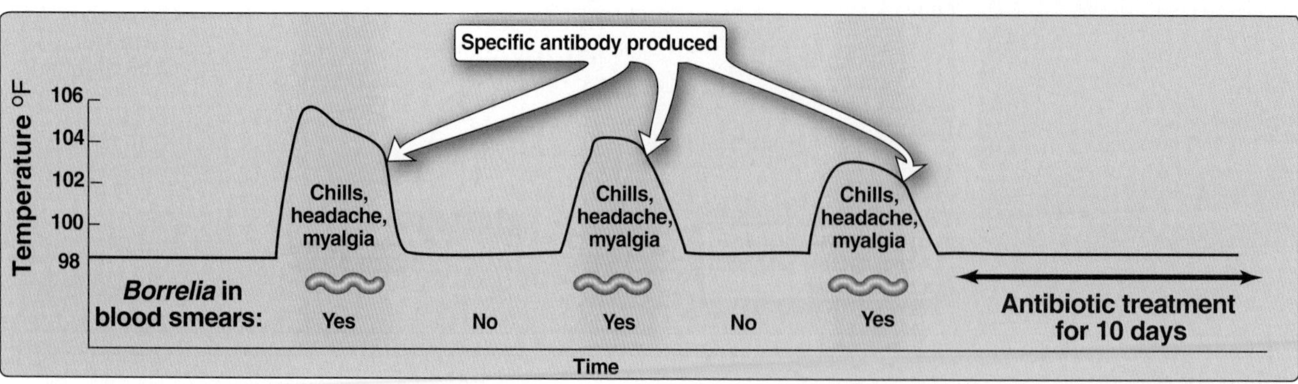

Figure 15.11
Clinical stages of relapsing fever.

louse-infested environments. In this situation, fatalities can be as high as 30 percent if untreated.

B. Clinical significance

The first symptoms of relapsing fever appear 3 to 10 days after exposure to an infected arthropod (Figure 15.11). These symptoms include an abrupt onset of high fever accompanied by severe headache, muscle pain, and general malaise. During this febrile period, which lasts 3 to 5 days, abundant spirochetes are present in the blood. The fever abates along with the number of spirochetes. Apparent recovery is experienced for a period of 4 to 10 days but is followed by a recurrence of the initial symptoms. There may be as many as ten such recurrences, generally with decreasing severity. In fatal cases, the spirochete invades many organs of the body (for example, heart, spleen, liver, and kidney), with death generally due to myocarditis with shock.

C. Diagnosis and treatment

Diagnosis is usually based on the appearance of Giemsa- or Wright-stainable, loosely coiled spirochetes in the blood during the febrile stage of the disease. Tetracyclines, erythromycin, and penicillin have proven effective treatments (Figure 15.12). However, the relapsing nature of the disease makes it difficult to distinguish spontaneous remissions from response to therapy. No vaccines are available.

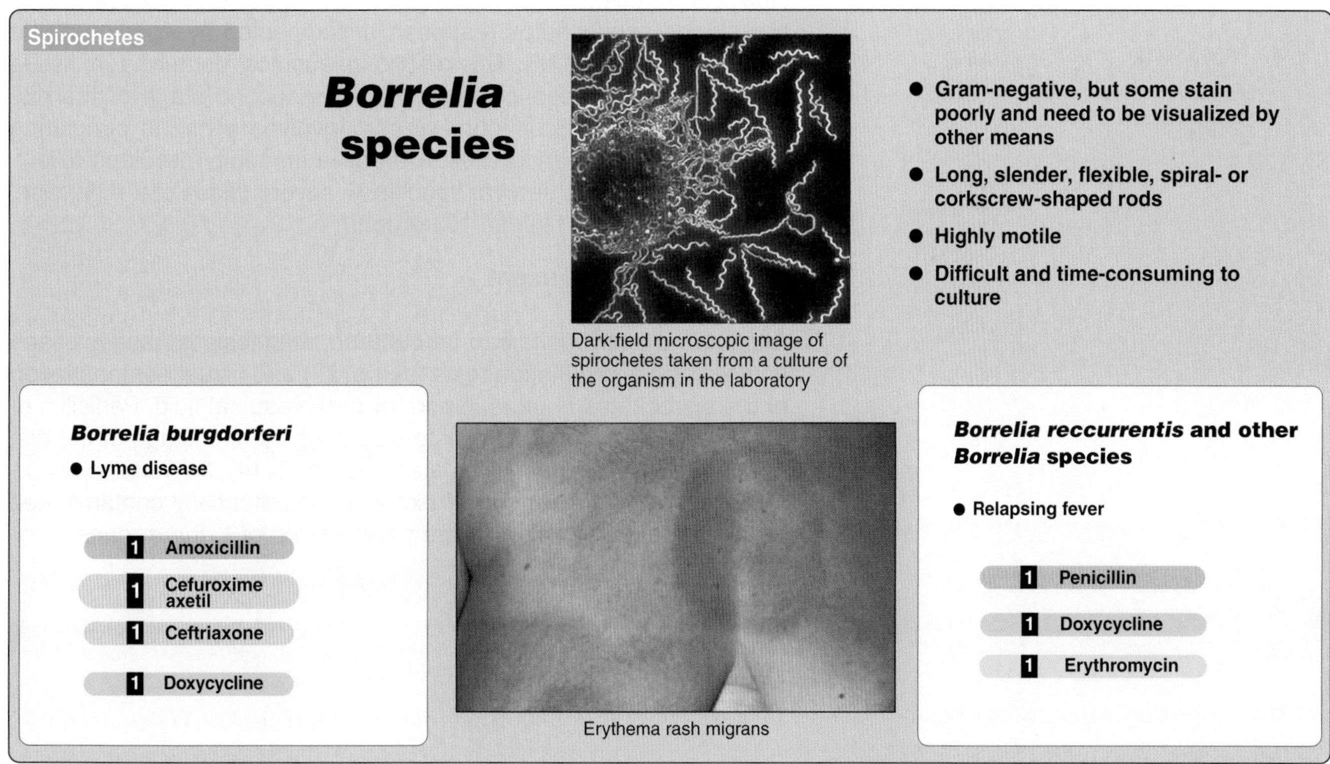

Figure 15.12
Summary of *Borrelia* species. 1 Indicates first-line drugs.

VI. LEPTOSPIRA INTERROGANS

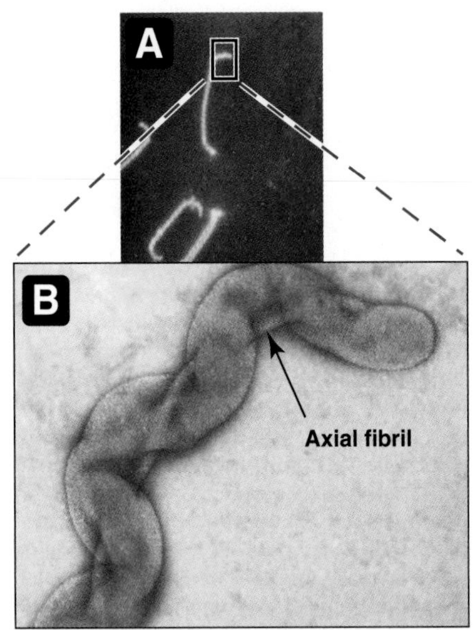

Figure 15.13
A. Dark-field micrograph of *Leptospira interrogans*. B. Electron micrograph of one end of a negatively stained *Leptospira interrogans* showing the axial fibril.

L. interrogans infection causes the disease leptospirosis. The organism is a slender (*lepto* = slender), tightly coiled, culturable spirochete with a single, thin, axial filament and hooked ends (Figure 15.13). *L. interrogans* is an obligate aerobe. Many serovars have been characterized based upon polysaccharide differences in the LPS component in the outer membrane, and these serovars are specific to distinct geographic locales. *L. interrogans* is sensitive to drying and a broad range of disinfectants. It can, however, survive for weeks in slightly alkaline water.

A. Epidemiology and pathogenesis

Leptospirosis is essentially an animal disease that is coincidentally transmitted to humans, primarily by water or food contaminated with animal urine. Entrance to the body can also occur via small skin abrasions or the conjunctiva. Although leptospirosis occurs worldwide (under various local names, such as infectious jaundice, marsh fever, Weil disease, and swineherd's disease), the incidence of the disease today in developed countries is very low. Less than 100 cases of clinically significant *L. interrogans* infections are reported annually in the United States.

B. Clinical significance

Fever occurs 1 to 2 weeks after infection, at which time spirochetes appear in the blood. These symptoms decrease after about 1 week. However, in cases of biphasic disease (that is, the disease having two stages), spirochetes reappear, accompanied by invasion of the liver, kidneys, and CNS. This results in jaundice, hemorrhage, tissue necrosis, and/or aseptic meningitis. This second stage of the disease, which lasts 3 or more weeks, involves a rise in circulating immunoglobulin M antibodies. Protective immunity develops following disease, but it is serovar specific. In severe cases of the disease, mortality can be as high as 10 percent.

C. Diagnosis and treatment

Although *L. interrogans* can be cultured, diagnosis is usually based on serologic agglutination tests (see p. 27) and visual demonstration of the spirochetes in urine, blood, or cerebrospinal fluid. Penicillin or doxycycline is useful if administered during the first stage of the disease, but both are ineffective later (Figure 15.14). No vaccine is currently available. Prevention of exposure to potentially contaminated water and food helps control the transmission of *L. interrogans*.

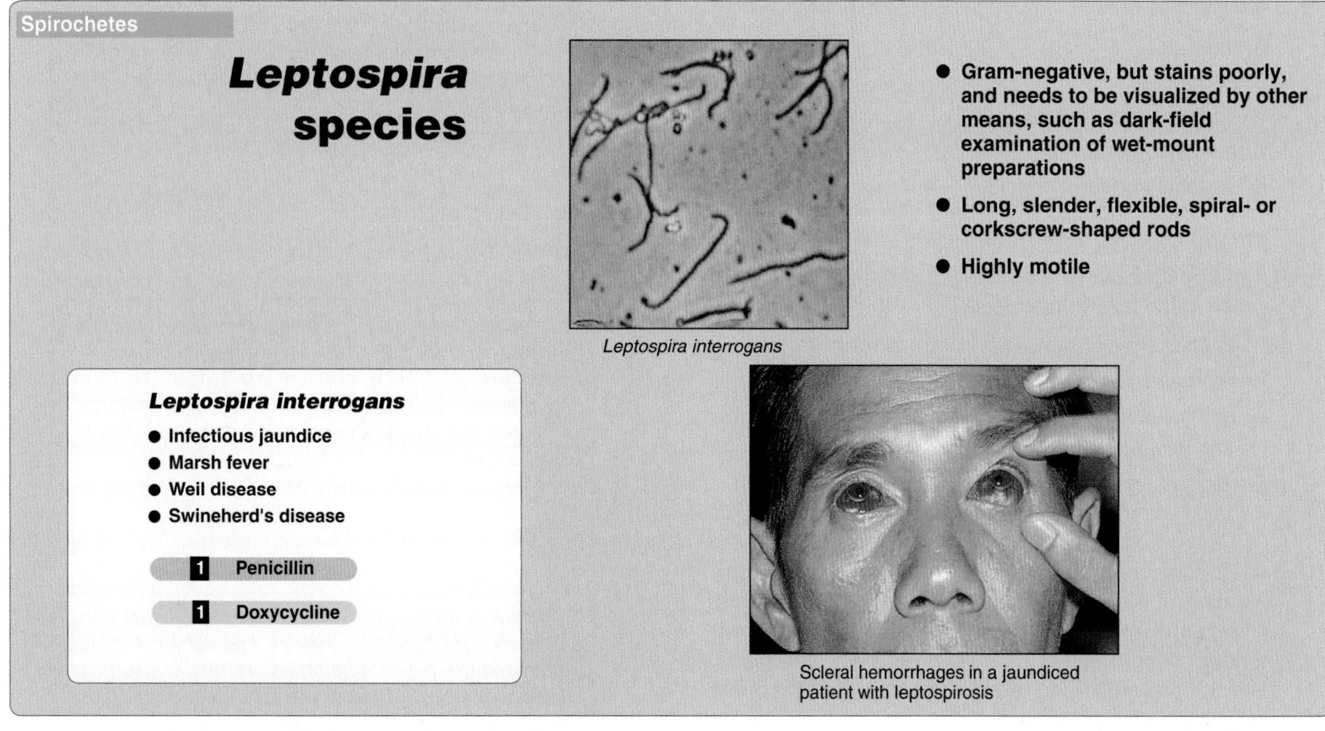

Figure 15.14
Summary of *Leptospira* species. **1** Indicates first-line drugs.

Study Questions

Choose the ONE correct answer

15.1 The probable cause for the relapsing nature of relapsing fever caused by *Borrelia recurrentis* is:

A. the sequential appearance of new antibiotic resistant variants.
B. periodic spore dormancy and activation.
C. successive appearance of antigenic variants.
D. periodic hormonal fluctuations in the host.
E. organisms that survive and propagate after spirochete-induced fever.

Correct answer = C. Any of these mechanisms are conceivable with various degrees of plausibility. The weight of evidence, however, favors the mechanism whereby new antigenic variants arise that elude, for a period, the host's immune defenses, to then be replaced by another variant.

15.2 Which of the following spirochete-caused diseases is transmitted by an arthropod?

A. Leptospirosis
B. Pinta
C. Relapsing fever
D. Yaws
E. Syphilis

Correct answer = C. *Borrelia hermsii* is one of several species of *Borrelia* that cause relapsing fever, when it is transmitted by ticks. Pinta, yaws, and syphilis are transmitted by direct human-to-human contact, whereas leptospirosis is transmitted via water contaminated with animal urine.

15.3 A distinctive feature of spirochetes is the presence of:

A. fimbriae.

B. endoflagella.

C. helically arranged pili.

D. nucleosomes.

E. variable surface antigens.

Correct answer = B. The endoflagella are thought to be responsible for the corkscrew motion of spirochetes. The other structural features are not specific to spirochetes.

15.4 Syphilis and Lyme disease are strikingly similar in which of the following aspects?

A. Their modes of transmission are similar.

B. Both diseases display three similar, distinct phases.

C. Both causative agents share many antigenic markers.

D. The diseases show cross-immunity.

E. Both causative agents can be cultured.

Correct answer = B. Syphilis, like Lyme disease, has three distinct phases. The other listed properties are either irrelevant or false. Unlike *Treponema pallidum*, *Borrelia burgdorferi* can be cultured, but the procedure is difficult and takes 6 to 8 weeks.

15.5 A 22-year-old male presents to his physician, complaining of a 2-week history of a sore on his penis. Physical examination shows a firm, raised, red, nontender chancre midway between the base and glans. Which of the following is the most appropriate course of action for the physician?

A. Test a serum sample for antibodies to herpes simplex virus.

B. Swab the chancre and culture on Thayer-Martin agar.

C. Swab the chancre and perform a Gram stain.

D. Perform a dark-field examination on a swab of the active lesion.

E. Swab the chancre and culture on blood agar.

Correct answer = D. The patient most likely has primary syphilis rather than herpes simplex virus because the penile chancre is not tender. Herpes lesions are typically very painful. *Treponema pallidum*, the etiologic agent of syphilis, cannot be readily cultured in the routine clinical microbiology laboratory. Treponemal spirochetes from primary and secondary lesions can be detected microscopically using immunofluorescent stain or dark-field illumination. However, syphilis is usually diagnosed serologically by detection of: 1) antitreponemal antibodies that are specific to the treponemal surface proteins and 2) nontreponemal antibodies (reagin) that are directed against normal phospholipid components.

15.6 A 13-year-old boy, previously healthy, developed flu-like symptoms including fever and malaise. These constitutional symptoms were accompanied by a spreading, circular rash on the child's back. Travel and recreational history indicated that the boy had recently been camping in rural Connecticut. The boy was unaware of any abrasions, bites, or other injury. Which of the following characteristics is unique to the organism that is the most likely cause of this infection?

A. The outer membrane contains lipopolysaccharide.

B. The outer surface is composed of mycolic acids.

C. The genome is composed of one linear chromosome and a series of circular and linear plasmids.

D. The disease is caused by elaboration of a potent exotoxin.

E. The disease is transmitted by the bite of a body louse.

Correct answer = C. *Borrelia burgdorferi*, the causative agent of Lyme disease, has a unique genome composed of a linear chromosome and a complement of circular and linear plasmids. The outer sheath of the spirochetes is also relatively unique in that it does not contain lipopolysaccharide, or endotoxin. The outer surface does not contain mycolic acids, which are found in the *Mycobacterium* species. *B. burgdorferi* does not produce any known exotoxins and is transmitted to humans by the bite of a tick. Many patients, however, do not know that they have been bitten by a tick until the characteristic rash appears. The highest incidence of Lyme disease caused by *B. burgdorferi* is in the Northeast and upper Midwestern United States.

Mycoplasma

16

I. OVERVIEW

Mycoplasmas are small, prokaryotic organisms with no peptidoglycan in their cell walls. Instead, they are enclosed in a single plasma membrane. Because of their extremely small size, mycoplasmas frequently pass through bacteriologic filters. The many *Mycoplasma* species are widely distributed in nature and include several commensals commonly found in the mouth and genitourinary (GU) tracts of humans and other mammals. For these reasons, mycoplasmas are often recovered as contaminants or adventitious flora from biologic materials, including clinical samples. Three *Mycoplasma* species are definitively associated with human disease, namely *Mycoplasma pneumoniae*, which is the cause of a atypical pneumonia, and *Mycoplasma hominis* and *Ureaplasma urealyticum*, which are associated with a variety of GU diseases, such as urethritis, pelvic inflammatory disease (PID), and intrapartum infections (Figure 16.1). *Mycoplasma genitalium* is a recently recognized sexually transmitted pathogen that causes nongonococcal urethritis (NGU). Lacking cell walls, mycoplasmas are insensitive to antibiotics that inhibit cell division by preventing cell wall synthesis (such as penicillin, see p. 42). However, they are susceptible to other inhibitors of prokaryotic metabolism.

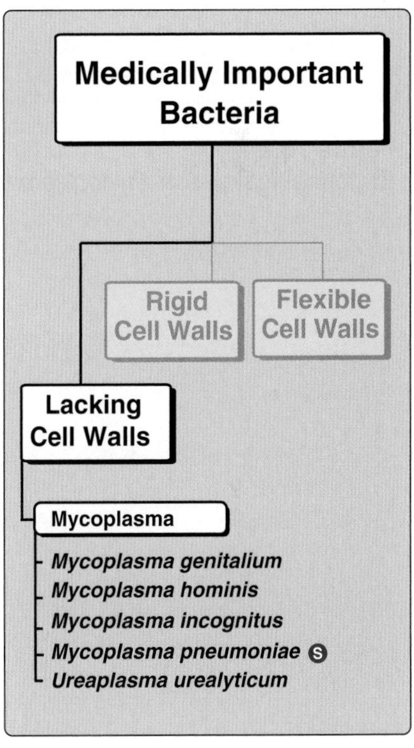

Figure 16.1
Classification of Mycoplasma.
S See p. 334 for a summary of this organism.

II. GENERAL FEATURES OF MYCOPLASMAS

Lacking cell walls, mycoplasmas are enclosed instead by a membrane composed of a lipid bilayer (Figure 16.2). They are, therefore, plastic and pleomorphic and thus cannot be classified as either cocci or rods. Mycoplasmas are also the smallest of known free-living, self-replicating prokaryotic cells. Their double-stranded DNA genomes are among the smallest known, containing less than 1,200 kilobase pairs (kbs). [Note: This may approach the minimum DNA coding capacity required for the free-living state.]

A. Physiology

Mycoplasmas have limited biosynthetic capabilities and require a variety of small, organic molecules for growth. Unlike other prokary-

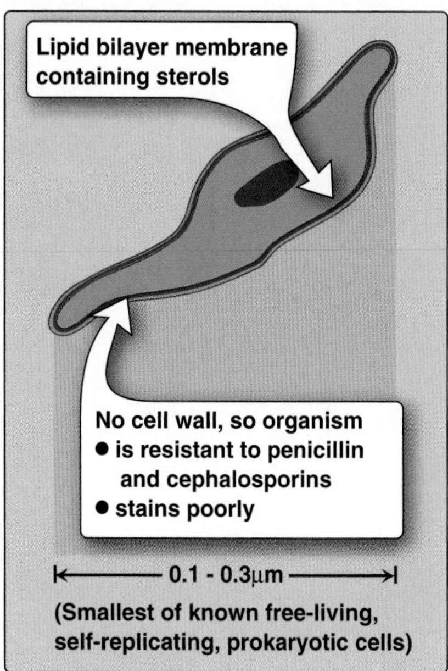

Figure 16.2
Structural features of *Mycoplasma*.

otes, mycoplasmas contain sterols in their cell membranes. Because most mycoplasma species cannot synthesize the sterol ring, they require an external source of cholesterol from serum or a similar medium supplement. Given appropriate supplementation, they can be grown in cell-free media. However, because of their fastidious growth requirements, these organisms are rarely cultured in the laboratory.

B. Colony production

Mycoplasmas produce minute colonies on specialized agar after several days of incubation. These are best visualized under 30× to 100× magnification. The central portion of the colony penetrates the agar, whereas the periphery spreads over the adjacent surface, in some cases giving the colony a characteristic "fried egg" appearance (see Figure 16.5).

III. MYCOPLASMA PNEUMONIAE

M. pneumoniae is transmitted by respiratory droplets and causes a lower respiratory tract infection (atypical pneumonia, so named because the signs and symptoms are unlike typical lobar pneumonia). The organism accounts for approximately 20 percent of pneumonia cases as well as causing milder infections such as bronchitis, pharyngitis, and nonpurulent otitis media. Infections occur worldwide and year round, with increased incidence in late fall and winter. Cases are usually sporadic, although occasional epidemics among individuals in close contact are reported in both civilian settings (for example, schools and prisons) and among military populations. The highest incidence of clinical disease is seen in older children and young adults (ages 6 to 20 years).

A. Pathogenesis

M. pneumoniae possesses a membrane-associated protein, P1, which functions as a cytoadhesin. It is concentrated in a specialized organelle visible under electron microscopy, which binds sialic acid-rich glycolipids found on certain host cell membranes. Among susceptible cell types are ciliated bronchial epithelial cells. The organisms grow closely attached to the host cell luminal surface and inhibit ciliary action. Eventually, patches of affected mucosa desquamate, and an inflammatory response develops in bronchial and adjacent tissues involving lymphocytes and other mononuclear cells. *M. pneumoniae* produces an exotoxin that is similar to pertussis toxin. The toxin is an adenosine diphosphate–ribosylase and results in extensive vacuolization and death of host cells. In infected individuals, organisms are shed in saliva for several days before onset of clinical illness. Reinfection is common, and symptoms are more severe in older children and young adults who have previously encountered the organism.

B. Clinical significance

Atypical pneumonia (lower respiratory tract disease) is the best-known form of *M. pneumoniae* infection. However, this disease accounts for a minority of the infectious episodes with this organism, upper respiratory tract and ear infection being much more frequent. Atypical pneumonia clinically resembles pneumonia caused by a number of viruses and bacteria such as *Chlamydia* species. The incubation period averages 3 weeks. Onset is usually gradual, beginning with nonspecific symptoms such as unrelenting headache, accompanied by fever, chills, and malaise. After 2 to 4 days, a dry or scantily productive cough develops. Earache is sometimes an accompanying complaint. Chest radiographs reveal a patchy, diffuse bronchopneumonia involving one or more lobes (Figure 16.3). Patients often remain ambulatory throughout the illness (hence, "walking pneumonia"). In the absence of preexisting compromise (for example, immunodeficiency or emphysema), the disease remits after 3 to 10 days without specific treatment. X-ray abnormalities resolve more slowly in 2 weeks to 2 months. Complications are rare, but include central nervous system (CNS) disturbances; a rash (erythema multiforme); and mild, hemolytic anemia (the latter associated with production of cold agglutinins, see below). The patient may complain of significant illness despite minimal abnormalities on physical examination.

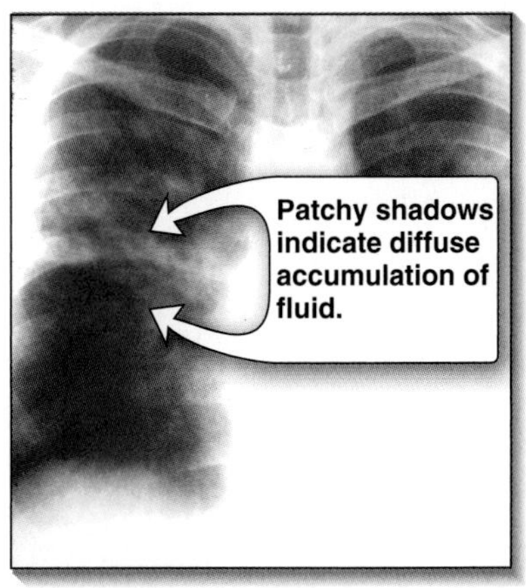
Patchy shadows indicate diffuse accumulation of fluid.

Figure 16.3
Radiograph of lung of an individual with *M. pneumoniae*–induced atypical pneumonia.

C. Immunity

Infection with *M. pneumoniae* elicits both local and systemic immune responses. Only one *M. pneumoniae* serotype has been described. Serum antibody to outer membrane glycolipids and to the P1 adhesin can be demonstrated, with antibody peaking 2 to 4 weeks after infection and gradually disappearing over the following year. An immunoglobulin M antibody, the cold agglutinin, is produced by approximately 60 percent of infected patients. [Note: This antibody's name derives from the fact that it reacts with the human erythrocyte antigen I, reversibly agglutinating I^+ red blood cells at temperatures of 0°C to 4°C but not at 37°C.] Some patients develop very high titers of cold agglutinins. With exposure to cold temperatures this may result in ischemia and even necrosis of distal extremities [hands and feet] because of *in vivo* clumping of red blood cells.

D. Laboratory identification

Direct microscopic examination of clinical material for *M. pneumoniae* is of limited value. Sputum is scanty and nonpurulent, and the pathogen stains poorly or not at all using standard bacteriologic stains. Sputum samples or throat swabs can be cultured on special media, but, because isolation of the organism usually requires 8 to 15 days, they cannot aid in early treatment decisions. *M. pneumoniae* grows under both aerobic and anaerobic conditions and can be isolated on specialized media supplemented with serum. However, the organism is fastidious, and isolation is not commonly performed in clinical laboratories. Serologic tests are the most widely used procedures for establishing a diagnosis of atypical pneumonia due to

M. pneumoniae. Specific antibody can be detected by complement fixation, using an extract of mycoplasmal glycolipids. A diagnosis is established by a fourfold rise in titer between acute and convalescent samples. Because symptoms of illness develop slowly, the initial serum sample may be positive. Molecular diagnostics, including polymerase chain reaction (PCR) amplification, are replacing serological tests.

E. Treatment

M. pneumoniae is sensitive to doxycycline, azithromycin, or levofoxacin (see Figure 16.5). When given early, antibiotic treatment shortens the course of disease, although symptoms may be eliminated only gradually. The organisms, however, may persist in the convalescent upper respiratory tract for weeks. Because there is no rapid way to make the diagnosis of *M. pneumoniae* pneumonia, treatment begins with empiric therapy (most often with macrolide antibiotics) for atypical pneumonia.

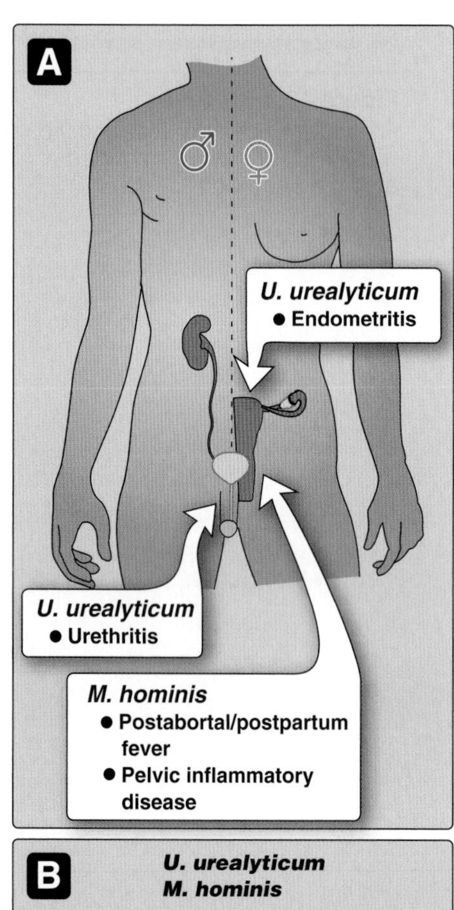

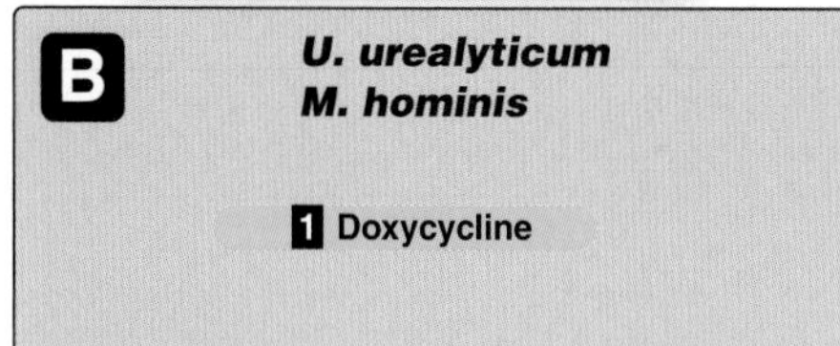

Figure 16.4
A. Diseases caused by *M. hominis* and *U. urealyticum*. B. The antibiotic used to treat these infections.
1 Indicates first-line drug.

IV. GENITAL MYCOPLASMAS

Three *Mycoplasma* species, *M. hominis*, *U. urealyticum*, and *M. genitalium,* are human urogenital pathogens. They are often associated with sexually transmitted infections, such as NGU or puerperal infections (that is, infections connected with, or occurring during childbirth or the period immediately following childbirth).

A. Mycoplasma hominis and Ureaplasma urealyticum

M. hominis and *U. urealyticum* are common inhabitants of the GU tract, particularly in sexually active adults. Because colonization rates in some populations are in excess of 50 percent, it is difficult to establish an unequivocal causal role in various disease states with which the organisms are associated. Both agents can be cultured. They grow more rapidly than *M. pneumoniae* and can be distinguished by their carbon utilization patterns: *M. hominis* degrades arginine, whereas *U. urealyticum* hydrolyses urea. [Note: *Ureaplasma* is sometimes referred to as a "T strain" of mycoplasma because it produces tiny colonies not visible to the naked eye.] The major clinical condition associated with *M. hominis* is postpartum or postabortal fever (Figure 16.4). The organism has been isolated from blood cultures in up to 10 percent of women so affected. It is also recovered locally in cases of PID, although sometimes in mixed culture. A number of serotypes of *M. hominis* have been described. It is important to note that *M. hominis* isolates are uniformly resistant to erythromycin, in contrast to other mycoplasmas. A tetracycline, such as doxycyline, is effective for specific treatment. *U. urealyticum* is a common cause of urethritis when neither gonococcus nor chlamydia can be demonstrated, particularly in men. In women, the organism has been isolated from the endometrium of patients with endometritis and from vaginal secretions of women who undergo premature labor or deliver low-birth-weight babies. The infants are often colonized, and *U. urealyticum* has been isolated from the infant's lower respiratory tract and CNS both with and without evidence of inflammatory response.

B. Mycoplasma genitalium

M. genitalium has been recognized as a sexually transmitted pathogen, resulting in a series of syndromes similar to those caused by *Neisseria gonorrhoeae* (see p. 103) and *Chlamydia trachomatis* (see p. 179). *M. genitalium* causes NGU in males and is associated with cervicitis and PID in women. The organisms appear to be resistant to doxycycline, which is the treatment of choice for NGU caused by *C. trachomatis*. Therefore, recommendations for testing for *M. genitalium* include cases in which the patient fails to respond to doxycycline treatment. PCR amplification is recommended for specific diagnosis of *M. genitalium* infections. Azithromycin is effective for treating *M. genitalium* infections.

V. OTHER MYCOPLASMAS

Several other species of mycoplasmas can be recovered from human sources. No pathogenic role has been established to date for these organisms. One such organism, AIDS-associated mycoplasma, or *Mycoplasma incognitus*, has been isolated in high frequency from HIV-positive patients, in which the organism may play a role, possibly as a secondary invader.

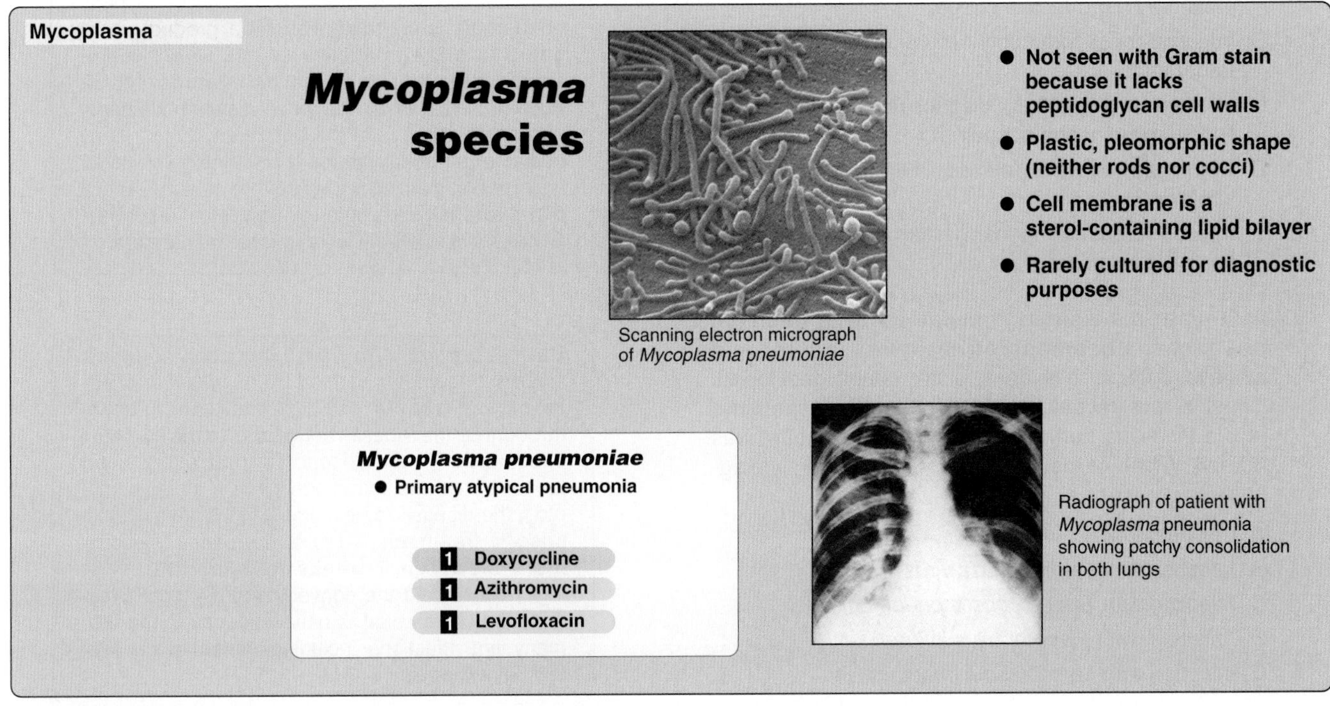

Figure 16.5
Summary of *Mycoplasma* species. **1** Indicates first-line drugs.

Study Questions

Choose the ONE correct answer

16.1 Postpartum fever due to *Mycoplasma hominis* is treated with:

A. tetracycline.
B. erythromycin.
C. penicillin G.
D. a second-generation cephalosporin.
E. vancomycin.

Correct answer = A. Mycoplasmas are small, prokaryotic organisms with no peptidoglycan cell walls. Thus inhibitors of cell wall synthesis, such as penicillins, cephalosporins, and vancomycin are not effective. *Mycoplasma hominis* isolates, in contrast to other mycoplasmas, are uniformly resistant to erythromycin. Tetracycline is effective for specific treatment.

16.2 A distinguishing feature of human *Mycoplasma* species is that they:

A. stain well with Giemsa but not by Gram stain.
B. contain no bacterial peptidoglycan.
C. are not immunogenic because they mimic host cell membrane components.
D. cannot be cultivated *in vitro.*
E. are dependent on host sources of adenosine triphosphate.

Correct answer = B. The distinguishing feature of mycoplasmas is their complete lack of a cell wall.

16.3 Which of the following is most characteristic of *Mycoplasma pneumoniae* infection?

A. Infection results in a fever of sudden onset accompanied by a productive cough.
B. Infection most commonly occurs in the upper respiratory tract.
C. Infection is definitively diagnosed by direct microscopic examination of sputum.
D. Reinfection is rare and less severe than primary infection.
E. Infection causes extensive scarring and calcification of affected lung tissue.

Correct answer = B. Atypical pneumonia is the best known form of *Mycoplasma pneumoniae* infection. However, upper respiratory tract and ear infection are much more frequent. Atypical pneumonia is characterized by a gradual onset and a scantily productive cough. Direct microscopic examination of clinical material for *M. pneumoniae* is of limited value. Sputum is scanty and nonpurulent, and the pathogen stains poorly or not at all using standard bacteriologic stains. Reinfection causes more severe lesions and a more extensive chronic inflammatory response. Recovery is slow, but without residual damage.

16.4 A 30-year-old woman complained of unrelenting headache, accompanied by fever, chills, and malaise. After 2 to 4 days, a dry cough developed. Chest X-rays reveal a patchy, diffuse bronchopneumonia involving both lobes. Her white cell count was normal. Which of the following is the most likely diagnosis?

A. Legionellosis
B. Infection with parainfluenza virus
C. Infection with *Streptococcus pneumoniae*
D. Infection with *Haemophilus influenzae*
E. Infection with *Mycoplasma pneumoniae*

Correct answer = E. The description suggests atypical pneumonia caused by *Myoplasma pneumoniae.* Patients often remain ambulatory throughout the illness, hence the name "walking pneumonia." In the absence of preexisting compromise (such as immunodeficiency, emphysema, etc.), the disease remits after 3 to 10 days without specific treatment. X-ray abnormalities resolve more slowly in 2 weeks to 2 months. With legionellosis and the conventional bacterial infections the white count is usually elevated and with many viral infections, including influenza, it is usually below normal.

Chlamydiae

17

I. OVERVIEW

The family Chlamydiaceae consists of small bacteria that are obligate intracellular parasites, depending on the host cell for energy in the forms of adenosine triphosphate (ATP) and nicotinamide adenine dinucleotide (NAD^+). They grow in cytoplasmic vacuoles in a limited number of host cell types. The family has three important human pathogens: *Chlamydia trachomatis, Chlamydophila psittaci,* and *Chlamydophila pneumoniae.* [Note: The recently described nomenclature separating these pathogens into two different genera (*Chlamydia* and *Chlamydophila*) has not been widely adopted. Furthermore, complete genome sequence analyses suggest separation of these bacteria into two genera is inconsistent with their evolutionary history.] *C. trachomatis* infections cause diseases of the genitourinary (GU) tract and the eye, including many cases of nongonococcal urethritis (NGU) and ocular infections such as trachoma. *C. psittaci* and *C. pneumoniae* infect the respiratory tract. *C. psittaci* causes psittacosis and is spread to the respiratory tract of humans via inhalation of infected bird feces or respiratory secretions. *C. pneumoniae* causes atypical pneumonia and is spread person to person via respiratory droplets. Figure 17.1 summarizes the clinically significant chlamydiae.

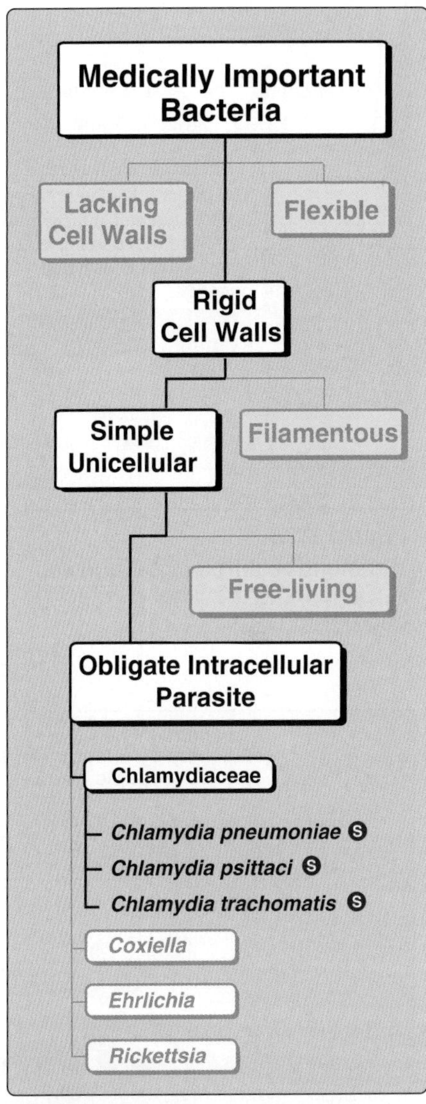

Figure 17.1
Classification of *Chlamydia.*
S See pp. 335–336 for summaries of these organisms.

II. GENERAL FEATURES OF CHLAMYDIAE

Chlamydiae are small, round-to-ovoid organisms that vary in size during the different stages of their replicative cycle (Figure 17.2). The chlamydial cell envelope consists of two lipid bilayers resembling a gram-negative envelope. Although the presence of peptidoglycan has never been directly demonstrated in isolated organisms, genes for the biosynthesis of peptidoglycan are universally present in the genomes of the family. Cell wall active antimicrobials have negative impacts on the life cycle of the chlamydiae, inducing a persistent state that may contribute to the chronicity of infection. The chlamydial DNA genome is small. For example, the genome of *C. pneumoniae* comprises 1,230 kilobase pairs (kbs), making it among the smallest found in prokaryotic cells. Chlamydiae possess ribosomes and synthesize their own proteins and, therefore, are sensitive to antibiotics that inhibit this process, such as tetracyclines and macrolides (see pp. 43–44).

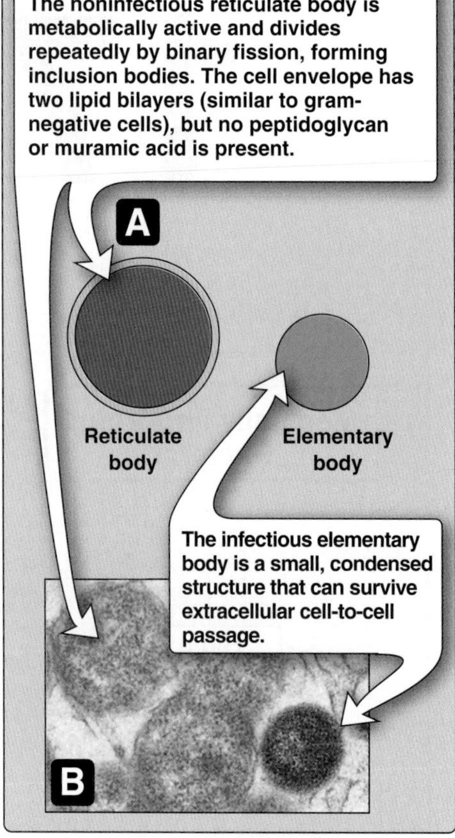
The noninfectious reticulate body is metabolically active and divides repeatedly by binary fission, forming inclusion bodies. The cell envelope has two lipid bilayers (similar to gram-negative cells), but no peptidoglycan or muramic acid is present.
A
Reticulate body
Elementary body
The infectious elementary body is a small, condensed structure that can survive extracellular cell-to-cell passage.
B

Figure 17.2
Structural features of *Chlamydia*. A. Schematic drawing. B. Electron micrograph.

A. Physiology

Chlamydiae are energy parasites, requiring living cells for growth. They are unable to synthesize their own pools of ATP or regenerate NAD^+ by oxidation. With these high-energy molecules exogenously supplied, chlamydiae produce CO_2 from compounds such as glucose, pyruvate, and glutamate and carry out the usual bacterial metabolic activities.

B. Pathogenesis

Chlamydiae have a unique life cycle, with morphologically distinct infectious and reproductive forms (Figure 17.3). The extracellular infectious form, the elementary body, is a tiny, condensed, apparently inert structure that can survive extracellular cell-to-cell passage and initiate an infection. The elementary body is taken up by phagocytosis into susceptible host cells, a process facilitated by proteins in the chlamydial cell envelope that function as adhesins, directing attachment to glycolipid or glycopolysaccharide receptors on the host cell membrane. Once inside the cell, the elementary body prevents fusion of the phagosome and lysosome, protecting itself from enzymatic destruction. The particle reorganizes over the next 8 hours into a larger, noninfectious reticulate body, which becomes metabolically active and divides repeatedly by binary fission within an inclusion in the cytoplasm of the host cell. As the reticulate body divides, it fills the endosome with its progeny, forming an inclusion body. After 48 hours, multiplication ceases, and reticulate bodies condense to become new infectious elementary bodies. The elementary bodies are then released from the cell by cytolysis, ending in host cell death.

C. Laboratory identification

1. **Useful stains:** Chlamydiae are not stained using the Gram stain but can be visualized under light microscopy by stains that pre-

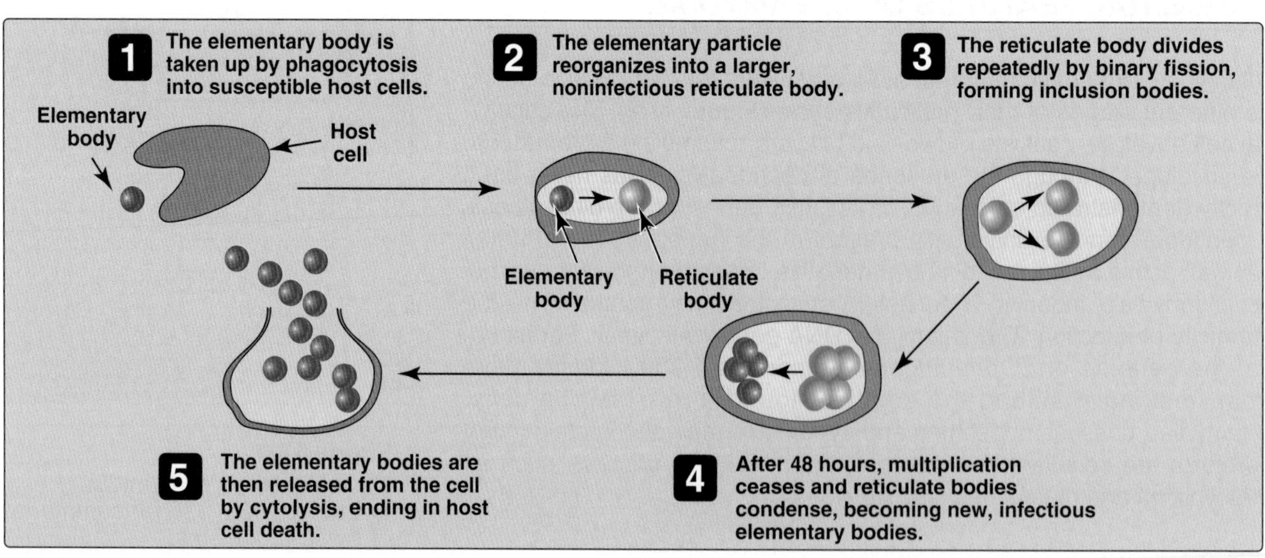
1 The elementary body is taken up by phagocytosis into susceptible host cells.
Elementary body
Host cell
2 The elementary particle reorganizes into a larger, noninfectious reticulate body.
Elementary body
Reticulate body
3 The reticulate body divides repeatedly by binary fission, forming inclusion bodies.
4 After 48 hours, multiplication ceases and reticulate bodies condense, becoming new, infectious elementary bodies.
5 The elementary bodies are then released from the cell by cytolysis, ending in host cell death.

Figure 17.3
Reproductive cycle of *Chlamydiaceae*.

serve the host cell architecture. Direct immunofluorescence is also a common and useful procedure. In *C. trachomatis* only, a matrix of glycogen-like material accumulates in the inclusions, which can be shown by staining with iodine. Other species do not produce this reaction.

2. **Chlamydial antigens:** Although DNA identity among the family Chlamydiaceae is less than 30 percent, they share lipopolysaccharide antigens. In addition, there is a class of abundant outer membrane proteins that have species or subspecies specificity and elicit protective antibodies. Antigenic classification in this genus is usually done by immunofluorescence, using monoclonal antibodies.

III. CHLAMYDIA TRACHOMATIS

C. trachomatis is divided into a number of serotypes, which correlate with the clinical syndrome they cause (Figure 17.4). For example, *C. trachomatis*, the major causal agent of the syndrome NGU, is currently the most common reportable infectious disease in the United States. *C. trachomatis* can also cause eye infections, with symptoms ranging from irritation to blindness. Trachoma, which is an ancient disease, was well described in Egyptian writings around 3800 B.C. It remains widely prevalent in developing areas of the world.

Species and serotype	Disease
C. trachomatis	
A, B, C	• Trachoma
D – K	• Cervicitis • Endometritis • Epididymitis • Inclusion conjunctivitis of the newborn or adult • Infant pneumonia syndrome • Nongonococcal urethritis • Proctitis • Salpingitis
L_1, L_2, L_3	• Lymphogranuloma venereum
C. psittaci Many	• Pneumonia (psittacosis)
C. pneumoniae One	Acute respiratory diseases, including: • Bronchitis • Pharyngitis • Pneumonia • Sinusitis

Figure 17.4
Correlation between chlamydial species/serotypes and disease.

A. Clinical significance

C. trachomatis causes a range of GU and eye infections.

1. **Nongonococcal urethritis:** Annually, more than 4 million urogenital *C. trachomatis* infections occur in the United States in young, sexually active individuals of all socioeconomic groups. In men, the urethra is the initial site of infection. Women may present with cervicitis and/or urethritis (see p. 182). Infections are often asymptomatic, although communicable. [Note: Among women, the asymptomatic rate is higher than 50 percent.] Whether locally symptomatic or not, the infection may ascend into the upper reproductive tract to involve the epididymis in men and fallopian tubes and adjacent tissues in women (pelvic inflammatory disease). Chlamydial NGU is symptomatically similar to infections caused by *Neisseria gonorrhoeae* (see p. 102), although the average incubation time is longer (2 to 3 weeks), and the discharge tends to be more mucoid and contains fewer pus cells. In addition, the two infections often occur simultaneously. Therefore, patients suspected of chlamydial infection should be treated for gonococcal infection. NGU is caused by serotypes D–K of *C. trachomatis* (see Figure 17.4). These serotypes also cause eye infections, for example, in infants born to genitally infected women (Figure 17.5). Infection with *C. trachomatis* confers little protection against reinfection, which commonly occurs. Repeated or chronic episodes may lead to infertility in both sexes and to ectopic pregnancies.

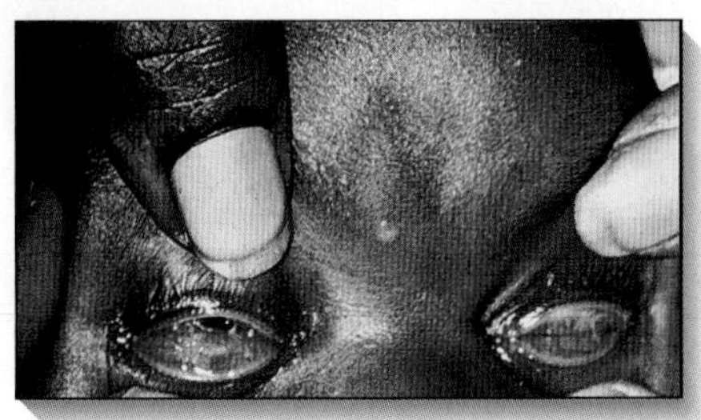

Figure 17.5
Neonatal conjunctivitis due to chlamydial infection.

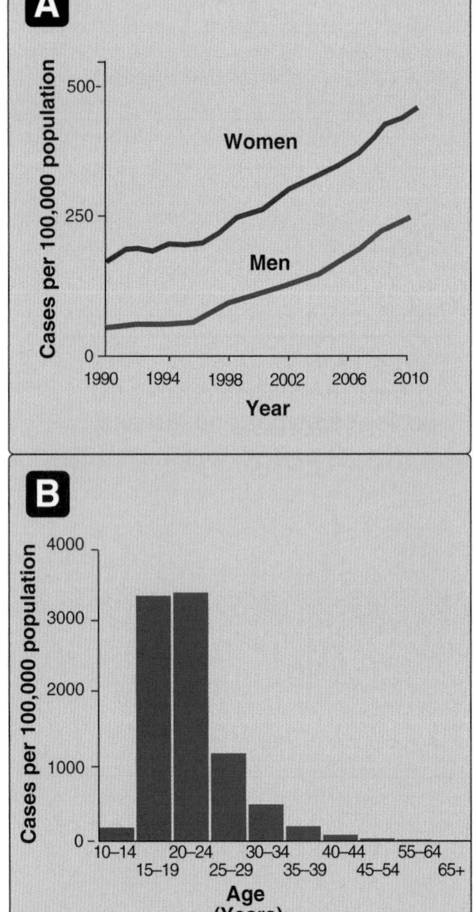

Figure 17.6
Prevalence of chlamydial infection in the United States (2010). A. by sex; B. Among females according to age.

2. **Lymphogranuloma venereum:** *C. trachomatis* serotypes L_1, L_2, and L_3 cause lymphogranuloma venereum (LGV), a more invasive sexually transmitted disease. It is uncommon in the United States but endemic in Asia, Africa, and South America. LGV is characterized by transient papules on the external genitalia, followed in 1 to 2 months by painful swelling of inguinal and perirectal lymph nodes. Adenopathy (swelling of the lymph nodes) is often accompanied by mild constitutional symptoms. The inguinal ligament often forms a cleft known as the "groove sign" between masses of inguinal lymph nodes. The affected lymph nodes suppurate (to form or discharge pus), and chronic inflammation and fibrosis lead to extensive ulceration and blockage of regional lymphatic drainage. (See pp. 367–371 for a summary of sexually transmitted diseases.)

3. **Trachoma:** *C. trachomatis*, serotypes A, B, B_a, and C cause a chronic keratoconjunctivitis that often results in blindness (see p. 182). Trachoma is transmitted by personal contact, for example, from eye to eye via droplets, by contaminated surfaces touched by hands and conveyed to the eye, or by flies. Because of persistent or repeated infection over several years, the inflammatory response with attendant scarring leads to permanent opacities of the cornea and distortion of eyelids.

4. **Neonatal conjunctivitis and other infections:** Over 50 percent of infants born to women infected with *C. trachomatis*, serotypes D–K (see Figure 17.4) will contract symptomatic infection on passage through the birth canal. The most common presentation is inclusion conjunctivitis of the newborn (see Figure 17.5). This acute, purulent conjunctivitis (named for the inclusion bodies [see p. 178] seen in infected conjunctival epithelial cells) usually heals after appropriate antimicrobial therapy, without permanent damage to the eye. If untreated, the infection can lead to permanent scarring of the cornea or conjunctiva. Approximately 1 of 10 infected infants will present with or develop pneumonia, which can be treated with erythromycin.

5. **Inclusion conjunctivitis in adults:** Individuals of any age may develop transient purulent conjunctivitis caused by *C. trachomatis* serotypes D–K (see Figure 17.4). Such individuals are often found to be genitally infected as well.

B. Laboratory identification

C. trachomatis can be demonstrated in clinical material by several direct procedures and by culturing in human cell lines. Samples, particularly from the urethra and cervix in GU infection and conjunctivae in ocular disease, should be obtained by cleaning away overlying exudate and gently scraping to collect infected epithelial cells.

1. **Direct tests:** Microscopic examination using direct fluorescent antibody staining reveals characteristic cellular cytoplasmic inclusions. *C. trachomatis* infections can be detected with high sensitivity and

specificity using DNA amplification performed on urine specimens. This permits cost-effective screening of large numbers of individuals without the need for access to a medical clinic and a pelvic examination. Figure 17.6 shows the high prevalence of infection among young females.

2. **Culturing methods:** *C. trachomatis* can be cultivated by tissue culture in several human cell lines. In the standard procedure using McCoy cells, addition to the culture medium of a eukaryotic metabolic inhibitor, such as cycloheximide, enhances growth of the parasite. The presence of chlamydial inclusions can be demonstrated after 2 to 7 days of incubation.

3. **Detection of serotypes:** Serotypes of *C. trachomatis* can be determined by immunofluorescence staining with monoclonal antibodies. However, the procedure is not widely used because it adds little to clinical impressions. Serologic testing for specific antibodies is similarly not helpful except in suspected LGV, in which a single high-titer response is diagnostic.

C. Treatment and prevention

Chlamydiae are sensitive to a number of broad-spectrum antibacterials. Azithromycin and tetracycline are currently the drugs of choice. Resistant strains have not been reported in the clinical setting. Erythromycin should be used in small children and pregnant women because of the effects of tetracyclines on teeth and bones (see Figure 17.8). The only recommended treatment for a concurrent gonococcal infection is with ceftriaxone. A topical ocular preparation containing erythromycin provides moderately effective prophylaxis in newborns. Detection (a particular problem in asymptomatic individuals) followed by specific treatment is the key means of control.

IV. CHLAMYDIA PSITTACI

Psittacosis, also known as ornithosis, denotes a zoonotic (animal) disease that is transmitted to humans by inhalation of dust contaminated with respiratory secretions or feces of infected birds. The human disease usually targets the lower respiratory tract (Figure 17.7). There is an acute onset of fever, hacking dry cough, and flulike symptoms. Bilateral patchy pulmonary infiltrates are observed. Enlargement of liver and spleen is a frequent accompanying feature. Frank hepatitis, encephalitis, or myocarditis sometimes ensues. The severity of illness ranges from essentially asymptomatic infection to, rarely, a fatal outcome, usually for older patients. A wide variety of bird species, including psittacines (the parrot family), carry *C. psittaci*, often latently, and whether contact occurred with either diseased or healthy birds is an important factor in formulating the differential diagnosis. Veterinarians, zookeepers, and poultry processing workers, who handle birds regularly, are particularly at risk. A specific diagnosis can be made by showing a fourfold rise in antibody titer with either complement fixation (see p. 274) or indirect immunofluorescence tests (see p. 27). Although the organism can be grown in tissue culture from sputum and other clinical materials, this is not routinely attempted.

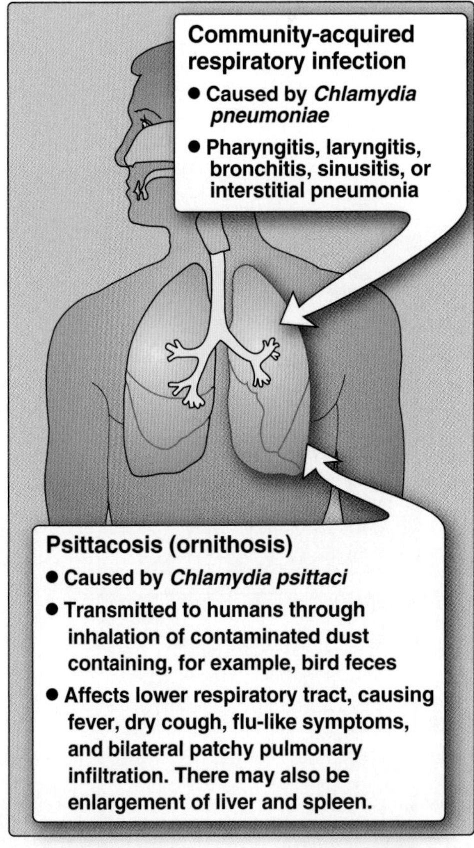

Community-acquired respiratory infection
• Caused by Chlamydia pneumoniae
• Pharyngitis, laryngitis, bronchitis, sinusitis, or interstitial pneumonia
Psittacosis (ornithosis)
• Caused by Chlamydia psittaci
• Transmitted to humans through inhalation of contaminated dust containing, for example, bird feces
• Affects lower respiratory tract, causing fever, dry cough, flu-like symptoms, and bilateral patchy pulmonary infiltration. There may also be enlargement of liver and spleen.

Figure 17.7
Diseases caused by *Chlamydia psittaci* and *Chlamydia pneumoniae*.

Chlamydia

Chlamydia species

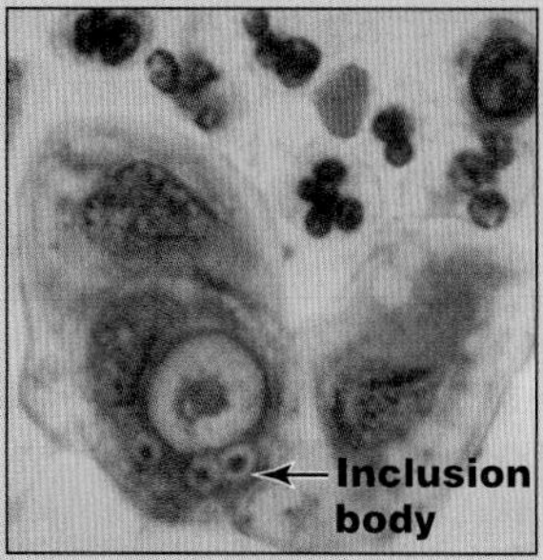

Chlamydia trachomatis inclusion bodies

- Not routinely stained with Gram stain
- Small, round-to-ovoid organisms
- Envelope consists of two lipid bilayers
- Obligate intracellular parasites; replicate in endocytic vacuoles, creating characteristic cytoplasmic inclusion bodies

Chlamydia pneumoniae

- Community-acquired respiratory infection

Chlamydia psittaci

- Psittacosis (ornithosis)

Chlamydia trachomatis

- Nongonococcal urethritis
- Trachoma
- Inclusion conjunctivitis of the newborn
- Lymphogranuloma venereum

1 Doxycycline

1 Azithromycin[1]

1 Erythromycin[1]

[1] Azithromycin or erythromycin should be substituted for doxycycline in small children and pregnant women because of the effects of tetracyclines on calcification of bones and teeth.

Non-gonococcal urethritis

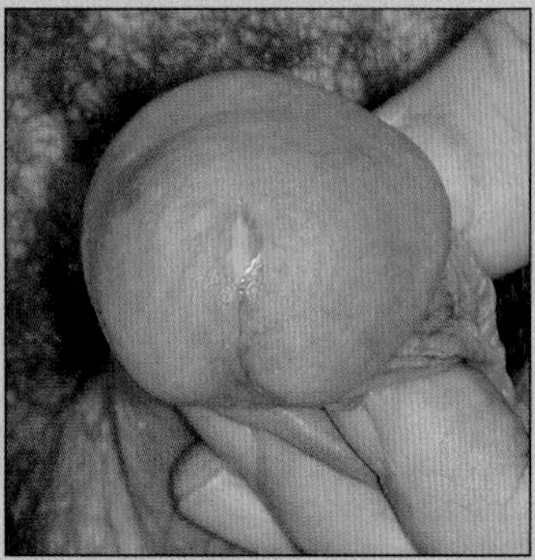

Trachoma

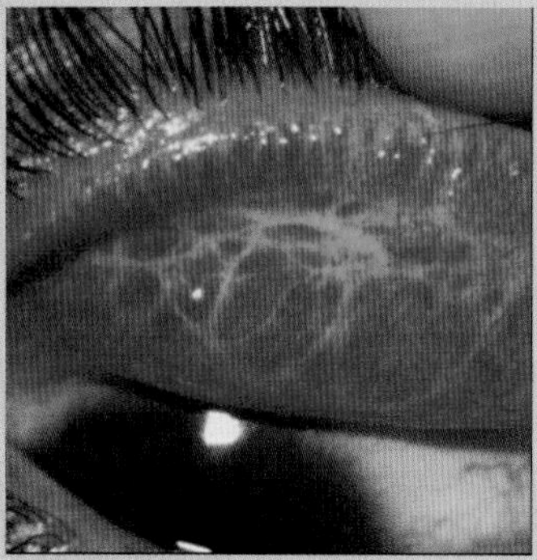

Lymphogranuloma venerium

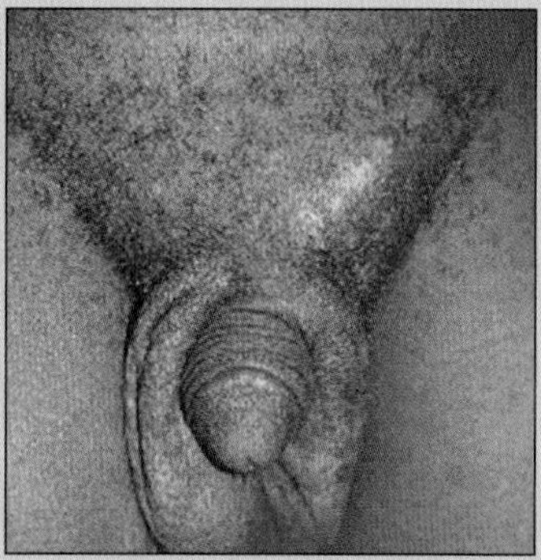

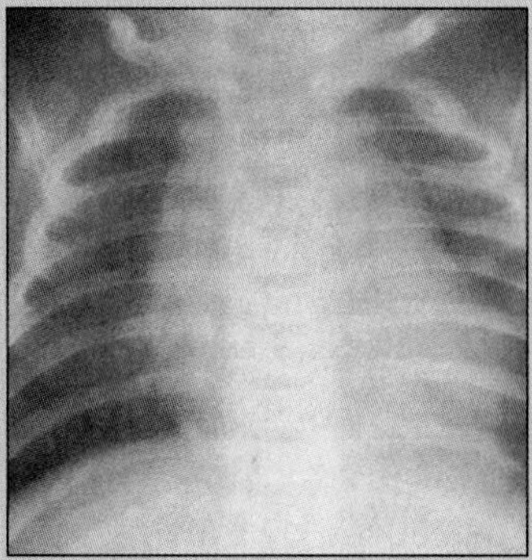

Respiratory infections

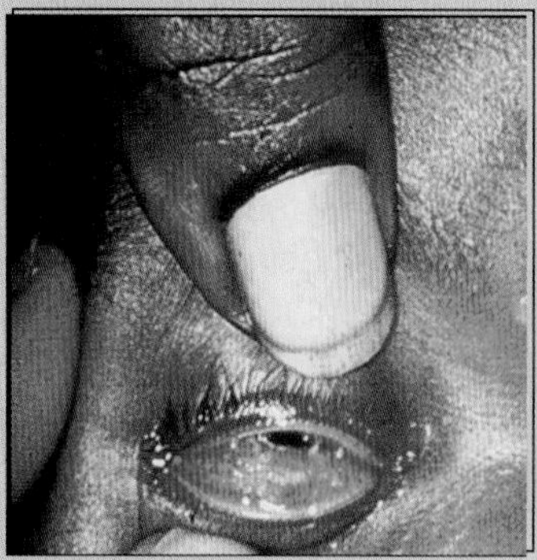

Inclusion conjunctivitis of the newborn

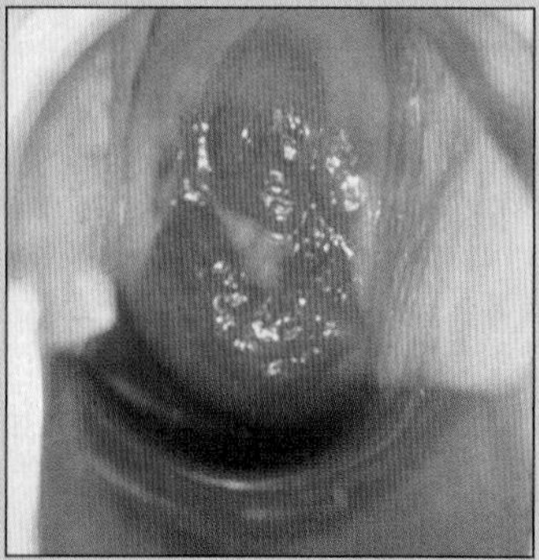

Chlamydial cervicitis

Figure 17.8
Summary of *Chlamydia* . 1 Indicates first-line drugs.

Some strains are highly contagious and impose a considerable laboratory risk. If given early in the disease, doxycycline or erythromycin is effective in eradicating symptoms, but the organisms sometimes persist well into convalescence, because the drugs are bacteriostatic, not bactericidal (see p. 31).

V. CHLAMYDIA PNEUMONIAE

C. pneumoniae is a respiratory pathogen causing pharyngitis, sometimes followed by laryngitis, bronchitis, or interstitial pneumonia. It is a significant cause of community-acquired respiratory infection, occurring worldwide and without seasonal incidence. Epidemic outbreaks have been reported. About 50 percent of adults in the United States have antibodies to *C. pneumoniae*. Nevertheless, reinfection is known to occur. Several recent studies have linked *C. pneumoniae* antigens (or higher antibody titers to the organism) with atherosclerotic processes and asthma. However, a role for the organism in these diseases has not been established. Neither serologic tests nor recovery by culturing is routinely available. The organism is sensitive to doxycycline and erythromycin. Some patients will have a clinical relapse after completing 10 – 14 days of antibiotic therapy. In these patients, a second course of treatment may be helpful in achieving more lasting improvement

Study Questions

Choose the ONE correct answer.

17.1 Which one of the following is characteristic of chlamydiae?

A. Reticulate bodies are an infectious, extracellular form of the organism.

B. Most genital tract infections are asymptomatic and undiagnosed and untreated.

C. They are sensitive to β-lactam antibiotics.

D. They stain gram-positive.

E. Inclusion bodies are formed from division of elementary bodies.

Correct answer = B. The extracellular infectious form is called the elementary body, not the reticulate body. Once inside the cell, the elementary body reorganizes into a larger, noninfectious reticulate body, which becomes metabolically active and divides repeatedly by binary fission within the cytoplasm of the host cell, forming an inclusion body. Chlamydiae are not stained using the Gram stain. The chlamydial cell envelope contains no peptidoglycan; thus β-lactam antibiotics have no effect on cell growth.

17.2 A feature of *chlamydiae* that is unique to this group is:

A. the requirement of an obligate intracellular habitat.
B. its replicative cycle is distinguished by two morphologic forms that develop within cytoplasmic vacuoles.
C. the lack of detectable peptidoglycan in its cell envelope.
D. its use of host coenzymes of energy metabolism.
E. all of the above.

Correct answer = B. Extracellularly, chlamydiae exist as small, dense elementary bodies that are highly infective but metabolically inert. In host cell cytoplasmic vacuoles, they develop into larger, metabolically active reticulate bodies that divide, and the progeny finally mature into elementary bodies that are released. Rickettsiae are also obligately intracellular and use certain host energy coenzymes. Certain other unrelated species appear to require living host cells for growth. Mycoplasmas also have no detectable peptidoglycan in their cell envelope.

17.3 A 19-year old male presents at an STD clinic with a urethral discharge and dysuria. A swab specimen was collected and examined by Gram stain followed by light microscopy. Polymorphonuclear leukocytes were detected in the exudate along with intracellular and extracellular Gram negative diplococci. How should this patient's infection be treated?

A. No treatment is necessary
B. With a tetracycline-based antibiotic such as doxycycline.
C. With a third-generation cephalosporin antibiotic such as ceftriaxone
D. With a combination of ceftriaxone and doxycycine
E. With penicillin

Correct answer = D. The presentation and microbiological findings suggest that the patient is suffering from gonococcal urethritis. However, chlamydial urethritis is also a possibility and the two infections are often co-resident in the same patient. Appropriate treatment for both infections includes ceftriaxone and doxycycline. Without treatment, the infection could spread to the upper genital tract leading to more serious sequelae. Use of doxycycline alone would not treat the gonococcal infection as many clinical isolates are resistant to tetracycline derivatives. Similarly, treatment with ceftriaxone alone would not be effective against a chlamydial infection. Penicillin is not recommended to treat infections with either pathogen.

17.4 A 35-year-old, small animal veterinarian presents with severe headache, myalgia, and splenomegaly in addition to pulmonary findings. A scanty sputum was obtained, containing a few mixed bacteria and scattered mononuclear cells on routine Gram staining. Which of the following organism is most likely to caause these symptoms?

A. *Chlamydophila pneumoniae*
B. *Chlamydophila psittaci*
C. *Chlamydia trachomatis*
D. *Legionella pneumophila*
E. *Mycoplasma pneumoniae*

Correct answer = B. The veterinarian probably has psittacosis, which is transmitted to humans by inhalation of dust contaminated with respiratory secretions from infected birds.

17.5 Which of the following antibiotics is most likely to be effective for chlamydial infections?

A. Penicillins
B. Vancomycin
C. Cephalosporins
D. Carbapenems
E Macrolides

Correct answer = E. Chlamydiae possess ribosomes and synthesize their own proteins and, therefore, are sensitive to antibiotics that inhibit this process, such as tetracyclines and macrolides. Chlamydiae lack detectable peptidoglycan in their cell wall even though genes that encode their peptidoglycan biosynthesis enzymes are encoded in their genomes. Antibitoics that interfere with peptidoglycan synthesis, such as penicillin and cephalosporins, are not effective in clearance of these intracellular organisms.

Mycobacteria and Actinomycetes

18

I. OVERVIEW

Mycobacteria are slender rods with lipid-rich cell walls that are resistant to penetration by chemical dyes such as those used in the Gram stain. They stain poorly but, once stained, cannot be easily decolorized by treatment with acidified organic solvents. Therefore, they are termed "acid-fast" (see p. 21). Mycobacteria survive and replicate intracellularly. Mycobacterial infections generally result in the formation of slow-growing granulomatous lesions that are responsible for major tissue destruction. For example, *Mycobacterium tuberculosis* causes tuberculosis, the principal chronic bacterial disease in humans and a leading cause worldwide of death from infection. This organism has increasingly become a cause for special concern in immunocompromised patients. Members of the genus *Mycobacterium* also cause leprosy as well as several tuberculosis-like human infections. This genus belongs to the order of organisms (Actinomycetales) that also includes the genera *Actinomyces* and *Nocardia*. These organisms all cause granulomatous lesions with various clinical presentations. Mycobacteria and other clinically significant Actinomycetales discussed in this chapter are listed in Figure 18.1.

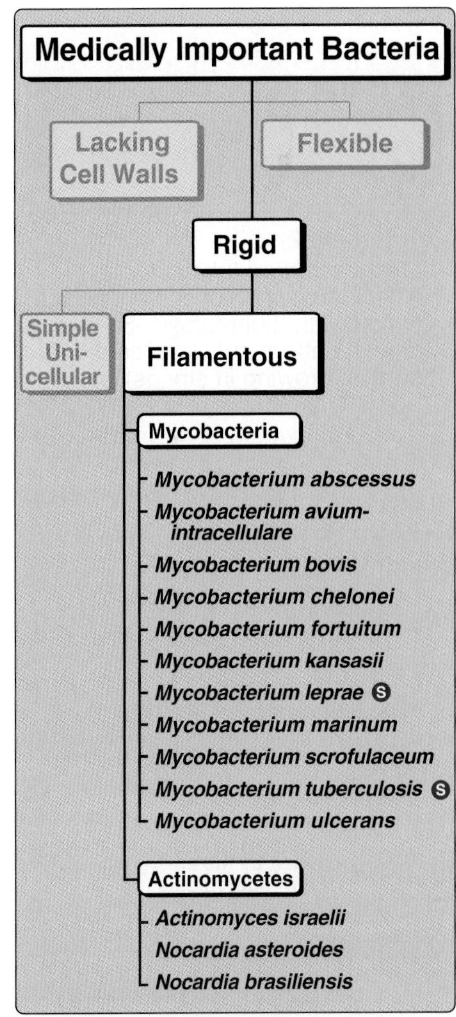

Figure 18.1
Classification of *Mycobacteria* and *Actinomycetes*.
S See pp. 343–344 for summaries of these organisms.

II. MYCOBACTERIA

Mycobacteria are long, slender rods that are nonmotile and do not form spores (Figure 18.2). Mycobacterial cell walls are unusual in that they are approximately 60 percent lipid, including a unique class of very long–chain (75 to 90 carbons), β-hydroxylated fatty acids (mycolic acids). These complex with a variety of polysaccharides and peptides, creating a waxy cell surface that makes mycobacteria strongly hydrophobic and accounts for their acid-fast staining characteristic. Their unusual cell walls make mycobacteria impervious to many chemical disinfectants and convey resistance to the corrosive action of strong acids or alkalis. Use is made of this fact in decontaminating clinical specimens, such as sputum, in which nonmycobacterial organisms are digested by such treatments. Mycobacteria are also resistant to drying but not to heat or ultraviolet irradiation. Mycobacteria are strictly aerobic. Most species grow slowly with generation times of 8 to 24 hours.

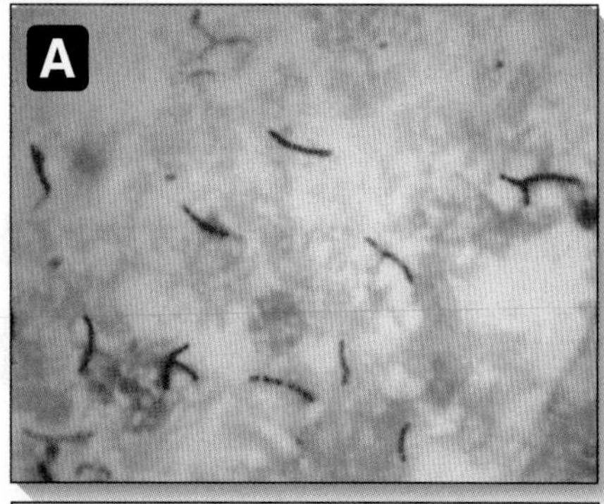

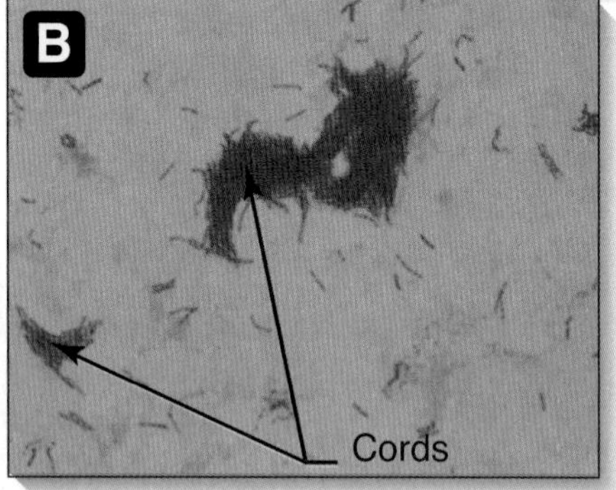

Figure 18.2
Mycobacterium tuberculosis.
A. Acid-fast stain of sputum from a patient with tuberculosis. B. Typical growth pattern showing "cording" (that is, growing in strings).

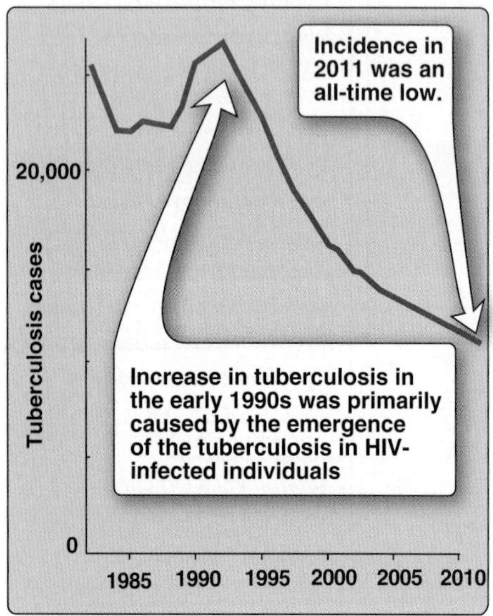

Figure 18.3
Incidence of new cases of tuberculosis (United States).

A. Mycobacterium tuberculosis

It is currently estimated that about one third of the world's population is infected with *M. tuberculosis* (tubercle bacillus), with 30 million people having active disease. The incidence of tuberculosis in the United States has declined for many years and is now at a historic low (Figure 18.3). In contrast to the decline of tuberculosis in the West, the incidence of the disease in some Asian and sub-Saharan African nations has dramatically increased. In some of these nations, nearly 50 percent of the HIV-infected population is co-infected with *M. tuberculosis.*

1. **Epidemiology:** Patients with active pulmonary tuberculosis shed large numbers of organisms by coughing, creating aerosol droplet nuclei. Because of resistance to dessication, the organisms can remain viable as droplet nuclei suspended in room air for at least 30 minutes. The principal mode of contagion is person-to-person transmission by inhalation of the aerosol. A single infected person can pass the organism to numerous people in an exposed group, such as a family, classroom, or hospital ward without proper isolation.

2. **Pathogenicity:** After being inhaled, mycobacteria reach the alveoli, where they multiply in the pulmonary epithelium or macrophages. Within 2 to 4 weeks, many bacilli are destroyed by the immune system, but some survive and are spread by the blood to extrapulmonary sites. The virulence of *M. tuberculosis* rests with its ability to survive and grow within host cells (Figure 18.4). Although the organism produces no demonstrable toxins, when engulfed by macrophages, bacterial sulfolipids inhibit the fusion of phagocytic vesicles with lysosomes. The ability of *M. tuberculosis* to grow even in immunologically activated macrophages and to remain viable within the host for decades is a unique characteristic of the pathogen.

3. **Immunity:** *M. tuberculosis* stimulates both a humoral and a cell-mediated immune response. Although circulating antibodies appear, they do not convey resistance to the organism. Instead, cellular immunity ($CD4^+$ T cells) and the accompanying delayed hypersensitivity directed against a number of bacterial protein antigens, develop in the course of infection and contribute to both the pathology of and immunity to the disease.

4. **Clinical significance:** Primary tuberculosis occurs in a person who has had no previous contact with the organism. For the majority of cases (about 95 percent), the infection becomes arrested, and most people are unaware of this initial encounter. The only evidence of tuberculosis may be a positive tuberculin test (see p. 189). Figure 18.4 illustrates the course of tuberculosis infection either remaining dormant or progressing to clinical disease. A chest radiograph sometimes shows the initial pulmonary nodule (a healing tubercle, see below), and some fibrosis as shown in Figure 18.5. Approximately 10 percent of those with an arrested primary infection develop clinical tuberculosis at some later time in their lives.

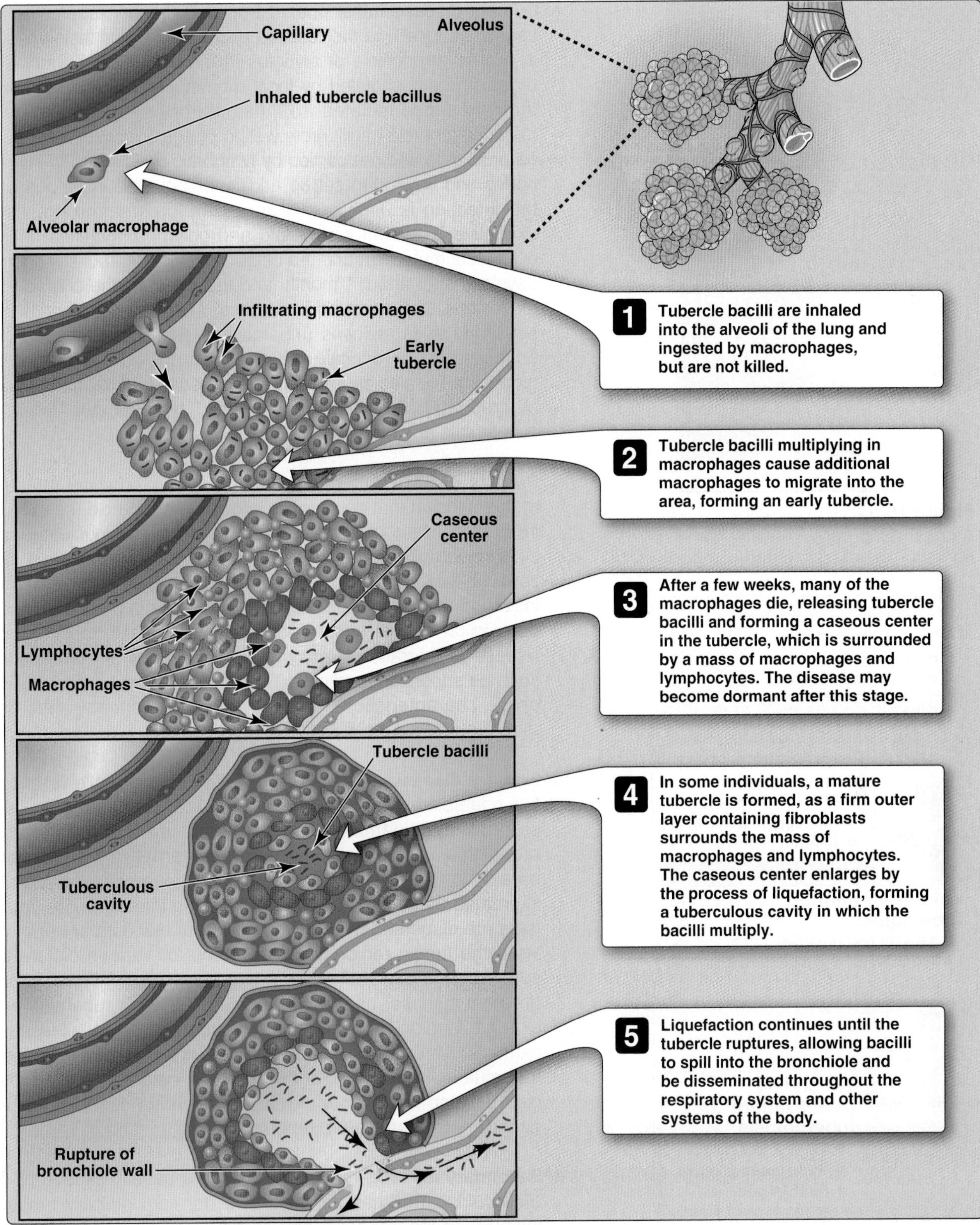

Figure 18.4
Progression of active tuberculosis infection.

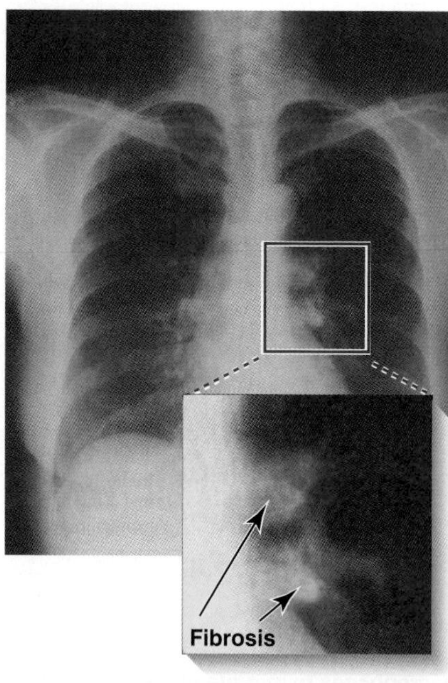

Figure 18.5
A chest radiograph showing some fibrosis—the classic Ghon complex.

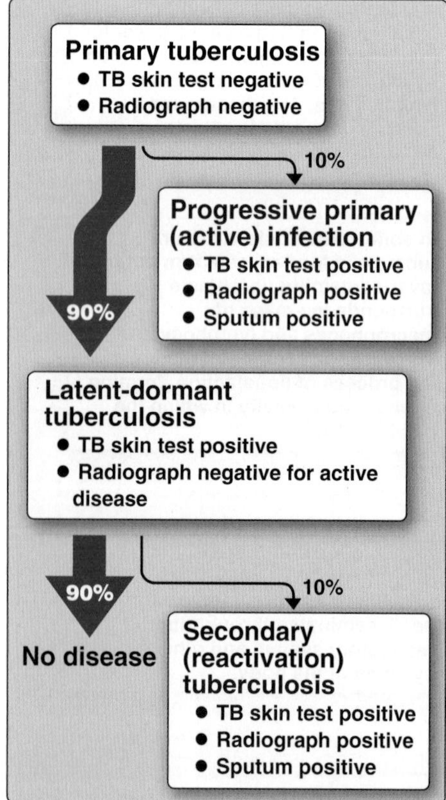

Figure 18.6
Stages in the pathogenesis of tuberculosis (TB).

a. **Primary disease–initial phase:** Because primary tuberculosis is usually acquired via the respiratory tract, the initial lesion occurs in a small bronchiole or alveolus in the midlung periphery. The organisms are engulfed by local mononuclear phagocytes, and their presence initiates an inflammatory reaction. However, because tubercle bacilli grow well in phagocytic cells, the bacteria proliferate and are carried by lymphatic drainage to the lymph nodes and beyond to set up additional foci. This initial phase of the infection is usually mild or asymptomatic and results in exudative lesions in which fluid and polymorphonuclear leukocytes accumulate around the bacilli. A specific immune response develops after about 1 month, and this changes the character of the lesions. Cell-mediated immunity to *M. tuberculosis* and hypersensitivity to its antigens (tuberculoproteins) not only confer an enhanced ability to localize the infection and curb growth of the organism, but also cause a greater capacity to damage the host. Macrophages, activated by specific T lymphocytes, begin to accumulate and destroy the bacilli.

b. **Primary disease–tubercle formation:** The productive (granulomatous) lesion that develops is known as a tubercle (see Figure 18.4). It consists of a central area of large, multinucleate giant cells (macrophage syncytia) containing tubercle bacilli, a midzone of pale epithelioid cells, and a peripheral collar of fibroblasts and mononuclear cells. Tissue damage is produced by the destruction of both bacilli and phagocytes, which results in the release of degradative enzymes and reactive oxygen species such as superoxide radicals. The center of the tubercle develops a characteristic expanding, caseous (cheesy) necrosis (see Figure 18.4).

c. **Primary disease–course:** Primary tuberculosis follows one of two courses: If the lesion arrests, the tubercle undergoes fibrosis and calcification, although viable but nonproliferating organisms may persist (Figure 18.6). Alternatively, if the lesion breaks down, the caseous material is discharged, and a cavity is created that can facilitate spread of the infection. The organisms are dispersed by the lymph and the bloodstream and can seed the lungs; regional lymph nodes; or various distant tissues, such as liver, spleen, kidneys, bone, or meninges. In progressive disease, one or more of the resulting tubercles may expand, leading to destruction of tissue and clinical illness (for example, chronic pneumonitis, tuberculous osteomyelitis, and tuberculous meningitis). In the extreme instance, active tubercles develop throughout the body, a serious condition known as miliary (disseminated) tuberculosis.

d. **Secondary disease–reactivation:** This is usually caused by *M. tuberculosis* that has survived in a dormant primary tubercle lesion (see Figure 18.6). Any of the preexisting tubercles may be involved, but pulmonary sites are most common, particularly the lung apices where high oxygen tension favors mycobacterial growth. The resulting pathology is known as

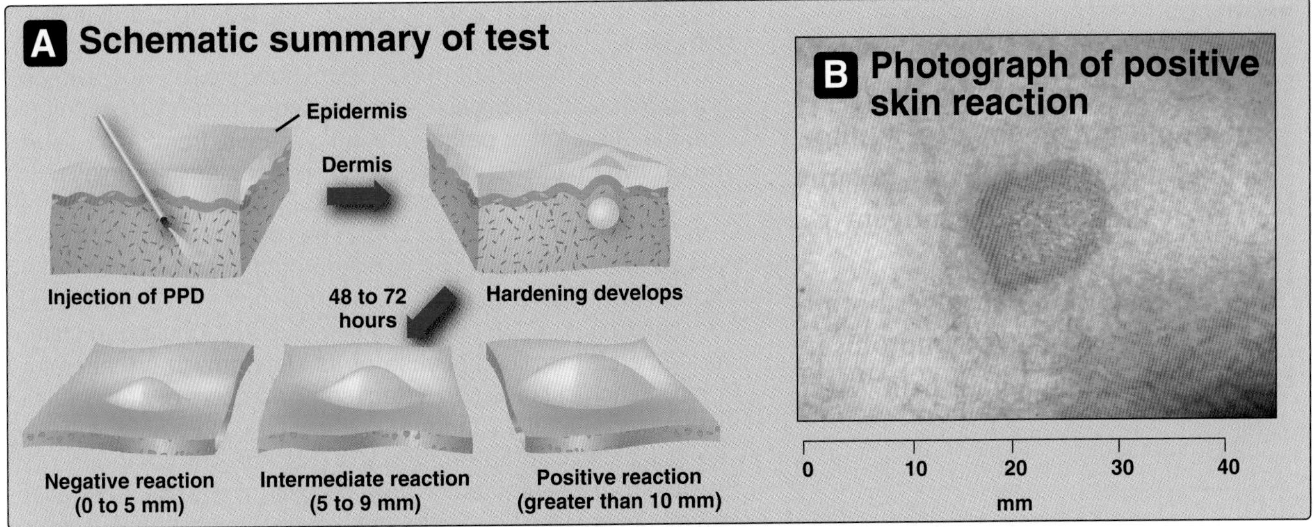

Figure 18.7
Mantoux skin test for tuberculosis. [Note: For some people, determination of a positive reaction may be interpreted more stringently (see Figure 18.8).] PPD = purified protein derivative

"caseation necrosis." Destruction of the lung tissue leads to air-filled cavities where the bacteria replicate actively. Bacterial populations in such lesions often become quite large, and many organisms are shed (for example, in sputum). The patient again becomes capable of exposing others to the disease. Reactivation is apparently caused by an impairment in immune status, often associated with malnutrition, alcoholism, advanced age, or severe stress. Immunosuppressive medication or diseases (such as diabetes and, particularly, AIDS) are common preconditions leading to reactivation.

5. **Tuberculin reaction:** The tuberculin reaction test is a manifestation of delayed hypersensitivity to protein antigens of *M. tuberculosis*. Although such tests can be used to document contact with the tubercle bacillus, they do not confirm that the patient currently has active disease. In the Mantoux test, purified protein derivative (PPD) is prepared from culture filtrates of the organism and biologically standardized. Activity is expressed in tuberculin units. In the routine procedure (Mantoux test), a measured amount of PPD is injected intradermally in the forearm (Figure 18.7). It is read 48 to 72 hours later for the presence and size of an area of induration (hardening) at the site of injection, which must be observed for the test to be positive (Figure 18.8). A positive reaction usually develops 4 to 6 weeks after initial contact with the organism. It remains positive for life, although it may wane after some years or in the presence of immunosuppression by medications or disease.

6. **Laboratory identification:** Diagnosis of active pulmonary tuberculosis includes demonstration of clinical symptoms and abnormal chest radiographs and confirmation by isolation of *M. tuberculosis* from relevant clinical material.

An induration of >5 mm is interpreted as positive in the following populations:

- Persons who have had contact with infectious individuals
- Persons with an abnormal chest radiograph
- HIV-infected and other immunosuppressed persons

An induration of >10 mm is interpreted as positive in the following populations:

- Foreign-born persons from high-prevalence countries
- Residents of prisons, nursing homes, and other institutions
- Healthcare workers
- Persons with other medical risk factors

An induration of >15 mm is interpreted as positive in the following populations:

- Persons with no risk factors

Figure 18.8
Interpretations of the Mantoux skin test for tuberculosis.

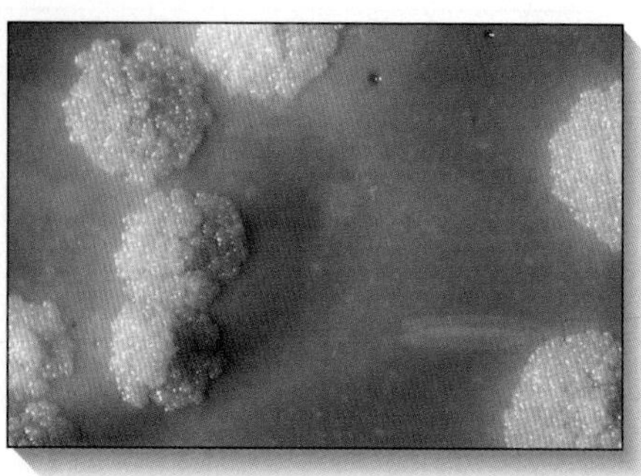

Figure 18.9
Mycobacterium tuberculosis colonies grown on Lowenstein-Jensen medium.

a. **Identification in clinical specimens:** A microscopic search for acid-fast bacilli using techniques such as the Ziehl-Neelsen stain is the most rapid test for mycobacteria. However, *M. tuberculosis* cannot be reliably distinguished on morphologic grounds from other pathogens in the genus, from some saprophytic mycobacterial species that may contaminate glassware and reagents in the laboratory, or from those mycobacteria that may be part of the normal flora. Therefore, a definitive identification of *M. tuberculosis* can only be obtained by culturing the organism or by using one of the newer molecular methods described below. Although 2 to 8 weeks are required to culture the tubercle bacillus because of its slow growth on laboratory media, such cultures can detect small numbers of organisms in the original sample. Figure 18.9 shows a culture of *M. tuberculosis*. Isolation of the organism is essential for determining its antibiotic sensitivity, in addition to confirming the specific identity of the bacillus by growth and biochemical characteristics.

b. **Nucleic acid amplification:** Molecular techniques are increasingly important in the diagnosis of tuberculosis because they have the potential to shorten the time required to detect and identify *M. tuberculosis* in clinical specimens. For example, the amplified *M. tuberculosis* direct test uses enzymes that rapidly make copies of *M. tuberculosis* 16S ribosomal RNA, which can be detected using genetic probes. The sensitivity of the test ranges from 75 to 100 percent, with a specificity of 95 to 100 percent, and it is used for patients whose clinical smears are positive for acid-fast bacilli and whose cultures are in progress. A second technique, the polymerase chain reaction (PCR), amplifies a small portion of a predetermined target region of the *M. tuberculosis* DNA. Using human sputum, commercial PCR kits can confirm the diagnosis of tuberculosis within 8 hours, with a sensitivity and specificity that rivals culture techniques. In addition, PCR analysis facilitates DNA fingerprinting of specific strains, allowing studies of the progress of epidemics.

7. **Treatment:** Several chemotherapeutic agents are effective against *M. tuberculosis*. Because strains of the organism resistant to a particular agent emerge during treatment, multiple drug therapy is employed to delay or prevent emergence. Isoniazid, rifampin, ethambutol, streptomycin, and pyrazinamide are the principal or "first-line" drugs because of their efficacy and acceptable degree of toxicity (see Figure 18.14).

a. **Drug resistance:** Mutants resistant to each of these agents have been isolated even prior to drug treatment. Therefore, the standard procedure is to begin treatment with two or more drugs to prevent outgrowth of resistant strains. Sensitivity tests, administered as soon as sufficient cultured organisms are available, are an important guide to modifying treatment. In most parts of the United States, 8 to 14 percent of *M. tuberculosis* strains are resistant to one or more of the primary drugs when initially isolated from new cases of tuberculosis. The higher incidence of multiple drug–resistant strains (MDR-TB) in some locations and patient populations (for example, prisons) is a cause for great concern.

b. Course of treatment: Clinical tuberculosis requires a long course of treatment because of the characteristics of the organisms and the lesions they produce. For example, as intracellular pathogens, the bacilli are shielded from drugs that do not penetrate host cells, and large cavities with avascular centers are penetrated by drugs with difficulty. Further, in chronic or arrested tubercles, the organisms are nonproliferating and, therefore, not susceptible to many antimicrobial agents. Until recently, 12 to 18 months of drug administration was thought to be required for a clinical cure. In recent years, short courses of 6 months, beginning with a daily dose of a combination of drugs and later by twice-weekly doses, have been successful in curing uncomplicated tuberculosis (Figure 18.10). If the drugs are effective in the pulmonary form of tuberculosis, sputum acid-fast bacteria smears become negative, and the patient becomes noninfectious in 2 to 3 weeks.

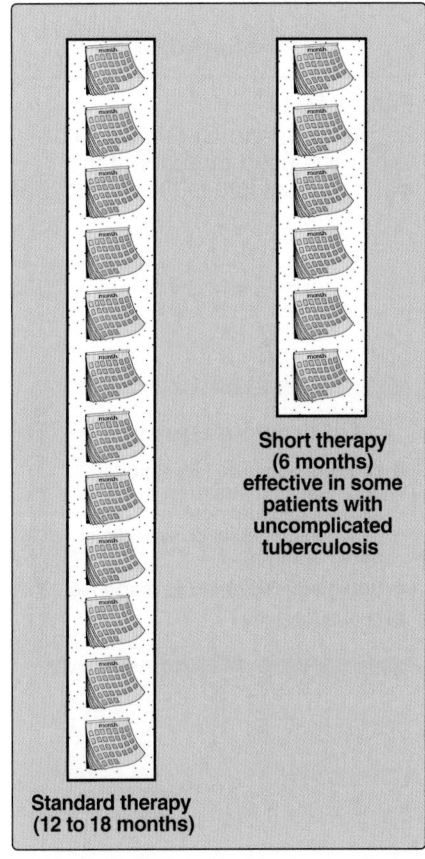

Figure 18.10
Duration of treatment for tuberculosis.

c. Directly observed therapy: Patient compliance is often low when multiple drug schedules last for 6 months or longer. One successful strategy for achieving better treatment completion rates is "directly observed therapy," in which patients take their medication while being supervised and observed. Some healthcare providers have embraced the concept of directly observed therapy, whereas others regard the strategy as expensive and intrusive, suitable only for individuals who have a history of noncompliance.

8. Prevention: Public health measures, such as tuberculin tests, chest radiographs, case registries, and contact tracing have done much to control tuberculosis at the population level.

a. Latent disease chemotherapy: For individuals who are tuberculin-positive but asymptomatic, chemotherapy is indicated in several situations, usually with the single antibiotic isoniazid. For example, people in whom a recent skin test conversion is documented or tuberculin-positive patients who need immunosuppressive therapy for another illness can be protected from active tuberculosis by this treatment.

b. Vaccines: A vaccine against tuberculosis has been available since early in the 20th century. It is produced from Bacille Calmette-Guérin (BCG), an attenuated strain of *Mycobacterium bovis*. When injected intradermally, it can confer tuberculin hypersensitivity and an enhanced ability to activate macrophages that kill the pathogen. This vaccine is about 80 percent protective against serious forms of tuberculosis, such as meningitis in children, and has been used in mass immunization campaigns by the World Health Organization

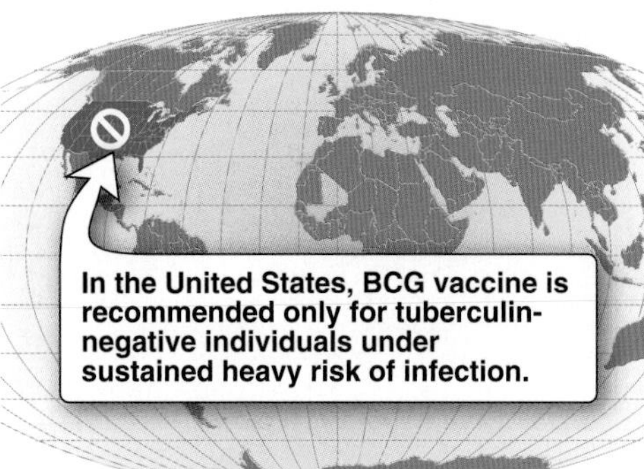

Figure 18.11
Bacille Calmette-Guérin (BCG) vaccine is used throughout the world, but seldom in the United States.

and in several European countries. However, public health officials in the United States recommend that vaccination be considered only for tuberculin-negative individuals under sustained heavy risk of infection, such as special groups of healthcare workers and those at high risk in areas where MDR-TB is common (Figure 18.11). Vaccination results in conversion from PPD negative to PPD positive, thus obviating the utility of the only available surveillance method.

B. Mycobacterium leprae

Leprosy, called Hansen's disease in publications of the United States Public Health Service, is rare in this country, but a small number of cases, both imported and domestically acquired, are reported each year. Worldwide, it is a much larger problem, with an estimated 10 to 12 million cases. Dozens of cases in the United States have been linked to contact with or ingestion of armadillos, a known reservoir of the pathogen.

1. **Pathogenicity:** *Mycobacterium leprae* is transmitted from human to human through prolonged contact, for example, between exudates of a leprosy patient's skin lesions and the abraded skin of another individual. The infectivity of *M. leprae* is low, and the incubation period protracted, so that clinical disease may develop years or even decades after initial contact with the organism.

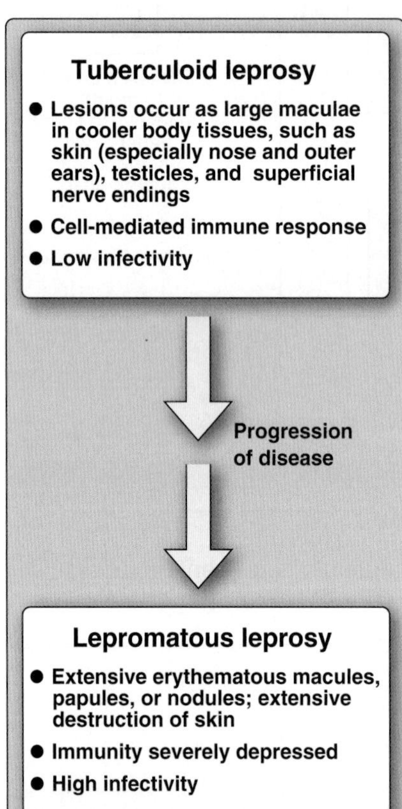

Figure 18.12
Classification of leprosy.

2. **Clinical significance:** Leprosy is a chronic granulomatous condition of peripheral nerves and mucocutaneous tissues, particularly the nasal mucosa. It occurs as a continuum between two clinical extremes: tuberculoid and lepromatous leprosy (Figure 18.12). In tuberculoid leprosy, the lesions occur as large maculae (spots) in cooler body tissues, such as skin (especially the nose, outer ears, and testicles), and in superficial nerve endings. Neuritis leads to patches of anesthesia in the skin. The lesions are heavily infiltrated by lymphocytes and giant and epithelioid cells, but caseation does not occur. The patient mounts a strong cell-mediated immune response and develops delayed hypersensitivity, which can be shown by a skin test with lepromin, a tuberculin-like extract of lepromatous tissue. There are few bacteria in the lesions (paucibacillary). The course of lepromatous leprosy is slow but progressive (Figure 18.13). Large numbers of organisms are present in the lesions and reticuloendothelial system (multibacillary), the results of a severely depressed immune system. No well-formed granulomas emerge.

3. **Laboratory identification:** *M. leprae* is an acid-fast bacillus. It has not been successfully maintained in artificial culture but can be grown in the footpads of mice and in the armadillo, which is a natural host and reservoir of the pathogen. Laboratory diagnosis of lepromatous leprosy, in which organisms are numerous, involves acid-fast stains of specimens from nasal mucosa or other infected areas. In tuberculoid leprosy, organisms are extremely rare, and diagnosis depends on clinical findings and the histology of biopsy material.

4. **Treatment and prevention:** Several drugs are effective in the treatment of leprosy, including sulfones such as dapsone, rifampin, and clofazamine (see Figure 18.14). Treatment is prolonged, and combined therapy is necessary to ensure the suppression of resistant mutants. The fact that vaccination with BCG (see p. 192) has shown some protective effect in leprosy has encouraged further interest in vaccine development. Thalidomide, an inhibitor of tumor necrosis factor-α, is being distributed under tight restrictions for use as a treatment for erythema nodosum leprosum, a serious and severe skin complication of leprosy.

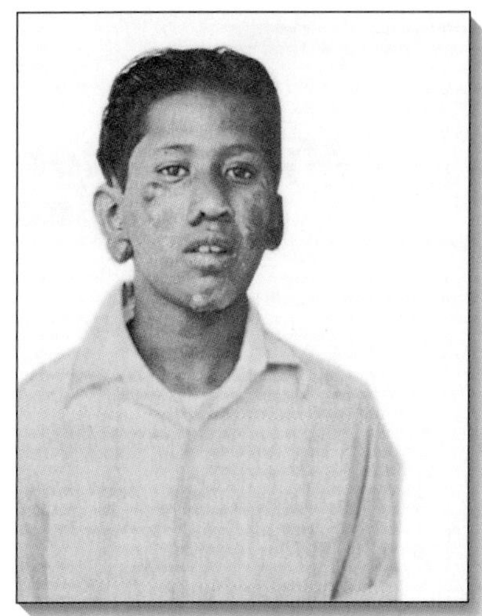

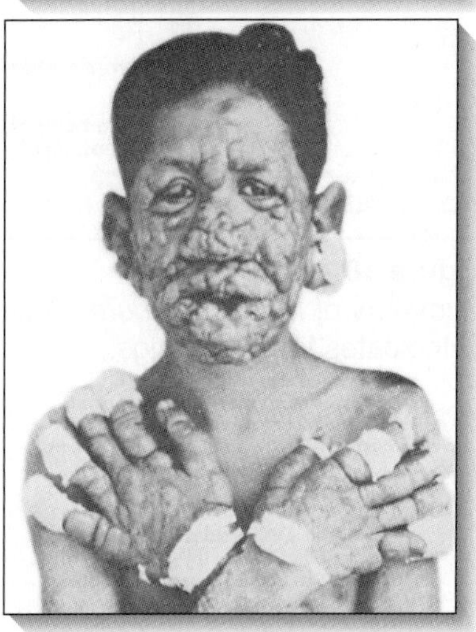

Figure 18.13
A. Leprosy in a 13-year-old Hawaiian boy in 1931. B. Same boy 2 years later. [Note: This patient had the misfortune of contracting leprosy before the era of effective antibiotics.]

III. ACTINOMYCETES

Actinomycetes are a group of filamentous, branching, gram-positive organisms that easily fragment into slender rods (Figure 18.15). Although they superficially resemble fungi on morphologic grounds, they are prokaryotes of bacterial size. They are free-living, mostly soil organisms that are related to corynebacteria and mycobacteria as well as to the streptomycetes that are sources of important antibiotics.

A. Actinomyces israelii

Actinomyces israelii is part of the normal oral and intestinal flora in humans. The organism is a strict anaerobe.

1. **Clinical significance:** Actinomycosis is an infection in which a chronic suppurative abscess leads to scarring and disfigurement. The infection is probably initiated by accidental introduction of organisms into the underlying soft tissue during conditions of sufficient anaerobiasis to support their growth. About half of the cases have a cervicofacial location and are associated with poor dental hygiene and/or tooth extraction ("lumpy jaw"). Other cases involve the lung and chest wall, cecum, appendix, abdominal wall, and pelvic organs. The lesion (mycetoma) begins as a hard, red, relatively nontender swelling that develops slowly, becomes filled with liquid, and ruptures to the surface, discharging quantities of pus. It also spreads laterally, draining pus through several sinus tracts.

2. **Laboratory identification:** The most typical and diagnostic finding in actinomycosis is the presence of "sulfur granules" in the draining pus. These are small, firm, usually yellowish particles, which, in fact, do not contain sulfur. When examined under the microscope, sulfur granules appear as microcolonies composed of filaments of the organism embedded in an amorphous, eosinophilic material thought to be antigen–antibody complexes. The organism can be grown anaerobically on enriched media, such as thioglycollate broth or blood agar. Growth is slow, often requiring 10 to 14 days for visible colonies.

3. **Treatment:** Penicillin G is the treatment of choice for actinomycosis, although a number of antibiotics (clindamycin, erythromycin, and tetracycline) have been shown to have clinical effect.

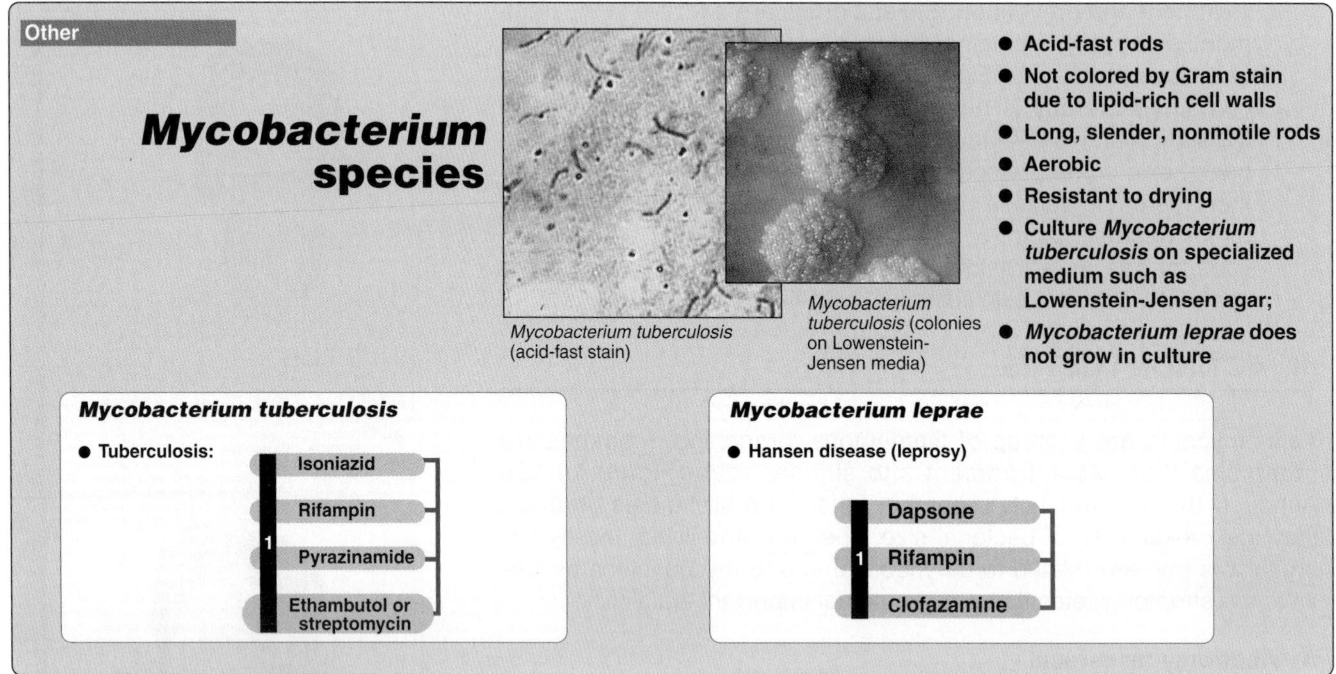

Figure 18.14
Summary of *Mycobacterium* species. Red lines connecting drugs indicates concomitant use of multiple drugs. **1** Indicates first-line drugs.

Treatment must be maintained for weeks to months and may be accompanied by surgical debridement and/or drainage. No significant resistance to penicillin G has been reported. [Note: Good oral hygiene is an important preventive measure.]

B. Nocardia asteroides and Nocardia brasiliensis

Nocardiae are aerobic soil organisms. Infections of humans and domestic animals are opportunistic and not transmissible from person to person. Instead, nocardiae are inhaled or acquired by contamination of skin wounds.

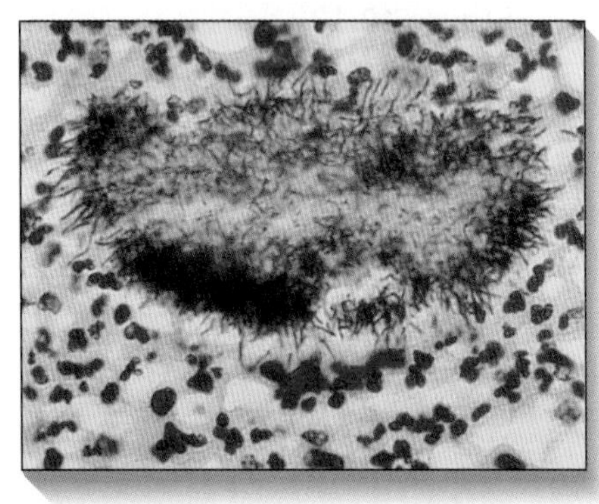

Figure 18.15
Actinomycetoma of the foot using a Brown-Brenn stain. Actinomycetoma is a chronic, granulomatous infection of the skin and subcutaneous tissue caused by *Actinomycetes*.

1. **Clinical significance:** The most common presentation of human **nocardiosis** is a pneumonia of rather chronic course with abscesses, extensive necrosis, and cavity formation. The organisms may metastasize, with the brain and kidneys the most common secondary locations. Important predisposing conditions are immunosuppression associated with lymphoma or other malignancy or with drugs. In the United States, *Nocardia asteroides* is the more common organism associated with this infection.

2. **Laboratory identification:** Nocardiae are gram-positive but irregularly staining, branched filaments (Figure 18.16). They are usually numerous in clinical material and do not form sulfur granules. They stain weakly acid-fast after decolorization with 1 percent sulfuric acid alcohol but fully decolorize with the routine Ziehl-

Neelsen procedure. Nocardiae are strictly aerobic. They grow slowly on a variety of simple media (such as fungal media without antibiotics) and on standard blood agar.

3. **Treatment:** Tmethoprim-sulfamethoxazole (TMP-SMX) is considered by most clinicians to be the drug of choice. Given that some isolates are resistant to TMP-SMX, formal antimicrobial susceptibility testing is always necessary to ensure optimal antibiotic therapy. Other antibiotics, such as ceftriaxone and minocycline, may be effective if *in vitro* susceptibility is demonstrated. The nocardiae are relatively resistant to penicillin. Surgical drainage of the lesions is important, and prolonged therapy may be required to eliminate the infection.

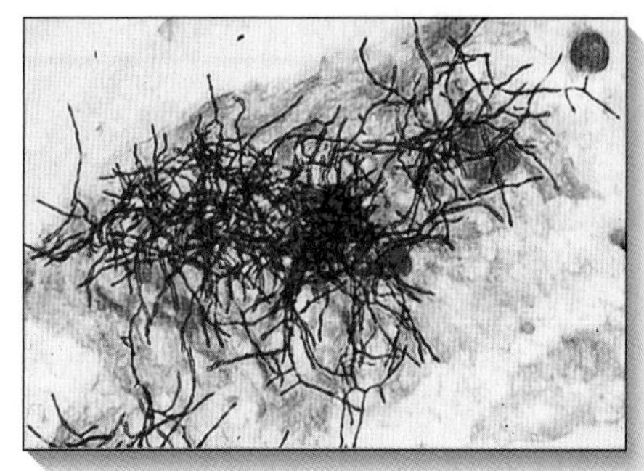

Figure 18.16
Nocardiae.

IV. ATYPICAL MYCOBACTERIA

The atypical mycobacteria are distinct from classical mycobacteria in that they are widespread in the environment and are not pathogenic in rodent animal models. The atypical mycobacteria are classified into four groups (Runyon groups I–IV) based upon several phenotypic characteristics, including pigment production and growth rate. Group I contains the photochromogens, which produce pigment in the light. This group grows very slowly and includes the species *Mycobacterium kansasii* and *Mycobacterium marinum. M. kansasii* causes a chronic pulmonary disease, which can spread within the lungs in a manner similar to tuberculosis. The organism is found in tapwater, primarily localized to the Midwestern states and Texas. *M. marinum* causes a cutaneous infection and is found in fresh- and saltwater habitats. Group II includes *Mycobacterium scrofulaceum*, which is a slow-growing atypical *Mycobacterium* species that produces pigment both in the light and in the dark. The pathogen causes cervical adenitis in children and is found in raw milk, dairy products, soil, and water. Clearance of this pathogen requires excision of the affected lymph nodes. Group III contains the slow-growing nonphotochromogens, including *Mycobacterium avium-intracellulare* complex and *Mycobacterium ulcerans. M. avium* and *M. intracellulare* are virtually indistinguishable diagnostically. They are both found ubiquitously in the environment and cause a serious disseminated disease, very similar to tuberculosis, in immunocompromised patients, in particular those with AIDS. These atypical mycobacteria are particularly resistant to antituberculosis drugs. *M. ulcerans* causes indolent cutaneous infections, known as Buruli ulcers in tropical countries, including those in Africa. The atypical mycobacteria within group IV grow rapidly but do not produce any pigment. This grouping includes three potential pathogens, although all are found ubiquitously in the environment. *Mycobacterium abscessus* causes a chronic lung disease, which can disseminate to skin, bone, and joints. *Mycobacterium fortuitum* and *Mycobacterium chelonei* primarily infect immunocompromised individuals to cause skin and soft tissue infections.

Study Questions

Choose the ONE correct answer

18.1 Which one of the following is characteristic of mycobacteria?

A. They contain mycolic acids.
B. They are resistant to inactivation by heat.
C. They grow extracellularly.
D. They are anaerobic.
E. They are spore forming.

Correct choice = A. Mycobacteria are unique in that their cell walls contain high concentrations of mycolic acids. Mycobacteria are not particularly heat resistant, as witnessed by their susceptibility to pasteurization. They are aerobic, intracellular organisms that do not form spores.

18.2 An acid-fast smear on a patient's sputum is positive. The tuberculin test, however, is negative. A more definitive diagnosis could be obtained by

A. paying attention to the patient's history.
B. a more extensive physical examination.
C. a chest radiograph.
D. repeat of the sputum smear.
E. laboratory culture and speciation.

Correct answer = E. Laboratory culture and speciation would best resolve the question, although any of the procedures listed might yield helpful information. The possibility of anergy could be investigated by skin testing for delayed hypersensitivity to unrelated antigens, but the patient might be anergic and still be infected with a mycobacterium.

18.3 Which of the following statements regarding *Actinomyces* and *Nocardia* is true?

A. Both organisms have branching growth but are prokaryotes.
B. Neither can be cultured in the laboratory
C. *Nocardia* infections are endogenous and often initiated by trauma.
D. *Actinomyces* usually causes infections in systemically compromised patients.
E. Neither is sensitive to antibacterial drugs.

Correct answer = A. Both species appear as filamentous rods or branching forms in stained preparations. *Actinomyces* are often seen in association with amorphous material from "sulfur granules" in such smears. Both *Actinomyces* and *Nocardia* can be cultured. Colonies produced by both genera have aerial hyphae that resemble those produced by fungi. *Actinomyces* infections can be endogenous, and often initiated by trauma. *Nocardia* usually causes infections in systemically compromised patients.

18.4 The treatment of tuberculosis

A. is initiated with a single "first-line" drug.
B. is initiated after the results of sensitivity testing is available.
C. is most effective in patients with chronic or arrested tubercles.
D. may last 2 to 3 weeks.
E. should be directly observed whenever possible.

Correct answer = E. Where directly observed therapy used, the incidence of new cases falls dramatiacally and success of therapy is much more likely. The standard procedure is to begin treatment with two or more drugs to prevent emergence of resistant strains. Sensitivity tests are an important guide to modifying treatment, but sensitivity data are not required to initiate therapy. In chronic or arrested tubercles, the organisms are nonproliferating, and therefore are not susceptible to many antimicrobial agents. Therapy may last from 6 to 18 months.

18.5 Virulence in mycobacteria is most strongly correlated with:

A. mycotoxin production.
B. slow growth.
C. composition of the cell envelope.
D. small size of cells.
E. dependence on oxygen for growth.

Correct answer = C: Several cell wall components promote the intracellular growth of the organisms, and their dissemination in the infected host.

Rickettsia, Erhlichia, Anaplasma and Coxiella 19

I. OVERVIEW

Rickettsia, *Ehrlichia*, *Anaplasma,* and *Coxiella* (Figure 19.1) have a number of features in common. For example: 1) They grow only inside living host cells. [Note: Many pathogenic bacteria grow well inside particular cell types but do not require this environment for multiplication. The organisms discussed here, like chlamydiae, are obligately intracellular parasites.] 2) Most infections are transmitted by infected arthropods vectors (for example, lice, ticks, fleas, and mites). 3) Diseases caused by these organisms, such as typhus, spotted fevers, human ehrlichiosis, and Q fever, are generalized infections, with rash sometimes being a prominent feature. Mortality rates of these diseases are variable but may be high in the absence of appropriate treatment.

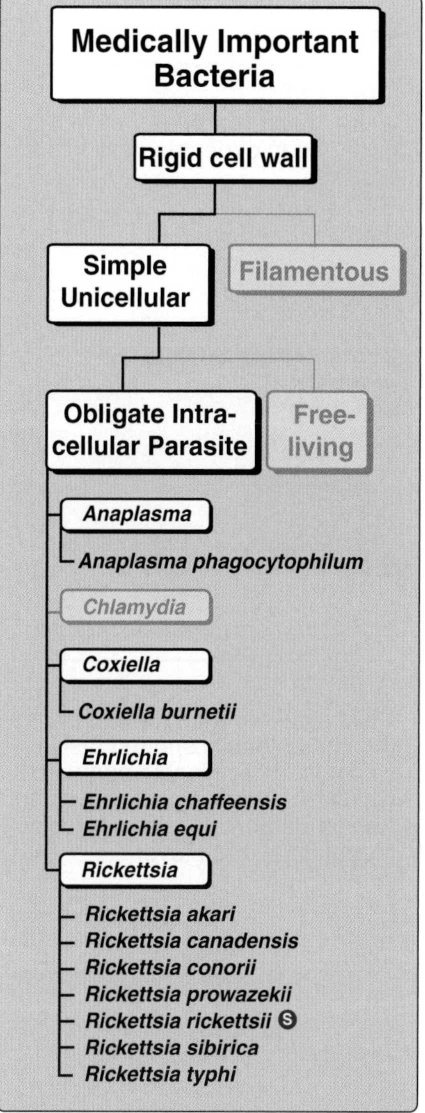

Figure 19.1
Classification of obligate intracellular parasites. See p. 347 for a summary of this organism.

II. RICKETTSIA

Rickettsia have the structural features of typical prokaryotic cells. They are small, rodlike or coccobacillary shaped (Figure 19.2), and have a typical double-layered, gram-negative cell wall. However, they stain poorly and, because of their usual occurrence inside host cells, are best visualized under the light microscope with one of the polychrome stains, such as Giemsa or Macchiavello.

A. Physiology

The obligate requirement for an intracellular environment for rickettsial replication is not fully understood, but its plasma membrane is leaky and, therefore, easily permeable to host cell nutrients and coenzymes. These intracellular parasites employ host-derived carbon sources, amino acids, and nucleosides for their own metabolism. They lack a glycolytic pathway but retain the enzymes necessary for the Krebs cycle. This genus is closely related to the ancestor of mitochondria, found within eukaryotic cells. The rickettsial electron transport chain and adenosine triphosphate–generating machinery closely resemble those found in current-day mitochondria. *Rickettsia* contain a number of antigens that convey both group and species specificity.

B. Pathogenesis

Rickettsia are transmitted to humans by arthropods, such as fleas, ticks, mites, and lice. Depending on the rickettsial species, rodents, humans, or arthropods can serve as reservoirs of infectious organisms. *Rickettsia* species have an affinity for endothelial cells located throughout the circulatory system. Following a bite by an infected

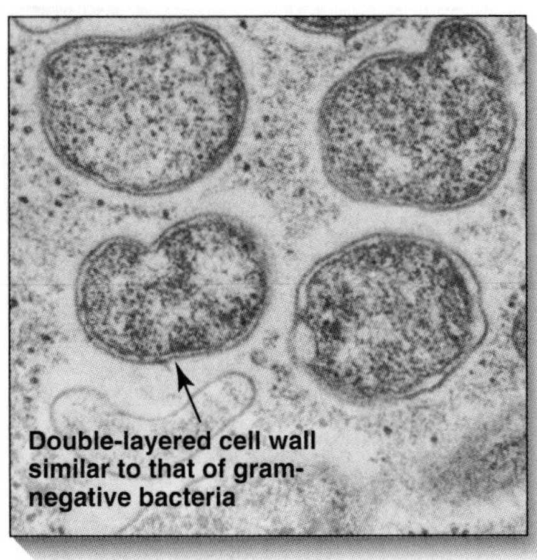

Figure 19.2
Electron micrograph of *Rickettsia prowazekii* in experimentally infected tick tissue.

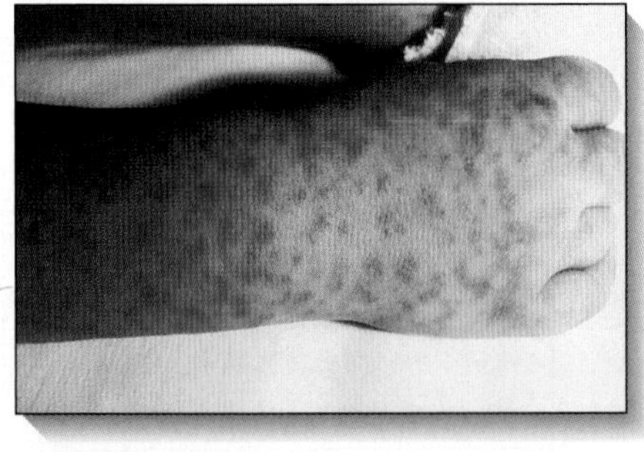

Figure 19.3
Child's right hand and wrist displaying the characteristic spotted rash with raised or palpable purpura, which is pathognomonic of vasiculitis (the fundamental lesion of Rocky Mountain spotted fever).

arthropod, the organisms are taken into cells by a process similar to phagocytosis. The organisms degrade the phagosome membrane by production of a phospholipase C. The *Rickettsia* in the spotted fever group multiply in both the nucleus and cytoplasm of host cells. They appear to mobilize host cell actin fibrils that facilitate their exit into adjacent cells in a manner similar to that of the genera *Listeria and Shigella* (see pp. 97, 119). The *Rickettsia* within the typhus group are not capable of actin-based motility; cannot escape the cell via cytoplasmic extensions; and, therefore, are limited to growth within the cytoplasm until the host cell eventually dies, releasing the bacteria. In both cases, the rickettsiae spread throughout the body via the bloodstream or lymphatics. Focal thrombi are formed in various organs including the skin (Figure 19.3), and a variety of small hemorrhages and hemodynamic disturbances create the symptoms of illness.

C. Clinical significance—spotted fever group

1. **Rocky Mountain spotted fever**: Rocky Mountain spotted fever is a potentially lethal, but usually curable tickborne disease, and is the most common rickettsial infection in the United States. The disease is caused by *Rickettsia rickettsii.* Human infection is initiated by the bite of an infected wood or dog tick. Ticks can transmit the organism transovarially to their progeny and, thereby, the organism can be maintained without mammalian hosts in specific geographic regions for many years. Currently in the United States, such infected tick populations are prevalent in south-central states and along the mid-Atlantic coast. The disease usually occurs with highest frequency during the warmer months when tick activity is greatest. Symptoms begin to develop an average of 7 days after infection. The disease is characterized by high fever and malaise, followed by a prominent rash that is initially macular but may become petechial or frankly hemorrhagic (see Figure 19.3). The rash typically begins on the extremities, involving the palms and soles, and develops rapidly to cover the body. In untreated cases, vascular disturbances leading to tissue infarction and maryocardial or renal failure may ensue. Two thirds of cases of Rocky Mountain spotted fever occur in children younger than age 15 years, with the peak incidence occurring between ages 5 and 9 years. A potential diagnostic problem occurs in those infected patients (approximately 10 percent) in whom a rash does not occur. These cases of "spotless" Rocky Mountain spotted fever may be severe and end fatally.

2. **Other spotted fevers:** Tickborne spotted fevers similar to Rocky Mountain spotted fever are found in several regions of the world. They vary in severity and are caused by organisms such as *Rickettsia conorii*, *Rickettsia canadensis*, and *Rickettsia sibirica*. A clinically different disease, rickettsialpox, is caused by *Rickettsia akari.* It has been reported in the United States and the former Soviet Union. The vector for *R. akari* is a mite, and its reservoir is the common house mouse or similar small rodents. Rickettsialpox is characterized by scattered papulovesicles that are preceded by an eschar at the site of the mite bite and with mild constitutional symptoms of a few days' duration. Figure 19.4 illustrates the spotted fevers caused by rickettsial organisms.

C. Clinical significance—typhus group

1. **Louseborne (epidemic) typhus:** Louseborne typhus is caused by *Rickettsia prowazekii*. [Note: Epidemic typhus is a different disease from salmonella-induced typhoid fever (see p. 86). Both were originally thought to be variations of the same disease, which was called "typhus" after the Greek word meaning "stupor." When the two diseases were determined to be caused by different organisms, the salmonella-induced disease was named "typhoid," meaning "typhuslike."] *R. prowazekii* is transmitted from person to person by an infected human body louse that excretes organisms in its feces. Scratching louse bites facilitates the introduction of the pathogen from louse feces into a bite wound. Infected lice are themselves eventually killed by the infecting bacterium. Thus, this disease is not maintained in the louse population, but, rather, lice serve as vectors, transmitting the organism between humans.

   a. **Typhus epidemics:** Typhus occurs most typically in large epidemics under conditions of displacement of people, crowding, and poor sanitation. Currently a major focus of such outbreaks is found in northeast Africa. The epidemic form of typhus has not occurred in the United States since early in the 20th century. However, sporadic cases of typhus have occurred in the eastern half of the United States, where the reservoir appears to be flying squirrels. The pathogen is probably transmitted from flying squirrels to humans via the bite of ectoparasites. Clinical symptoms of typhus develop an average of 8 days after infection and include high fever; chills; severe headache; and, often, a considerable degree of prostration and stupor. Although rash may be observed, unlike the rash associated with Rocky Mountain spotted fever, the epidemic typhus rash spreads centrifugally from trunk to extremities. The disease lasts 2 weeks or longer,and tends to be more severe in older individuals. Complications of epidemic typhus may include central nervous system dysfunction, myocarditis, and death.

   b. **Brill-Zinsser disease (recrudescent typhus):** This is a usually milder form of typhus that occurs in persons who previously recovered from primary infections (10 to 40 years earlier). Latent infection is thought to be maintained in the reticuloendothelial system and probably serves as a reservoir for the organism in interepidemic periods.

2. **Other forms of typhuslike fever:** Murine (endemic) typhus, caused by *Rickettsia typhi*, is a clinically similar but usually milder disease than that caused by *R. prowazekii*. Human infections are initiated by the bites of infected rat fleas, and a worldwide reservoir for *R. typhi* exists in urban rodents. Murine typhus was endemic in rat-infested areas, particularly in the southeastern United States and in the Gulf of Mexico region. However, with improving rodent control, it has become rare in this country. [Note: The cat flea, which also resides on skunks, opossums, and raccoons, is still a significant vector of murine typhus in the United States.]

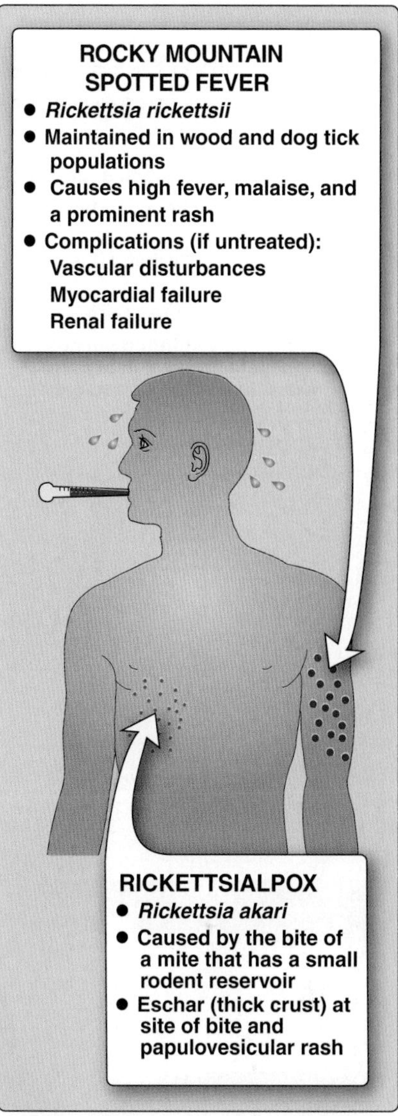

Figure 19.4
Spotted fevers caused by *Rickettsia*.

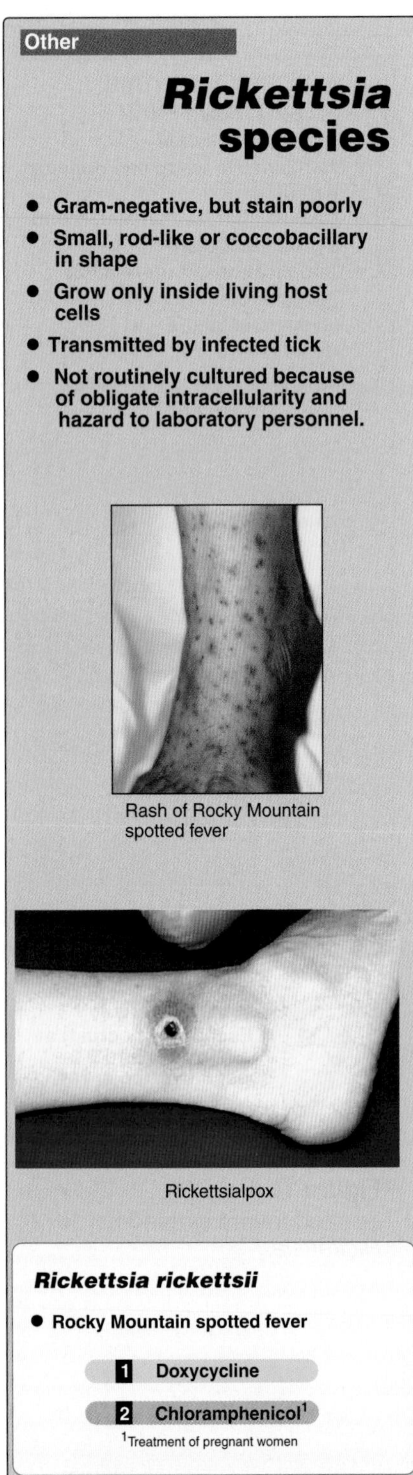

Other
Rickettsia species
• Gram-negative, but stain poorly
• Small, rod-like or coccobacillary in shape
• Grow only inside living host cells
• Transmitted by infected tick
• Not routinely cultured because of obligate intracellularity and hazard to laboratory personnel.
Rash of Rocky Mountain spotted fever
Rickettsialpox
Rickettsia rickettsii
• Rocky Mountain spotted fever
1 Doxycycline
2 Chloramphenicol[1]
[1]Treatment of pregnant women

Figure 19.5
Summary of *Richettsia* disease. 1 Indicates first-line drug; 2 indicates alternative drug.

D. Laboratory identification

A variety of serologic procedures have been developed, most of which rely on the demonstration of a rickettsia-specific antibody response during the course of infection. Suspensions or soluble extracts of rickettsia are used to demonstrate group- and species-specific antibodies by indirect immunofluorescence. Alternatively, although not widely available, infected cells can be detected by immunofluorescence or histochemical procedures on some clinical samples such as punch biopsies from areas of rash. Polymerase chain reaction (PCR) amplification can also be employed for the specific diagnosis of rickettsial diseases.

E. Treatment

Doxycycline is the drug of choice for the treatment of Rocky Mountain spotted fever in both adults and children, except for pregnant women who should be treated with chloramphenicol (Figure 19.5). The risk of dental staining with doxycycline is minimal if a short course is administered. The decision to treat must be made on clinical grounds, together with a history or suspicion of contact with an appropriate arthropod vector, before the seroconversion data are available. Early therapy for Rocky Mountain spotted fever is important, because delay beyond the 5th day of illness is associated with an increased mortality rate.

F. Prevention of infection

Prevention depends on vector control, for example, delousing, rodent-proofing buildings, or clearing brush in tick- or mite-infested areas as appropriate. Personal protection should include wearing clothes that cover exposed skin, use of tick repellents, and frequent inspection of the body and removal of attached ticks. It is of interest that infected ticks do not transmit the infection until several hours of feeding have elapsed. Prophylactic therapy with doxycycline or another tetracycline is not recommended following tick exposure because less than 1 percent of ticks in endemic areas is infected with *R. rickettsii.* Patients who experience tick bites should seek treatment if any systemic symptoms, especially fever and headache, occur in the following 14 days. Vaccines are not currently licensed for use in the United States.

III. EHRLICHIA AND ANAPLASMA

Ehrlichia and *Anaplasma* resemble *Rickettsia* in appearance and behavior. However, these organisms parasitize monocytes and neutrophils, respectively, and grow exclusively within host-derived cytoplasmic vacuoles, creating characteristic inclusions called morulae.

A. Clinical significance

Human monocytic ehrlichiosis (HME) is caused by *Ehrlichia chaffeensis.* Human granulocytic anaplasmosis (HGA) is caused by the organism *Anaplasma phagocytophilum* (Figure 19.6). The symptoms of HME and HGA are similar and often nonspecific. Common symptoms include fever, chills, headache, myalgia, and arthralgia. HME often presents with nausea, which is rare with HGA. More severe manifestations of HME include meningoencephalitis, myocarditis, and acute renal failure. Serious manifestations of HGA include severe leukocytopenia and thrombocytopenia due to damage of the infected cell populations. Rash is seldom seen for either HME or HGA, and deaths from HGA and HME have occurred. HME has been confirmed in some thirty states in the southeastern and south-central United States and has been most commonly associated with bites of the Lone Star tick. HGA has been associated with the bites of deer and dog ticks and has been reported in North and South America, Europe, and Asia.

B. Laboratory identification

Antibody assays and a PCR method have been diagnostically useful in investigative laboratories. Occasionally, the characteristic morulae can be seen in peripheral blood smears during acute illness.

C. Treatment

The treatment of choice is doxycycline.

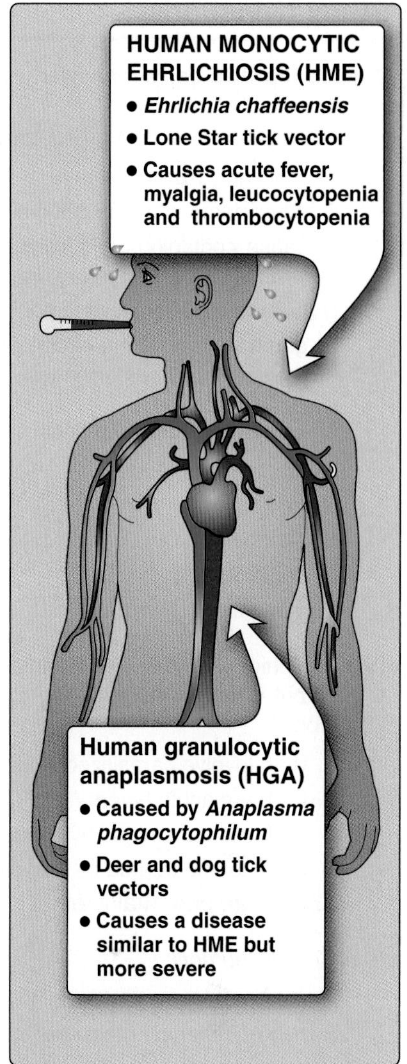

HUMAN MONOCYTIC EHRLICHIOSIS (HME)
• *Ehrlichia chaffeensis*
• Lone Star tick vector
• Causes acute fever, myalgia, leucocytopenia and thrombocytopenia
Human granulocytic anaplasmosis (HGA)
• Caused by *Anaplasma phagocytophilum*
• Deer and dog tick vectors
• Causes a disease similar to HME but more severe

Figure 19.6
Diseases caused by *Ehrlichia* and *Anaplasma*.

IV. COXIELLA

Coxiella burnetii, the causal agent of Q fever, is found worldwide (the "Q" stands for "query" because the cause of the fever was unknown for many years). It has several features that distinguish it from other rickettsia. For example: 1) It grows in cytoplasmic vacuoles and seems to be stimulated by the low pH of a phagolysosome, being resistant to the host degradative enzymes within that structure; 2) it is extremely resistant to heat and drying and can persist outside its host for long periods; and 3) it causes disease in livestock, such as cattle and in other mammals, but is not transmitted to humans by arthropods. Although the organism has been reported to be recovered from ticks, human infection usually occurs following inhalation of infected dust in, for example, barnyards and slaughterhouses (a transmission route made possible because of the ability of *C. burnetii* to withstand drying). [Note: *C. burnetii* has also been known to enter the body via other mucous membranes, abrasions, and the gastrointestinal tract through consumption of milk from infected animals.]

A. Clinical significance

C. burnetii reproduces in the respiratory tract and then (in the absence of treatment) is disseminated to other organs. Clinical illness takes several forms. Classic Q fever is an interstitial pneumonitis (not unlike some viral or mycoplasmal illnesses) that may be complicated by hepatitis, myocarditis, or encephalitis. *C. burnetii* should also be considered as a potential causative agent in culture-negative endocarditis. Infections are usually self-limiting but, in rare instances (especially endocarditis), can become chronic.

B. Laboratory identification

Serologic assays are the principal means of specific diagnosis, and serologic surveys indicate that inapparent infections are common.

C. Treatment and prevention

Doxycycline is the drug of choice for treatment. A vaccine has been reported to be of limited use in occupationally exposed individuals, but it is not readily available in the United States.

Study Questions

Choose the ONE correct answer.

19.1 Pathogens in the genus *Rickettsia*:

A. grow only extracellularly.
B. have eukaryotic-type cell organization.
C. cause contagious infections because they are disseminated by respiratory droplets.
D. are clinically sensitive to penicillin.
E. generally invade the endothelial lining of capillaries, causing small hemorrhages.

Correct answer = E. Most *Rickettsia* cause rashes resulting from damage to the vascular system. They are obligate intracellular, prokaryotic parasites. *Rickettsia* species are transmitted by the bite of an arthropod. They are sensitive to tetracyclines but not to penicillin.

19.2 The vector of Rocky Mountain spotted fever is the:

A. human body louse.
B. rat flea.
C. deer tick.
D. dog tick.
E. mosquito.

Correct answer = D. Rocky Mountain spotted fever is initiated by the bite of an infected wood or dog tick. The human louse is involved in the transmission of *Rickettsia prowazekii,* causing thypus. Deer ticks are involved in the transmission of Lyme disease (see p. 165). Mosquito-borne diseases include dengue fever, malaria, and yellow fever.

19.3 Ehrlichiosis and Rocky Mountain spotted fever have all but which of the following clinical features in common?

A. Both involve parasitized blood cells.
B. Both are acute fevers.
C. Both are transmitted by the same vector.
D. Both can be treated by doxycycline.
E. Both are potentially lethal.

Correct answer = A. *Ehrlichia* parasitizes leukocytes, whereas *Rickettsia rickettsii* invades capillary linings, causing the "spotted" rash of Rocky Mountain spotted fever.

19.4 *Coxiella burnetii:*

A. cannot survive outside its host.
B. has no reservoir other than humans.
C. causes a pneumonitis called Q fever.
D. causes symptomatic disease only in the lower respiratory tract.
E. is found only in the United States.

Correct answer = C. Whereas lower respiratory tract disease is most characteristic, the organism fairly frequently causes hepatitis, myocarditis or endocarditis, and other visceral infections. It is resistant to drying and heat and infects a variety of animals (including ticks, but they play no role in human disease). Its distribution is worldwide.

19.5 A 14-year-old male presents to the emergency room in North Carolina with fever and a distinctive rash on his extremities. The rash is most prominent on the palms of his hands, but has spread to his lower arms as well. The patient was well before a camping trip 1 week prior to symptom onset. Which of the following bacterial pathogens is the most likely causative agent of this disease?

A. *Coxiella burnetii*
B. *Ehrlichia chaffeensis*
C. *Rickettsia rickettsii*
D. *Anaplasma phagocytophilum*
E. *Rickettsia prowazekii*

Correct answer: C. The symptoms and presentation of this disease are most consistent with Rocky Mountain spotted fever, caused by *Rickettsia rickettsii.* The rash is the most prominent symptom of infection, which typically begins on the extremities and spreads towards the trunk. The infection is transmitted to humans by the bite of a tick, which is common during outdoor activities. Q fever, caused by *Coxiella burnetii,* generally presents with respiratory symptoms and most likely follows recent contact with livestock. *Ehrlichia chaffeensis* causes human monocytic ehrlichiosis, which presents with systemic signs but no rash. Presentation of human granulocytic anaplasmosis, caused by *Anaplasma phagocytophilum,* similarly does not include a distinctive rash. *Rickettsia prowazekii* causes epidemic typhus, which is rare in the United States. However, if it occurs, the rash is different from that caused by *R. rickettsii* in that it spreads from the trunk.

UNIT III: Fungi and Parasites

Fungi 20

I. OVERVIEW

Fungi are a diverse group of saprophytic (deriving nourishment from dead organic matter) and parasitic eukaryotic organisms. Although formerly considered to be plants, they are now assigned their own kingdom, Mycota. Virtually all organisms are subject to fungal infection. Of some 200,000 fungal species, only about 100 have pathogenic potential for humans. Of these, only a few species account for most clinically important fungal infections (Figure 20.1). Human fungal diseases (mycoses) are classified by the location on or in the body where the infection occurs. They are called cutaneous when limited to the epidermis, subcutaneous when the infection penetrates significantly beneath the skin, and systemic when the infection is deep within the body or disseminated to internal organs. Systemic mycoses can be further divided into those that are caused by true pathogenic fungi capable of infecting healthy individuals and those that are opportunistic, infecting primarily those individuals who have predisposing conditions, such as immunodeficiency or debilitating diseases (for example, diabetes, leukemia, and Hodgkin and other lymphomas). Fungi produce and secrete a variety of unusual metabolic products, some of which, when ingested, are highly toxic to animals, including humans. Thus, fungi can cause poisoning as well as infection. Lastly, fungal spores, which are critical for dispersal and transmission of the fungus, are also important as human allergenic agents.

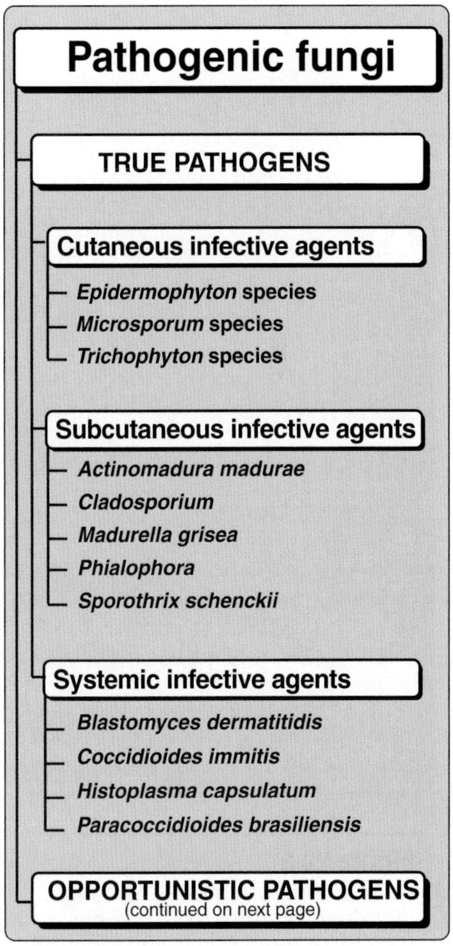

Pathogenic fungi

- **TRUE PATHOGENS**
  - **Cutaneous infective agents**
    - *Epidermophyton* species
    - *Microsporum* species
    - *Trichophyton* species
  - **Subcutaneous infective agents**
    - *Actinomadura madurae*
    - *Cladosporium*
    - *Madurella grisea*
    - *Phialophora*
    - *Sporothrix schenckii*
  - **Systemic infective agents**
    - *Blastomyces dermatitidis*
    - *Coccidioides immitis*
    - *Histoplasma capsulatum*
    - *Paracoccidioides brasiliensis*
- **OPPORTUNISTIC PATHOGENS**

(continued on next page)

Figure 20.1
Classification of pathogenic fungi (figure continues on next page).

II. CHARACTERISTICS OF MAJOR FUNGAL GROUPS

Fungi can be distinguished from other infectious organisms such as bacteria or viruses because they are eukaryotes (that is, they have a membrane-enclosed nucleus and other organelles). Fungi have no chlorophyll or chloroplasts, thus distinguishing them from plants. Their characteristic structures, habitats, and modes of growth and reproduction are used to distinguish different groups among fungi.

Pathogenic fungi (continued)

OPPORTUNISTIC PATHOGENS

- *Absidia corymbifera*
- *Aspergillus fumigatus*
- *Candida albicans*
- *Cryptococcus neoformans*
- *Pneumocystis jiroveci*
- *Rhizomucor pusillus*
- *Rhizopus oryzae (R. arrhizus)*

Figure 20.1 (continued)
Classification of pathogenic fungi.

A. Cell wall and membrane components

The fungal cell wall and cell membrane are fundamentally different from those of bacteria and other eukaryotes. Fungal cell walls are composed largely of chitin, a polymer of N-acetylglucosamine, rather than peptidoglycan, which is a characteristic component of bacterial cell walls. Fungi are, therefore, unaffected by antibiotics (for example, penicillin) that inhibit peptidoglycan synthesis. The fungal membrane contains ergosterol rather than the cholesterol found in mammalian membranes. These chemical characteristics are useful in targeting chemotherapeutic agents against fungal infections. Many such agents interfere with fungal membrane synthesis or function. For example, amphotericin B and nystatin bind to ergosterol present in fungal cell membranes. There they form pores that disrupt membrane function, resulting in cell death. Imidazole antifungal drugs (clotrimazole, ketoconazole, miconazole) and triazole antifungal agents (fluconazole and itraconazole) interact with the P450 enzyme 14 α-sterol-demethylase to block demethylation of lanosterol to ergosterol. Because ergosterol is a vital component of fungal cell membranes, disruption of its biosynthesis results in cell death.

B. Habitat and nutrition

All fungi are chemoheterotrophs, requiring some preformed organic carbon source for growth. Fungi do not ingest food particles as do organisms such as protozoa (see p. 217) but depend upon transport of soluble nutrients across their cell membranes. To obtain these soluble nutrients, fungi secrete degradative enzymes (for example, cellulases, proteases, nucleases) into their immediate environment, which enable them to live saprophytically on organic waste. Therefore, the natural habitat of almost all fungi is soil or water containing decaying organic matter. Some fungi can be parasitic on living organisms. However, these parasitic infections usually originate from the individual's contact with fungus-contaminated soil, an exception being *Candida*, which is part of the normal human mucosal flora (see p. 7).

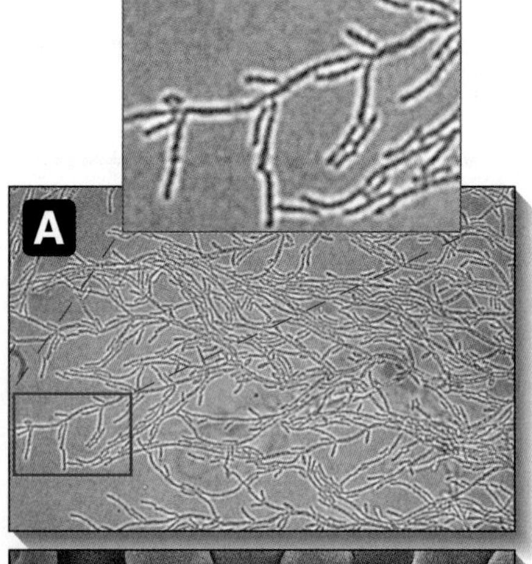

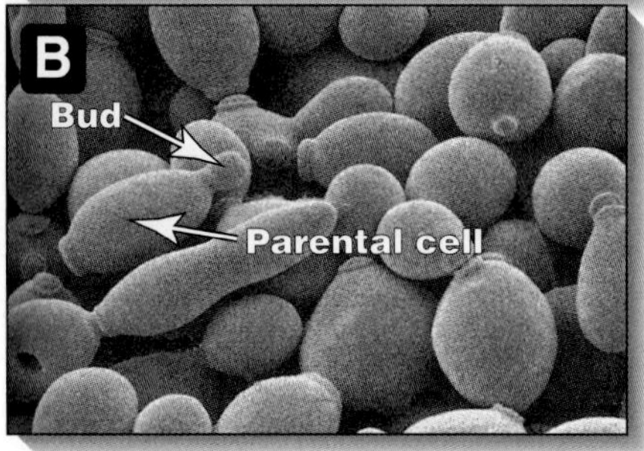

Figure 20.2
A. Filamentous (mold-like) fungi (light micrograph). B. Budding yeast-like fungi (scanning electron micrograph).

C. Modes of fungal growth

Most fungi exist in one of two basic morphologic forms (that is, either as filamentous mold or unicellular yeast). However, some fungi are dimorphic and can switch between these two forms in response to environmental conditions.

1. **Filamentous (mold-like) fungi:** The vegetative body, or thallus, of mold-like fungi is typically a mass of threads with many branches (Figure 20.2A). This mass is called a mycelium, which grows by branching and tip elongation. The threads (hyphae) are actually tubular cells that, in some fungi, are partitioned into segments (septate), whereas, in other fungi, the hyphae are uninterrupted by crosswalls (nonseptate). Even in septate fungi, however, the septae are perforated so that the cytoplasm of the hyphae is continuous. When hyphal filaments become densely packed, the mycelium may have the appearance of a cohesive tissue (for example, as seen in the body of a mushroom).

2. **Yeast-like fungi:** These fungi exist as populations of single, unconnected, spheroid cells, not unlike many bacteria, although they are some 10 times larger than a typical bacterial cell (see Figure 20.2B). Yeast-like fungi generally reproduce by budding.

3. **Dimorphic fungi:** Some fungal species, especially those that cause systemic mycoses, are dimorphic, being yeast-like in one environment and mold-like in another. Conditions that can affect morphology include temperature and carbon dioxide level. Examples of dimorphic fungi include *Blastomyces dermatiditis* and *Histoplasma capsulatum*.

D. Sporulation

Sporulation is the principal means by which fungi reproduce and spread through the environment. Fungal spores are metabolically dormant, protected cells, released by the mycelium in enormous numbers. They can be borne by air or water to new sites, where they germinate and establish colonies. Spores can be generated either asexually or sexually (Figure 20.3).

1. **Asexual sporulation:** Asexual spores (conidia) are formed by mitosis in or on specialized hyphae (conidiophores) as shown in

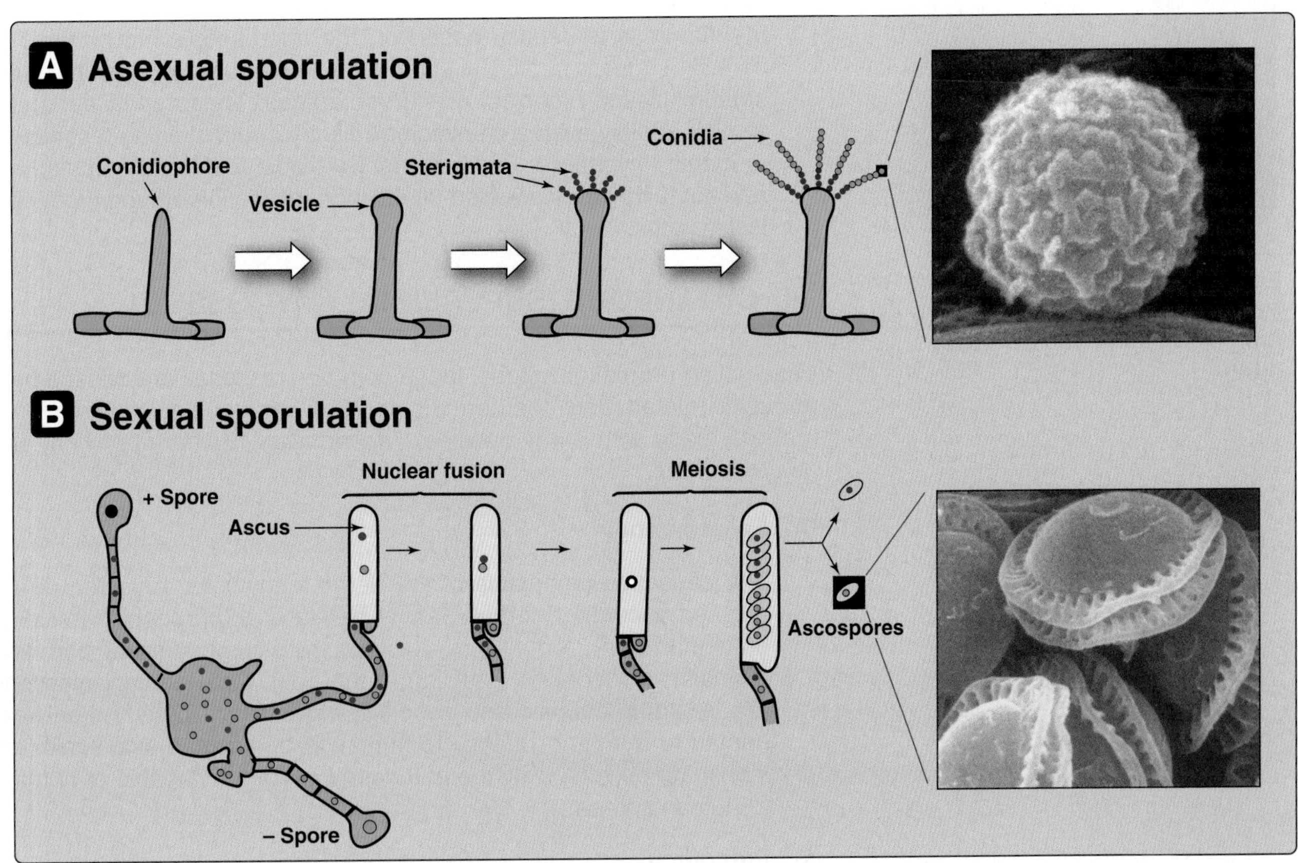

Figure 20.3
Sporulation among *Aspergillus nidulans*. A. Asexual. B. Sexual.

Figure 20.3A. The color of a typical fungal colony seen on bread, fruit, or culture plate is caused by the conidia, which can number tens of millions per cm^3 of surface. Because they are easily detached from their underlying mycelial mats, conidia can become airborne and, therefore, are a major source of fungal infection (see p. 209).

2. **Sexual sporulation:** This process is initiated when a haploid nucleus from each of two compatible strains of the same species fuse to form a transient diploid (see Figure 20.3B). The products of meiosis of this transient diploid become sexual spores (ascospores). Compared to asexual sporulation, sexual sporulation is relatively rare among human fungal pathogens. Spores, especially sexual spores, often have a characteristic shape and surface ornamentation pattern that may serve as the primary or only means of species identification.

E. Laboratory identification

Most fungi can be propagated on any nutrient agar surface. The standard medium is Sabouraud dextrose agar, which, because of its low pH (5.0), inhibits bacterial growth while allowing fungal colonies to form (Figure 20.4). Various antibacterial antibiotics can also be added to the medium to further inhibit bacterial colony formation. Cultures can be started from spores or hyphal fragments. Identification is usually based on the microscopic morphology of conidial structures. Clinical samples may be pus, blood, spinal fluid, sputum, tissue biopsies, or skin scrapings. These specimens can also be rapidly evaluated histologically by direct staining techniques to identify hyphae or yeast forms. Serologic tests and immunofluorescent techniques are also useful in identification of fungi from clinical isolates.

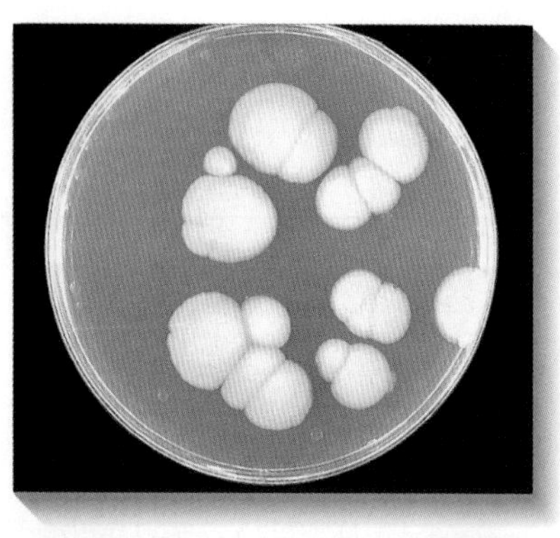

Figure 20.4
Colonies of *Candida albicans* grown on Sabouraud dextrose agar.

III. CUTANEOUS (SUPERFICIAL) MYCOSES

Also called dermatophytoses, these common diseases are caused by a group of related fungi, the dermatophytes. Dermatophytes fall into three genera, each with many species: *Trichophyton*, *Epidermophyton*, and *Microsporum*.

A. Epidemiology

The causative organisms of the dermatophytoses are often distinguished according to their natural habitats: anthropophilic (residing on human skin), zoophilic (residing on the skin of domestic and farm animals), or geophilic (residing in the soil). Most human infections are by anthropophilic and zoophilic organisms. Transmission from human to human or animal to human is by infected skin scales on inanimate objects. Only the pathogenic fungi are capable of human-to-human spread.

B. Pathology

A defining characteristic of the dermatophytes is their ability to use keratin as a source of nutrition. This ability allows them to infect keratinized tissues and structures, such as skin, hair, and nails. There is some specificity, however. Although all three genera attack the skin, *Microsporum* does not infect nails, and *Epidermophyton* does not infect hair. None invades underlying, nonkeratinized tissue.

C. Clinical significance

Dermatophytoses are characterized by itching, scaling skin patches that can become inflamed and weeping. Specific diseases are usually identified according to affected tissue (for example, scalp, pubic area, or feet), but a given disease can be caused by any one of several organisms, and some organisms can cause more than one disease, depending, for example, on the site of infection or condition of the skin. The following are the most commonly encountered dermatophytoses.

1. **Tinea pedis ("athlete's foot"):** Organisms most often isolated from infected tissue are *Trichophyton rubrum*, *Trichophyton mentagrophytes*, and *Epidermophyton floccosum*. The infected tissue is initially between the toes but can spread to the nails, which become yellow and brittle. Skin fissures can lead to secondary bacterial infections with consequent lymph node inflammation (Figure 20.5A).

2. **Tinea corporis ("ringworm"):** Organisms most often isolated are *E. floccosum* and several species of *Trichophyton* and *Microsporum*. Lesions appear as advancing rings with scaly centers (see Figure 20.5B). The periphery of the ring, which is the site of active fungal growth, is usually inflamed and vesiculated. Although any site on the body can be affected, lesions most often occur on nonhairy areas of the trunk.

3. **Tinea capitis ("scalp ringworm"):** Several species of *Trichophyton* and *Microsporum* have been isolated from scalp ringworm lesions, the predominant infecting species depending on the geographic location of the patient. In the United States, for example, the predominant infecting species is *Trichophyton tonsurans*. Disease manifestations range from small, scaling patches, to involvement of the entire scalp with extensive hair loss (see Figure 20.5C). The hair shafts can become invaded by *Microsporum* hyphae, as demonstrated by their green fluorescence in long-wave ultraviolet light (Wood lamp).

4. **Tinea cruris ("jock itch"):** Causative organisms are *E. floccosum* and *T. rubrum*. Disease manifestations are similar to ringworm, except that lesions occur in the moist groin area, where they can spread from the upper thighs to the genitals (see Figure 20.5D).

5. **Tinea unguium (onychomycosis):** The causative organism is most often *T. rubrum*. Nails thicken and become discolored and brittle. Treatment must continue for 3 to 4 months until all infected portions of the nail have grown out and are trimmed off (see Figure 20.5E).

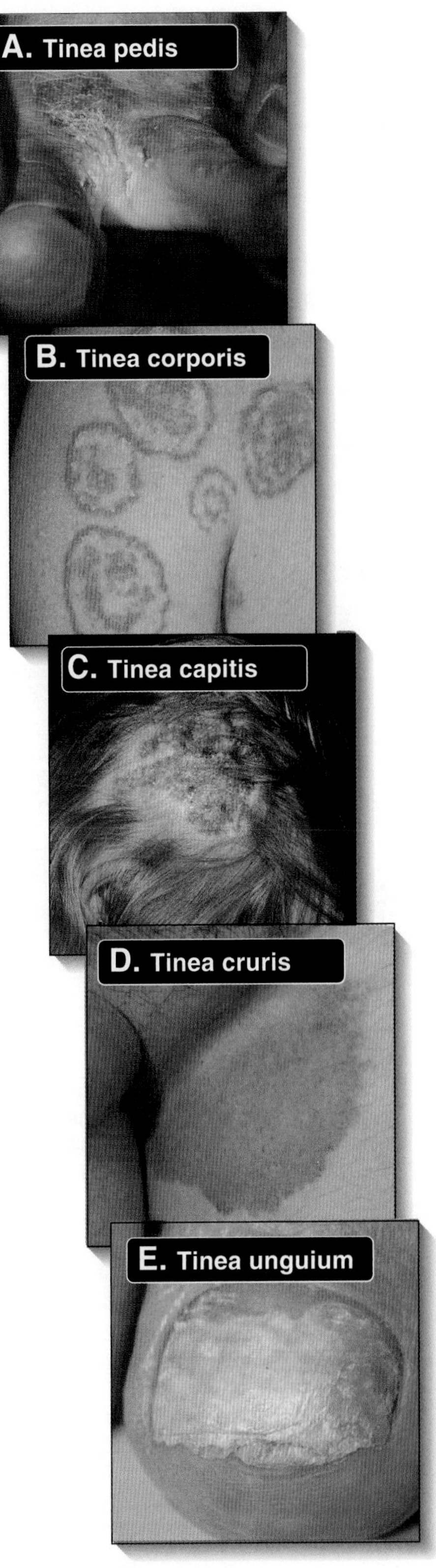

Figure 20.5
Cutaneous mycoses.

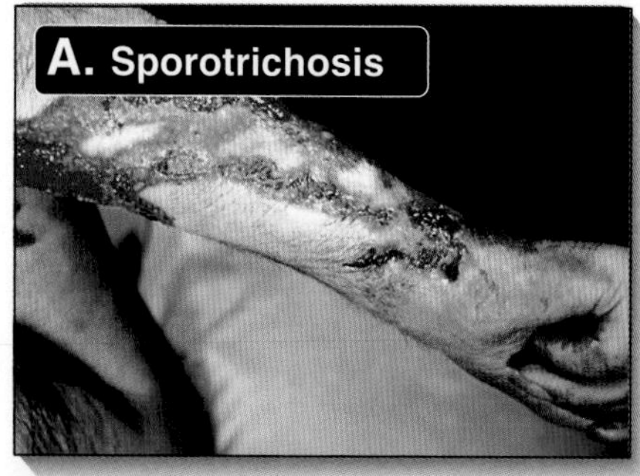

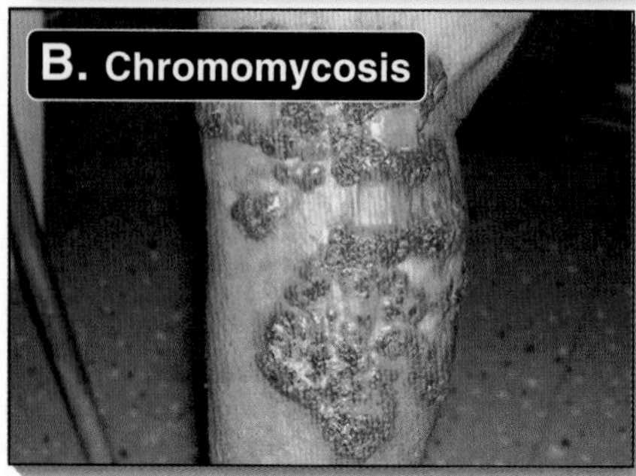

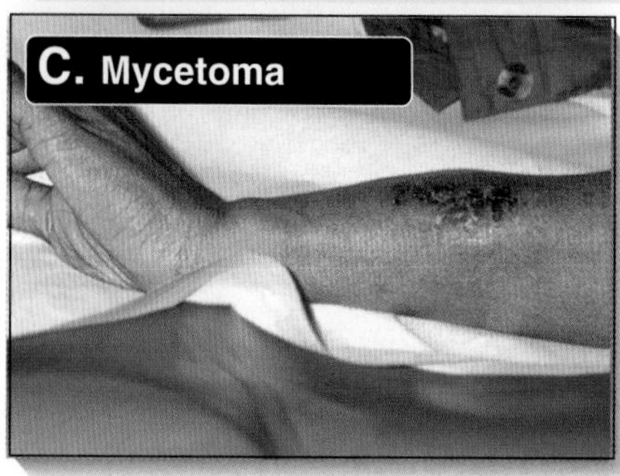

Figure 20.6
Subcutaneous mycoses.
A. Sporotrichosis. The forearm of a gardener exhibiting the cutaneous-lymphatic form of sporotrichosis.
B. Chromomycosis showing multiple plaques on the lower leg.
C. Mycetoma of the arm.

D. Treatment

Removal of infected skin, followed by topical application of antifungal antibiotics, such as miconazole and clotrimazole, is the first course of treatment. Refractory infections usually respond well to oral griseofulvin and itraconazole. Infections of the hair and nails usually require systemic (oral) therapy. Terbinafine is the drug of choice for onychomycosis.

IV. SUBCUTANEOUS MYCOSES

Subcutaneous mycoses are fungal infections of the dermis, subcutaneous tissue, and bone. Causative organisms reside in the soil and decaying or live vegetation.

A. Epidemiology

Subcutaneous fungal infections are almost always acquired through traumatic lacerations or puncture wounds. Sporotrichosis, for example, is often acquired from the prick of a thorn. As expected, these infections are more common in individuals who have frequent contact with soil and vegetation and wear inadequate protective clothing. The subcutaneous mycoses are not transmissible from human to human.

B. Clinical significance

With the rare exception of sporotrichosis, which shows a broad geographic distribution in the United States, the common subcutaneous mycoses discussed below are confined to tropical and subtropical regions.

1. **Sporotrichosis:** This infection, characterized by a granulomatous ulcer at the puncture site, may produce secondary lesions along the draining lymphatics (Figure 20.6A). The causative organism, *Sporothrix schenckii*, is a dimorphic fungus that exhibits the yeast form in infected tissue (see Figure 20.7) and the mycelial form upon laboratory culture. In most patients, the disease is self-limiting but may persist in a chronic form. Dissemination to distant sites is possible in patients with deficiencies in T-cell function (such as in AIDS and lymphomas). Oral itraconazole is the drug of choice.

2. **Chromomycosis:** Also called chromoblastomycosis, this infection is characterized by warty nodules that spread slowly along the lymphatics and develop crusty abscesses (see Figure 20.6B). Pathogens causing this mycosis include several species of pigmented soil fungi (for example, *Phialophora* and *Cladosporium)*, and the infection is most commonly seen in the tropics. Treatment is difficult. Surgical removal of small lesions is effective but must be performed cautiously and with wide margins to prevent dissemination. More advanced stages of the disease are treated with itraconazole and terbinafine.

3. **Mycetoma ("Madura foot"):** Mycetoma appears as a localized abscess, usually on the feet, but is not limited to the lower extremity (see Figure 20.6C). The abscess discharges pus, serum, and blood through sinuses (in this usage, sinus means "abnormal channel"). The infection can spread to the underlying bone and results in crippling deformities . The pathogenic agents are various soil fungi. Most common are *Madurella grisea* and *Exophiala jeanselmei.* Mycetomas appear similar to the lesions of chromomycosis, but the defining characteristic of mycetoma is the presence of colored grains, composed of compacted hyphae, in the exudate. The color of the grains (black, white, red, or yellow) is characteristic of the causative organism and, therefore, useful in identifying the particular pathogen. There is no effective chemotherapy for fungal mycetoma. Treatment is usually surgical excision.

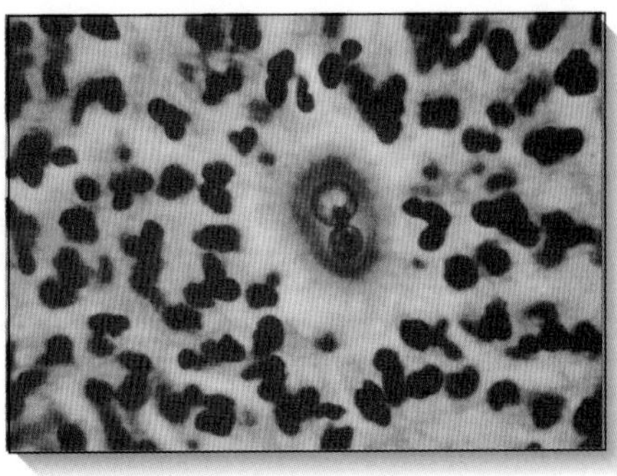

Figure 20.7
Tissue section showing the budding yeast *Sporothrix schenckii.*

V. SYSTEMIC MYCOSES

The organisms responsible for systemic mycoses fall into two general categories: 1) those that infect normal healthy individuals ("true" pathogens) and 2) those that primarily infect debilitated, and/or immunocompromised individuals ("opportunistic pathogens," see p. 385). In the United States, coccidioidomycosis, histoplasmosis, and blastomycosis are the most common systemic mycotic infections in the immunocompetent host. These infections occur in defined geographic areas where fungal pathogens are found in the soil and can be aerosolized. Clinical manifestations closely resemble those seen in tuberculosis in that asymptomatic primary pulmonary infection is common, whereas chronic pulmonary or disseminated infection is rare. The fungi causing these diseases are uniformly dimorphic, exhibiting the yeast form in infected tissue and the mycelial form in culture or in their natural environment.

A. Epidemiology and pathology

Entry into the host is by inhalation of airborne spores, which germinate in the lungs. From the lungs, dissemination can occur to any organ of the body, where the fungi can invade and destroy tissue (Figure 20.8).

B. Clinical significance

In spite of the seemingly grave nature of potentially systemic disease, most cases of coccidioidomycosis, histoplasmosis, and paracoccidioidomycosis in otherwise healthy patients present only mild symptoms and are self-limiting. In immunosuppressed patients, however, the same infections can be life threatening.

1. **Coccidioidomycosis:** Caused by *Coccidioides immitis*, most cases of coccidioidomycosis occur in the arid areas of southwestern United States (Figure 20.9) and Central and South America. Initial infection with *C. immitis* can cause fever with varying degrees of respiratory illness (called "Valley fever" because of its prevalence in the San Joaquin Valley of the southwestern United States). In the soil, the fungus generates spores by septation of

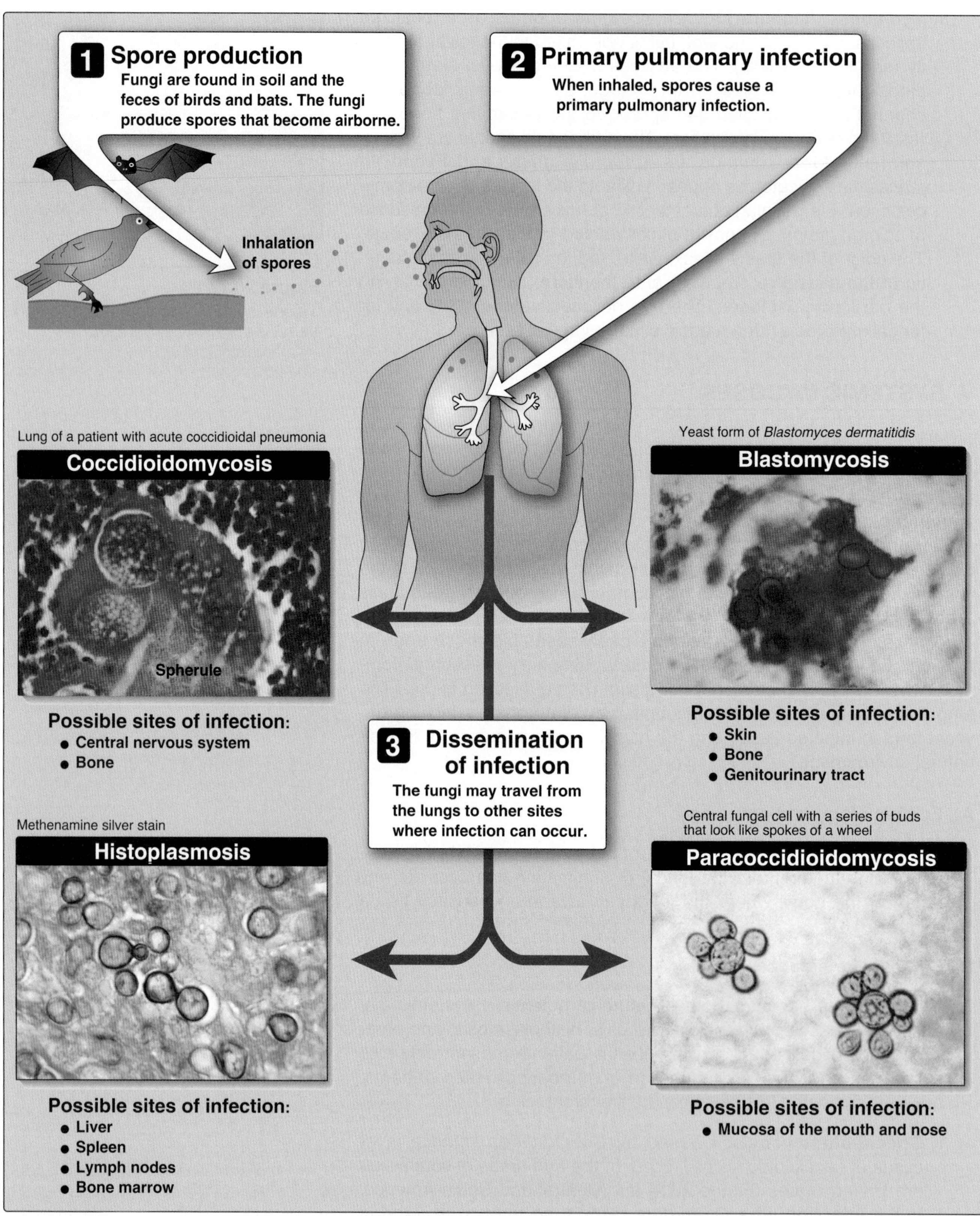

Figure 20.8
Systemic mycoses.

hyphal filaments (arthrospores). These spores become readily airborne and enter the lungs, where they germinate and develop into large (20 to 40 μm) spherules filled with many endospores. Rupture of the spherule releases the endospores, each of which can spread by the bloodstream and then form a new spherule. In cases of disseminated disease, lesions occur most often in the bones and the central nervous system, where they result in meningitis. The spores from the hyphal filaments are easily spread, so cultivation carries a significant risk of accidental infection of laboratory personnel.

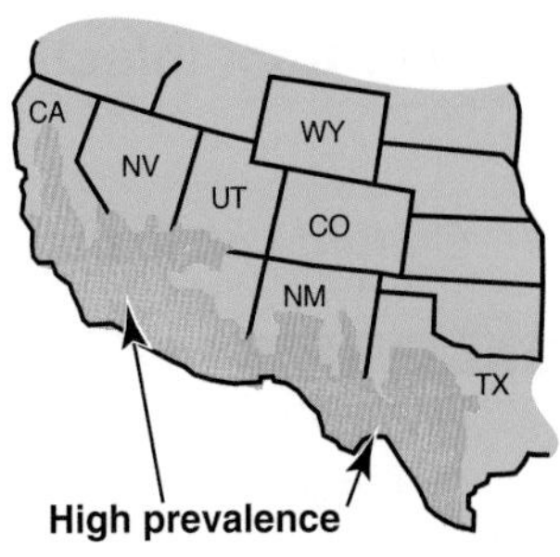

Figure 20.9
Geographic prevalence of coccidioidomycosis in the United States.

2. **Histoplasmosis:** Histoplasmosis is caused by *Histoplasma capsulatum.* In the soil, the fungus generates conidia, which, when airborne, enter the lungs and germinate into yeast-like cells. These yeast cells are engulfed by macrophages, in which they multiply. Pulmonary infections may be acute but relatively benign and self-limiting, or they can be chronic, progressive, and fatal. Dissemination is rare but can occur in older adults, the very young, and patients with deficiencies in T-cell function. Disseminated disease results in invasion of cells of the reticuloendothelial system, which distinguishes this organism as the only fungus to exhibit intracellular parasitism. Definitive diagnosis is by isolation and culture of the organism, which is a slow process (4 to 6 weeks), or by detection of exoantigen in urine specimens. The disease occurs worldwide but is most prevalent in central North America, especially the Ohio and Mississippi River Valleys (Figure 20.10). Soils that are laden with bird, chicken, or bat droppings are a rich source of *H. capsulatum* spores. Local epidemics of the disease can occur, in particular, in areas where construction has disturbed bird, chicken, and bat roosts. AIDS patients who live in or travel through endemic areas are especially at risk. The wide range of clinical manifestations of histoplasmosis makes it a particularly complex disease, often resembling tuberculosis.

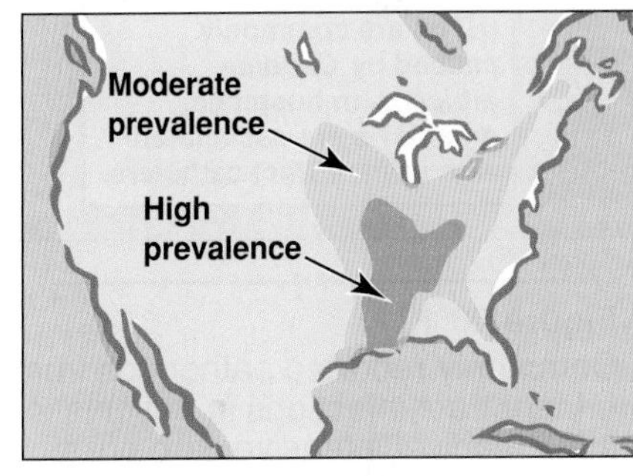

Figure 20.10
Endemic areas of histoplasmosis in North America.

3. **Blastomycosis:** *Blastomyces dermatitidis* causes blastomycosis. Like *Histoplasma,* the fungus produces microconidia, most often in the soil, which become airborne and enter the lungs. There they germinate into thick-walled yeast cells that often appear with unipolar, broad-based buds. Although initial pulmonary infections (Figure 20.11) rarely disseminate to other sites, when dissemination does occur, secondary sites include skin (70 percent), bone (30 percent), and the genitourinary tract (20 percent), where they manifest as ulcerated granulomas. Definitive diagnosis is accomplished by isolation and culture of the organism. Identifiable colonies can be obtained in 1 to 3 weeks, but identity can be established more rapidly by subjecting the young mycelial colonies to an exoantigen test. Infections are most common in the South Central and South Eastern United States and are much more common in adult males than in females or children.

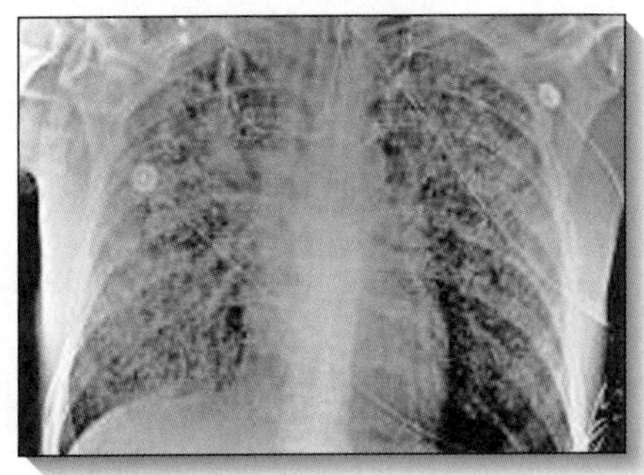

Figure 20.11
Chest radiograph showing a diffuse reticulonodular infiltrate of the lungs in a male landscaper. Broncho-alveolar lavage recovered *Blastomyces dermatitidis.*

4. **Paracoccidioidomycosis**: Also called South American blastomycosis, paracoccidioidomycosis is caused by *Paracoccidioides brasiliensis.* The clinical presentation is much like that of histoplasmosis and blastomycosis except that the most common sec-

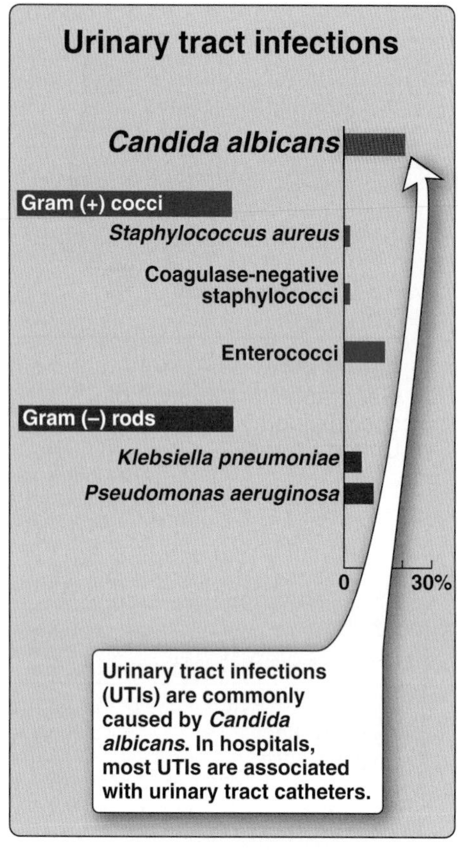

Figure 20.12
Commonly reported pathogens from urinary tract infections in patients in adult medical intensive care units.

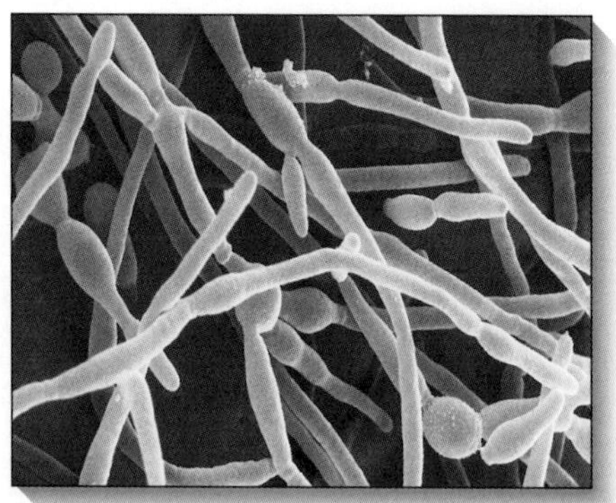

Figure 20.13
Candida albicans.

ondary site of infection is the mucosa of the mouth and nose, where painful, destructive lesions may develop. Like other dimorphic pathogens, morphologic identification via conidia is slow, but the yeast form observed in infected tissue or exudates has a characteristic appearance resembling a ship's steering wheel, caused by the presence of multiple buds (see Figure 20.8). The disease is restricted to Central and South America, and over 90 percent of patients with symptomatic disease are mature males. It is speculated that estrogen may inhibit formation of the yeast form.

C. Laboratory identification

These diseases are not communicable from one person to another. However, laboratory cultures should be handled cautiously, especially those of *C. immitis*, because, under culture conditions, the fungi revert to the spore-bearing, infectious form. Because these organisms have slow growth rates, morphologic identification of the characteristic conidia can take several weeks. Histological examination of body fluids (sputum, pus, draining fistulas) for the presence of yeasts, hyphae, or conidia allows for rapid identification of the fungal etiological agent prior to the availability of culture results. A rapid method for identifying the four systemic pathogens discussed above is the exoantigen test in which cell-free antigens produced by young mycelial colonies (or liquid cultures) are detected by immunodiffusion assay. The exoantigen test can also be applied to urine specimens collected from patients suffering from histoplasmosis. Polymerase chain reaction is another rapid, accurate diagnostic method that detects specific fungal DNA sequences.

D. Treatment

Systemic mycoses are usually treated with amphotericin B, sometimes in combination with flucytosine. Ketoconazole, fluconazole and intraconazole are also used, depending on the infecting organism and the stage and site of the disease.

VI. OPPORTUNISTIC MYCOSES

Opportunistic mycoses afflict debilitated or immunocompromised individuals but are rare in healthy individuals. The use of immunosuppressive drugs for organ transplantation and chemotherapy in cancer treatment, and the high number of immunodeficient individuals caused by the AIDS epidemic have resulted in significant expansion of the immunocompromised population as well as increased spectrum of opportunistic fungal pathogens. Fungal infections represent approximately 15 percent of all nosocomial infections (infections that are a result of treatment in a hospital) in intensive care units in the United States, with *Candida* species being the most commonly occurring fungal nosocomial pathogen (Figure 20.12). The opportunistic mycoses most commonly encountered today include the following.

A. Candidiasis (candidosis)

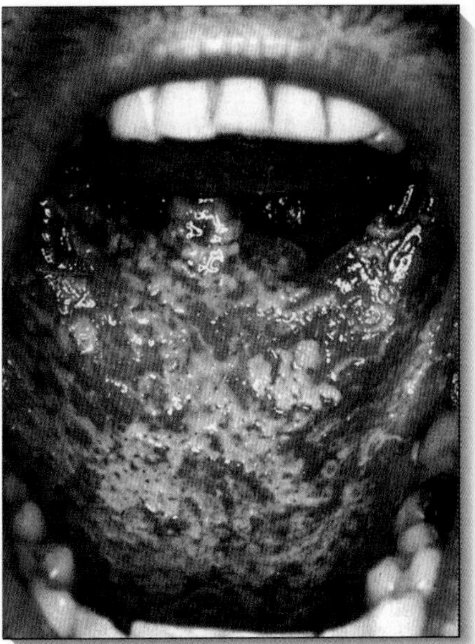

Figure 20.14
Oral candidiasis (thrush).

Candidiasis is caused by the yeast *Candida albicans* and other *Candida* species, which are normal body flora found in the skin, mouth, vagina, and intestines. Although considered a yeast, *C. albicans* is dimorphic and can form a true mycelium (Figure 20.13). Infections occur when competing bacterial flora are eliminated, for example, by antibacterial antibiotics, allowing the yeast to overgrow. *Candida* infections have various manifestations, depending on the site and the degree of immunoincompetence of the patient. For example, oral candidiasis (thrush) presents as raised, white plaques on the oral mucosa, tongue, or gums (Figure 20.14). The plaques can become confluent and ulcerated and spread to the throat. Most HIV-positive individuals eventually develop oral candidiasis, which often spreads to the esophagus. The latter condition is considered an indicator of full-blown AIDS. Vaginal candidiasis presents as itching and burning pain of the vulva and vagina, accompanied by a white discharge. Systemic candidiasis is a potentially life-threatening infection that occurs in debilitated individuals, cancer patients (with neutropenia secondary to chemotherapy), individuals on systemic corticosteroids, and patients treated with broad-spectrum antibiotics, especially those with long intravenous catheters. Systemic candidiasis may involve the gastrointestinal (GI) tract, kidneys, liver, and spleen. Both oral and vaginal infections are treated topically with nystatin or clotrimazole. Depending on the severity and extent of a candidal infection, treatment with an azole drug, such as ketoconazole, fluconazole, and itraconazole, may be given orally or intravenously. Amphotericin B by itself or in combination with flucytosine is used in systemic disease. Echinocandins, such as caspofungin, micafungin and anidulafungin are active against *Aspergillus* and most *Candida*, including those species resistant to azoles.

B. Cryptococcosis

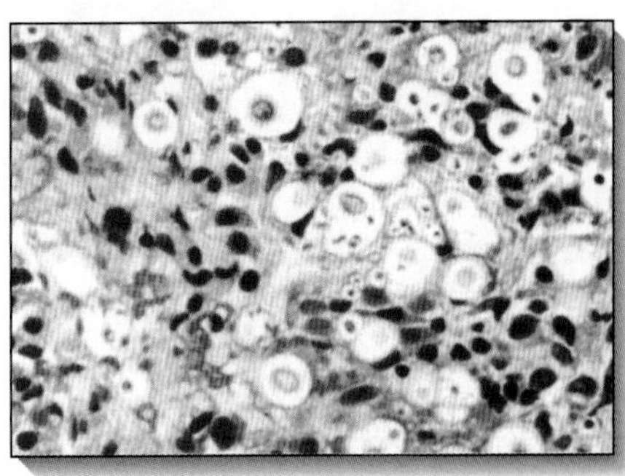

Figure 20.15
Cryptococcus neoformans. [Note: Capsules are visible because they do not take up the hematoxylin and eosin stain].

Cryptococcosis is caused by the yeast *Cryptococcus neoformans* (Figure 20.15), which is found worldwide. The organism is especially abundant in soil containing bird (especially pigeon) droppings, although the birds are not infected. The organism has a characteristic polysaccharide capsule that surrounds the budding yeast cell, which is observable on a background of India ink (see Figure 34.26). A positive capsule stain on cerebrospinal fluid can give a quick diagnosis of cryptococcal meningitis, but false negatives are common. A latex agglutination test is also available. The most common form of cryptococcosis is a mild, subclinical lung infection. In immunocompromised patients, the infection often disseminates to the brain and meninges, with fatal consequences. However, about 20% of patients with cryptococcal meningitis have no obvious immunologic defect. In AIDS patients, cryptococcosis is the second most common fungal infection (after candidiasis) and is potentially the most serious. The antifungal drugs used to treat cryptococcosis are amphotericin B and flucytosine, the precise treatment regimen depending on the stage of disease, site of infection, and whether the patient has AIDS. When the CD4 cell count in an AIDS patient falls below 100 cells per µl, cryptococcal infection is so likely that fluconazole is used prophylactically.

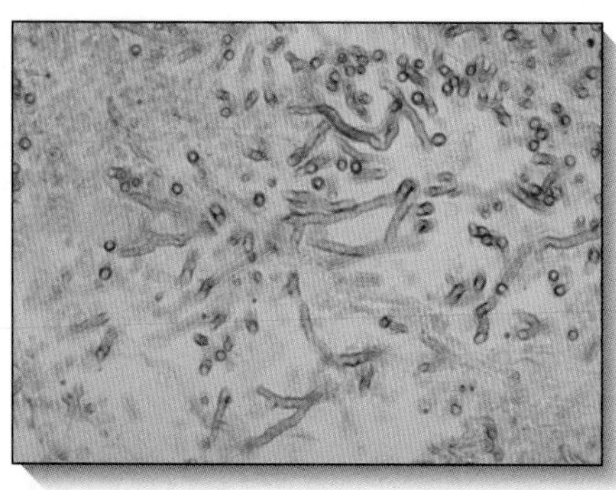

Figure 20.16
Aspergillus species.

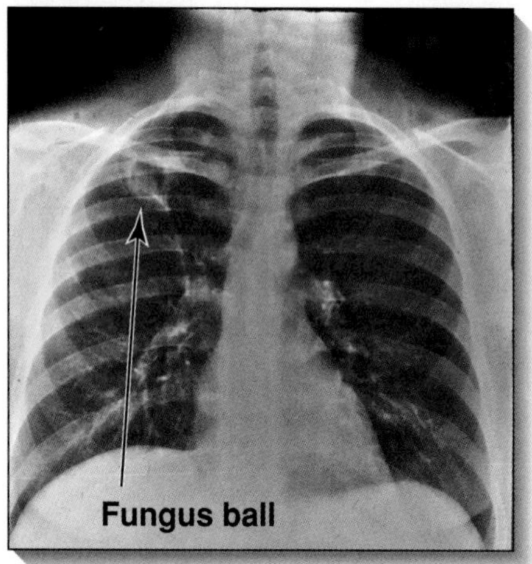

Figure 20.17
Fungus ball.

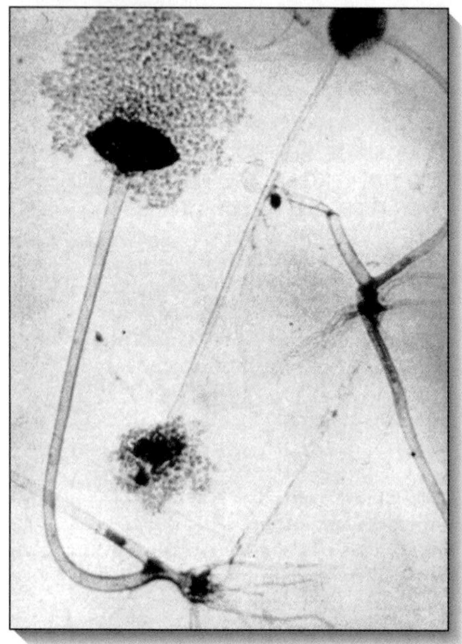

Figure 20.18
Rhizopus oryzae.

C. Aspergillosis

Aspergillosis is caused by several species of the genus *Aspergillus* but primarily by *Aspergillus fumigatus. Aspergillus* is rarely pathogenic in the normal host but can produce disease in immunosuppressed individuals and patients treated with broad-spectrum antibiotics. The disease has a worldwide distribution. Aspergilli are ubiquitous, growing only as filamentous molds (Figure 20.16) and producing prodigious numbers of conidiospores. They reside in dust soil, and decomposing organic matter. In fact, hospital outbreaks affecting neutropenic patients (that is, those with decreased neutrophils in their blood) have been traced to dust from neighboring construction work. Aspergillosis manifests itself in several forms, depending in part on the patient's immunologic status.

1. **Acute aspergillus infections:** The most severe, and often fatal, form of aspergillosis is acute invasive infection of the lung, from which the infection can be disseminated to the brain, GI tract, and other organs. A less severe, noninvasive lung infection gives rise to a fungus ball (aspergilloma), a mass of hyphal tissue that can form in lung cavities derived from prior diseases such as tuberculosis (Figure 20.17). Although the lung is the most common primary site of infection, the eye, ear, nasal sinuses, and skin can also be primary sites.

2. **Diagnosis and treatment:** Definitive diagnosis of an aspergillus infection is afforded by detection of hyphal masses and isolation of the organism from clinical samples. *Aspergillus* hyphae characteristically form V-shaped branches (septate hyphae that branch at a 45-degree angle, see Figure 20.16) that are distinguished from *Mucor* species, which form right-angle branches. Also, septa are present in *Aspergillus* hyphae but absent from those of *Mucor.* In culture, the spore-bearing structures of the aspergilli are unmistakable, but, because these organisms are so ubiquitous, external contamination of clinical samples can give false-positives. Treatment of *Aspergillus* infections is typically by amphotericin B and surgical removal of fungal masses or infected tissue. The antifungal drugs miconazole, ketoconazole, and fluconazole have not proven useful, although itraconazole has been used with some effectiveness for *Aspergillus* osteomyelitis.

D. Mucormycosis

Mucormycosis is caused most often by *Rhizopus oryzae* (also called *R. arrhizus*), as shown in Figure 20.18, and less often by other members of the order Mucorales, such as *Absidia corymbifera* and *Rhizomucor pusillus.* Like the aspergilli, these organisms are ubiquitous in nature, and their spores are found in great abundance on rotting fruit and old bread. *Mucor* infections occur worldwide but are almost entirely restricted to individuals with some underlying predisposing condition, such as burns, leukemias, or acidotic states such as diabetes mellitus. The most common form of the disease, which can be fatal within 1 week, is rhinocerebral mucormycosis, in which the infection begins in the nasal mucosa or sinuses and progresses to the orbits, palate, and brain. Because the disease is so aggressive, many cases are not diagnosed until after death. Treatment is based on high-dose amphotericin B but must be accompanied, when possible, by surgical debridement of necrotic tissue and correction of the underlying predisposing condition. Antifungal drugs other than amphotericin have not proven useful. With early diagnosis and optimal treatment, about half of diabetic patients survive rhinocerebral mucormycosis, but prognosis is very poor for leukemic patients.

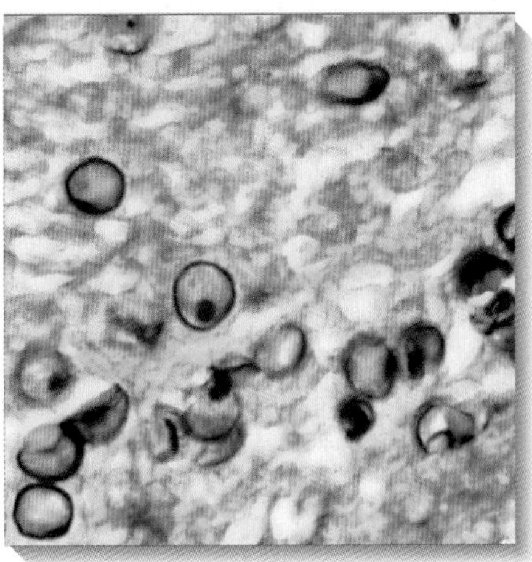

Figure 20.19
Silver stain of *Pneumocystis jiroveci* cysts in tissue from a patient with AIDS.

E. Pneumocystis jiroveci

Pneumocystis jiroveci pneumonia is caused by a yeast-like fungus called *P. jiroveci* (formerly, *P. carinii*) as shown in Figure 20.19. The disease is still often referred to as PCP, for *P. carinii* pneumonia. Before the use of immunosuppressive drugs and the onset of the AIDS epidemic, infection with this organism was a rare occurrence. It is one of the most common opportunistic diseases of individuals infected with HIV-1 (see Figure 33.10) and almost 100 percent fatal if untreated.

1. **Classification:** Previously, *P. jiroveci* was considered a protozoan, but recent molecular homology studies of both protein and nucleic acid sequences indicate that *P. jiroveci* is a fungus related to the ascomycetous yeasts. However, ergosterol, which is an essential component of most fungal membranes, is lacking in *P. jiroveci*. It has so far not been possible to cultivate *P. jiroveci in vitro*, limiting understanding of its life cycle.

2. **Pathology:** The infectious form and the natural reservoir of this organism have not been identified, but they must be ubiquitous in nature because almost 100 percent of children worldwide have antipneumocystis antibodies. The disease is not transmitted from person to person. Instead, development of *P. jiroveci* in immunodeficient patients is thought to be by activation of preexisting dormant cells in the lungs. The encysted forms induce inflammation of alveoli, resulting in production of an exudate that blocks gas exchange. Figure 20.20 shows typical radiographic findings in *Pneumocystis* pneumonia.

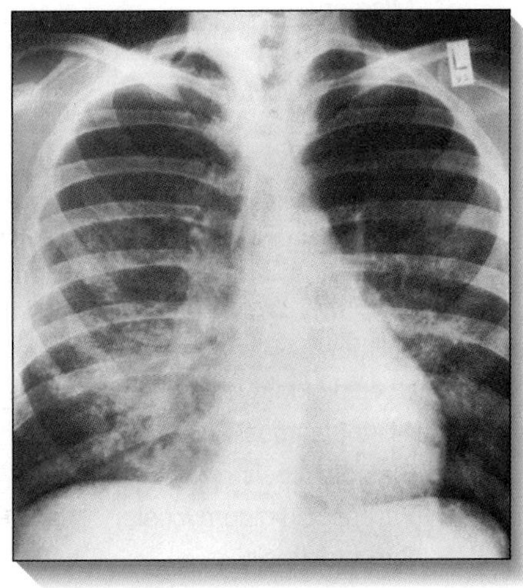

Figure 20.20
Pneumocystis pneumonia.

3. **Diagnosis and treatment:** Because *P. jiroveci* cannot be cultivated, diagnosis is based on microscopic examination of biopsied lung tissue or washings. The most effective therapy is a combination of sulfamethoxazole and trimethoprim, which is also used prophylactically to prevent infection in AIDS patients. Aggressive treatment can spare about half of patients. Because the mechanism of action of many antifungal drugs, such as amphotericin, involves interfering with ergosterol synthesis or function, these drugs are useless for fungi that lack ergosterol.

Study Questions

Choose the ONE correct answer.

20.1 A component of the cell membrane of most fungi is:

A. cholesterol.
B. chitin.
C. ergosterol.
D. peptidoglycan.
E. keratin.

Correct answer = C. Ergosterol in fungi is the functional equivalent of cholesterol in higher organisms. Peptidoglycan is a component of the bacterial cell wall, whereas chitin is a component of the cell wall of fungi. [Note: Chitin also comprises the exoskeletons of insects and crustacea.] Keratin is the major protein of hair and nails

20.2 A physician visiting a rural Latin American village finds that many mature males but few immature males or females of any age are afflicted by a particular fungal disease. What is likely to be the diagnosis?

A. Mycetoma
B. Blastomycosis
C. Paracoccidioidomycosis
D. Mucormycosis
E. Histoplasmosis

Correct answer = C. For some reason, possibly hormonal, this disease favors mature males.

20.3 A fungus that can attack hair is:

A. *Trichophyton.*
B. *Rhizopus.*
C. *Microsporum.*
D. *Sporothrix.*
E. *Epidermophyton.*

Correct answer = C. All attack skin, but only *Microsporum* attacks hair.

20.4 A farmer in Mississippi presents with a chronic cough. Chest radiograph reveals an opaque mass, and biopsy of the lung shows macrophages with multiple yeast forms. Which one of the following diagnoses is most likely?

A. Coccidioidomycosis
B. Histoplasmosis
C. Blastomycosis
D. Paracoccidioidomycosis
E. Sporotrichosis

Correct answer = B. Histoplasmosis is caused by *Histoplasma capsulatum.* In the soil, the fungus generates conidia, which, when airborne, enter the lungs and germinate into yeast-like cells. These yeast cells are engulfed by macrophages, in which they multiply. Pulmonary infections may be acute but relatively benign and self-limiting, or it may be chronic, progressive, and fatal. Dissemination is rare but results in invasion of reticuloendothelial system cells, which distinguishes this organism as the only fungus to exhibit intracellular parasitism. The disease occurs worldwide but is most prevalent in central North America, especially the Ohio and Mississippi River Valleys.

Protozoa

21

I. OVERVIEW

Protozoa are a diverse group of unicellular, eukaryotic organisms. Many have evolved structural features (organelles) that mimic the organs of multicellular organisms. Reproduction is generally by mitotic binary fission, although in some protozoal species, sexual (meiotic) reproduction with several variations occurs as well. Only a few of the many tens of thousands of protozoan species are pathogenic for humans. Those discussed in this chapter are listed in Figure 21.1. These pathogens are of two general kinds: those that parasitize the intestinal and urogenital tracts and those that parasitize blood cells and tissues. Protozoal infections are common in developing tropical and subtropical regions where sanitary conditions and control of the vectors of transmission are poor. However, with increased world travel and immigration, protozoal diseases are no longer confined to specific geographic locales. Because they are eukaryotes, protozoa, like fungi, have metabolic processes closer to those of the human host than to prokaryotic bacterial pathogens. Protozoal diseases are, therefore, less easily treated than bacterial infections because many antiprotozoal drugs are toxic to the human host.

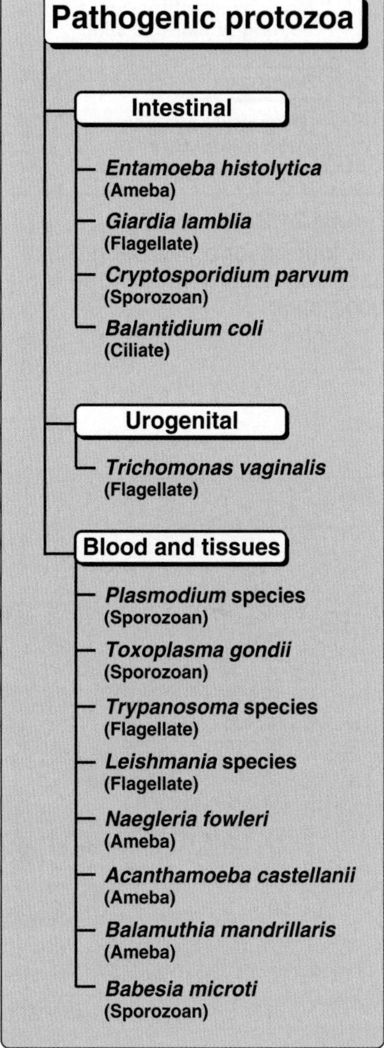

Figure 21.1
Clinically relevant protozoa, classified according to site of infection.

II. CLASSIFICATION OF CLINICALLY IMPORTANT PROTOZOA

Among the pathogenic protozoa, there are important common features that are clinically relevant. For example, many protozoa have both a dormant, immotile cyst stage that permits survival when environmental conditions are hostile and a motile, actively feeding and reproducing, vegetative (trophozoite) stage. For convenience, protozoa are classified according to mode of locomotion. The clinically relevant protozoa are divided into four groups (Figure 21.2).

A. Amebas

Amebas move by extending cytoplasmic projections (pseudopodia) outward from the main cell body. A single cell can have several pseudopodia projecting in the same general direction, with the remainder of the cytoplasm flowing into the pseudopodia. Amebas feed by engulfing food particles with their pseudopodia. Some amebas have flagella as well.

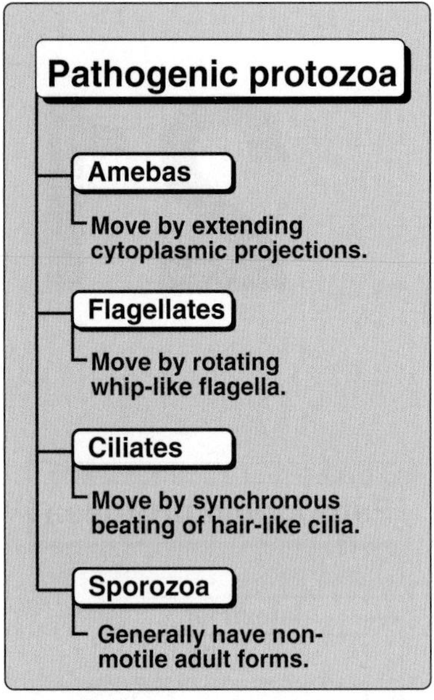

Figure 21.2
The four major protozoal groups, classified according to mode of locomotion.

B. Flagellates

Flagellates move by means of two or more whiplike projections (flagella) that rotate and propel the cells through their liquid environment. Some flagellates, for example *Trichomonas vaginalis*, also have undulating membranes that assist in swimming. Flagellates ingest food particles through an oral groove called a cytostome.

C. Ciliates

Ciliates move by means of many hairlike projections (cilia) arranged in rows that cover the cell surface and beat in synchrony, propelling the cell much like a row boat. Most ciliates have cytostomes that pass food particles through a cytopharynyx and finally into vacuoles where digestion takes place. Although there are some 7,000 species of ciliates, only *Balantidium coli* is pathogenic for humans, and the disease, balantidiasis, is rare.

D. Sporozoa

Sporozoans (also called apicomplexa) are obligate, intracellular parasites. Although they generally have nonmotile adult forms, in some species, male gametes have flagella. An example of a sporozoan is *Plasmodium vivax* (see p. 221), which causes malaria. Sporozoans can have complex life cycles with more than one host. The definitive host is that which harbors the sexually reproducing stage, whereas the intermediate host provides the environment in which asexual reproduction occurs.

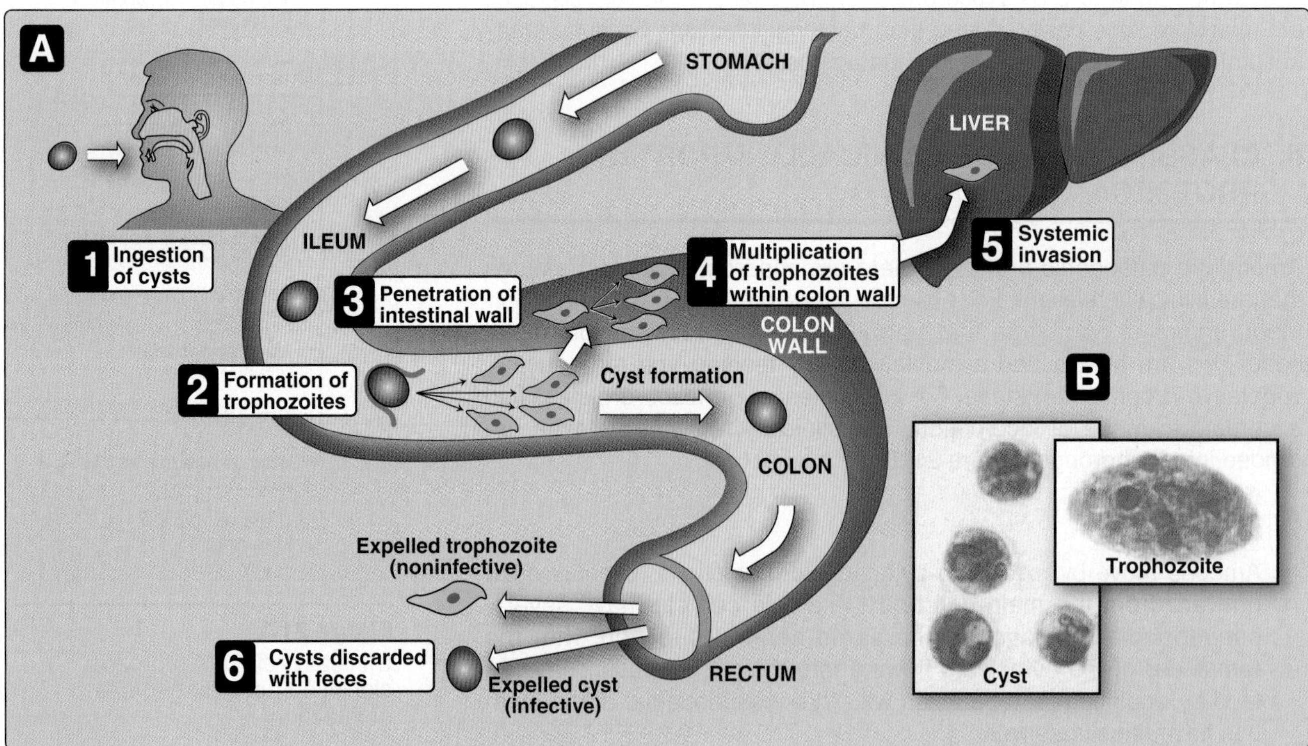

Figure 21.3
A. Life cycle of *Entamoeba histolytica*. B. Photomicrographs of trophozoite and cyst forms.

III. INTESTINAL PROTOZOAL INFECTIONS

There are four principal protozoal intestinal parasites: the ameba, *Entamoeba histolytica*; the flagellate, *Giardia lamblia*; the sporozoan, *Cryptosporidium* (several species); and *Balantidium coli* (the only ciliate protozoan to cause human disease). Each pathogen causes diarrhea, which, although similar, differ in the site of infection, its severity, and secondary consequences.

A. Amebic dysentery (*Entamoeba histolytica*)

Ingested cysts from contaminated food or water form trophozoites in the small intestine (Figure 21.3). These pass to the colon, where they feed on intestinal bacteria, and may invade the epithelium, potentially inducing ulceration. The parasite can further spread to the liver and cause abscesses. In the colon, trophozoites form cysts that pass in the feces. Amebic cysts are resistant to chlorine concentrations used in most water treatment facilities. Diagnosis is made by examination of fecal samples for motile trophozoites or cysts (Figure 21.4). Serologic test kits are useful when microscopic examination is negative. Liver abscesses should be biopsied from the abscess edge where the active amebas accumulate. Mild cases of luminal amebic dysentery are treated with iodoquinol, paromomycin, or diloxanide furoate. More severe cases, including liver infections, are treated with metronidazole (which also has antibacterial activity) in combination with chloroquine and/or diloxamide furoate or emetine. Up to 80% of infections due to *E. histolytica* are asymptomatic. These asymptomatic cyst-passers are a source of infection to others and may not be detected because they are asymptomatic.

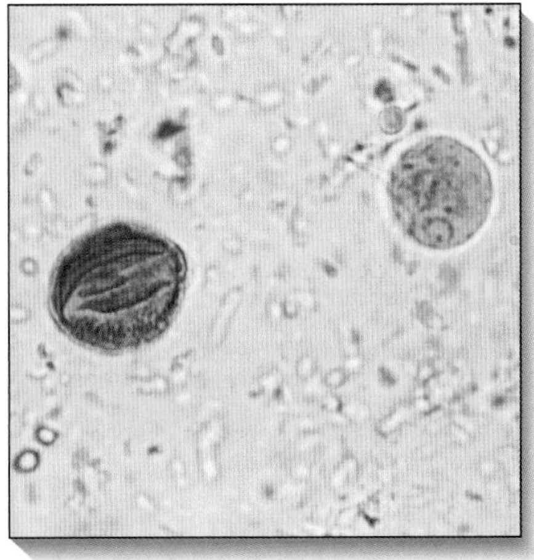

Figure 21.4
Entamoeba histolytica cysts.

B. Giardiasis (*Giardia lamblia*)

Giardiasis is the most commonly diagnosed parasitic intestinal disease in the United States. Similar to *E. histolytica*, *G. lamblia* has two life-cycle stages: the binucleate trophozoite that has four flagella and the drug-resistant, four-nucleate cyst. Ingested cysts form trophozoites in the duodenum, where they attach to the wall but do not invade (Figure 21.5). *Giardia* infections are often clinically mild, although in some individuals, massive infection may damage the duodenal mucosa. Because the *Giardia* parasite preferentially inhabits the duodenum, fecal examination may be negative. A commercial enzyme-linked immunosorbent assay to measure *Giardia* antigen in fecal material has proven useful. Metronidazole is an effective treatment. *G. lamblia* cysts are resistant to chlorine concentrations used in most water treatment facilities, as is true for *E. histolytica*.

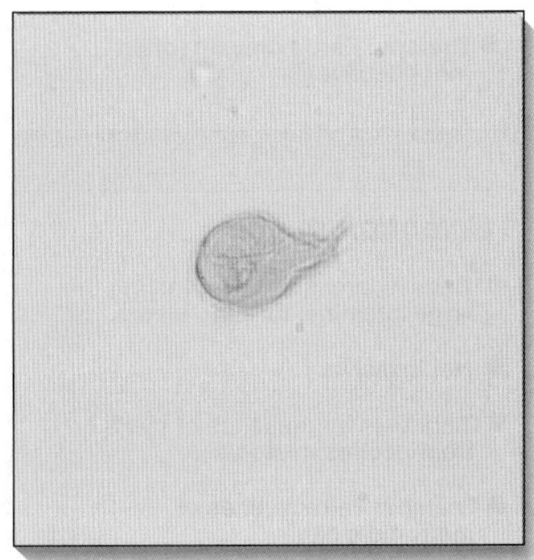

Figure 21.5
Giardia lamblia trophozoite in stool sample.

C. Cryptosporidiosis (*Cryptosporidium* species)

Cryptosporidium is an intracellular parasite that inhabits the epithelial cells of the villi of the lower small intestine. The source of infection is often the feces of domestic animals, and farm run-off has been implicated as a source of *Cryptosporidium* contamination of drinking water. Asymptomatic to mild cases are common, and, if the immune system of the patient is normal, the disease usually

Entamoeba histolytica

- Infects colon with secondary infection of liver.
- Infected patients pass noninfectious trophozoites as well as infectious cysts in stools.
- Diagnosis by presence of characteristic cysts (containing one to four nuclei) in stools.
- Therapy: Iodoquinol, metronidazole.

Giardia lamblia

- Infection usually results from drinking contaminated water.
- Infects duodenum, with incubation time of about 10 days.
- Acute infection shows sudden onset with foul smelling, watery diarrhea.
- Diagnosis by presence of cysts or trophozoites in stools.
- Therapy: Metronidazole.

Cryptosporidium parvum

- Infects lower small intestine.
- Organisms are intracellular parasites in epithelial cells of intestinal villi.
- Diagnosis by modified acid-fast stain of stool sample.
- Therapy: Paromomycin (often not effective).

Balantidium coli

- Causes dysentery by infecting the large intestine, forming ulcers.
- Not invasive.
- Diagnosis by presence of cysts or trophozoites in stools.
- Therapy: Tetracyclines or metronidazole.

Figure 21.6
Summary of intestinal protozoal infections.

resolves without therapy. However, in immunocompromised individuals (for example, those with AIDS), infection may be severe and intractable, although paromomycin has provided some improvement. Diagnosis is made by acid-fast staining of the tiny (4 to 6 μm) oocysts in fresh stool samples.

D. Balantidiasis (*Balantidium coli*)

Balantidiasis is caused by the ciliate protozoon *B. coli*, which causes dysentery by infecting the large intestine. *B. coli* is locally invasive, causing colonic ulcers. Although these may perforate, leading to peritonitis, it is unlike *E. histolytica* in that it is very rarely associated with spread to distant organs. Manifestations can range from asymptomatic carriage to abdominal discomfort and mild diarrhea to acute dysentery with blood and pus in the stool. The life cycle includes both trophozoite and cyst forms, and identification of either in the stool can be diagnostic. The cysts, which are the infective stage, can be found in contaminated water and are not inactivated by chlorination. Pigs are the natural reservoir of *B. coli*. The infection can be treated with tetracyclines or metronidizole. A summary of intestinal protozoal infections is shown in Figure 21.6.

IV. UROGENITAL TRACT INFECTION: TRICHOMONIASIS

Trichomoniasis is caused by *Trichomonas vaginalis* (Figure 21.7). Trichomoniasis is the most common protozoal urogenital tract infection of humans. The trichomonads are pear-shaped flagellates, with undulating membranes. There is no cyst form in the life cycle of Trichomonas. Several nonpathogenic species, including *Trichomonas tenax* and *Trichomonas hominis*, can be found in the human mouth and intestines, respectively. These species, which are part of the normal flora, are not easily distinguished morphologically from the pathogenic species, *T. vaginalis*. In females, it causes inflammation of the mucosal tissue of the vagina, vulva, and cervix, accompanied by a copious, yellowish, malodorous discharge. Less commonly, it infects the male urethra, prostate, and seminal vesicles, producing a white discharge. The disease is largely sexually transmitted, and both (or all) sexual partners should be treated. Because the optimum pH for growth of this organism is about 6.0, *T. vaginalis* does not thrive in the normal, acidic vagina, which has a pH of about 4.0. Abnormal alkalinity of the vagina, therefore, favors acquisition of the disease. Diagnosis is made by detection of motile trophozoites in vaginal or urethral secretions. If the concentration of parasites is too low to be observed directly, laboratory culture can be used to obtain observable organisms. Effective treatment is afforded by metronidazole. Figure 21.8 summarizes urogenital infections caused by *T. vaginalis*.

V. BLOOD AND TISSUE PROTOZOAL INFECTIONS

The major protozoal diseases that involve the blood and internal organs are malaria (*Plasmodium* species), toxoplasmosis (*Toxoplasma* species), trypanosomiasis (*Trypanosoma* species), and leishmaniasis (*Leishmania* species). *Plasmodium* and *Toxoplasma* are sporozoans (apicomplexa), whereas *Trypanosoma* and *Leishmania* are flagellates, sometimes referred to as hemoflagellates. Three free-living amebas cause amoebic encephalitis in humans. *Babesia microcoti* causes babesiosis, which is transmitted to humans by the bite of an *Ixodes* tick and results in a red blood cell (RBC) infection, similar to that caused by *Plasmodium* species.

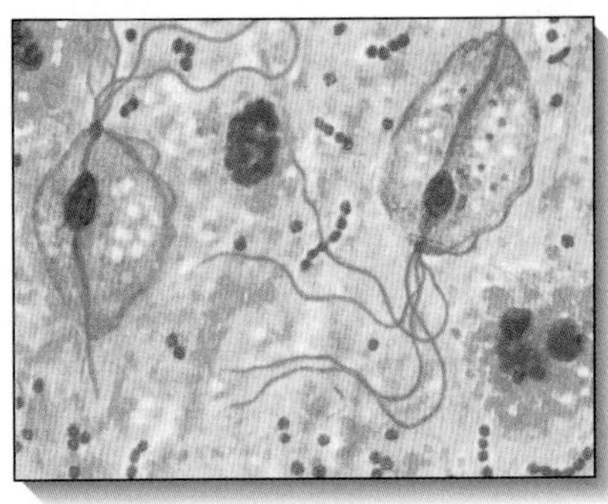

Figure 21.7
Trichomonas vaginalis.

A. Malaria (*Plasmodium falciparum* and other species)

Malaria is an acute infectious disease of the blood, caused by one of five species of the protozoal genus, *Plasmodium*, which is a sporozoan. *P. falciparum* accounts for some 15 percent of all malaria cases, and *P. vivax* for 80 percent of malarial cases. The plasmodial parasite is transmitted to humans through the bite of a female *Anopheles* mosquito or by an infected, blood-contaminated, needle. Sporozoans reproduce asexually in human cells by a process called schizogony, in which multiple nuclear divisions are followed by envelopment of the nuclei by cell walls producing merozoites. These, in turn, become trophozoites. Sexual reproduction occurs in the mosquito, where new spores (sporozoites) are formed. *Plasmodium knowlesi* causes malaria, at least in some parts of Asia. In addition to mosquito bites and blood-contaminate needles, blood transfusion is a potentially important mode of transmission, at least in parts of the world in which screening of bank blood may not be as assiduous as it is in the United States.

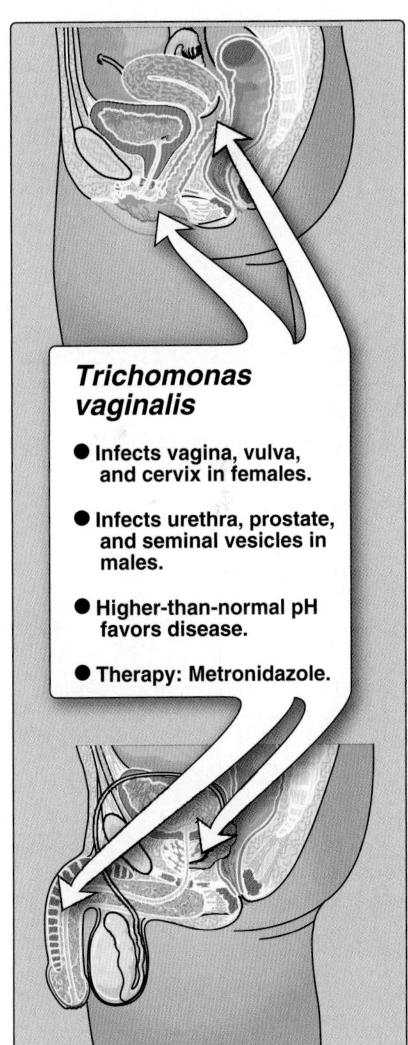

Figure 21.8
Summary of urogenital infection.

1. **Pathology and clinical significance:** Plasmodium sporozoites are injected into the bloodstream, where they rapidly migrate to the liver. There they form cyst-like structures containing thousands of merozoites. Upon release, the merozoites invade RBCs, using hemoglobin as a nutrient. Eventually, the infected RBCs rupture, releasing merozoites that can invade other erythrocytes. If large numbers of RBCs rupture at roughly the same time, a paroxysm (sudden onset) of fever can result from the massive release of toxic substances. A predictable consequence of RBC lysis is anemia, which is typical of *Plasmodium* infections. *P. falciparum* is the most dangerous plasmodial species. It can cause a rapidly fulminating disease, characterized by persistent high fever and orthostatic hypotension. Infection can lead to capillary obstruction and death if treatment is not prompt. *P. malariae*, *P. vivax*, and *P. ovale* cause milder forms of the disease, probably because they invade either young or old red cells, but not both. This is in contrast to *P. falciparum*, which invades cells of all ages. Even today, malarial infection is a common and serious disease and in 2010 is estimated to have caused about 655,000 deaths worldwide. A summary of the life cycle of *Plasmodium* is shown in Figure 21.9.

2. **Diagnosis and treatment:** Diagnosis depends on detection of the parasite inside RBCs (Figure 21.10). Thick blood smears stained with Giemsa stain provide the most sensitive visual test. Thin blood smears, in which more detail can be discerned, are used to determine the species involved, which is important in planning a course of therapy. Serologic tests are usually too slow for diagnosis of acute disease. Drug treatment is determined by the *Plasmodium* species that is causing the infection.

Figure 21.9
Life cycle of the malarial parasite, *Plasmodium falciparum*.

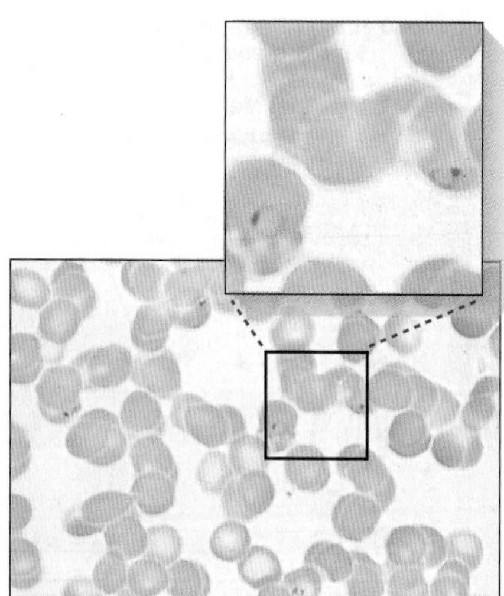

Figure 21.10
Ring form of *Plasmodium falciparum* in red blood cell.

Because *P. falciparum* has no exoerythrocytic phase, it needs only to be treated with quinine, artemisin, mefloquine or doxycycline, depending on resistance patterns in the given geographic location. Chloroquine resistance is so prevalent among *P. falciparum* that it is almost never used for this organism any more. For *ovale* or *vivax* infections, after treatment with chloroquine, a two-week course of primaquine is necessary to achieve a "radical cure" by eliminating exoerythrocytic organisms that persist in the liver. If, in the geographic location of infection, there is chloroquine resistance among *P. vivax* or *P. ovale*, then an alternative drug must be used prior to radical cure. Before treatment with primaquine, patients should be screened for glucose 6-phosphate dehydrogenase deficiency as individuals with deficiency of this enzyme develop hemolytic anemia, sometimes very severe, when treated with primaquine.

B. Toxoplasmosis (*Toxoplasma gondii*)

Toxoplasma gondii is an intracellular sporozoan, distributed worldwide, that infects all vertebrate species, although the definitive host is the cat. Humans can become infected by the accidental ingestion of oocysts present in cat feces, by eating raw or undercooked meat, congenitally from an infected mother, or from a blood transfusion.

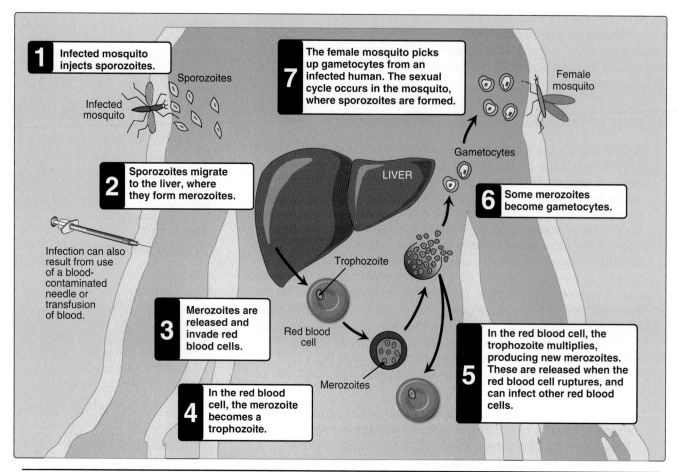

1. **Pathology and clinical significance:** There are two kinds of *Toxoplasma* trophozoites found in human infections: rapidly growing tachyzoites ("tachy-" = rapid) that are seen in body fluids in early, acute infections, and slowly growing bradyzoites ("brady-" = slow) that are contained in cysts in muscle and brain tissue and in the eye. Tachyzoites directly destroy cells, particularly parenchymal and reticuloendothelial cells, whereas bradyzoites released from ruptured tissue cysts cause local inflammation with blockage of blood vessels and necrosis. Infections of normal human hosts are common and usually asymptomatic. However, they can be very severe in immunocompromised individuals, who may also suffer recrudescence (relapse) of the infection. Congenital infections can also be severe, resulting in stillbirths, brain lesions, and hydrocephaly, and they are a major cause of blindness in newborns.

2. **Diagnosis and treatment:** The initial diagnostic approach involves detection of parasites in tissue specimens, but this may often be inconclusive. With the recent availability of commercial diagnostic kits, serologic tests to identify toxoplasma are now routinely used. These include tests for *Toxoplasma*-specific immunoglobulin (Ig) G and IgM. The treatment of choice for this infection is the antifolate drug pyrimethamine, given in combination with sulfadiazine. For patients who can not receive sulfa drugs, clindamycin can be added to pyrimethamine.

C. Trypanosomiasis (various trypanosome species)

Trypanosomiasis refers to two chronic, eventually fatal, diseases (African sleeping sickness and American trypanosomiasis) caused by several trypanosome species. Some of the differences between these diseases and the available chemotherapeutic agents are summarized in Figure 21.11.

1. **Pathology and clinical significance:** African sleeping sickness is caused by the closely related flagellates, *Trypanosoma brucei gambiense* or *Trypanosoma brucei rhodesiense* (Figure 21.12). These parasites are injected into humans by the bite of the tsetse fly, producing a primary lesion, or chancre. The organism then spreads to lymphoid tissue and reproduces extracellularly in the blood. Later, the parasite invades the central nervous system (CNS), causing inflammation of the brain and spinal cord, mediated by released toxins. This inflammation produces the characteristic lethargy and, eventually, continuous sleep and death. American trypanosomiasis (Chagas disease), caused by *Trypanosoma cruzi*, occurs in Central and South America. Unlike African forms of the disease, infection is not transmitted by insect bite but rather by insect feces contaminating the conjunctiva or a break in the skin. The first symptom is a granulomatous lesion at the site of entry by the pathogen, followed by an acute disease characterized by fever and hepatosplenomegaly. Subsequently the disease may go into remission but reappear as digestive system problems. Potential, long term complications include cardiomyopathy and megacolon.

TRYPANOSOMIASIS

AMERICAN (also called Chagas disease) caused by *Trypanosoma cruzi*
- **Acute infection is common in children.**
- **Chronic infection causes cardiomyopathy.**
- **Transmitted by insect feces contaminating the eye or a break in the skin.**
- **Treated with nifurtimox.**

AFRICAN caused by *Trypanosoma brucei*
- **Transmitted by the bite of the tsetse fly.**
- **Causes "sleeping sickness."**

Trypanosoma brucei gambiense
- **Slow to enter CNS.**
- **Suramin and pentamidine are used only in the early stages of disease.**

Trypanosoma brucei rhodesiense
- **Early invasion of CNS.**
- **Usually fatal if not treated.**
- **Melarsoprol used when there is CNS involvement.**

Figure 21.11
Summary of trypanosomiasis. CNS = central nervous system.

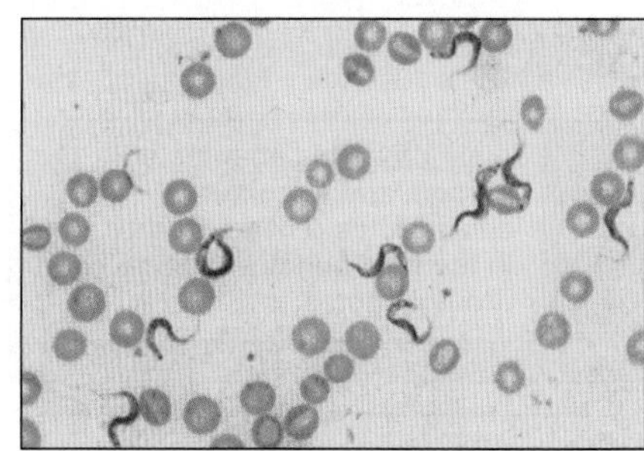

Figure 21.12
Trypanosoma brucei.

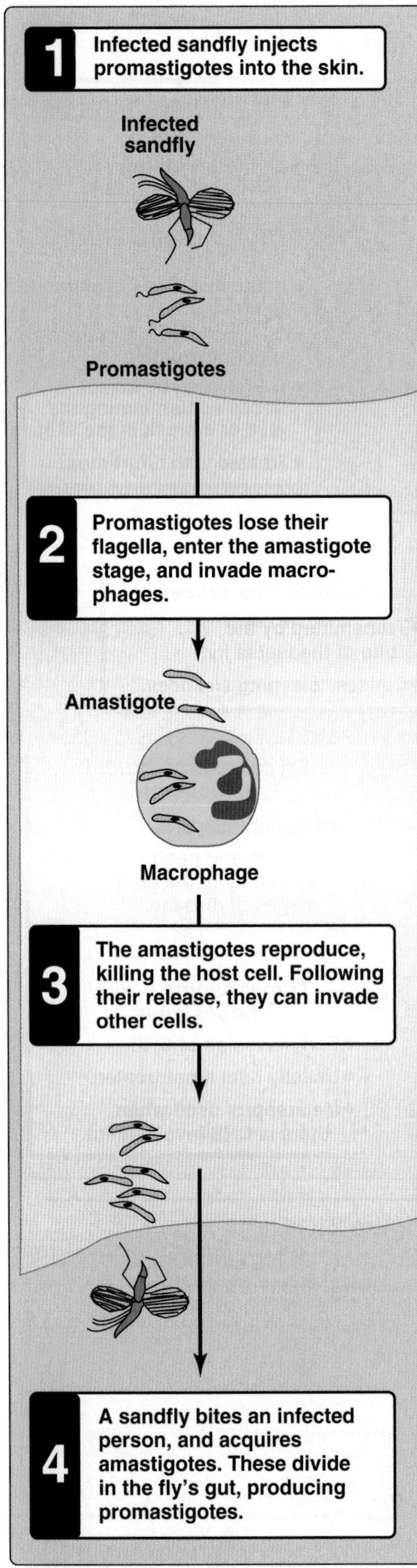

1
Infected sandfly injects promastigotes into the skin.
Infected sandfly
Promastigotes
2
Promastigotes lose their flagella, enter the amastigote stage, and invade macrophages.
Amastigote
Macrophage
3
The amastigotes reproduce, killing the host cell. Following their release, they can invade other cells.
4
A sandfly bites an infected person, and acquires amastigotes. These divide in the fly's gut, producing promastigotes.

Figure 21.13
Life cycle of *Leishmania*.

2. **Diagnosis and treatment:** Diagnosis of African trypanosomiasis is made primarily by detection of motile trypanosomes in Giemsa-stained smears of body fluids (for example, blood, cerebrospinal fluid, and lymph node aspirates). Highly specific serologic tests are also available for diagnostic confirmation. Early-stage African trypanosomiasis is treated with suramin or pentamidine. Melarsoprol is used in late-stage disease when the CNS is involved. American trypanosomiasis is treated with nifurtimox, but the drug's effectiveness is limited.

D. Leishmaniasis (various *Leishmania* species)

Leishmaniasis refers to a group of infections caused by the flagellate protozoa of the genus *Leishmania.* About half a million new cases are reported each year, and it is estimated that 12 million people are currently infected with this parasite. There are three clinical types of leishmaniasis: cutaneous, mucocutaneous, and visceral. The various infective organisms are indistinguishable morphologically but can be differentiated biochemically. Two subgenera are recognized (*Leishmania leishmania* and *Leishmania viannia*), each with several species. Any species has the potential to cause one of three clinical manifestations. The natural reservoir of the parasite varies with geography and species but is usually wild rodents, dogs, and humans. Transmission to humans is by the bite of the female sandfly of the genus *Phlebotomus* or *Lutzomyia*. The life cycle of *Leishmania* is shown in Figure 21.13.

1. **Cutaneous leishmaniasis (local name, "oriental sore"):** This disease is caused by *Leishmania tropica* in North and West Africa, Iran, and Iraq. The cutaneous form of the disease is characterized by ulcerating single or multiple skin sores (Figure 21.14). Most cases spontaneously heal, but the ulcers leave unsightly scars. In Mexico and Guatemala, the cutaneous form is due to *Leishmania mexicana*, which produces single lesions that rapidly heal.

2. **Mucocutaneous leishmaniasis (local name, espundia):** This disease is caused by *Leishmania viannia brasiliensis* in Central and South America, especially the Amazon regions. In this form of the disease, the parasite attacks tissue at the mucosal-dermal junctions of the nose and mouth, producing multiple lesions. Extensive spreading into mucosal tissue can obliterate the nasal septum and the buccal cavity, ending in death from secondary infection.

3. **Visceral leishmaniasis (local name, kala-azar):** This disease is caused by *Leishmania donovani* in India, East Africa, and China. In the visceral disease, the parasite initially infects macrophages, which, in turn, migrate to the spleen, liver, and bone marrow, where the parasite rapidly multiplies. Symptoms include intermittent fevers and weight loss. The spleen and liver enlarge, and jaundice may develop. Mortality is nearly 100% within 2 years if the disease is untreated. In some cases, complications resulting from secondary infection and emaciation result in death.

4. **Diagnosis and treatment:** Diagnosis is made by examination of Giemsa-stained tissue and fluid samples for the nonflagellated

form (amastigote), which is the only form of the organism that occurs in humans and other mammals. Cutaneous and mucocutaneous disease can be diagnosed from tissue samples taken from the edges of lesions or lymph node aspirates. Visceral disease is more difficult to diagnose, requiring liver, spleen, or bone marrow biopsy. Serologic tests (for example, indirect fluorescent antibody, see p. 28, and complement fixation, see p. 26) are used by the Centers for Disease Control and Prevention. The treatment of leishmaniasis is difficult because the available drugs have considerable toxicity and high failure rates. Pentavalent antimonials, such as sodium stibogluconate, are the conventional therapy, with pentamidine and amphotericin B as second-line agents.

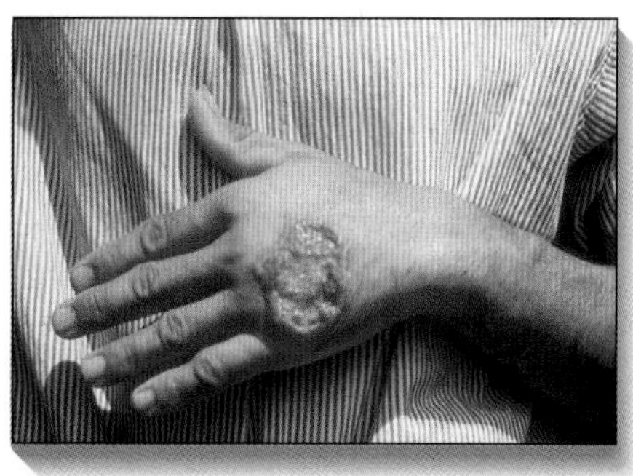

Figure 21.14
Skin ulcer due to leishmaniasis, on the hand of a Central American adult.

E. Amebic encephalitis (*Naegleria fowleri*, *Acanthamoeba castellanii,* and *Balamuthia mandrillaris*)

Several environmental amebae are capable of causing fatal CNS infections in humans. *Naegleria fowleri* can cause primary amebic meningoencephalitis (PAM) in immunocompetent individuals. The ameba exists in one of three morphological forms: flagellate, trophozoite, or cyst. The trophozoite (the infectious form found in fresh water) enters via the nasal cavity, generally infecting swimming children. From the nasal passages, the ameba directly invades the brain by way of the cribriform plate. The pathogen causes necrotic lesions in the brain, and the infection results in death within a few days of symptom onset. Symptoms initially include headache, fever, and nausea. More than 95 percent of cases are fatal, despite appropriate therapy with amphotericin B. *Acanthamoeba* species, also free-living amebas, cause granulomatous amebic encephalitis (GAE), which is not as rapidly progressing as PAM. However, like PAM, GAE is often fatal. *Acanthamoeba* species also cause cutaneous acanthamoebiasis, particularly in immunocompromised individuals. Acanthamoeba keratitis is an infection of the cornea, which is most often seen in contact lens wearers who suffer a traumatic eye injury. The source of the ameba is the contact lens solution, but, in immunocompetent persons, damage to the cornea is a prerequisite to infection. *Balamuthia mandrillaris* is also a free-living ameba capable of causing encephalitis (BAE). Acquisition of the pathogen is thought to be from water or soil with subsequent hematogenous spread to the brain. As with the other amebic encephalitides, infection in both immunocompetent and immunocompromised persons is likely to be fatal. Several cases of BAE were reported in 2010 in recipients of solid organ transplants.

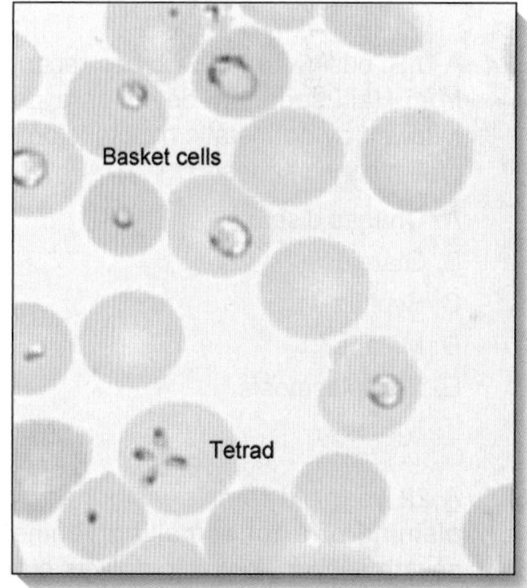

Figure 21.15
Wright-stained peripheral blood smear from a newborn with probable congenital *Babesia microti* infection.The smear shows parasites of variable size and morphologic appearance.

F. Babesiosis (*Babesia microti*)

B. microti is a protozoan transmitted by the bite of an *Ixodes* tick, which is the same arthropod vector that transmits Lyme disease. The reservoirs for both pathogens are small mammals and deer. *Babesia* infects RBCs in the human accidental host, multiplying within these cells and ultimately causing RBC lysis. Similar to *Plasmodium* species, *Babesia* species generate ring-like trophozoites within erythrocytes (Figure 21.15), which are diagnostic. The infection does not spread beyond the erythrocytes, but symptoms are related to loss of RBCs (anemia) and clearance of the cell debris (hepatosplenomegaly and jaundice).

Study Questions

Choose the ONE correct answer.

21.1 The protozoal trophozoite phase is characterized by:

A. metabolic dormancy.
B. toxin production.
C. active feeding and reproduction.
D. flagellar locomotion.
E. residence in the intermediate host.

Correct answer = C. The trophozoite is, generally speaking, the active phase, in contrast to the cyst, which is the dormant phase. In some species, several varieties of trophozoites are recognized, such as the tachyzoites and bradyzoites of *Toxoplasma gondii*.

21.2 The definitive host of a parasite is the host:

A. in which asexual reproduction occurs.
B. in which sexual reproduction occurs.
C. that is obligatory for the parasite.
D. that is capable of destroying the parasite.
E. that is the vector organism that transports a parasite from an uninfected to an infected host.

Correct answer = B. Sexual reproduction occurs in the definitive host, whereas asexual reproduction occurs in the intermediate host. For example, in the case of malarial *Plasmodium*, the definitive host is the mosquito, and the intermediate host is the human. In most cases, both hosts are obligatory for propagation of the parasite.

21.3 *Plasmodium falciparum*, which causes malaria, is an example of:

A. an ameboid protozoan.
B. a sporozoan.
C. a flagellate.
D. a ciliate.
E. a schizont.

Correct answer = B. The sporozoans are also called apicomplexa because of the presence of a complex of organelles at the cell tip that facilitates penetration of the parasite into host tissue. A schizont is not a taxonomic group but a mass of trophozoites.

21.4 A U.S. businessman who has recently returned home from Haiti suddenly develops a periodic high fever followed by orthostatic hypotension. What is the likely preliminary diagnosis?

A. Chagas disease
B. Giardiasis
C. Syphilis
D. Malaria
E. Toxoplasmosis

Correct answer = D. All of the signs point to malaria, especially the periodicity of the fever that results from synchronous rupturing of large numbers of red blood cells.

21.5 A 22 year old female visits her gynecologist complaining of a foul-smelling vaginal discharge and severe itching. A specimen was collected and examined it by light microscopy revealing highly motile, nucleated cells with multiple flagella. What is the most likely causative agent of this infection?

A. *Balantidium coli*
B. *Plasmodium falciparum*
C. *Toxoplasma gondii*
D. *Giardia lamblia*

Correct answer = E. The symptoms are consistent with the sexually transmitted infection caused by *Trichomonas vaginalis*. This protozoal flagellate is highly motile and easily distinguished from other sexually transmitted disease pathogens by light microscopy. The other protozoal pathogens listed do not cause diseases that present with genitourinary tract symptoms.

Helminths

22

I. OVERVIEW

Helminths are worms, some of which are parasitic to humans. These parasites belong to one of three groups: cestodes (tapeworms), trematodes (flukes), or nematodes (roundworms) as shown in Figure 22.1. Although individual species may have preferred primary sites of infestation (often the intestines where they generally do little damage) these organisms may disseminate to vital organs (for example, the brain, lungs, or liver) where they can cause severe damage. It is estimated that at least 70 percent of the world's population is infected with a parasitic helminth. The mode of transmission to humans varies from species to species but includes ingestion of larvae in raw or undercooked pork, beef, or fish; ingestion of helminth eggs in feces; transmission by insect bites; or by direct skin penetration. In North America, helminthic diseases are becoming rare, whereas they are endemic in regions of the world where community sanitary conditions are poor, and human feceal material is used as fertilizer.

II. CESTODES

Cestodes (tapeworms) are ribbon-like, segmented worms that are primarily intestinal parasites. They lack a digestive system and do not ingest particulate matter but, instead, absorb soluble nutrients directly through their cuticles. In the small intestine, some species (for example, the tapeworm *Diphyllobothrium latum)* can attain enormous lengths of up to 15 meters. Cestodes cause clinical injury by sequestering the host's nutrients; by excreting toxic waste; and, in massive infestations, by causing mechanical blockage of the intestine. The anterior end of the worm consists of a scolex, a bulbous structure with hooks and suckers that functions to attach the worm to the intestinal wall (Figure 22.2). The body (strobila) is composed of many segments (proglottids), which form continuously in the region just behind the scolex. Each proglottid has a complete set of sexual organs (that, both male and female) that generate fertilized eggs. The mature, egg-filled proglottids are located at the posterior end of the organism. These can break off the chain and pass out of the body in the stool. Characteristics of infections by the four medically important cestodes are summarized in Figure 22.3. Note that *Taenia solium* has two different disease manifestations, depending on whether transmission is by ingestion of larvae from undercooked pork or by ingestion of its eggs. In the former case, infestation is limited to the intestines, whereas, in the latter case, the eggs develop into larvae that form cysts (cysticerci) in the brain and other tissues.

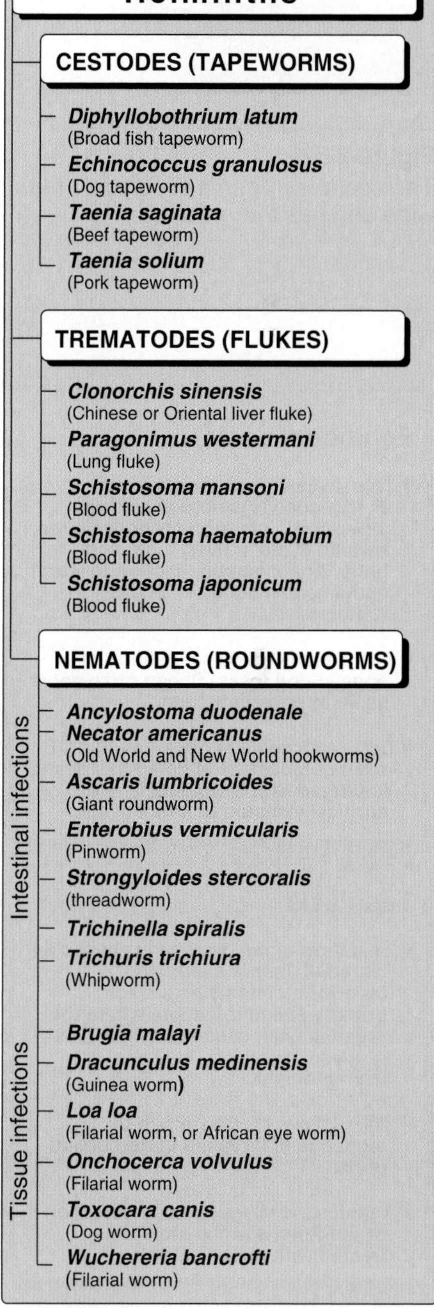

Figure 22.1
Clinically important helminths.

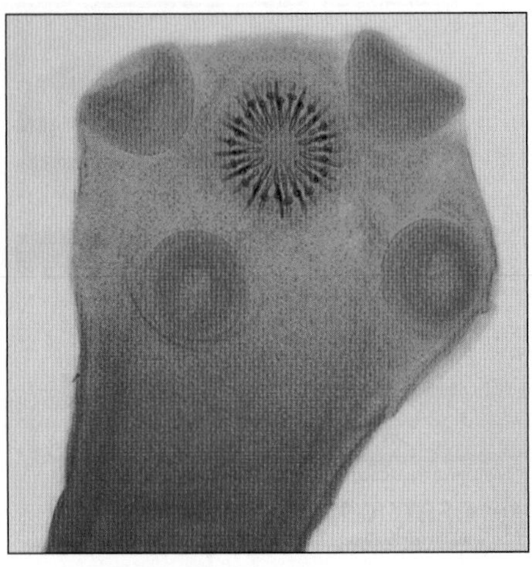

Figure 22.2
The scolex of *Taenia solium* is 1 mm wide and has four suckers.

III. TREMATODES

Trematodes, commonly called flukes, are small (about 1 cm), flat, leaf-like worms that, depending on the species, infest various organs of the human host (for example, intestinal veins, urinary bladder, liver, or lung). All parasitic trematodes use freshwater snails as an intermediate host.

A. Hermaphroditic flukes

Developmental events in the life cycle of a typical fluke begin when the adult fluke, which is hermaphroditic, produces eggs in the human (the definitive host). The eggs are then excreted into the environment. The first larval stage (miracidium) develops inside the eggs. These larvae seek out and infect suitable snail species, which are the first intermediate host. In the snail, asexual reproduction occurs, during which several intermediate developmental forms can be distinguished, including sporocyst; redia (an early larval stage); and, eventually, large numbers of the final larval stage, called cercariae, which leave the snail and seek out a second intermediate host (a fish or crustacean, depending on the species of fluke). In this

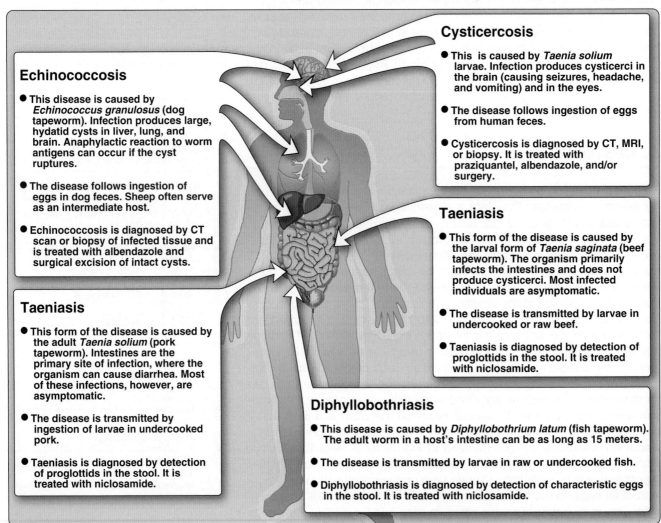

Echinococcosis

- **This disease is caused by *Echinococcus granulosus* (dog tapeworm). Infection produces large, hydatid cysts in liver, lung, and brain. Anaphylactic reaction to worm antigens can occur if the cyst ruptures.**
- **The disease follows ingestion of eggs in dog feces. Sheep often serve as an intermediate host.**
- **Echinococcosis is diagnosed by CT scan or biopsy of infected tissue and is treated with albendazole and surgical excision of intact cysts.**

Cysticercosis

- **This is caused by *Taenia solium* larvae. Infection produces cysticerci in the brain (causing seizures, headache, and vomiting) and in the eyes.**
- **The disease follows ingestion of eggs from human feces.**
- **Cysticercosis is diagnosed by CT, MRI, or biopsy. It is treated with praziquantel, albendazole, and/or surgery.**

Taeniasis

- **This form of the disease is caused by the adult *Taenia solium* (pork tapeworm). Intestines are the primary site of infection, where the organism can cause diarrhea. Most of these infections, however, are asymptomatic.**
- **The disease is transmitted by ingestion of larvae in undercooked pork.**
- **Taeniasis is diagnosed by detection of proglottids in the stool. It is treated with niclosamide.**

Taeniasis

- **This form of the disease is caused by the larval form of *Taenia saginata* (beef tapeworm). The organism primarily infects the intestines and does not produce cysticerci. Most infected individuals are asymptomatic.**
- **The disease is transmitted by larvae in undercooked or raw beef.**
- **Taeniasis is diagnosed by detection of proglottids in the stool. It is treated with niclosamide.**

Diphyllobothriasis

- **This disease is caused by *Diphyllobothrium latum* (fish tapeworm). The adult worm in a host's intestine can be as long as 15 meters.**
- **The disease is transmitted by larvae in raw or undercooked fish.**
- **Diphyllobothriasis is diagnosed by detection of characteristic eggs in the stool. It is treated with niclosamide.**

Figure 22.3
Characteristics and therapy for commonly encountered cestode infections. CT = computed tomography; MRI = magnetic resonance imaging.

second intermediate host, the cercariae form cysts called metacercariae that can remain viable indefinitely. Finally, if the infected raw or undercooked fish or crustacean is eaten by a human, the metacercaria excysts (emerges from cysts), and the fluke invades tissues such as the lung or the liver and begins producing eggs, thus completing the life cycle.

B. Sexual flukes (schistosomes)

The life cycle of schistosomes is similar to that of hermaphroditic flukes. One difference is that schistosomes have only one intermediate host, the snail. Another difference is that schistosomiasis is not acquired by ingestion of contaminated food, but rather from schistosome cercariae directly penetrating the skin of waders or swimmers in contaminated rivers and lakes. After dissemination and development in the human host, adult schistosomes take up residence in various abdominal veins, depending on the species and are, therefore, called "blood flukes." Also in contrast to the "typical" hermaph

roditic flukes described above, schistosomes have separate, distinctive sexes. A remarkable anatomic feature is the long groove or schist on the ventral surface of the large male in which the smaller female resides and continuously mates with the male (Figure 22.4).

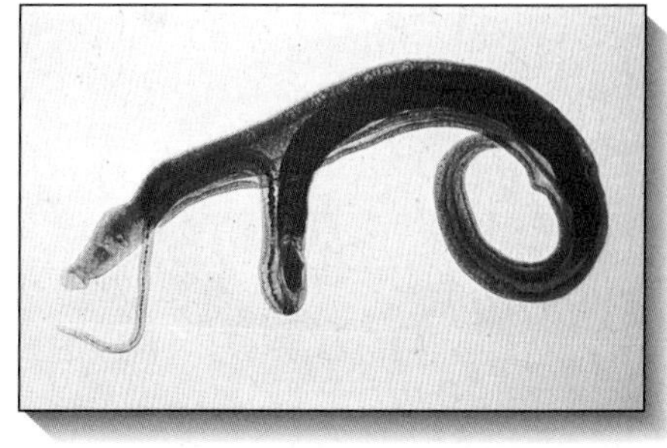

Figure 22.4
Male schistosome has a long groove in which the smaller female resides and continuously mates with the male.

Paragonimiasis

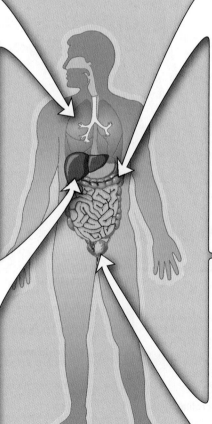

- This disease is caused by *Paragonimus westermani* (lung fluke). The organisms reach the lung by penetrating the duodenum, migrating into the peritoneal cavity and through the diaphragm into the pleural cavities. From there they enter the lungs which are the primary site of damage. The inflammatory response to the adults and eggs in the lungs results in cough that often produces bloody sputum.
- The disease is transmitted by ingestion of encysted larvae in raw or rare crab meat or crayfish.
- Paragonimiasis is diagnosed by identifying eggs in the sputum and stool. It is treated with praziquantel.

Clonorchiasis

- This disease is caused by *Clonorchis sinensis* (Oriental liver fluke). The primary site of infection is the biliary tract, where the resulting inflammatory response can cause fibrosis and hyperplasia.
- The disease is transmitted by eating raw freshwater fish.
- Clonorchiasis is diagnosed by identifying eggs in the stool. It is treated with praziquantel.

Schistosomiasis

- This disease is caused by *Schistosoma mansoni* and *Schistosoma japonicum*. The primary site of infection is the gastrointestinal tract. Damage to the intestinal wall is caused by the host's inflammatory response to eggs deposited at that site. The eggs also secrete proteolytic enzymes that further damage the tissue.
- Clinical presentation includes GI bleeding, diarrhea, and liver damage. Periportal fibrosis leads to portal hypertension and massive splenomegaly.
- The disease is transmitted by direct skin penetration.
- This form of schistosomiasis is diagnosed by identification of characteristic eggs in the stool. It is treated with praziquantel.

Schistosomiasis

- This disease is caused by *Schistosoma haematobium.* The primary sites of infection are veins of the urinary bladder, where the organism's eggs can induce fibrosis, granulomas, and hematuria.
- The disease is transmitted by direct skin penetration.
- This form of schistosomiasis is diagnosed by identifying characteristic eggs in the urine or bladder wall. It is treated with praziquantel.

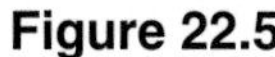

Figure 22.5
Characteristics and therapy for commonly encountered trematode infections.

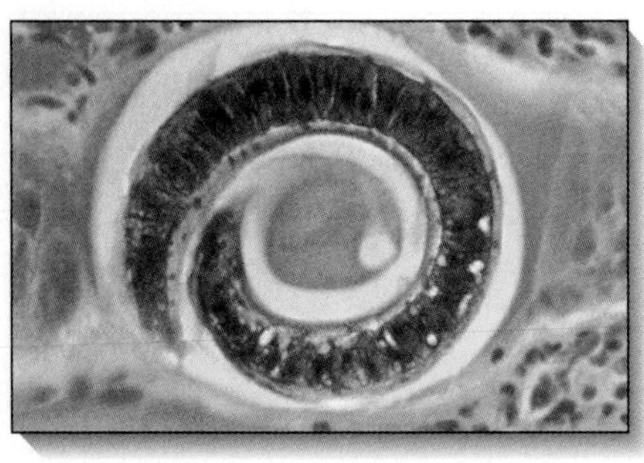

Figure 22.6
Coiled larva of *Trichinella spiralis* in skeletal muscle.

This mating takes place in the human liver. Fertilized eggs penetrate the human host's vascular walls and enter the intestine or bladder, emerging from the body in feces or urine. In fresh water, the organisms infect snails in which they multiply, producing cercariae (the final, free-swimming larval stage), which are released into the fresh water to complete the cycle. Characteristics of clinically important trematodes are summarized in Figure 22.5.

IV. NEMATODES

The nematodes (roundworms) are elongated, nonsegmented worms that are tapered at both ends (Figure 22.6). Unlike other helminths,

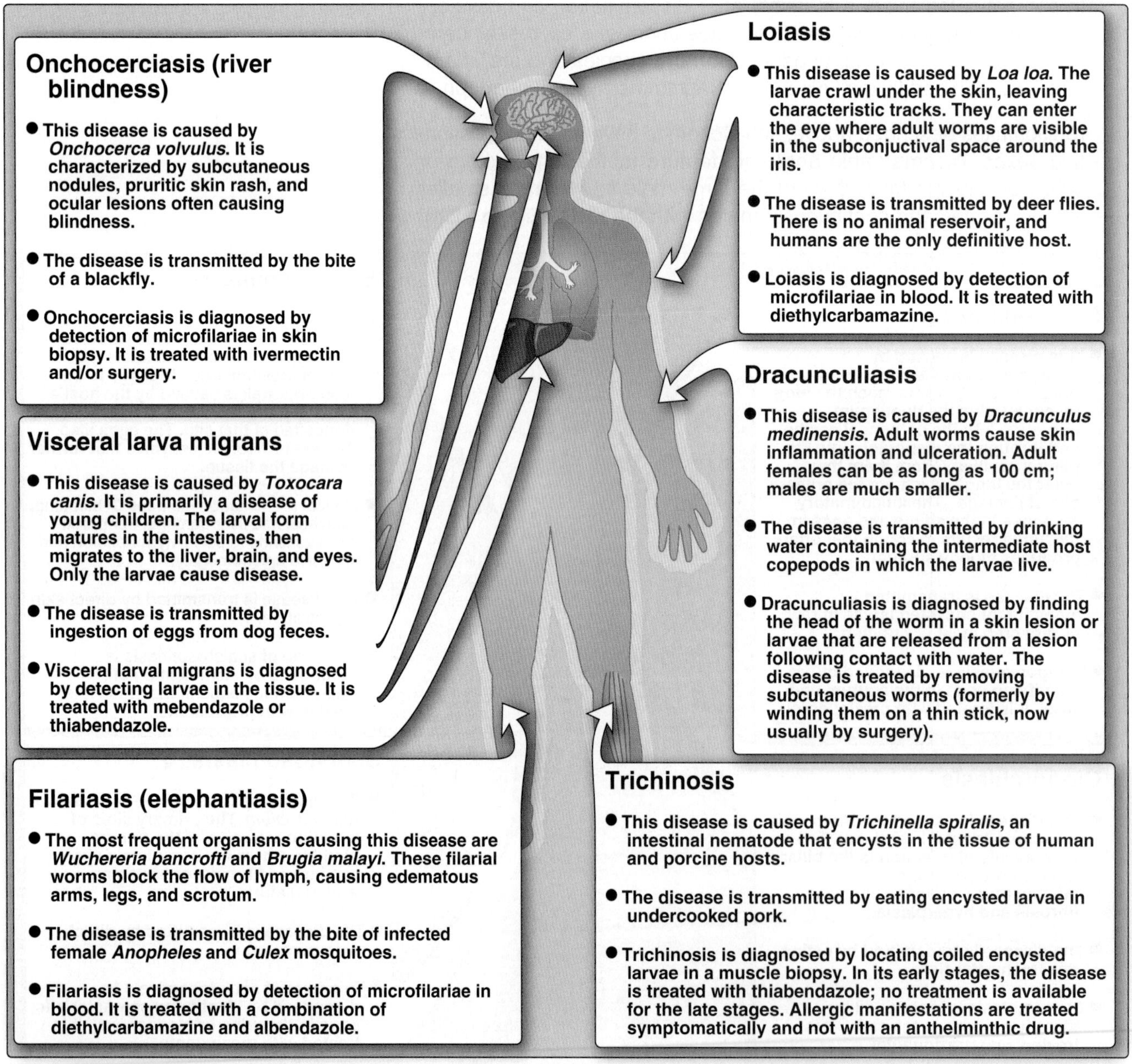

Onchocerciasis (river blindness)

- This disease is caused by *Onchocerca volvulus*. It is characterized by subcutaneous nodules, pruritic skin rash, and ocular lesions often causing blindness.
- The disease is transmitted by the bite of a blackfly.
- Onchocerciasis is diagnosed by detection of microfilariae in skin biopsy. It is treated with ivermectin and/or surgery.

Visceral larva migrans

- This disease is caused by *Toxocara canis*. It is primarily a disease of young children. The larval form matures in the intestines, then migrates to the liver, brain, and eyes. Only the larvae cause disease.
- The disease is transmitted by ingestion of eggs from dog feces.
- Visceral larval migrans is diagnosed by detecting larvae in the tissue. It is treated with mebendazole or thiabendazole.

Filariasis (elephantiasis)

- The most frequent organisms causing this disease are *Wuchereria bancrofti* and *Brugia malayi*. These filarial worms block the flow of lymph, causing edematous arms, legs, and scrotum.
- The disease is transmitted by the bite of infected female *Anopheles* and *Culex* mosquitoes.
- Filariasis is diagnosed by detection of microfilariae in blood. It is treated with a combination of diethylcarbamazine and albendazole.

Loiasis

- This disease is caused by *Loa loa*. The larvae crawl under the skin, leaving characteristic tracks. They can enter the eye where adult worms are visible in the subconjuctival space around the iris.
- The disease is transmitted by deer flies. There is no animal reservoir, and humans are the only definitive host.
- Loiasis is diagnosed by detection of microfilariae in blood. It is treated with diethylcarbamazine.

Dracunculiasis

- This disease is caused by *Dracunculus medinensis*. Adult worms cause skin inflammation and ulceration. Adult females can be as long as 100 cm; males are much smaller.
- The disease is transmitted by drinking water containing the intermediate host copepods in which the larvae live.
- Dracunculiasis is diagnosed by finding the head of the worm in a skin lesion or larvae that are released from a lesion following contact with water. The disease is treated by removing subcutaneous worms (formerly by winding them on a thin stick, now usually by surgery).

Trichinosis

- This disease is caused by *Trichinella spiralis*, an intestinal nematode that encysts in the tissue of human and porcine hosts.
- The disease is transmitted by eating encysted larvae in undercooked pork.
- Trichinosis is diagnosed by locating coiled encysted larvae in a muscle biopsy. In its early stages, the disease is treated with thiabendazole; no treatment is available for the late stages. Allergic manifestations are treated symptomatically and not with an anthelminthic drug.

Figure 22.7
Characteristics and therapy for commonly encountered nematode infections of tissues other than intestine.

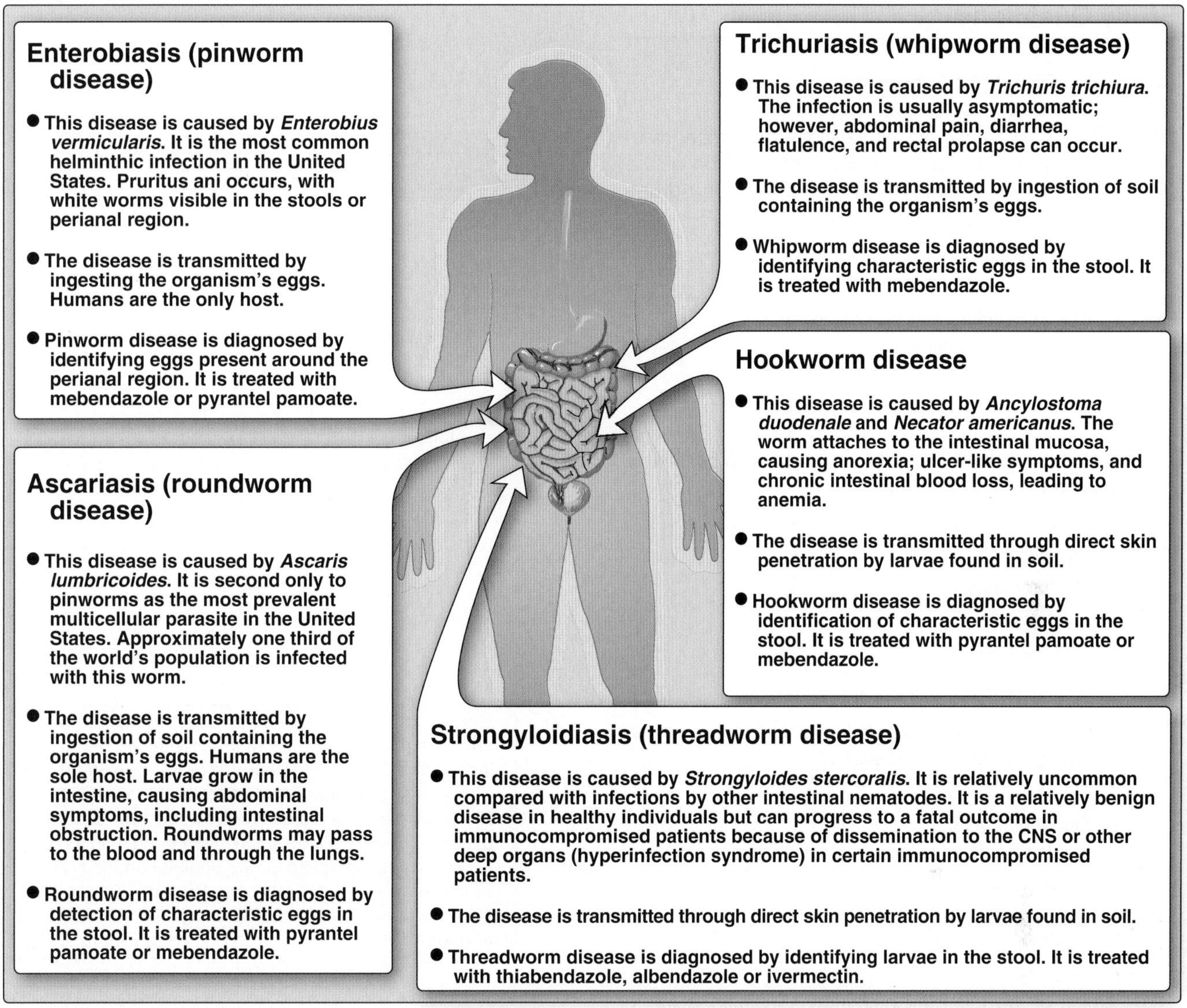

Enterobiasis (pinworm disease)

- This disease is caused by *Enterobius vermicularis.* It is the most common helminthic infection in the United States. Pruritus ani occurs, with white worms visible in the stools or perianal region.
- The disease is transmitted by ingesting the organism's eggs. Humans are the only host.
- Pinworm disease is diagnosed by identifying eggs present around the perianal region. It is treated with mebendazole or pyrantel pamoate.

Ascariasis (roundworm disease)

- This disease is caused by *Ascaris lumbricoides.* It is second only to pinworms as the most prevalent multicellular parasite in the United States. Approximately one third of the world's population is infected with this worm.
- The disease is transmitted by ingestion of soil containing the organism's eggs. Humans are the sole host. Larvae grow in the intestine, causing abdominal symptoms, including intestinal obstruction. Roundworms may pass to the blood and through the lungs.
- Roundworm disease is diagnosed by detection of characteristic eggs in the stool. It is treated with pyrantel pamoate or mebendazole.

Trichuriasis (whipworm disease)

- This disease is caused by *Trichuris trichiura.* The infection is usually asymptomatic; however, abdominal pain, diarrhea, flatulence, and rectal prolapse can occur.
- The disease is transmitted by ingestion of soil containing the organism's eggs.
- Whipworm disease is diagnosed by identifying characteristic eggs in the stool. It is treated with mebendazole.

Hookworm disease

- This disease is caused by *Ancylostoma duodenale* and *Necator americanus.* The worm attaches to the intestinal mucosa, causing anorexia; ulcer-like symptoms, and chronic intestinal blood loss, leading to anemia.
- The disease is transmitted through direct skin penetration by larvae found in soil.
- Hookworm disease is diagnosed by identification of characteristic eggs in the stool. It is treated with pyrantel pamoate or mebendazole.

Strongyloidiasis (threadworm disease)

- This disease is caused by *Strongyloides stercoralis.* It is relatively uncommon compared with infections by other intestinal nematodes. It is a relatively benign disease in healthy individuals but can progress to a fatal outcome in immunocompromised patients because of dissemination to the CNS or other deep organs (hyperinfection syndrome) in certain immunocompromised patients.
- The disease is transmitted through direct skin penetration by larvae found in soil.
- Threadworm disease is diagnosed by identifying larvae in the stool. It is treated with thiabendazole, albendazole or ivermectin.

Figure 22.8
Characteristics and therapy for commonly encountered intestinal nematode infections.

nematodes have a complete digestive system, including a mouth, an intestine that spans most of the body length, and an anus. The body is protected by a tough, noncellular cuticle. Most nematodes have separate, anatomically distinctive sexes. The mode of transmission varies widely, depending on the species, and includes direct skin penetration by infectious larvae, ingestion of contaminated soil, eating undercooked pork, and insect bites. The parasites can invade almost any part of the body: liver, kidneys, intestines, subcutaneous tissue, and eyes. Generally, nematodes are categorized by whether they infect the intestine or other tissues (Figures 22.7 and 22.8). Alternatively, they can be divided into those for which the eggs are infectious and those for which the larvae are infectious. The most common nematode infection in the United States is enterobiasis (pinworm disease), which causes anal itching (Figure 22.9) but otherwise does little damage. A more serious disease of worldwide occurrence is ascariasis, caused by *Ascaris lumbricoides* (see Figure 22.8).

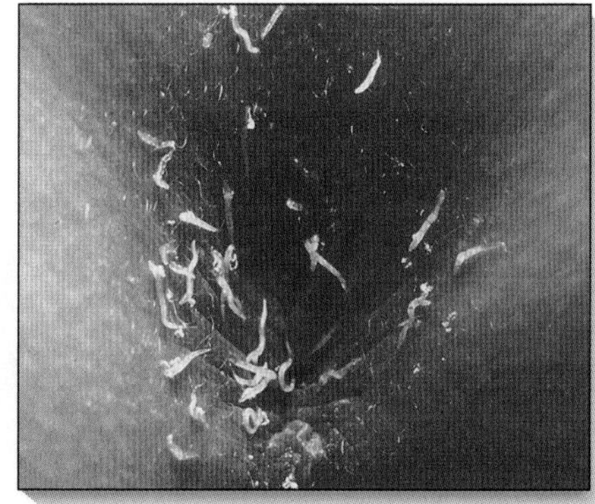

Figure 22.9
Pinworms leaving the anus of a five-year-old child.

Study Questions

Choose the ONE correct answer.

22.1 A patient is diagnosed as having a trematode infection. Lacking a more specific identification of the causative organism, which of the following drugs would most likely be effective?

A. Niclosamide
B. Thiabendazole
C. Praziquantel
D. Diethylcarbamazine
E. Tetracycline

Correct answer = C. Praziquantel is the drug of choice for most trematode infections.

22.2 Which of the following is the most common helminthic infection in the United States?

A. Schistosomiasis
B. Diphyllothriasis
C. Clonorchiasis
D. Trichinosis
E. Enterobiasis

Correct answer = E. Enterobiasis is known as pinworm disease.

22.3 Which of the following helminthic diseases is transmitted by the bite of a mosquito?

A. Filariasis
B. Onchocerciasis
C. Taeniasis
D. Schistosomiasis
E. Visceral larva migrans

Correct answer = A. Mosquitoes ingest filarial embryos (microfilariae) from infected blood. In the insect, the embryos develop into infective filariform larvae that are injected into the human host. Onchocerciasis is transmitted by the bite of the blackfly. Taeniasis is transmitted by ingestion of larvae in undercooked pork. Schistosomiasis is transmitted by direct skin penetration. Visceral larva migrans is transmitted by ingestion of eggs from dog feces.

22.4 Which of the following helminthic diseases is transmitted by direct skin penetration by helminth larvae?

A. Filariasis
B. Onchocerciasis
C. Dracunculiasis
D. Schistosomiasis
E. Visceral larva migrans

Correct answer = D. *Schistosome cercariae* released from snails in fresh water are capable of penetrating human skin. Filariasis is transmitted by mosquitoes. Onchocerciasis is transmitted by the bite of the blackfly. Dracunculiasis is transmitted by drinking water containing the intermediate host copepods in which the larvae live. Visceral larva migrans is transmitted by ingestion of eggs from dog feces.

UNIT IV:
Viruses

Introduction to the Viruses

23

I. OVERVIEW

A virus is an infectious agent that is minimally constructed of two components: 1) a genome consisting of either ribonucleic acid (RNA) or deoxyribonucleic acid (DNA), but not both, and 2) a protein-containing structure (capsid) designed to protect the genome (Figure 23.1A). Many viruses have additional structural features, for example, an envelope composed of a protein-containing lipid bilayer, whose presence or absence further distinguishes one virus group from another (Figure 23.1B). A complete virus particle combining these structural elements is called a virion. In functional terms, a virion can be envisioned as a delivery system that surrounds a nucleic acid payload. The delivery system is designed to protect the genome and enable the virus to bind to host cells. The payload is the viral genome and may also include enzymes required for the initial steps in viral replication—a process that is obligately intracellular. The pathogenicity of a virus depends on a great variety of structural and functional characteristics. Therefore, even within a closely related group of viruses, different species may produce significantly distinct clinical pathologies.

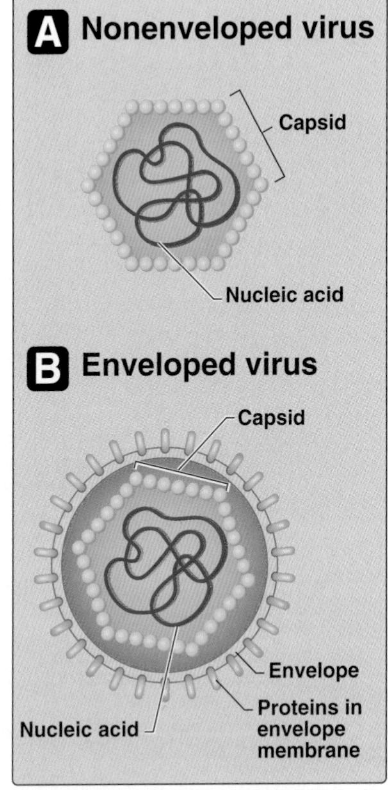

Figure 23.1
General structure: A. nonenveloped; B. enveloped viruses.

II. CHARACTERISTICS USED TO DEFINE VIRUS FAMILIES, GENERA, AND SPECIES

Viruses are divided into related groups, or families, and, sometimes into subfamilies based on: 1) type and structure of the viral nucleic acid, 2) the strategy used in its replication, 3) type of symmetry of the virus capsid (helical versus icosahedral), and 4) presence or absence of a lipid envelope. Within a virus family, differences in additional specific properties, such as host range, serologic reactions, amino acid sequences of

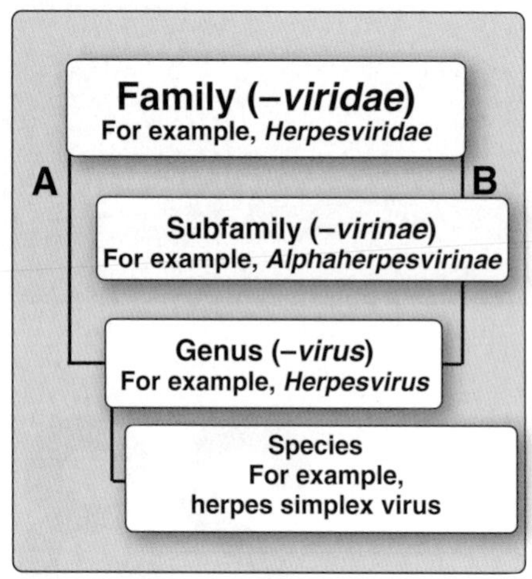

Figure 23.2
Classification of viruses: A. No subfamilies present. B. Subfamilies present.

viral proteins, degree of nucleic acid homology, among others, form the basis for division into genera (singular, genus) and species (Figure 23.2). Species of the same virus isolated from different geographic locations may differ from each other in nucleotide sequence. In this case, they are referred to as strains of the same species.

A. Genome

The type of nucleic acid found in the virus particle is perhaps the most fundamental and straightforward of viral properties. It may be RNA or DNA, either of which may be single stranded (ss) or double stranded (ds). The most common forms of viral genomes found in nature are ssRNA and dsDNA. However, both dsRNA and ssDNA genomes are found in viruses of medical significance (Figure 23.3). Single-stranded viral RNA genomes are further subdivided into those of "positive polarity" (that is, of messenger RNA sense, which can, therefore, be used as a template for protein synthesis) and those of "negative polarity" or are antisense (that is, complementary to messenger RNA sense, which cannot, therefore, be used directly as a template for protein synthesis). Viruses containing these two types of RNA genomes are commonly referred to as positive-strand and negative-strand RNA viruses, respectively.

B. Capsid symmetry

The protein shell enclosing the genome is, for most virus families, found in either of two geometric configurations (see Figure 23.3):

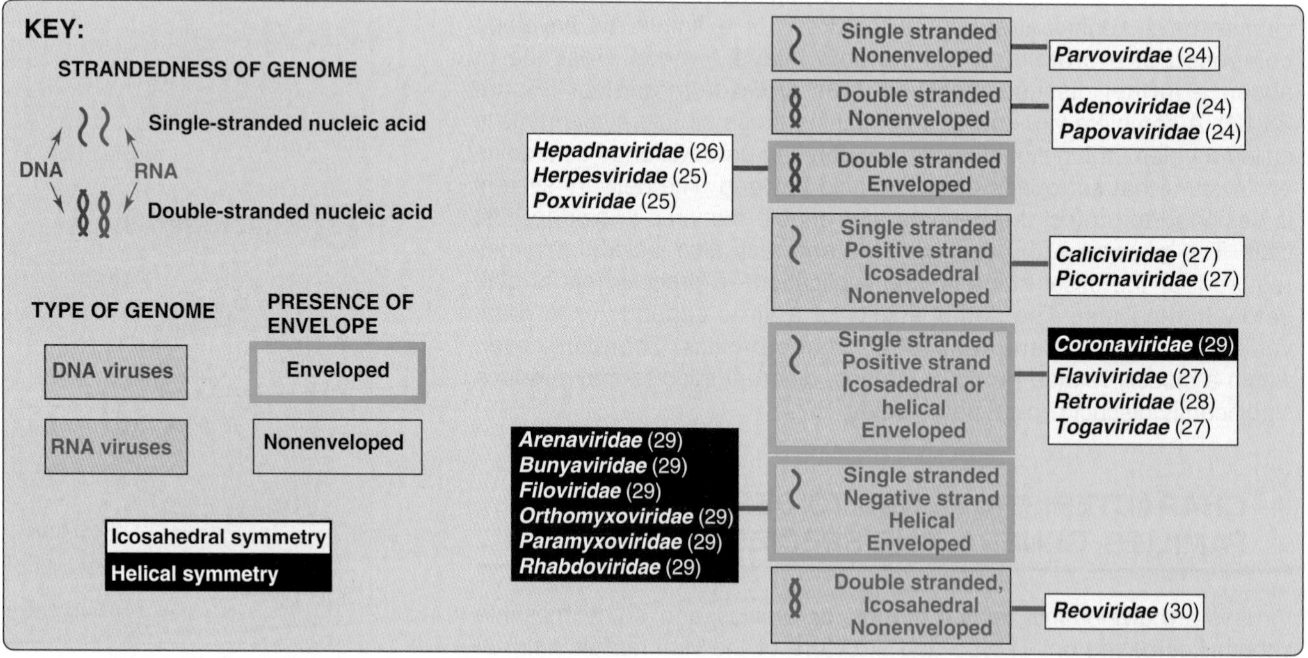

Figure 23.3
Viral families classified according to type of genome, capsid symmetry, and presence or absence of an envelope. RNA is shown in blue, DNA in red, and viral envelope in green. [Note: Numbers indicate chapters where detailed information is presented.]

helical (rod shaped or coiled) or icosahedral (spherical or symmetric). The capsid is constructed of multiple copies of a single polypeptide type (found in helical capsids) or a small number of different polypeptides (found in icosahedral capsids), requiring only a limited amount of genetic information to code for these structural components.

1. **Helical symmetry:** Capsids with helical symmetry, such as the paramyxoviridae (see p. 312), consist of repeated units of a single polypeptide species that—in association with the viral nucleic acid—self-assemble into a helical cylinder (Figure 23.4). Each polypeptide unit (protomer) is hydrogen-bonded to neighboring protomers. The complex of protomers and nucleic acid is called the nucleocapsid. Because the nucleic acid of a virus is surrounded by the capsid, it is protected from environmental damage.

2. **Icosahedral symmetry:** Capsids with icosahedral symmetry are more complex than those with helical symmetry, in that they consist of several different polypeptides grouped into structural subassemblies called capsomers. These, in turn, are hydrogen-bonded to each other to form an icosahedron (Figure 23.5). The nucleic acid genome is located within the empty space created by the rigid, icosahedral structure.

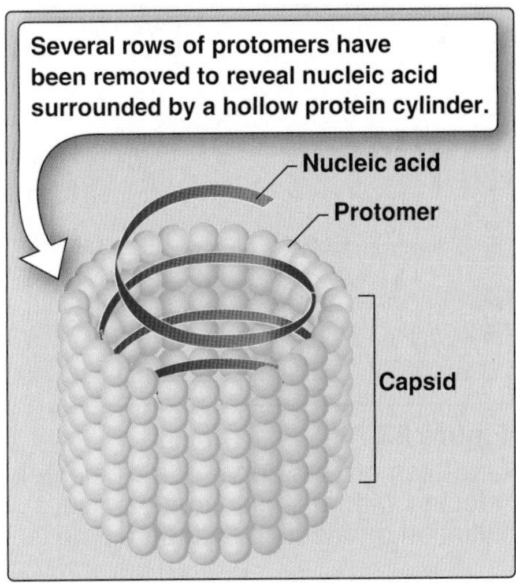

Figure 23.4
Nucleocapsid of a helical virus.

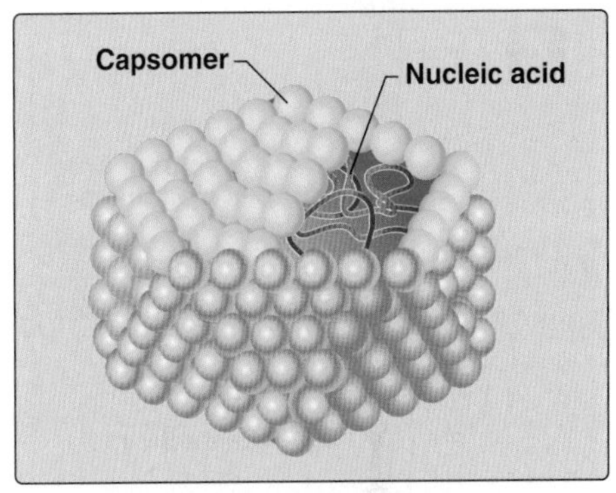

Figure 23.5
Structure of a nonenveloped virus showing icosahedral symmetry.

C. Envelope

An important structural feature used in defining a viral family is the presence or absence of a lipid-containing membrane surrounding the nucleocapsid. This membrane is referred to as the envelope. A virus that is not enveloped is referred to as a naked virus. In enveloped viruses, the nucleocapsid is flexible and coiled within the envelope, resulting in most such viruses appearing to be roughly spherical (Figure 23.6). The envelope is derived from host cell membranes. However, the cellular membrane proteins are replaced by virus-specific proteins, conferring virus-specific antigenicity upon the particle. Among viruses of medical importance, there are both naked and enveloped icosahedral viruses, but all the helical viruses of animals are enveloped and contain RNA.

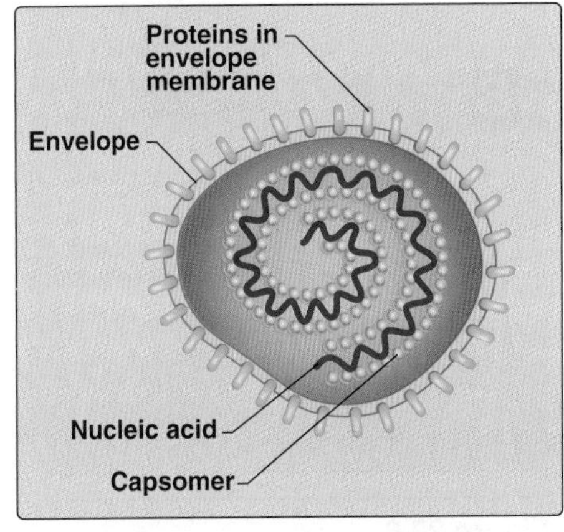

Figure 23.6
Structure of an enveloped helical virus.

III. VIRAL REPLICATION: THE ONE-STEP GROWTH CURVE

The one-step growth curve is a representation of the overall change, with time, in the amount of infectious virus in a single cell that has been infected by a single virus particle. In practice, this is determined by following events in a large population of infected cells in which the infection is proceeding as nearly synchronously as can be achieved by manipulating the experimental conditions. Whereas the time scale and yield of progeny virus vary greatly among virus families, the basic features of the infectious cycle are similar for all viruses. The one-step growth curve begins with the eclipse period, which is followed by a period of exponential growth (Figure 23.7).

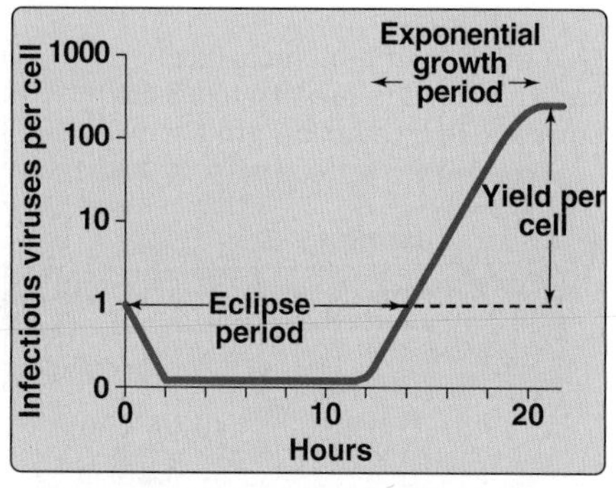

Figure 23.7
One-step growth curve of a single cell infected with a single virus particle. Initiation of infection is at zero time.

A. Eclipse period

Following initial attachment of a virus to the host cell, the ability of that virus to infect other cells disappears. This is the eclipse period, and it represents the time elapsed from initial entry and disassembly of the parental virus to the assembly of the first progeny virion. During this period, active synthesis of virus components is occurring. The eclipse period for most human viruses falls within a range of 1 to 20 hours.

B. Exponential growth

The number of progeny virus produced within the infected cell increases exponentially for a period of time, then reaches a plateau, after which no additional increase in virus yield occurs. The maximum yield per cell is characteristic for each virus-cell system and reflects the balance between the rate at which virus components continue to be synthesized and assembled into virions, and the rate at which the cell loses the synthetic capacity and structural integrity needed to produce new virus particles. This may be from 8 to 72 hours or longer, with yields of 100 to 10,000 virions per cell.

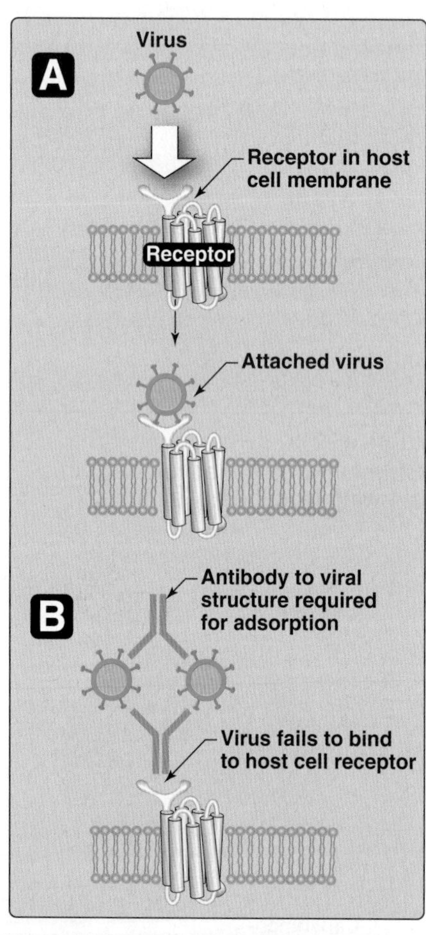

Figure 23.8
A. Attachment of virus to receptor on host cell membrane. B. Antibody prevents adsorption of virus.

IV. STEPS IN THE REPLICATION CYCLES OF VIRUSES

The individual steps in the virus replication cycle are presented below in sequence, beginning with virus attachment to the host cell and leading to penetration and uncoating of the viral genome. Gene expression and replication are followed by assembly and release of viral progeny.

A. Adsorption

The initial attachment of a virus particle to a host cell involves an interaction between specific molecular structures on the virion surface and receptor molecules in the host cell membrane that recognize these viral structures (Figure 23.8A).

1. **Attachment sites on the viral surface:** Some viruses have specialized attachment structures such as the glycoprotein spikes found in viral envelopes (for example, rhabdoviruses, see p. 310), whereas, for others, the unique folding of the capsid proteins forms the attachment sites (for example, picornaviruses, see p 284). In both cases, multiple copies of these molecular attachment structures are distributed around the surface of the virion. [Note: In some cases, the mechanism by which antibodies neutralize viral infectivity is through antibody binding to the viral structures that are required for adsorption (Figure 23.8B).]

2. **Host cell receptor molecules:** The receptor molecules on the host cell membrane are specific for each virus family. Not surprisingly, these receptors have been found to be molecular structures that usually carry out normal cell functions. For example, cellular membrane receptors for compounds such as growth factors may

also inadvertently serve as receptors for a particular virus. Many of the compounds that serve as virus receptors are present only on specifically differentiated cells or are unique for one animal species. Therefore, the presence or absence of host cell receptors is one important determinant of tissue specificity within a susceptible host species and also for the susceptibility or resistance of a species to a given virus. Information about the three-dimensional structure of virus-binding sites is being used to design antiviral drugs that specifically interact with these sites, blocking viral adsorption.

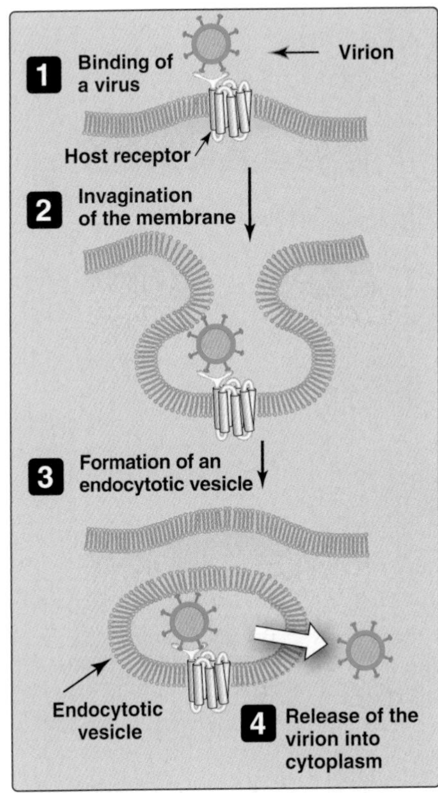

Figure 23.9
Receptor-mediated endocytosis of virus particle.

B. Penetration

Penetration is the passage of the virion from the surface of the cell across the cell membrane and into the cytoplasm. There are two principal mechanisms by which viruses enter animal cells: receptor-mediated endocytosis and direct membrane fusion.

1. **Receptor-mediated endocytosis:** This is basically the same process by which the cell internalizes compounds, such as growth regulatory molecules and serum lipoproteins, except that the infecting virus particle is bound to the host cell surface receptor in place of the normal ligand (Figure 23.9). The cell membrane invaginates, enclosing the virion in an endocytotic vesicle (endosome). Release of the virion into the cytoplasm occurs by various routes, depending on the virus, but, in general, it is facilitated by one or more viral molecules. In the case of an enveloped virus, its membrane may fuse with the membrane of the endosome, resulting in the release of the nucleocapsid into the cytoplasm. Failure to exit the endosome before fusion with a lysosome generally results in degradation of the virion by lysosomal enzymes. Therefore, not all potentially infectious particles are successful in establishing infection.

2. **Membrane fusion:** Some enveloped viruses (for example, human immunodeficiency virus, see p. 297) enter a host cell by fusion of their envelope with the plasma membrane of the cell (Figure 23.10). One or more of the glycoproteins in the envelope of these viruses promotes the fusion. The end result of this process is that the nucleocapsid is free in the cytoplasm, whereas the viral membrane remains associated with the plasma membrane of the host cell.

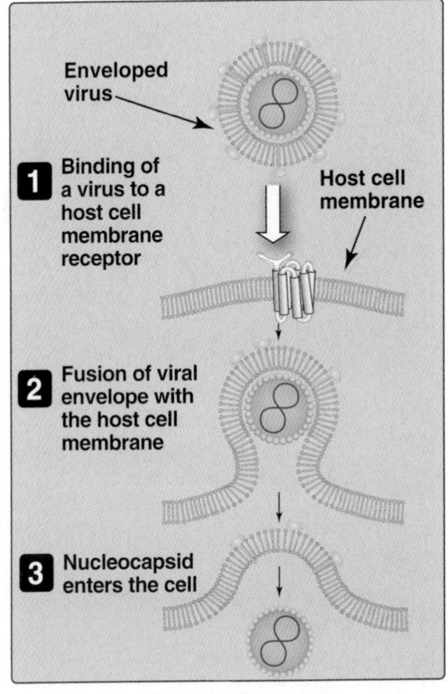

Figure 23.10
Fusion of viral envelope with membrane of host cell.

C. Uncoating

"Uncoating" refers to the stepwise process of disassembly of the virion that enables the expression of the viral genes that carry out replication. For enveloped viruses, the penetration process itself is the first step in uncoating. In general, most steps of the uncoating process occur within the cell and depend on cellular enzymes. However, in some of the more complex viruses, newly synthesized viral proteins are required to complete the process. The loss of one or more structural components of the virion during uncoating predictably leads to a loss of the ability of that particle to infect other cells, which is the basis for the eclipse period of the growth curve (see Figure 23.7). It is during this phase in the replication cycle that viral gene expression begins.

D. Mechanisms of DNA virus genome replication

Each virus family differs in significant ways from all others in terms of the details of the macromolecular events comprising the replication cycle. The wide range of viral genome sizes gives rise to great differences in the number of proteins for which the virus can code. In general, the smaller the viral genome, the more the virus must depend on the host cell to provide the functions needed for viral replication. For example, some small DNA viruses, such as Polyomaviruses (see p. 249), produce only one or two replication-related gene products, which function to divert host cell processes to those of viral replication. Other larger DNA viruses, such as poxviruses (see p. 270), provide virtually all enzymatic and regulatory molecules needed for a complete replication cycle. Most DNA

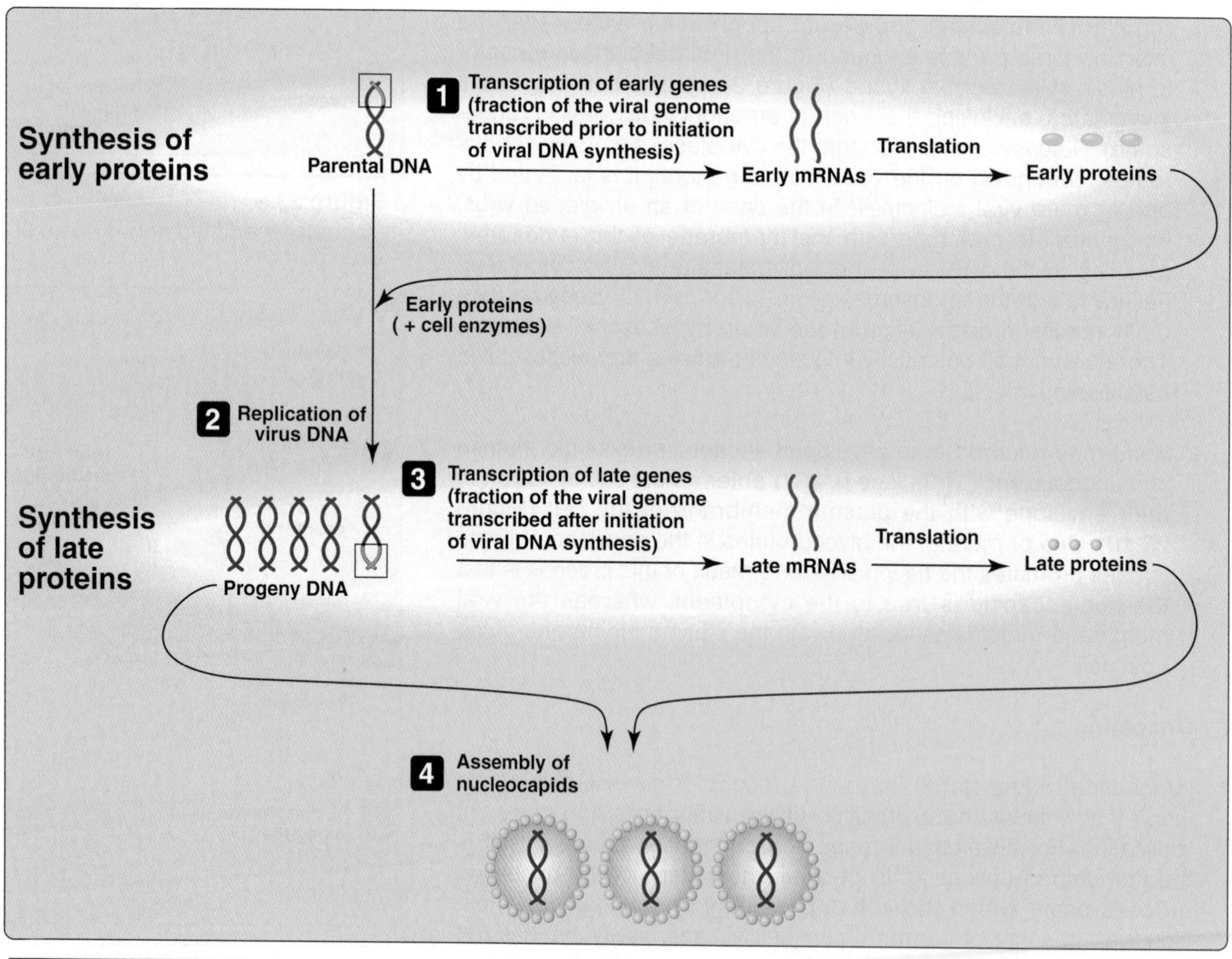

Figure 23.11
Replication of DNA viruses.

viruses assemble in the nucleus, whereas most RNA viruses develop solely in the cytoplasm. Figure 23.11 outlines the essential features of gene expression and replication of DNA viruses.

E. Mechanisms of RNA virus genome replication

Viruses with RNA genomes must overcome two specific problems that arise from the need to replicate the viral genome and to produce a number of viral proteins in eukaryotic host cells. First, there is no host cell RNA polymerase that can use the viral parental RNA as a template for synthesis of complementary RNA strands. Second, translation of eukaryotic mRNAs begins at only a single initiation site, and they are, therefore, translated into only a single polypeptide. However, RNA viruses, which frequently contain only a single molecule of RNA, must express the genetic information for at least two proteins: an RNA-dependent RNA polymerase and a minimum of one type of capsid protein. Although the replication of each RNA virus family has unique features, the mechanisms evolved to surmount these restrictions can be grouped into four broad patterns (or "types") of replication.

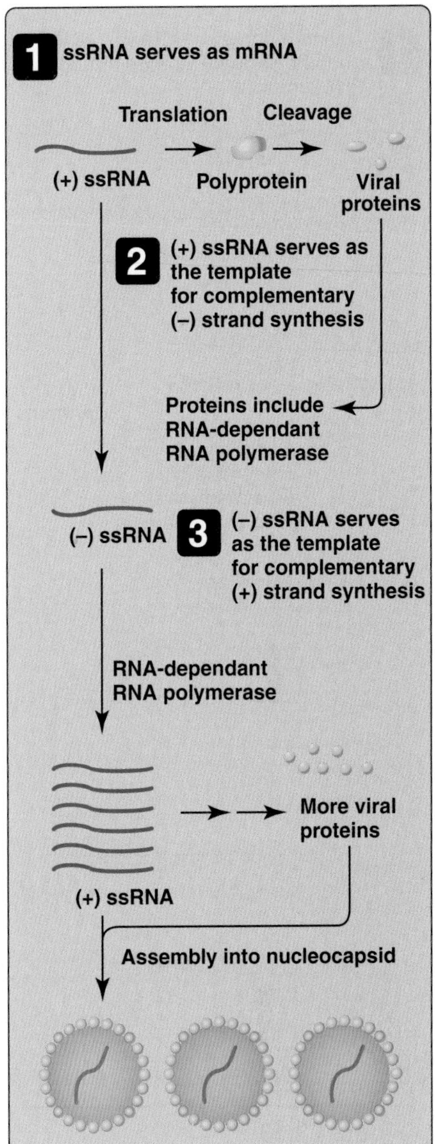

Figure 23.12
Type I virus with a ssRNA genome of (+) polarity replicates via a complementary (–) strand intermediate.

1. **Type I—RNA viruses with a single-stranded genome (ssRNA) of (+) polarity that replicates via a complementary (–) strand intermediate:** In Type I viral replication, the infecting parental RNA molecule serves both as mRNA and, later, as a template for synthesis of the complementary (–) strand (Figure 23.12).

   a. **Role of (+) ssRNA as mRNA:** Because the parental RNA genome is of (+), or messenger, polarity, it can be translated directly upon uncoating and associating with cellular ribosomes. The product is usually a single polyprotein from which individual polypeptides, such as RNA-dependent RNA polymerase and various proteins of the virion, are cleaved by a series of proteolytic processing events carried out by a protease domain of the polyprotein (see Figure 23.12).

   b. **Role of (+) ssRNA as the template for complementary (–) strand synthesis:** The viral (+) ssRNA functions early in infection, not only as mRNA for translation of polyproteins but also as a template for virus-encoded RNA-dependent RNA polymerase to synthesize complementary (–) ssRNA (see Figure 23.12). The progeny (–) strands, in turn, serve as templates for synthesis of progeny (+) strands, which can serve as additional mRNAs, amplifying the capacity to produce virion proteins for progeny virus. When a sufficient quantity of capsid proteins has accumulated later in the infection, progeny (+) ssRNAs begin to be assembled into newly formed nucleocapsids.

2. **Type II—viruses with a ssRNA genome of (–) polarity that replicate via a complementary (+) strand intermediate:** Viral genomes with (–) polarity, similar to the (+) strand genomes, also have two functions: 1) to provide information for protein synthesis and 2) to serve as templates for replication. Unlike (+) strand genomes,

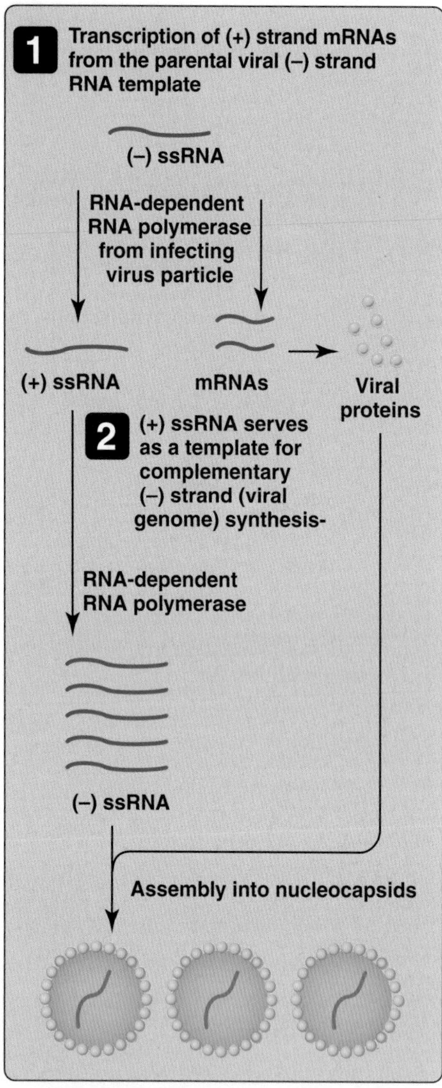

Figure 23.13
Type II virus with an ssRNA genome of (–) polarity that replicates via a complementary (+) strand intermediate.

however, the (–) strand genomes cannot accomplish these goals without prior construction of a complementary (+) strand intermediate (Figure 23.13).

a. **Mechanism of replication of viral ssRNA with (–) polarity:** The replication problems for these viruses are twofold. First, the (–) strand genome cannot be translated, and, therefore, the required viral RNA polymerase cannot be synthesized immediately following infection. Second, the host cell has no enzyme capable of transcribing the (–) strand RNA genome into (+) strand RNAs capable of being translated. The solution to these problems is for the infecting virus particle to contain viral RNA-dependent RNA polymerase and to bring this enzyme into the host cell along with the viral genome. As a consequence, the first synthetic event after infection is generation of (+) strand mRNAs from the parental viral (–) strand RNA template.

b. **Mechanisms for multiple viral protein synthesis in Type II viruses:** The synthesis of multiple proteins is achieved in one of two ways among the (–) strand virus families: 1) The viral genome may be transcribed into a number of individual mRNAs, each specifying a single, polypeptide. 2) Alternatively, the (–) strand viral genome may be segmented (that is, composed of a number of different RNA molecules, most of which code for a single polypeptide).

c. **Production of infectious virus particles:** Although the details differ, the flow of information in both segmented and unsegmented genome viruses is basically the same. In the Type II replication scheme, an important control point is the shift from synthesis of (+) strand mRNA to progeny (–) strand RNA molecules that can be packaged in the virions. This shift is not a result of activity of a different polymerase, but rather a result of interaction of (+) strand RNA molecules with one or more newly synthesized proteins. This enhances the availability of the (+) strands as templates for the synthesis of genomic (–) strands.

3. **Type III—viruses with a dsRNA genome:** The dsRNA genome is segmented, with each segment coding for one polypeptide (Figure 23.14). However, eukaryotic cells do not have an enzyme capable of transcribing dsRNA. Type III viral mRNA transcripts are, therefore, produced by virus-coded, RNA-dependent RNA polymerase (transcriptase) located in a subviral core particle. This particle consists of the dsRNA genome and associated virion proteins, including the transcriptase. The mechanism of replication of the dsRNA is unique, in that the (+) RNA transcripts are not only used for translation but also as templates for complementary (–) strand synthesis, resulting in the formation of dsRNA progeny.

4. **Type IV—viruses with a genome of ssRNA of (+) polarity that is replicated via a DNA intermediate:** The conversion of a (+) strand RNA to a double-stranded DNA is accomplished by an RNA-dependent DNA polymerase, commonly referred to as a "reverse transcriptase," that is contained in the virion. The resulting dsDNA becomes integrated into the cell genome by the action of a viral "integrase." Viral mRNAs and progeny (+) strand RNA genomes are transcribed from this integrated DNA by the host cell RNA polymerase (Figure 23.15).

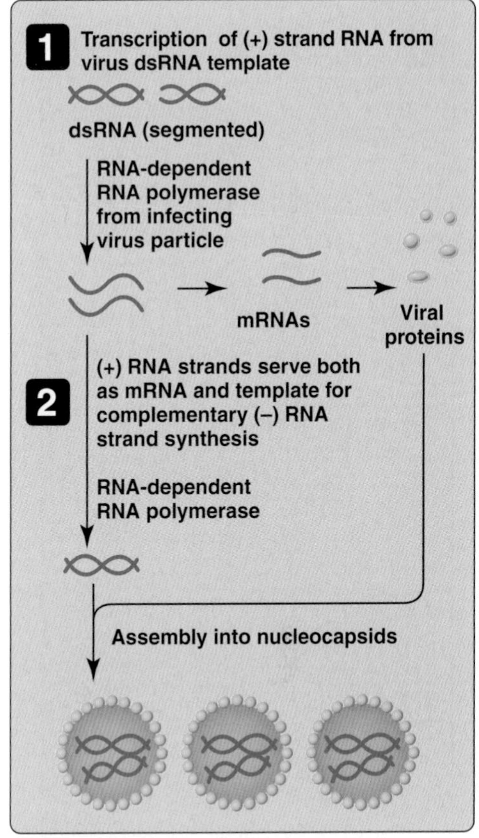

Figure 23.14
Type III virus with a dsRNA genome.

F. Assembly and release of progeny viruses

Assembly of nucleocapsids generally takes place in the host cell compartment where the viral nucleic acid replication occurs (that is, in the cytoplasm for most RNA viruses and in the nucleus for most DNA viruses). For DNA viruses, this requires that capsid proteins be transported from their site of synthesis (cytoplasm) to the nucleus. The various capsid components begin to self-assemble, eventually associating with the nucleic acid to complete the nucleocapsid.

1. **Naked viruses:** In naked (unenveloped) viruses, the virion is complete at this point. Release of progeny is usually a passive event resulting from the disintegration of the dying cell and, therefore, may be at a relatively late time after infection.

2. **Enveloped viruses:** In enveloped viruses, virus-specific glycoproteins are synthesized and transported to the host cell membrane

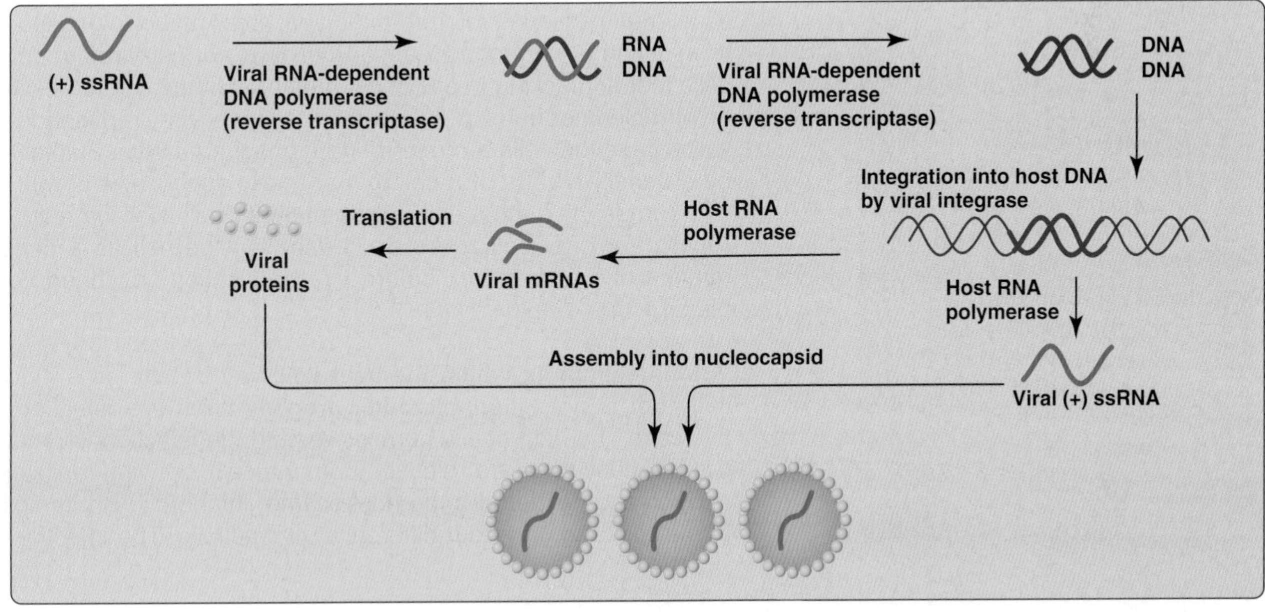

Figure 23.15
Type IV virus with a ssRNA genome of (+) polarity that replicates via a DNA intermediate.

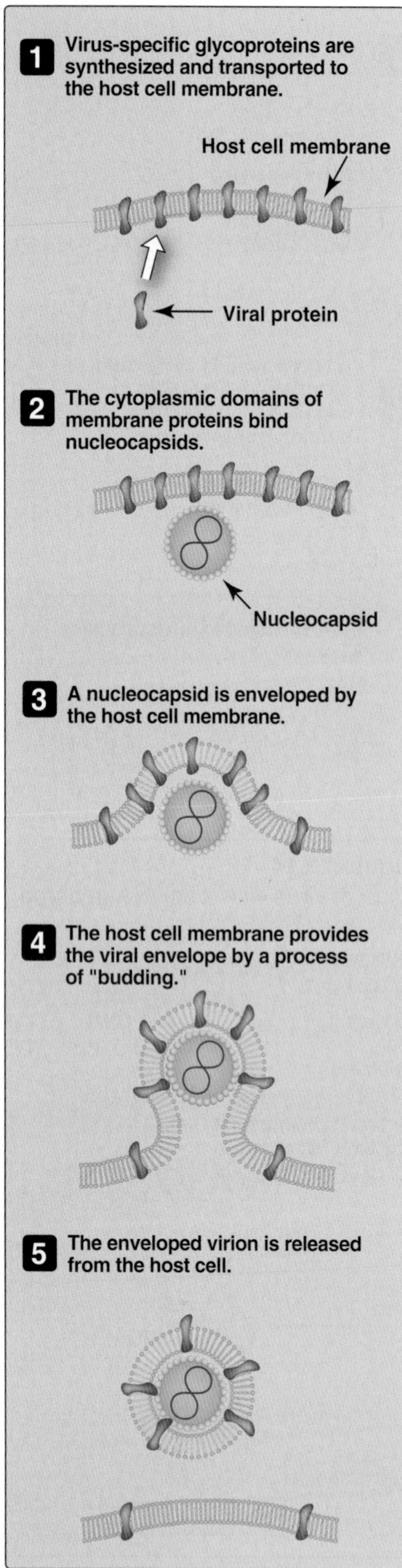

1 Virus-specific glycoproteins are synthesized and transported to the host cell membrane.
Host cell membrane
Viral protein
2 The cytoplasmic domains of membrane proteins bind nucleocapsids.
Nucleocapsid
3 A nucleocapsid is enveloped by the host cell membrane.
4 The host cell membrane provides the viral envelope by a process of "budding."
5 The enveloped virion is released from the host cell.

Figure 23.16
Release of enveloped virus from a host cell by the process of "budding."

in the same manner as cellular membrane proteins.[1] When inserted into the membrane, they displace the cellular glycoproteins, resulting in patches on the cell surface that have viral antigenic specificity. The cytoplasmic domains of these proteins associate specifically with one or more additional viral proteins (matrix proteins) to which the nucleocapsids bind. Final maturation then involves envelopment of the nucleocapsid by a process of "budding" (Figure 23.16). A consequence of this mechanism of viral replication is that progeny virus are released continuously while replication is proceeding within the cell and ends when the cell loses its ability to maintain the integrity of the plasma membrane. A second consequence is that, with most enveloped viruses, all infectious progeny are extracellular. The exceptions are those viruses that acquire their envelopes by budding through internal cell membranes such as those of the endoplasmic reticulum or nucleus. Viruses containing lipid envelopes are sensitive to damage by harsh environments and, therefore, tend to be transmitted by the respiratory, parenteral, and sexual routes. Nonenveloped viruses are more stable to hostile environmental conditions and often transmitted by the fecal–oral route.

G. Effects of viral infection on the host cell

The response of a host cell to infection by a virus ranges from: 1) little or no detectable effect; to 2) alteration of the antigenic specificity of the cell surface due to presence of virus glycoproteins; to 3) latent infections that, in some cases, cause cell transformation; or, ultimately, to 4) cell death due to expression of viral genes that shut off essential host cell functions (Figure 23.17).

1. **Viral infections in which no progeny virus are produced:** In this case, the infection is referred to as abortive. An abortive response to infection is commonly caused by: 1) a normal virus infecting cells that are lacking in enzymes, promoters, transcription factors, or other compounds required for complete viral replication, in which case the cells are referred to as nonpermissive; 2) infection by a defective virus of a cell that normally supports viral replication (that is, by a virus that itself has genetically lost the ability to replicate in that cell type); or 3) death of the cell as a consequence of the infection, before viral replication has been completed.

2. **Viral infections in which the host cell may be altered antigenically but is not killed, although progeny virus are released:** In this case, the host cell is permissive, and the infection is productive (progeny virus are released from the cell), but viral replication and release neither kills the host cell nor interferes with its ability to multiply and carry out differentiated functions. The infection is,

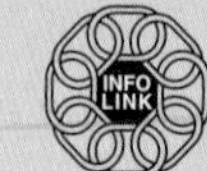

[1]See Chapter 14 in ***Lippincott's Illustrated Reviews: Biochemistry*** for a discussion of the mechanism of insertion of glycoproteins into cell membranes.

therefore, said to be persistent. The antigenic specificity of the cell surface may be altered as a result of the insertion of viral glycoproteins.

3. **Viral infections that result in a latent viral state in the host cell:** Some viral infections result in the persistence of the viral genome inside a host cell with no production of progeny virus. Such latent viruses can be reactivated months or years in the future, leading to a productive infection. Some latently infected cells contain viral genomes that are stably integrated into a host cell chromosome. This can cause alterations in the host cell surface; cellular metabolic functions; and, significantly, cell growth and replication patterns. Such viruses may induce tumors in animals, in which case they are said to be tumor viruses, and the cells they infect are transformed.

4. **Viral infections resulting in host cell death and production of progeny virus:** Eliminating host cell competition for synthetic enzymes and precursor molecules increases the efficiency with which virus constituents can be synthesized. Therefore, the typical result of a productive (progeny-yielding) infection by a cytocidal virus is the shutoff of much of the cell's macromolecular syntheses by one or more of the virus gene products, causing the death of the cell. Such an infection is said to be lytic. The mechanism of the shutoff varies among the viral families.

In summary, all viruses:

- are small;
- contain only one species of nucleic acid, either DNA or RNA;
- attach to their host cell with a specific receptor-binding protein; and
- express the information contained in the viral genome (DNA or RNA) using the cellular machinery of the host cell

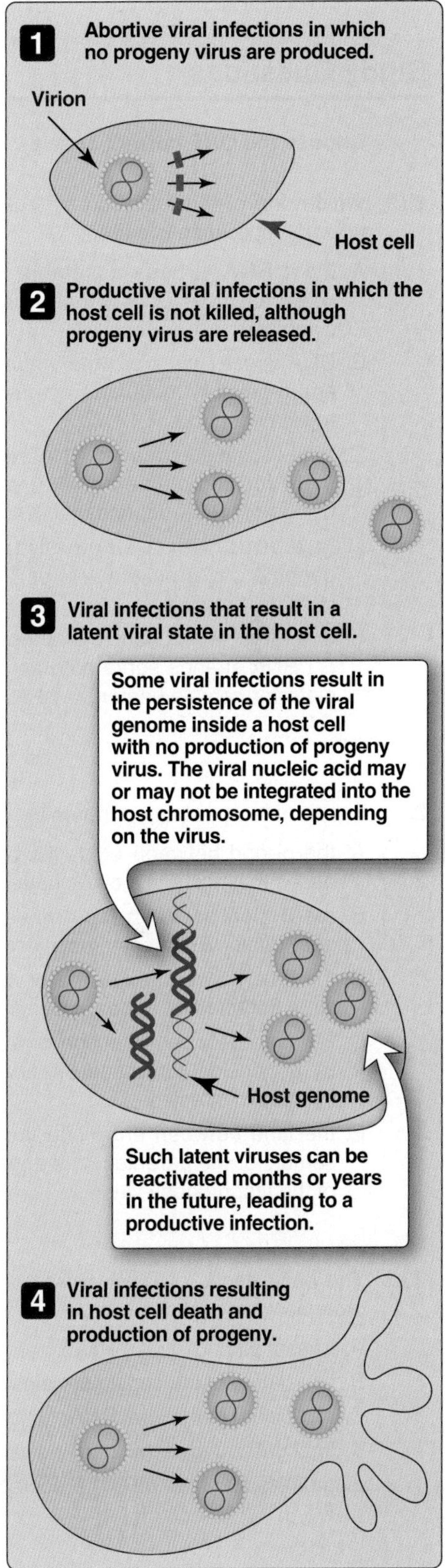

Figure 23.17
Effects of viral infection on a host cell.

Study Questions

Choose the ONE correct answer.

23.1 Which one of the following statements concerning the viral replication is correct?

A. Most RNA viruses assemble in the nucleus, whereas most DNA viruses develop solely in cytoplasm.

B. DNA viruses must provide virtually all enzymatic and regulatory molecules needed for a complete replication cycle.

C. Viral (+) single-stranded RNA serves as the template for complementary (–) strand synthesis using host RNA-dependant RNA polymerase.

D. In a virus with a single-stranded (ss) RNA genome of (–) polarity, (–) ssRNA is translated into viral proteins.

E. In a virus with a double-stranded RNA genome, (+) RNA strands serve both as mRNA and template for complementary (–) RNA strand synthesis.

Correct answer = E. The dual role for (+) RNA strands allows both the synthesis of double-stranded RNA and capsid proteins. Most DNA viruses assemble in the nucleus, whereas most RNA viruses develop solely in cytoplasm. Some DNA viruses may provide only one or two replication-related gene products which function to divert host cell processes to those of viral replication. (–) RNA cannot serve as mRNA. (+) Single-stranded RNA serves as the template for complementary (–) strand synthesis using viral (not host) RNA-dependant RNA polymerase.

23.2 The term "eclipse period" refers to:

A. the period between epidemic outbreaks of diseases that occur in a cyclic pattern.

B. the period between recurrences of disease in individuals with latent virus infections.

C. the time between exposure of an individual to a virus and the first appearance of disease.

D. the time between infection of a susceptible cell by a cytocidal virus and the first appearance of cytopathic effects.

E. the time between entry into the cell and disassembly of the parental virus and the appearance of the first progeny virion.

Correct answer = E. Following initial attachment of a virus to the host cell, the ability of that virus to infect other cells disappears. This is the eclipse period. During this period, active synthesis of virus components is occurring. The time between exposure of an individual to a virus and the first appearance of disease is referred to as the incubation period (choice C). There is no specific term applied to the time periods described by A, B, and D.

23.3 The early genes of DNA viruses code primarily for proteins whose functions are required for:

A. transcription of viral mRNA.

B. translation of the capsid proteins.

C. replication of the viral DNA.

D. final uncoating of the infecting virions.

E. processing of the mRNA precursors

Correct answer = C. Depending on the virus family, this may consist of a DNA polymerase and other enzymes directly involved in DNA replication or, alternatively, may be a product that stimulates the cell to produce all of the enzymes and precursors needed for DNA synthesis. Transcription, for the most part, is carried out by cellular RNA polymerase. Similarly, translation is done with the cell's translation system. The poxviruses do code for proteins that are involved in completion of uncoating, but this is an exception. mRNA processing is accomplished by cell enzymes.

Nonenveloped DNA Viruses

24

I. OVERVIEW

The DNA viruses discussed in this chapter—*Papovaviridae*, *Adenoviridae*, and *Parvoviridae* (Figure 24.1)—share the properties of lacking an envelope and having relatively simple structures and genome organization. However, the diseases commonly associated with these viruses and their mechanisms of pathogenesis are quite different, ranging from upper respiratory infections to tumors.

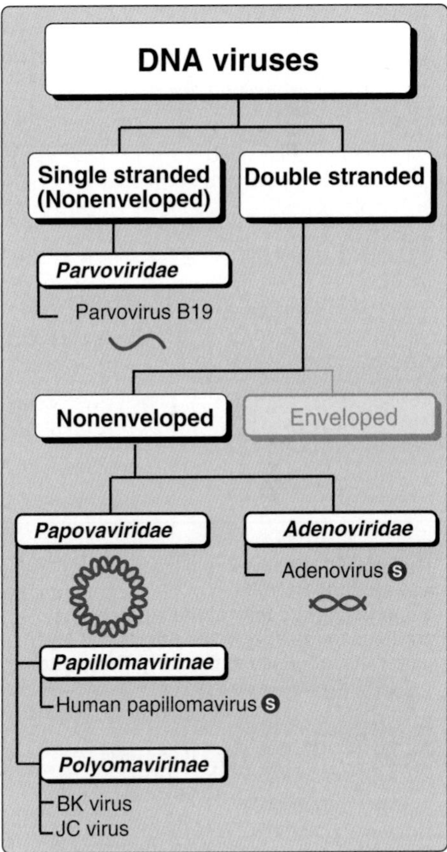

Figure 24.1
Classification of non-enveloped DNA viruses. See pp. 354, 361 for summaries of these viruses.
= Single-stranded, linear DNA
= Double-stranded, linear DNA
= Double-stranded, circular DNA

II. INTRODUCTION TO THE PAPOVAVIRDAE

Papovaviruses are nonenveloped (naked); have icosahedral nucleocapsids; and contain supercoiled, double-stranded, circular DNA. However, basic differences in genome complexity and regulation of gene expression led to division of this family into two subfamilies: the Papillomavirinae and the Polyomavirinae. Papovaviruses induce both lytic infections and either benign or malignant tumors, depending on infected cell type.

III. PAPOVAVIRIDAE: SUBFAMILY PAPILLOMAVIRINAE

All papillomaviruses induce hyperplastic epithelial lesions in their host species. Over 150 types of human papillomaviruses (HPVs) are now recognized, based on differences in the DNA sequences of certain well-characterized virus genes. HPVs exhibit great tissue and cell specificity, infecting only surface epithelia of skin and mucous membranes. The HPVs within each of these tissue-specific groups have varying potential for causing malignancies. For example, there are: 1) a small number of virus types (specifically, types 16 and 18) that produce lesions with a high risk of progression to malignancy such as in cervical carcinoma; 2) other virus types produce mucosal lesions that progress to malignancy with lower frequency, causing, for example, anogenital warts (condyloma acuminata, a common sexually transmitted disease) and laryngeal papillomas (the most common benign epithelial tumors of the larynx); and 3) still other virus types that are associated only with benign lesions (for example, common, flat, and plantar warts).

A. Epidemiology

Transmission of HPV infection requires direct contact with infected individuals (for example, sexual contact) or with contaminated surfaces (fomites) such as communal bathroom floors. HPV can also be transmitted from mother to infant during passage down the birth canal. Because the initial phase, as well as the maintenance of infection, occurs in cells of the basal layer of the skin, access to these cells is presumably via epithelial surface lesions such as abrasions.

B. Pathogenesis

The most striking characteristics of HPV multiplication and pathogenesis are its specificity for epithelial cells and its dependence on the differentiation state of the epithelial host cell.

1. **Wart formation:** The development of a typical wart results from cell multiplication and delayed differentiation induced by certain papillomavirus early proteins. In cutaneous tissues, for example, infected cells leave the basal layer and migrate toward the surface of the skin. The virus replication cycle proceeds in parallel with the steps of keratinocyte differentiation, which end with the terminally differentiated cornified layer of the growing wart. An important function of two early viral proteins is the activation of host cells, causing them to divide. This activation involves interaction between these viral proteins and cellular proteins (antioncoproteins) that normally function to regulate the cell cycle. Two of these antioncogenic cellular proteins are p53 (cellular growth suppressor protein) and pRb (retinoblastoma gene product). The viral genome is maintained in low copy numbers as an autonomously replicating episome in the nuclei of multiplying basal cells. Expression of only one early gene appears to be required for maintaining this balance between episome persistence and basal cell division. (See Figure 24.2 for a summary of papillomavirus replication and wart formation.)

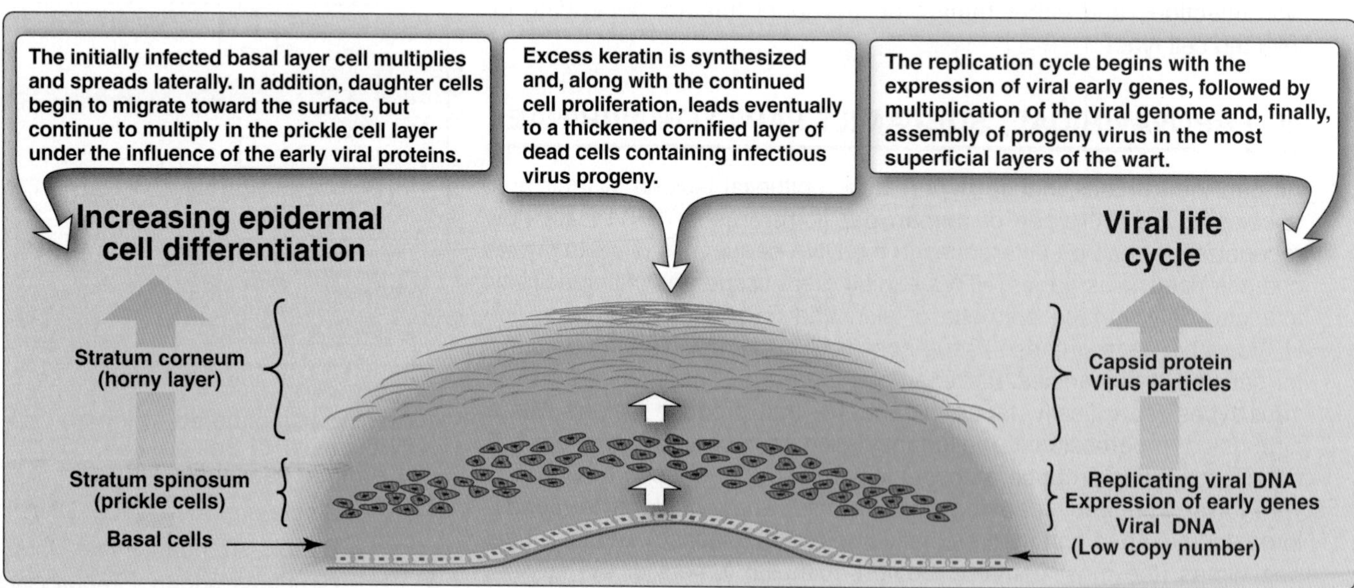

Figure 24.2
Relationship between steps in the development of a skin wart and the life cycle of papilloma virus.

2. **Development of malignancies:** Progression to malignancy occurs primarily in warts located on mucosal surfaces, particularly those of the genital tract, and is associated with a limited number of papillomavirus types. The affinity of binding between virus early proteins and cellular antioncoproteins p53 and pRb (which inactivate these cellular regulatory proteins) correlates with a high risk for malignant progression. However, it is clear that this interaction is only the first step in a multistep process involving alterations in expression of other cell oncoproteins and antioncoproteins and including, at some point, the non–site-specific integration of part of the viral genome into a host cell chromosome.

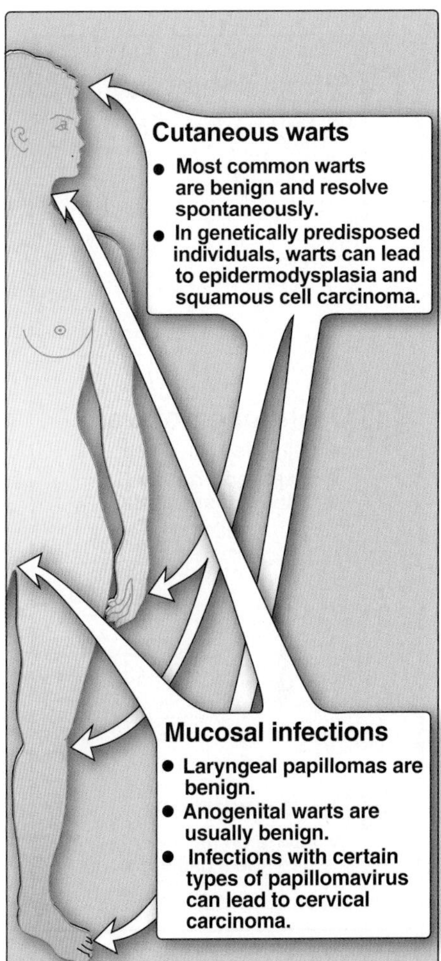

Cutaneous warts
• Most common warts are benign and resolve spontaneously.
• In genetically predisposed individuals, warts can lead to epidermodysplasia and squamous cell carcinoma.
Mucosal infections
• Laryngeal papillomas are benign.
• Anogenital warts are usually benign.
• Infections with certain types of papillomavirus can lead to cervical carcinoma.

Figure 24.3
Location and properties of papilloma infections.

C. Clinical significance

HPVs cause diseases that cover the spectrum from simple warts to malignancies. Warts can occur on any part of the body, including both cutaneous and mucosal surfaces (Figure 24.3). Specific HPV types tend to be associated with specific wart morphology, although a wart's morphologic type is also related to its location (Figure 24.4).

1. **Cutaneous warts (primarily caused by types 1 through 4):** These warts may be classified as common (fingers and hands), plantar (sole of foot), or flat (arms, face, and knee). Another category of cutaneous lesion occurs in patients with what appears to be an inherited predisposition for multiple warts that do not regress but, instead, spread to many body sites (epidermodysplasia verruciformis). Of particular interest is that these lesions frequently give rise to squamous cell carcinomas several years after initial appearance of the original warts, especially in areas of skin exposed to sunlight.

2. **Oral infections (caused by types 13 and 32):** Oral and nasopharyngeal mucosal surfaces can be infected by some HPV types. Most of these infections result in benign papillomas.

3. **Genital tract infections:** Approximately 30 different types of HPV can infect the genital tract, but types 6 and 11 cause 90 percent of genital papillomas. All of the genital tract HPV infections are acquired via sexual contact. HPV types 6 and 11 can also be spread to the oral mucosa via sexual contact. HPV infections caused by these virus types produce anogenital warts (condyloma acuminata), which are occasionally large (but usually

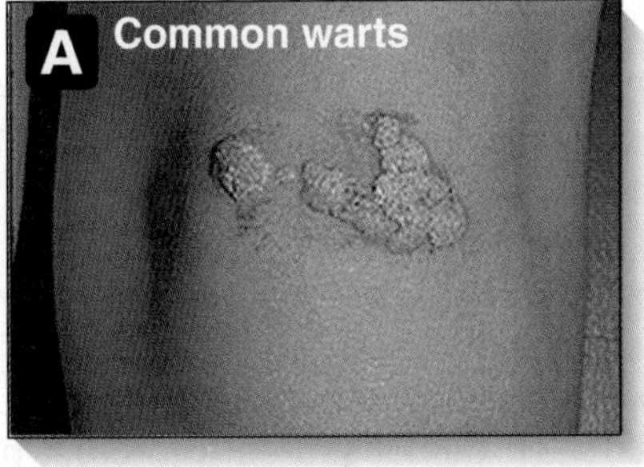

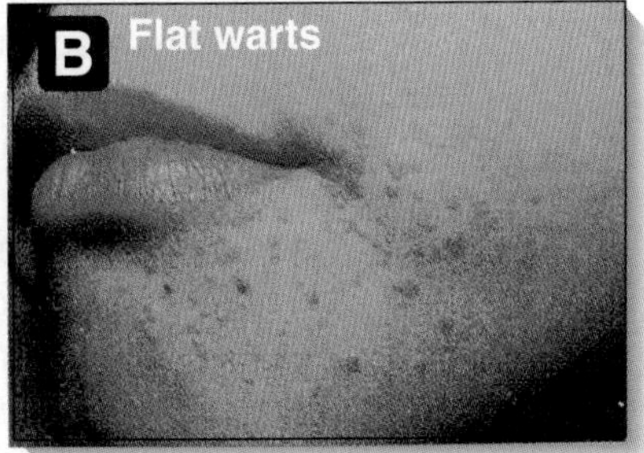

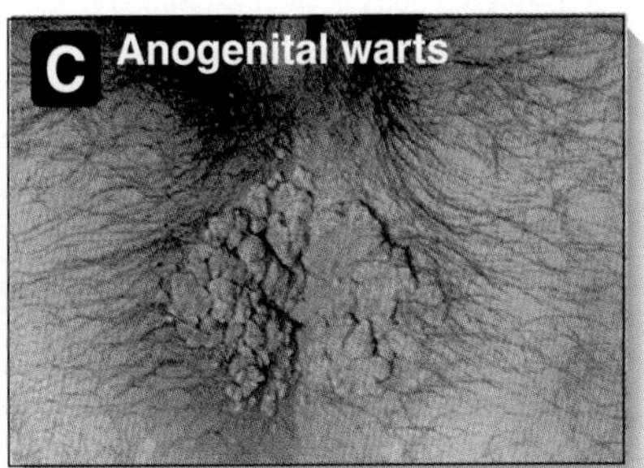

Figure 24.4
Warts caused by papillomavirus.

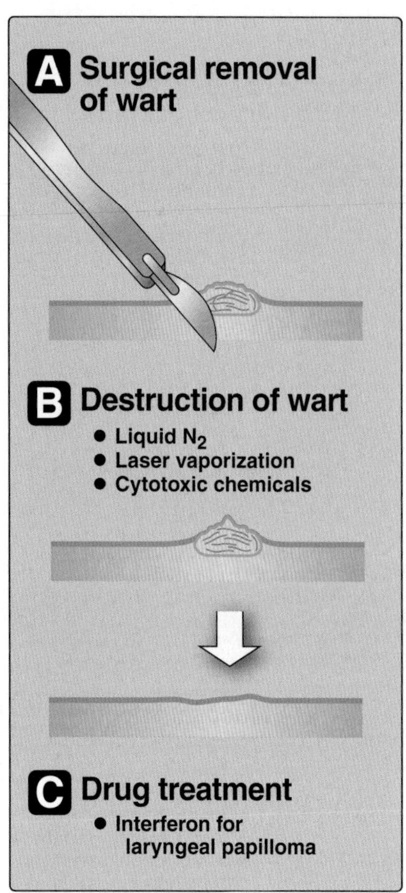

Figure 24.5
Treatment of papilloma.

benign) lesions that often regress spontaneously. Infections with other types of HPV do not lead to overt wart formation but have a high risk of progressing to malignancy. In fact, HPV has been established as the primary cause of cervical cancer in the majority of cases. HPV types 16 and 18 are associated with up to 70 percent of all cervical cancers. There are approximately 13 other, infrequently encountered types of HPV that are also associated with cancer development. Cumulatively, it is estimated that more than 95 percent of all cervical cancers are caused by these high-risk types of HPV. In addition to cervical cancer, the high-risk HPV types are linked to the development of anal, penile, vaginal, vulvar, and oropharyngeal cancers.

D. Laboratory identification

Diagnosis of cutaneous warts generally involves no more than visual inspection. The major role of laboratory identification in papillomavirus infections is to: 1) determine whether HPV is present in abnormal tissue recovered by biopsy or cervical swab and 2) whether the HPV type detected is one considered a high risk for progression to malignancy (the latter applying primarily to infections of the genital tract). The lack of any tissue culture system for recovery of the virus, and the fact that HPV types are defined by molecular criteria, means that typing is done by quantitative DNA amplification techniques (polymerase chain reaction), using defined, type-specific oligonucleotide primers (see p. 30). In addition, immunohistochemistry can be employed to detect viral protein expression *in situ*.

E. Treatment and prevention

Treatment of warts generally involves surgical removal or destruction of the wart tissue with liquid nitrogen, laser vaporization, or cytotoxic chemicals such as podophyllin or trichloroacetic acid (Figure 24.5). Although such treatments remove the wart, HPV often remains present in cells of the surrounding tissue, and recurrence rates of 50 percent have been reported. Common warts often regress spontaneously, and removal is not usually warranted unless there is unusual pain caused by the location or for cosmetic reasons. Cidofovir, an inhibitor of DNA synthesis, appears to be effective when applied topically. Interferon, given orally, has been shown to cause regression of laryngeal papillomas. When injected directly into genital warts, it has given positive results in about one half of patients. Because transmission of the infection is by direct inoculation, avoiding contact with wart tissue is the primary means of prevention. In genital tract warts, all of the procedures for prevention of sexually transmitted diseases are appropriate. In 2006, the Food and Drug Administration approved a vaccine against the four most common HPV types. The vaccine, called Gardasil, contains viral capsids from HPV types 6, 11, 16, and 18. The first two types cause most genital warts, and the latter two types cause the majority of cervical cancers. The vaccine was originally recommended for young females as a protection against cervical cancer. However, the vaccine is now recommended for young males, as well, because it has been demonstrated to protect both males and females against genital warts and specific types of cancer. A second vaccine, Cervarix, contains only two capsid types and is protective against infection with the high-risk HPV types, 16 and 18.

IV. PAPOVAVIRIDAE: SUBFAMILY POLYOMAVIRINAE

All members of this virus subfamily have the capacity to transform normal cells in culture and to induce tumors in species other than those in which they are normally found in nature. "Polyoma" means many (poly-) tumor (-oma). However, Polyomavirus has not yet been shown to cause tumors in humans. There are three human polyomaviruses: BK, JC, and Merkel cell polyomaviruses (BKV, JCV, and MCV, respectively). JCV has been associated with progressive multifocal leukoencephalopathy (PML), a rare, fatal, demyelinating disease that occurs only in patients with impaired immune function (for example, those with AIDS). BKV can cause cystitis in this same population. MCV was discovered in 2008 by molecular technologies. MCV DNA can be detected in the majority of cases of Merkel cell carcinoma, a rare and aggressive form of skin cancer.

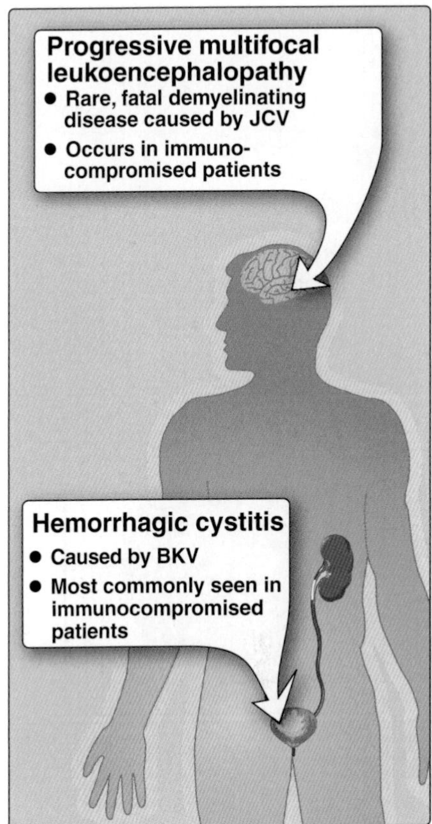

Figure 24.6
Location and properties of polyomavirus infections. JCV = JC polyomavirus; BKV = BK polyomavirus.

A. Epidemiology and pathogenesis

The human polyomaviruses BKV and JCV are transmitted by droplets from the upper respiratory tract of infected persons and, possibly, through contact with their urine. Infection with these viruses usually occurs in childhood. Specific antibody to one or both human polyomaviruses is present in 70 to 80 percent of the adult population. There is evidence that both BKV and JCV spread from the upper respiratory tract to the kidneys, where they may persist in an inactive state in the tubular epithelium of healthy individuals. Polyomaviruses follow the basic pattern of DNA virus genome replication and gene expression in the nucleus. The enzymes and precursors synthesized in preparation for cellular DNA synthesis are made available for synthesis of viral DNA. This productive cycle leads to viral multiplication and, ultimately, to death of the host cell.

B. Clinical significance

Immune compromise of various types can be associated with the development of PML, so named because the lesions are restricted to white matter (Figure 24.6). PML, thought to be caused by reactivated JCV that has entered the central nervous system via the blood, occurs as a complication of a number of lymphoproliferative disorders and chronic diseases that affect immune competence. [Note: In recent years, PML has been seen especially in patients with AIDS.] In PML, JCV carries out a cytocidal infection of the brain, specifically of oligodendrocytes, leading to demyelination resulting from myelinated cells losing their capacity to maintain their myelin sheaths. Early development of impaired speech and mental capacity is rapidly followed by paralysis and sensory abnormalities, with death commonly occurring within 3 to 6 months of onset of the initial symptoms. [Note: BKV is also found in the urine (Figure 24.7) but rarely has pathologic consequences except in immunocompromised patients, who may develop hemorrhagic cystitis.] Merkel cell carcinomas are relatively rare, but aggressive, and develop more frequently in older individuals. These carcinomas also develop more often in persons who are immunocompromised due to AIDS or other immunodeficiency or following organ transplant.

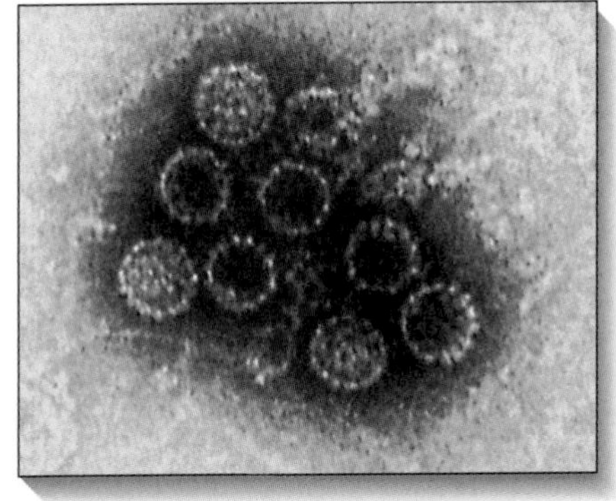

Figure 24.7
Electron micrograph of BK virions from the urine of an infected patient.

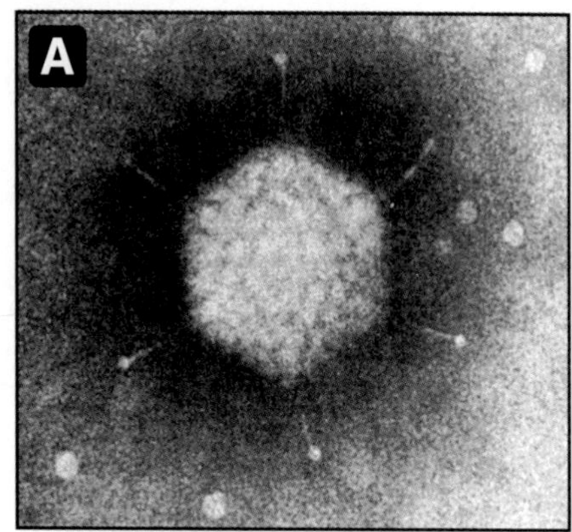

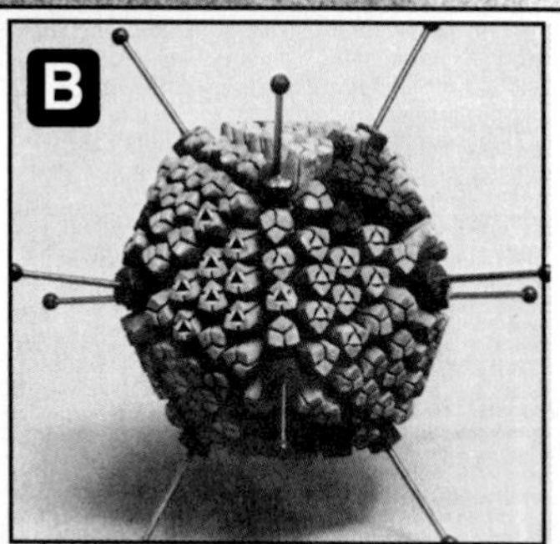

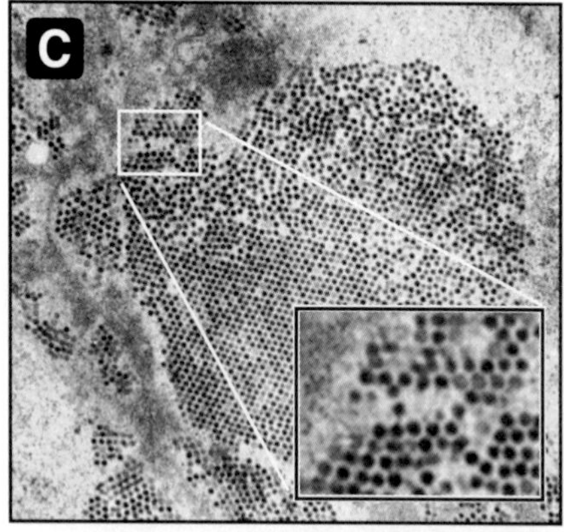

Figure 24.8
A. Electron micrograph of an adenovirus virion with fibers. B. Model of adenovirus. C. Crystalline aggregate of adenovirus in the nucleus of a cell.

C. Laboratory identification

Because most people have antibodies to these viruses, serologic techniques are not generally useful in the diagnosis of acute infections. Identification by DNA hybridization of BKV in the urine or JCV in PML lesions in brain tissue is the most sensitive and specific technique for diagnosis of these infections. MCV viral DNA and protein antigens can be detected by molecular techniques in Merkel cell tumors.

D. Treatment and prevention

No successful, specific, antiviral therapy is available. Because polyomavirus infection is nearly universal and asymptomatic, and PML represents reactivation of "latent" virus, there are currently no viable preventive measures.

V. ADENOVIRIDAE

Adenoviruses are nonenveloped, icosahedral viruses containing double-stranded linear DNA (Figure 24.8). They commonly cause diseases such as respiratory tract infections, gastroenteritis, and conjunctivitis. Adenoviruses were first discovered during screenings of throat washings and cultures of adenoids and tonsils, performed in the search for the common cold virus. They are now recognized as a large group of related viruses commonly infecting humans, other mammals, and birds. Over fifty serotypes of human adenoviruses are known, and antibody surveys have shown that most individuals have been infected by several different types by adulthood. Although some human serotypes are highly oncogenic in experimental animals, none have been associated with human malignancies.

A. Epidemiology and pathogenesis

The site of the clinical syndrome caused by an adenovirus infection is generally related to the mode of virus transmission. For example, most adenoviruses are primarily agents of respiratory disease, which are transmitted via the respiratory route. However, most adenoviruses also replicate efficiently and asymptomatically in the intestine, and can be isolated from stool well after respiratory disease symptoms have ended as well as from the stools of healthy persons. Similarly, ocular infections are transmitted by direct inoculation of the eye by virus-contaminated hands, ophthalmologic instruments, or bodies of water in which groups of children swim together.

B. Structure and replication

The adenovirus capsid is composed of hexon capsomers making up the triangular faces of the icosahedron, with a penton capsomer at each of the vertices (see Figure 24.8). Replication of adenoviruses essentially follows the general model for DNA viruses (see p. 238). Attachment to a host cell receptor occurs via knobs on the tips of the viral fibers, which is followed by entry into the cell by receptor-mediated endocytosis. The viral genome is then progressively uncoated while it is transported to the nucleus, where all transcription of viral genes, genome replication, and assembly occurs. Two early viral genes have the same function as the early proteins of the Papovaviridae [that is, inactivating cellular regulatory proteins (including p53 and pRb) that normally prevent progression through the cell cycle]. However, the considerably larger adenovirus genome encodes a number of additional early proteins, including a DNA polymerase and others that affect transcription and replication of the viral genome. The productive cycle kills the host cell, as cellular DNA, RNA, and protein synthesis are all shut off during the course of infection. Release of infectious virus from the cell occurs by slow disintegration of the dying cell.

C. Clinical significance

Adenoviruses all replicate well in epithelial cells. The observed disease symptoms are related primarily to the killing of these cells, and systemic infections are rare. Most adenovirus infections are asymptomatic, but certain types are more commonly associated with disease than others. These diseases can be conveniently grouped into those affecting the: 1) respiratory tract; 2) eye; 3) gastrointestinal (GI) tract; and, less commonly, 4) other tissues, including the urinary tract and heart (Figure 24.9).

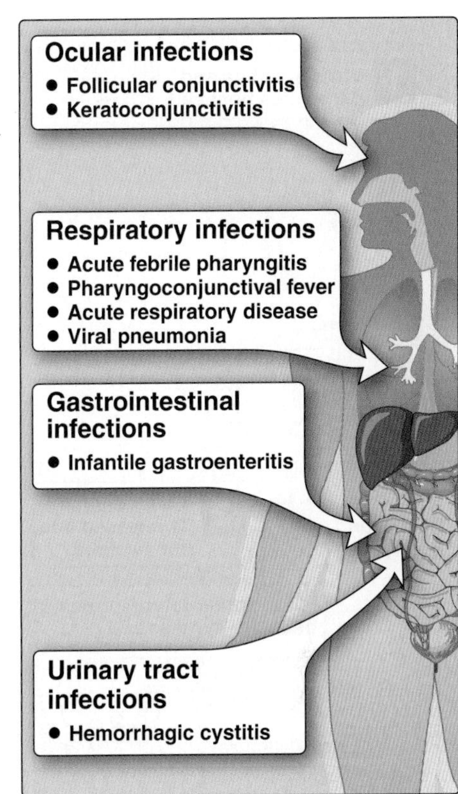

Figure 24.9
Adenovirus infections.

1. **Respiratory tract diseases:** The most common manifestation of adenovirus infection of infants and young children is acute febrile pharyngitis, characterized by a cough, sore throat, nasal congestion, and fever. Isolated cases may be indistinguishable from other common viral respiratory infections. Some adenovirus types tend additionally to produce conjunctivitis, in which case the syndrome is referred to as pharyngoconjunctival fever. This entity is more prevalent in school-aged children and occurs both sporadically and in outbreaks, often within family groups or in groups using the same swimming facility ("swimming pool conjunctivitis"). The syndrome referred to as acute respiratory disease occurs primarily in epidemics among new military recruits. It is thought to reflect the lowered resistance brought on by exposure to new strains, fatigue, and crowded living conditions, promoting efficient spread of the infection. Lastly, the respiratory syndromes described above may progress to true viral pneumonia, which has a mortality rate of about 10 percent in infants.

2. **Ocular diseases:** In addition to the conjunctivitis that sometimes accompanies the upper respiratory syndrome described above, a similar follicular conjunctivitis may occur as a separate disease. It is self-limiting and has no permanent sequelae. A more serious infection is epidemic keratoconjunctivitis, which involves the corneal epithelium, and may be followed by corneal opacity lasting several years. The epidemic nature of this disease partly results from transmission via shared towels or ophthalmic solutions, person-to-person contact, and improperly sterilized ophthalmologic instruments.

3. **Gastrointestinal diseases:** Most human adenoviruses multiply in the GI tract and can be found in stools. However, these are generally asymptomatic infections. Two serotypes have been associated specifically with infantile gastroenteritis. Adenovirus infections have been estimated to account for 5 to 15 percent of all viral diarrheal disease in children.

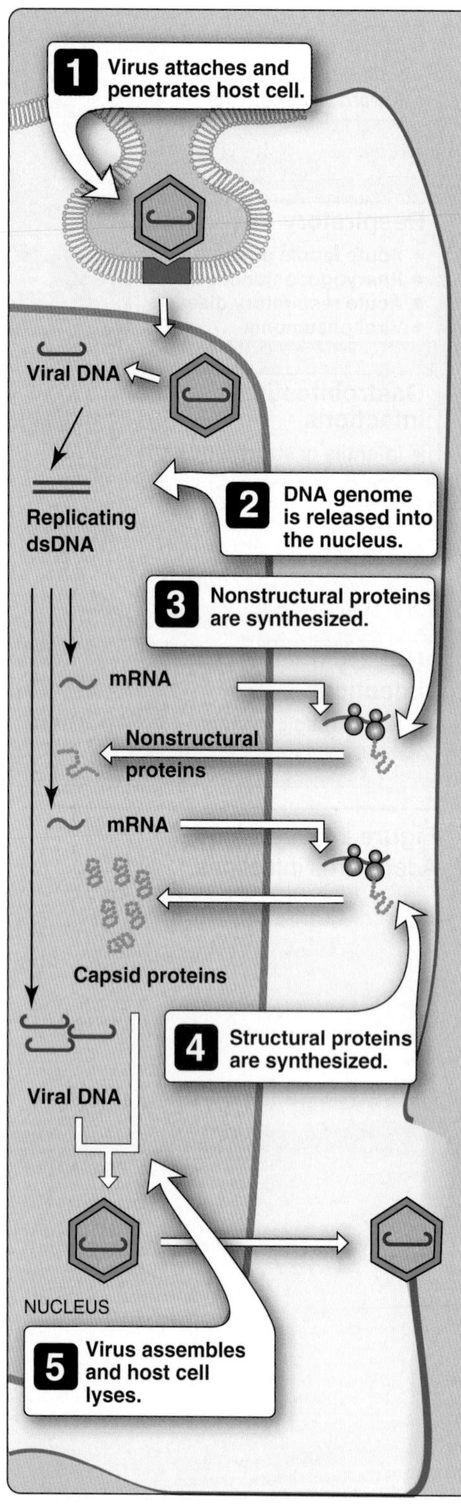

Figure 24.10
Replication of B19 parvovirus.

4. **Less common diseases:** Several adenovirus serotypes have been associated with an acute, self-limited, hemorrhagic cystitis, which occurs primarily in boys. It is characterized by hematuria, and virus can usually be recovered from the urine. Similarly, adenovirus infection of heart muscle has recently been shown to be one cause of left ventricular dysfunction in both children and adults. In immunocompromised patients, such as those with AIDS, the common respiratory adenovirus infections have a greater risk of proceeding to serious, often fatal, pneumonia. Other disseminated infections leading to a fatal outcome have been reported in patients with a compromised immune system or those immunosuppressed from drug therapy.

D. Laboratory identification

Isolation of virus for identification is not done on a routine basis but may be desirable in cases of epidemic disease or nosocomial outbreak, especially in the nursery. Identification of the adenovirus serotype can be done by neutralization or hemagglutination inhibition using type-specific antisera. The virus is more commonly detected by direct test of stool specimens by ELISA (enzyme-linked immunosorbent assay).

E. Treatment and prevention

No antiviral agents are currently available for treating adenovirus infections. Prevention of epidemic respiratory disease by immunization has been used only for protection of the military population. A live, attenuated adenovirus vaccine is used for this purpose that produces a good neutralizing antibody response. In 2011, a new vaccine was licensed for use among U.S. military personnel. This vaccine contains live, unattenuated adenovirus types 4 and 7, formulated for oral administration.

VI. PARVOVIRIDAE

Parvoviruses are the smallest of the DNA viruses. They are nonenveloped and icosahedral, with single-stranded, linear DNA. A human parvovirus, B19, has been isolated and identified as the cause of transient aplastic crisis in patients with sickle cell disease and implicated in adult acute polyarthritis. This virus is also the cause of the common childhood disease erythema infectiosum and is associated with fetal death in pregnant women experiencing a primary infection. The parvovirus family is divided into two genera, based on whether their ability to replicate requires coinfection with a helper DNA virus, or if they are capable of independent replication ("autonomous parvoviruses"). Members of the first group are referred to as adenoassociated viruses (AAVs), because they are usually found in infected cells in combination with a helper adenovirus.

A. Epidemiology and pathogenesis

Transmission of parvoviruses is by the respiratory route. A high-titered viremia lasting a few days follows about 1 week after infection, during which time virus is also present in throat secretions. A specific antibody response occurs rapidly, resulting in suppression of the viremia. Replication of parvoviruses requires a host cell in which

DNA synthesis is in progress. Therefore, damage is limited primarily to specific tissues that are mitotically active. [Note: In the case of B19 virus, these are primarily tissues of erythroid origin.] Because of the single-stranded nature of the genome, conversion to a double-stranded DNA molecule by a cellular DNA polymerase must occur before production of additional single-stranded viral DNA genomes or viral mRNA transcription can begin. Despite the limited amount of genetic material, two or three capsid proteins and two nonstructural regulatory proteins are produced by a combination of alternative RNA splicing patterns and posttranslational processing. The parvovirus life cycle is summarized in Figure 24.10.

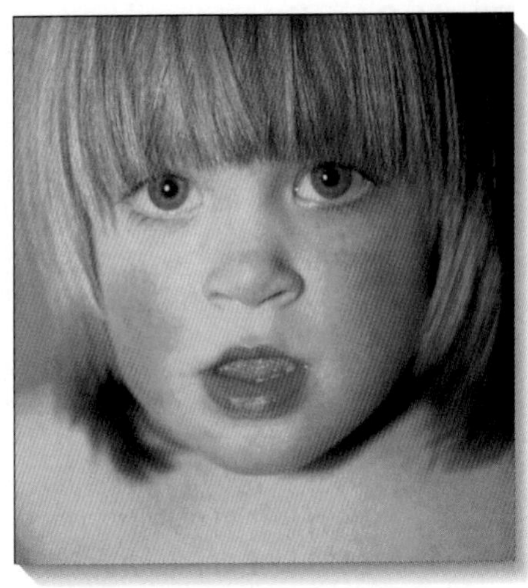

Figure 24.11
Typical "slapped cheek" appearance of a child infected with parvovirus B19 ("fifth disease").

B. Clinical significance

The single human pathogen in this family is the autonomous parvovirus, B19. The spectrum of illnesses caused by this virus is related to its unique tropism for cycling erythroid progenitor cells. Although B19 was initially isolated from sickle cell disease patients undergoing a transient aplastic crisis, it has since been recognized that chronic, progressive bone marrow suppression results from B19 infection of immunocompromised patients unable to mount an immune response capable of eliminating the virus.

1. **Erythema infectiosum:** The observation that 30 to 60 percent of some human populations have antibodies to B19 led eventually to the identification of this virus as the causative agent of the common childhood rash, erythema infectiosum ("fifth disease") as shown in Figure 24.11. The characteristic rash ("slapped cheek" appearance) occurs about 2 weeks after initial exposure, when the virus is no longer detectable. The rash is apparently immune-system mediated. Another complication accompanying B19 infection is an acute arthritis that usually involves joints symmetrically. This is considerably more frequent in adults than in children and usually resolves within several weeks.

2. **Birth defects:** Spontaneous abortion rate is elevated in women having a primary infection during the first trimester, and primary infection during the second or third trimester is associated with some instances of hydrops fetalis.

C. Laboratory identification

Laboratory identification of B19 infection is not routinely done. The large amount of virus present during the viremic (usually asymptomatic) phase permits detection of viral proteins by immunologic methods or of viral DNA by various amplification techniques. Retrospective diagnosis can be made by any of the usual procedures used to demonstrate a specific antibody response.

D. Treatment and prevention

No antiviral agent or vaccine is available for treating human B19 infections. Isolation of patients with signs of parvovirus disease is not a useful approach to control because subclinical infections occur, and infected individuals shed virus before symptoms appear. Intraveneously administered immunoglobulin G specific for B19 virus may be helpful in immunocompromised patients with chronic infections.

Study Questions

Choose the ONE correct answer.

24.1 An important step in the mechanism proposed for oncogenesis by human papillomaviruses is:

A. inactivation of a cellular regulatory gene by human papillomavirus integration into the coding region of the gene.

B. transactivation of a normally silent cellular oncogene by a human papillomavirus early protein.

C. reversal of keratinocyte differentiation caused by continued active replication and production of progeny human papillomavirus.

D. specific binding of certain human papillomavirus early proteins to cellular antioncoproteins.

E. induction of a specific chromosome translocation that results in activation of a cellular oncogene.

Correct answer = D. The early proteins of both adenoviruses and *Papovaviridae* required for immortalization and transformation of normal cells have been shown to bind specifically to cellular proteins p53 and pRb, which are important in maintaining regulation of the mitotic cycle. Interaction with viral proteins is believed to result in loss of their normal functions, as do the mutations that are commonly associated with spontaneously occurring cancers. A, B: Neither gene inactivation by integration nor transcriptional activation by an early protein has been observed. C: Virus replication occurs only in differentiated keratinocytes, but dedifferentiation does not occur. E: Multiple chromosome rearrangements are observed late in progression to malignancy, but none are specific for human papillomavirus–transformed cells.

24.2 The characteristic spectrum of diseases caused by autonomous parvoviruses is related to the fact that they:

A. integrate into a specific chromosomal site that disrupts an essential gene and leads to death of the cell.

B. require host cells that are actively progressing through the mitotic cycle.

C. infect only terminally differentiated cells.

D. code for an early protein that shuts off cellular protein synthesis.

E. increase the severity of the disease normally caused by their associated helper virus.

Correct answer = B. The diseases caused by the autonomous parvoviruses all result from the effects of killing multiplying cells that are essential for normal functions. For example, B19 specifically infects erythroblasts, leading to anemia in the fetus or in immunodeficient patients. A, C, D: Parvoviruses are not observed to integrate during the replicative cycle, they cannot replicate in terminally differentiated cells, and they do not shut off cell syntheses. E: By definition, the autonomous parvoviruses do not require a helper virus for replication.

24.3 The characteristic rash of erythema infectiosum is due to:

A. virion/antibody immune complex formation.

B. bone marrow suppression caused by killing of erythrocyte precursors by B19 infection.

C. damage to the liver.

D. B19 infection of epithelial cells.

E. the inflammatory response to B19 infection of capillary endothelium.

Correct answer = A. The appearance of the rash coincides with production of antibodies to B19, which occurs several days after the peak of viremia. B: Infection in immunodeficient individuals can lead to chronic, progressive depletion of erythrocyte precursors and severe anemia but not rash. C: The host range of B19 is restricted to erythroid precursors, including those found in the fetal liver. Although this may be a factor in causing hydrops fetalis due to B19 infection of a pregnant woman, it is not related to the rash. D and E: Again, B19 is not known to infect other than erythroid precursor cells.

Enveloped DNA Viruses

25

I. OVERVIEW

Two of the three enveloped DNA virus families, the *Herpesviridae* and the *Poxviridae*, are discussed in this chapter. [Note: *Hepadnaviridae*, the third enveloped DNA virus family, is discussed in Chapter 26.] The *Herpesviridae* and the *Poxviridae* are both structurally and genetically more complex than the DNA viruses discussed in Chapter 24. For example, there is less dependence on host cell–supplied functions, with a correspondingly greater number of virus-encoded proteins involved in viral replication. This latter characteristic contributes to the greater success in developing antiviral drugs against these viruses, because there are more virus-specific enzymes that can serve as targets for inhibitors (in contrast to viruses that are more dependent on host cell function). Replication of herpesviruses and poxviruses is also independent of the host cell cycle. The *Herpesviridae* family includes important human pathogens (Figure 25.1). The one highly virulent member of the *Poxviridae* family, variola (the cause of smallpox), is the only human pathogen that has been successfully eradicated. This triumph serves as a model for attempts to control and potentially eradicate other infectious diseases.

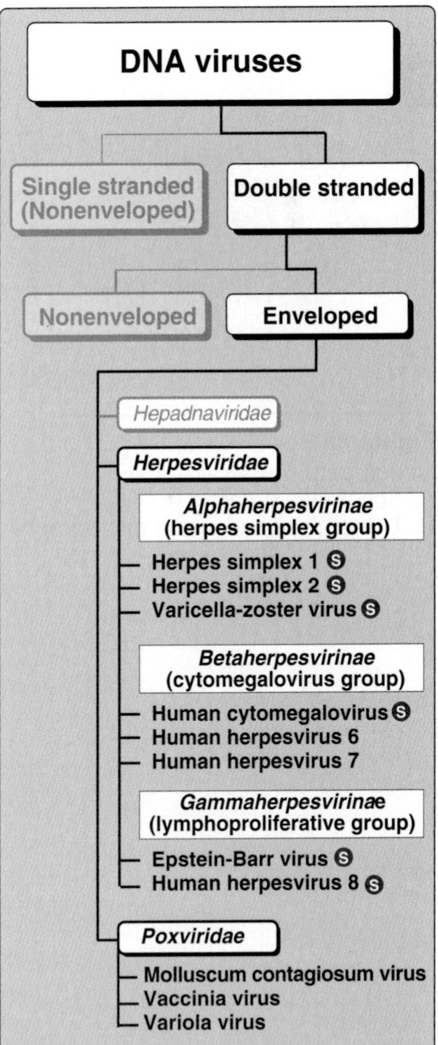

Figure 25.1
Classification of enveloped DNA viruses. S See p. 356 for summaries of these viruses.

II. HERPESVIRIDAE: STRUCTURE AND REPLICATION

Eight human herpesvirus species are known. All have the ability to enter a latent state following primary infection of their natural host and be reactivated at a later time. However, the exact molecular nature of the latency and the frequency and manifestation of reactivation vary with the type of herpesvirus.

A. Structure of herpesviruses

Herpesvirus virions consist of an icosahedral capsid enclosed in an envelope derived from the host's nuclear membrane (Figure 25.2). Between the envelope and the capsid lies an amorphous proteinaceous material called tegument, which contains virus-encoded enzymes and transcription factors essential for initiation of the infectious cycle, although none of these is a polymerase. The genome is a single molecule of linear, double-stranded DNA, encoding from 70 to 200 proteins, depending on the species. Although all members of the family have some genes with homologous functions, there is little nucleotide sequence conservation and little antigenic relatedness between species.

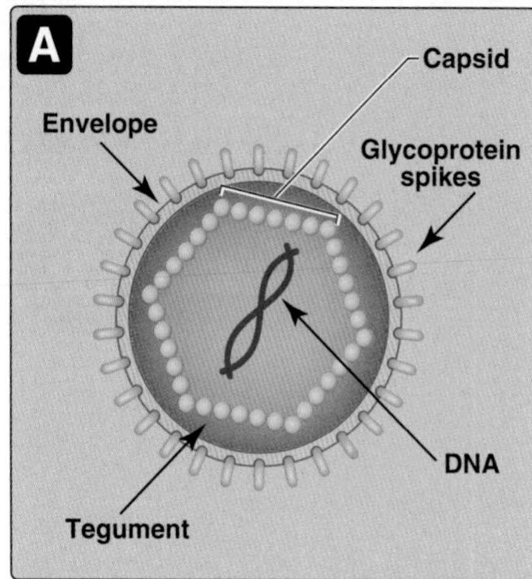

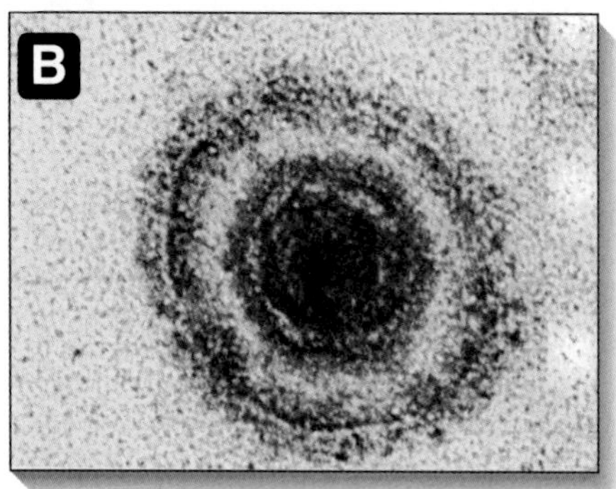

Figure 25.2
Structure of herpesvirus.
A. Schematic drawing.
B. Transmission electron micrograph.

B. Classification of herpesviruses

Herpesviridae cannot readily be differentiated by morphology in the electron microscope, because they all have similar appearances. However, *Herpesviridae* have been divided into three subfamilies, based primarily on biologic characteristics (see Figure 25.1).

1. ***Alphaherpesvirinae* (herpes simplex virus group):** These viruses have a relatively rapid, cytocidal or lytic growth cycle and establish dormant or latent infections in nerve ganglia. Herpes simplex virus types 1 and 2 (HSV-1 and HSV-2) and varicella-zoster virus (VZV) belong to this group. HSV-1 and HSV-2 share significant nucleotide homology and, therefore, share many common features in replication and pathogenesis. VZV has a smaller genome than HSV, but the two viruses have many genes that share sequence identity.

2. ***Betaherpesvirinae* (cytomegalovirus group):** These viruses have a relatively slow replication cycle that results in the formation of characteristic, multinucleated, giant host cells. Latency is established in nonneural tissues, primarily lymphoreticular cells and glandular tissues. Human cytomegalovirus (HCMV) and human herpesviruses types 6 and 7 (HHV-6 and HHV-7) are in this group.

3. ***Gammaherpesvirinae* (lymphoproliferative group):** These viruses replicate in mucosal epithelium and establish latent infections primarily in B cells. They induce cell proliferation in and immortalize lymphoblastoid cells. Epstein-Barr virus (EBV) was previously the only well-characterized human gammaherpesvirus. However, genome analysis of a virus recovered from cells of Kaposi sarcoma (KS) revealed it to also be a human member of the Gammaherpesvirinae. It has been designated human herpesvirus type 8 (HHV-8). HHV-8 can also establish latency and immortalize endothelial cells.

C. Replication of the herpesviruses

Herpesviruses replicate in the nucleus, following the basic pattern of DNA virus replication (see p. 238). Regulation of herpesvirus transcription is referred to as "cascade control," in that expression of a first set of genes is required for expression of a second set, which, in turn, is required for expression of a third set of genes. [Note: A similar pattern is found in some other DNA virus families in which the genes are referred to as immediate early, delayed early, and late.] The general features of herpesvirus replication are summarized in Figure 25.3.

1. **Virus adsorption and penetration:** Herpesviruses adsorb to host cell receptors that can differ according to the virus species and the tissue type being infected. Viral envelope glycoproteins promote fusion of the envelope with the cell's plasma membrane, depositing the nucleocapsid and tegument proteins in the cytosol. One of the tegument proteins is a general RNase that efficiently degrades all mRNAs, effectively shutting off host cell protein syn-

thesis. Because this protein's nucleolytic activity occurs prior to the onset of viral mRNA synthesis, it is selective for host RNAs.

2. **Viral DNA replication and nucleocapsid assembly:** The nucleocapsid is transported to a nuclear pore, through which viral DNA is released into the nucleus. Another tegument protein is an activator of cellular RNA polymerase that causes the enzyme to initiate transcription of the set of viral immediate early genes, which code for a variety of regulatory functions, including initiation of further gene transcription. Delayed early genes are expressed next, and they code primarily for enzymes that are required for replication of viral DNA, such as viral DNA polymerase, helicase, and thymidine kinase. Because these enzymes are virus specific, they provide excellent targets for antiherpes agents (such as acyclovir), which are relatively nontoxic for the cell. As is the case with other DNA viruses, late genes code for structural proteins of the virion and proteins involved in assembly and maturation of viral progeny.

3. **Viral envelope acquisition:** Newly synthesized envelope proteins accumulate in patches on the nuclear membrane, and nucleocapsids that have been assembled in the nucleus acquire their envelopes by budding through these patches. The completed virus is transported by a vacuole to the surface of the cell. Additional copies of the envelope glycoproteins are also transported to the plasma membrane, which acquires herpesvirus antigenic determinants. These glycoproteins may also cause fusion of neighboring cells, in some cases producing characteristic multinucleated giant cells. The end result of this productive, lytic cycle is cell death because most cellular synthetic pathways are effectively turned off during viral replication.

4. **Latency:** All herpesviruses can undergo an alternative infection cycle, entering a quiescent, dormant state (latency) from which they can subsequently be reactivated. The cell type in which this occurs is usually not the same cell type in which productive, lytic infection occurs. For each of the herpesviruses, the mechanism of latency, nature of the host cells, frequency of reactivation, and the nature of the recurrent disease are characteristic. Therefore, the topic of latency is discussed in this chapter in the context of the individual virus species.

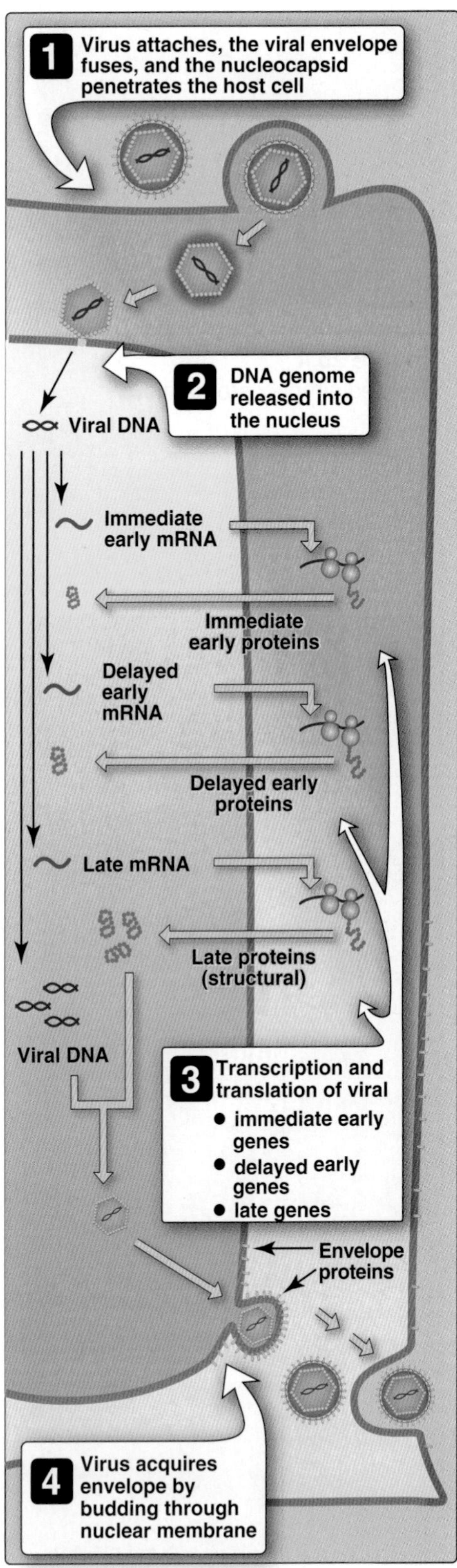

Figure 25.3
Replication of herpesviruses.

III. Herpes simplex virus, types 1 and 2

HSV-1 and HSV-2 are the only human herpesviruses that have a significant degree of nucleotide sequence identity (about 50 percent). Therefore, they share many common features in replication, disease production, and latency.

A. Epidemiology and pathogenesis

Transmission of both HSV types is by direct contact with virus-containing secretions or with lesions on mucosal or cutaneous surfaces. Primary or recurrent infections in the oropharyngeal region, caused

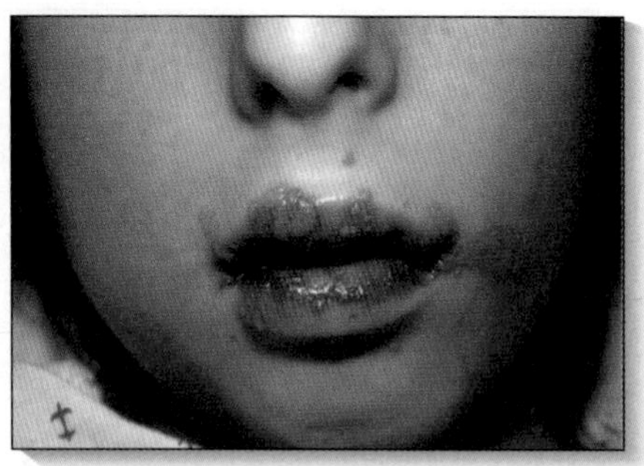

Figure 25.4
Herpes simplex stomatitis.

primarily by HSV-1, are accompanied by virus release into saliva, and kissing and saliva-contaminated fingers are major modes of transmission. In genital tract infections, caused primarily by HSV-2, virus is present in genital tract secretions. Consequently, sexual intercourse and passage of newborns through the birth canal of infected mothers are major modes of transmission. Both HSV-1 and HSV-2 multiply in epithelial cells of the mucosal surface onto which they have been inoculated, resulting in production of vesicles or shallow ulcers containing infectious virus. In immunocompetent individuals, epithelial infection remains localized because cytotoxic T lymphocytes recognize the HSV-specific antigens on the surface of infected cells and kill these cells before progeny virus has been produced. A lifelong latent infection is usually established in the regional ganglia as a result of entry of infectious virions into sensory neurons that terminate at the site of the infection.

B. Clinical significance

A generality (albeit of limited use) is that HSV-1 is most commonly found in lesions above the waist, and HSV-2 is more commonly the cause of lesions below the waist. However, HSV-1 can infect the genital tract, causing similar lesions, and, similarly, HSV-2 can cause lesions in the oral cavity.

1. **Primary infections of the upper body:** Many primary HSV infections are subclinical, but the most common symptomatic infections of the upper body are gingivostomatitis in young children (Figure 25.4) and pharyngitis or tonsillitis in adults. The painful lesions typically consist of vesicles and shallow ulcers, which are often accompanied by systemic symptoms, such as fever, malaise, and myalgia. Another clinically important site of infection is the eye, in which keratoconjunctivitis can lead to corneal scarring and eventual blindness. If HSV infection spreads to the central nervous system (CNS), it can cause encephalitis, which, if untreated, has a mortality rate estimated to be 70 percent. Survivors are usually left with neurologic deficits. In the United States, HSV-1 infection of the eye is the second most common cause of corneal blindness (after trauma). HSV infections of the CNS account for up to 20 percent of encephalitis viral infections.

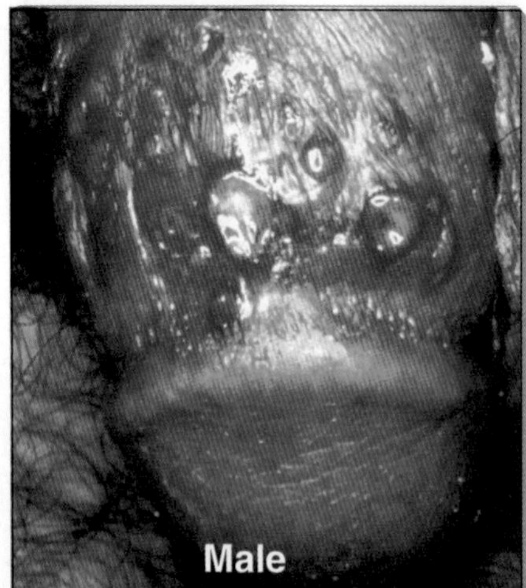

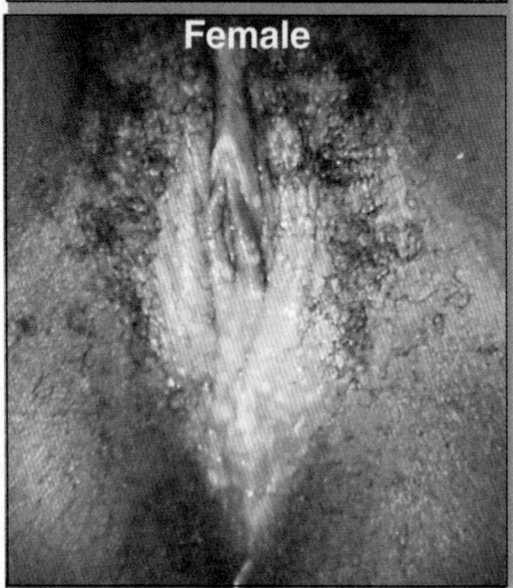

Figure 25.5
Genital herpes simplex infections.

2. **Primary infections of the genital tract:** Primary genital tract lesions are similar to those of the oropharynx. However, based on the frequency of antibody in the population, the majority of these infections are asymptomatic. When symptomatic (genital herpes), local symptoms include painful vesiculo-ulcerative lesions on the vulva, cervix, and vagina in women and the penis in men (Figure 25.5). Systemic symptoms of fever, malaise, and myalgia may be more severe than those that accompany primary oral cavity infections. In pregnant women with a primary genital HSV infection, the risk of infecting the newborn during birth is estimated to be 30 to 40 percent (neonatal herpes). Because such infants have no protective maternal antibody, a disseminated infection, often involving the CNS, may result. There is a high mortality rate if untreated, and survivors are likely to have permanent neurologic sequelae. A newborn is also at risk of acquiring infection from an infected

mother by transfer on contaminated fingers or in saliva. However, infection *in utero* appears to occur only rarely.

3. **Latency:** In latently infected cells of the ganglia—HSV-1 in trigeminal ganglia and HSV-2 in sacral or lumbar ganglia—from one to thousands of copies of the viral genome are present as nonintegrated, circular molecules of DNA in the nuclei (Figure 25.6). A limited number of viral genes are expressed during latency. These transcripts (called LATS for latency-associated transcripts) suppress production of progeny virus.

4. **Reactivation:** Several factors, such as hormonal changes, fever, and physical damage to the neurons, are known to induce reactivation and replication of the latent virus (see Figure 25.6). The newly synthesized virions are transported down the axon to the nerve endings from which the virus is released, infecting the adjoining epithelial cells. Characteristic lesions are thus produced in the same general area as the primary lesions. [Note: Virus replication occurs in only a fraction of the latently infected neurons, and these nerve cells eventually die.] The presence of circulating antibody does not prevent this recurrence but does limit the spread of virus to surrounding tissue. Sensory nerve symptoms, such as pain and tingling, often precede and accompany the appearance of lesions. In general, the severity of any systemic symptoms is considerably less than that of a primary infection, and many recurrences are characterized by shedding of infectious virus in the absence of visible lesions.

   a. **Herpes simplex virus type 1:** The frequency of oropharyngeal symptomatic recurrences is variable, ranging from none to several a year. The lesions occur as clusters of vesicles at the border of the lips (herpes labialis, or "cold sores" or "fever blisters") and heal without scarring in 8 to 10 days.

   b. **Herpes simplex virus type 2:** Reactivation of HSV-2 genital infections can occur with considerably greater frequency (for example, monthly) and is often asymptomatic but still results in viral shedding. Consequently, sexual partners or newborn infants may be at increased risk of becoming infected resulting from lack of precautions against transmission. The risk of transmission to the newborn is much less than in a primary infection because considerably less virus is shed and the baby has some maternal anti-HSV antibody. This antibody also lessens the severity of the disease if infection does occur.

C. Laboratory identification

Laboratory identification is not required for diagnosis of characteristic HSV lesions in normal individuals. Identification is important, however, to prevent neonatal infection and HSV encephalitis and keratoconjunctivitis, in which early initiation of therapy is essential, yet characteristic lesions are not present. Further, for purposes of therapy in the immunocompromised patient, HSV infection must be distinguished from that of VZV (see p. 261). It must also be distinguished from simi-

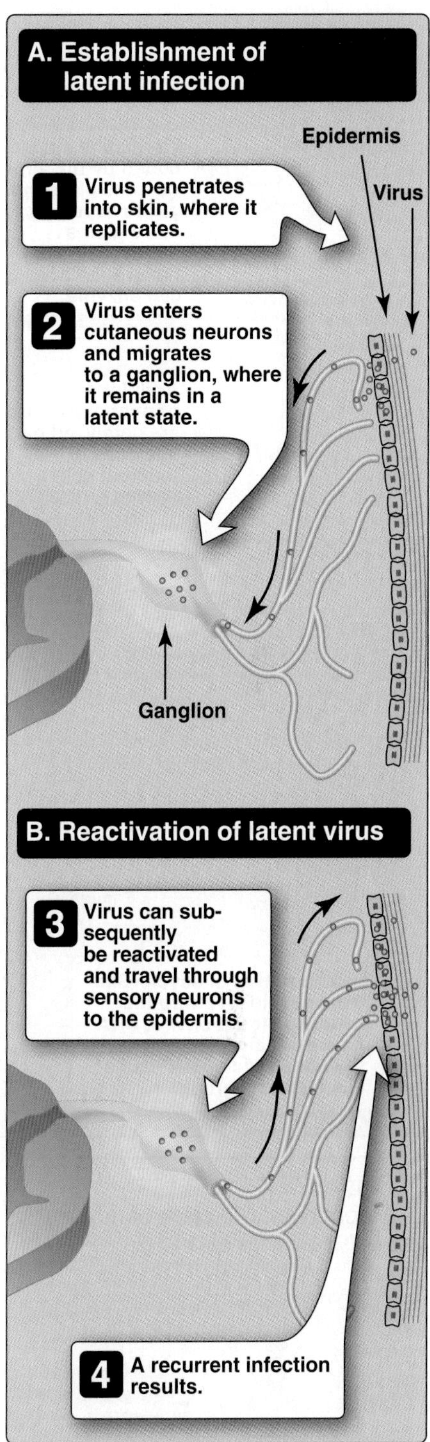

A. Establishment of latent infection
Epidermis
Virus
1 Virus penetrates into skin, where it replicates.
2 Virus enters cutaneous neurons and migrates to a ganglion, where it remains in a latent state.
Ganglion
B. Reactivation of latent virus
3 Virus can subsequently be reactivated and travel through sensory neurons to the epidermis.
4 A recurrent infection results.

Figure 25.6
Primary and recurrent herpes simplex infections.

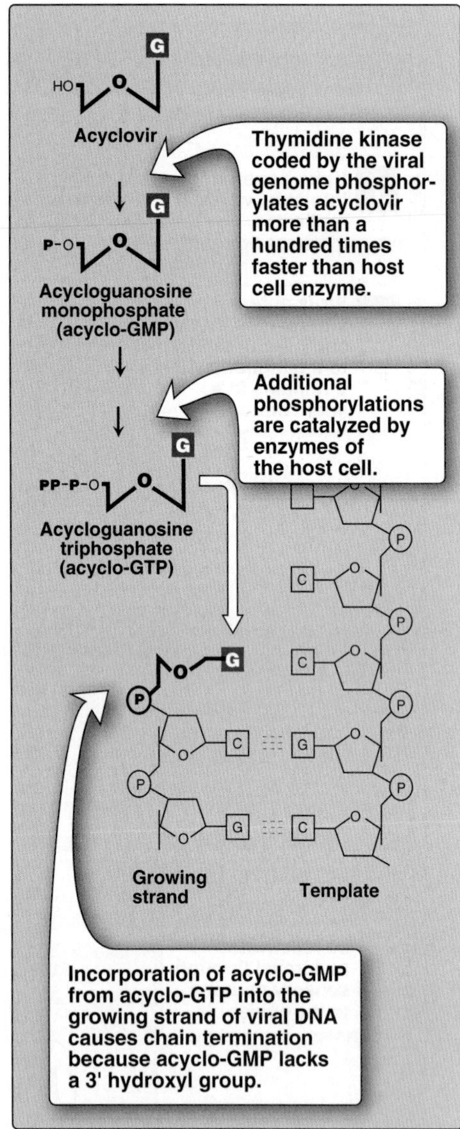

Figure 25.7
Mechanism of action of acyclovir.

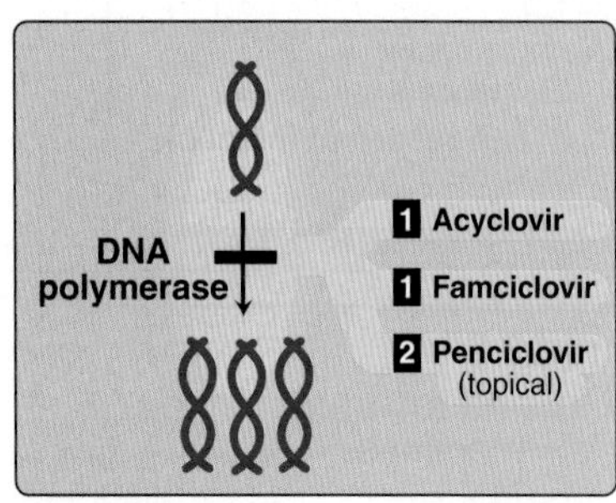

Figure 25.8
Drug therapy for herpes simplex infection. 1 Indicates first-line drugs; 2 indicates alternative drugs.

lar exanthems (skin eruptions) caused by other viruses or, in some cases, by bacteria or noninfectious, allergy-based reactions. Demonstration of HSV by inoculation of human cell tissue culture with a sample of vesicle scraping, fluid, or genital swab is the definitive method for demonstrating infection. The presence of the virus can result in syncytia formation between cells and the formation of Cowdry type A bodies within the host cell nucleus. Gross cytopathic changes may require several days to appear, but individual infected cells can be detected within 24 hours by use of immunofluorescence (see p. 28) or immunoperoxidase staining with antibodies directed against viral early proteins. Using these same techniques, infected cells can also be demonstrated directly in clinical specimens, although this approach is generally less sensitive than virus isolation in tissue culture. Direct detection of viral DNA by hybridization techniques complements these procedures and, after amplification of the DNA by polymerase chain reaction ([PCR] see p. 29), is considerably more sensitive. For example, in patients with encephalitis, HSV etiology can be confirmed by demonstration of viral DNA in the cerebral spinal fluid (CSF) instead of by brain biopsy.

D. Treatment

The guanine analog, acycloguanosine (acyclovir), is selectively effective against HSV because it becomes an active inhibitor of DNA synthesis only after initially being phosphorylated by the HSV thymidine kinase (Figure 25.7). The drug of choice for any primary HSV infection, acyclovir is especially important in treating herpes encephalitis, neonatal herpes, and disseminated infections in immunocompromised patients. Other drugs effective in treating herpes simplex infection include famciclovir and topical penciclovir (Figure 25.8). Famciclovir is a prodrug that is metabolized to the active penciclovir. It provides more convenient dosing and greater bioavailability than oral acyclovir. Penciclovir is active against HSV-1, HSV-2, and VZV. None of these drugs can cure a latent infection, but they can minimize asymptomatic viral shedding and recurrences of symptoms (Figure 25.9).

E. Prevention

Prevention of HSV transmission is enhanced by avoidance of contact with potential virus-shedding lesions and by safe sexual practice. Although prevention of neonatal HSV infections is important, genital infection of the mother can be difficult to detect because it is often asymptomatic. When overt genital tract lesions are detected at the time of delivery, cesarean section is usually warranted. Prophylactic therapy of the mother and the newborn with acyclovir can be employed if the presence of HSV is detected just before or at the time of birth. Measures to prevent physical transmission following birth are also important. A vaccine is not currently available.

IV. VARICELLA-ZOSTER VIRUS

VZV has biologic and genetic similarities to HSV and is classified with HSVs in the *Alphaherpesvirinae* subfamily. Biologic similarities between VZV and HSV include that latency is established in sensory ganglia and infections are rapidly cytocidal. Primary infections with VZV cause varicella ("chickenpox"), whereas reactivation of the latent virus causes herpes zoster ("shingles").

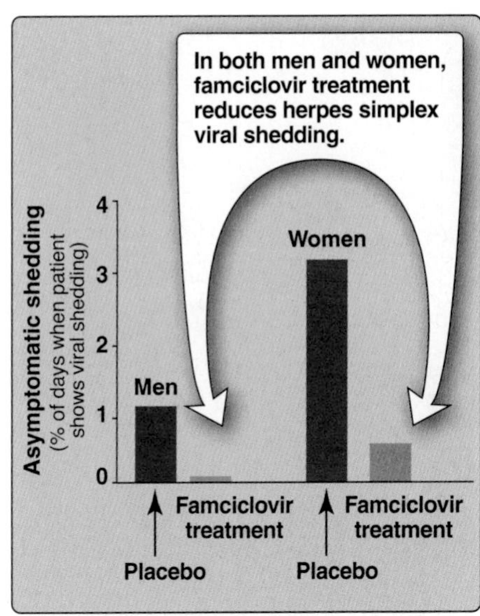

Figure 25.9
Chronic suppressive antiviral therapy reduces the frequency of asymptomatic herpes simplex virus shedding.

A. Epidemiology and pathogenesis

VZV is the only herpesvirus that can be easily spread from person to person by casual contact. Transmission of VZV is usually via respiratory droplets and results in initial infection of the respiratory mucosa, followed by spread to regional lymph nodes (Figure 25.10). Progeny virus enter the bloodstream, undergo a second round of multiplication in cells of the liver and spleen, and are disseminated throughout the body by infected mononuclear leukocytes. Endothelial cells of the capillaries and, ultimately, skin epithelial cells become infected, resulting in the characteristic, virus-containing vesicles of chickenpox that appear from 14 to 21 days after exposure. The infected individual is contagious from 1 to 2 days before the appearance of the exanthem, implying that viruses reinfect cells of the respiratory mucosa near the end of the incubation period. The vesicular fluid from the chickenpox rash is also highly contagious and can be spread to nonimmune individuals if it becomes airborne."

B. Clinical significance

In contrast to HSV infections, the primary and recurrent diseases (varicella and zoster) due to VZV are quite distinct. Whereas neither is usually life threatening in the normal, healthy individual, both can have severe complications in immunocompromised patients.

1. **Primary infection (varicella, or chickenpox):** In a normal, healthy child, the incubation period is most commonly from 14 to 16 days. The first appearance of exanthem is often preceded by 1 to 2 days of a prodrome of fever, malaise, headache, and abdominal pain. The exanthem begins on the scalp, face, or trunk as erythe-

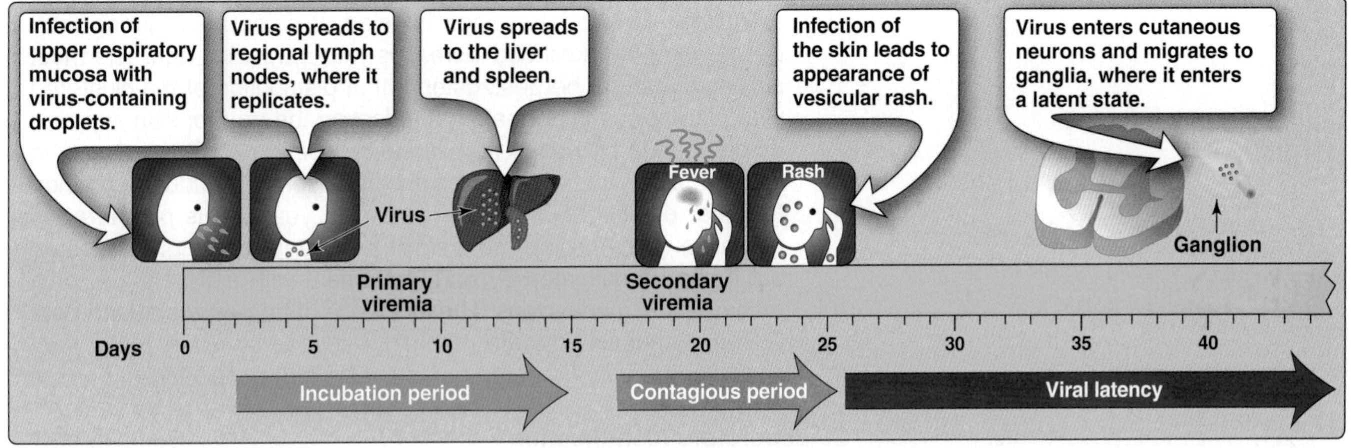

Figure 25.10
Time course of varicella (chickenpox) in children. In adults, the disease shows a longer time course and is more severe.

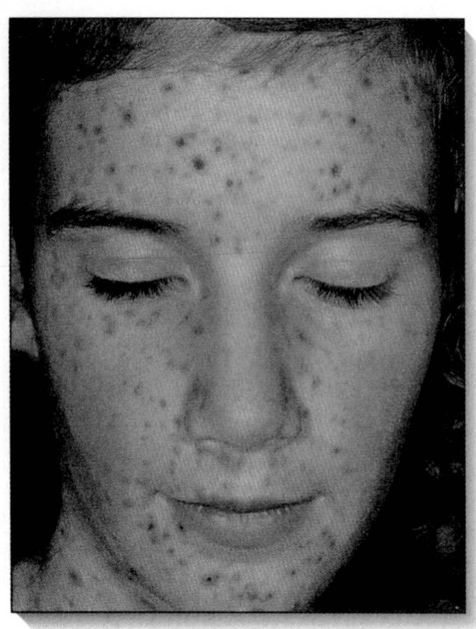

Figure 25.11
Appearance of chickenpox with lesions at all stages of development.

matous macules, which evolve into virus-containing vesicles that begin to crust over after about 48 hours (Figure 25.11). Itching is most severe during the early stage of vesicle development. While the first crop of lesions is evolving, new crops appear on the trunk and extremities. In older adults and the immunocompromised, lesions may also appear on mucous membranes, such as in the oropharynx, conjunctivae, and vagina. New lesions continue to appear over a period of up to 6 or 7 days. Healing usually occurs without long-term consequences, but crater-like scars can remain after the lesions heal. Varicella is a more serious disease in both healthy and immunocompromised adults than it is in children. Varicella pneumonia is the most common of the serious complications, but fulminant hepatic failure and varicella encephalitis may also result. Primary infection of a pregnant woman may cause her to contract the more severe adult form of varicella and may affect the fetus or neonate as well. Fetal infection early in pregnancy is uncommon but can result in multiple developmental anomalies. More commonly, a fetus infected near the time of delivery may exhibit typical varicella at birth or shortly thereafter. The severity of the disease depends on whether the mother has begun to produce anti-VZV immunoglobulin (Ig) G by the time of delivery.

2. **Reye syndrome:** Reye syndrome, an acute encephalopathy accompanied by fatty liver, can sometimes follow VZV or influenza infections in children. Epidemiological evidence suggests that use of aspirin or other salicylate-containing compounds to treat pain and fever during the viral illness is associated with the development of Reye syndrome. It is also important to avoid aspirin following vaccination against chickenpox.

3. **Recurrent infection (herpes zoster, or shingles):** Due to the disseminated nature of the primary infection, latency is established in multiple sensory ganglia, the trigeminal, and thoracic and lumbar dorsal root ganglia being most common. Unlike most of the herpesviruses, asymptomatic virus shedding is a rare event. Herpes zoster results from reactivation of the latent virus, rather than from new, exogenous exposure. Reactivation occurs in up to 30 percent of individuals who have been infected at some point during their lifetime, and the likelihood increases with advancing age. The most striking feature of herpes zoster is that distribution of the clustered vesicular lesions is dermatomal (affecting the area of skin supplied by cutaneous branches from a single spinal nerve) as shown in Figure 25.12. Even after the lesions heal, some individuals continue to suffer debilitating pain for months to years. This postherpetic neuralgia (PHN) is the most significant sequela of herpes zoster, but it can be mitigated by early treatment with antivirals and pain management medications. The incidence of herpes zoster and postherpetic neuralgia can be markedly reduced by using zoster vaccine in appropriate (greater than 50 years old) populations.

C. Laboratory identification

Laboratory diagnosis of uncomplicated varicella or zoster is generally not necessary and not usually done because of the typical clinical appearance and distribution of lesions. However, in the immunocompromised patient in whom therapy is warranted, it is important to distinguish VZV infection from other similar exanthems. Cell tissue cultures inoculated with a sample of vesicle fluid show gross cytopathic changes in several days. Individual infected cells can be detected within 24 hours by use of immunofluorescence or immunoperoxidase staining with antibodies against viral early proteins. More rapid diagnosis can be made by reacting epithelial cells scraped from the base of vesicles with the stains described above or by doing *in situ* hybridization with VZV-specific DNA probes.

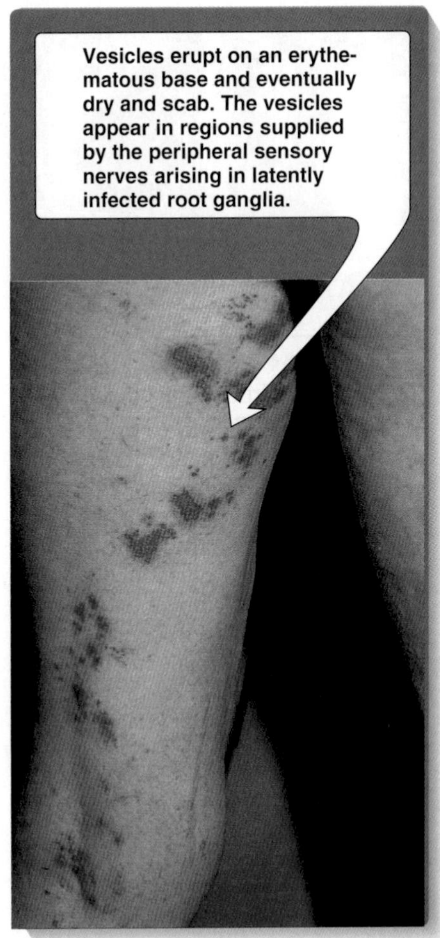

Vesicles erupt on an erythematous base and eventually dry and scab. The vesicles appear in regions supplied by the peripheral sensory nerves arising in latently infected root ganglia.

Figure 25.12
Cutaneous manifestations of acute herpes zoster in the territory of a cervical dorsal root ganglion (dermatome).

D. Treatment

Treatment of primary varicella in immunocompromised patients, adults, and neonates is warranted by the severity of the disease (Figure 25.13). Acyclovir has been the drug of choice in such patients but requires intravenous administration to achieve effective serum levels. Early administration of oral acyclovir reduces the time course and acute pain of zoster. Famciclovir and valacyclovir (base analogs similar to acyclovir) have greater activity against VZV.

E. Prevention

Certain susceptible individuals (for example, neonates born to mothers with active chickenpox from 2 days before to 5 days after delivery, and severely immunocompromised patients) can be protected by administration of varicella-zoster immunoglobulin (VariZIG). Administration of VariZIG has no effect on the occurrence of zoster. A live, attenuated vaccine that was approved in 1995 for use in the United States by children age 1 year or older is now recommended as one of the routine childhood vaccines. Mild, breakthrough cases of chickenpox have been reported as a side effect of vaccine administration. The vaccine is also indicated for nonimmune adults at risk of being exposed to contagious individuals. Zostavax is a high-potency version of the chickenpox vaccine, which also contains live, attenuated virus. Zostavax has been approved by the Food and Drug Administration for use in adults over age 50 years for prevention of zoster and, with it, the debilitating effects of PHN.

V. HUMAN CYTOMEGALOVIRUS

HCMV is a member of the Betaherpesvirinae subfamily and, as such, differs from HSV and VZV in several ways. Its replication cycle is significantly longer, and infected cells typically are greatly enlarged and multinucleated (hence, "cytomegalo-") as shown in Figure 25.14. There is only one recognized human species of HCMV, but there are many distinct strains that can be distinguished by antigenic differences as well as by restriction fragment analysis of their genomes. HCMV is the most common cause of intrauterine infections and congenital abnormalities in the United States. It also represents a serious threat to immunodeficient and immunosuppressed patients.

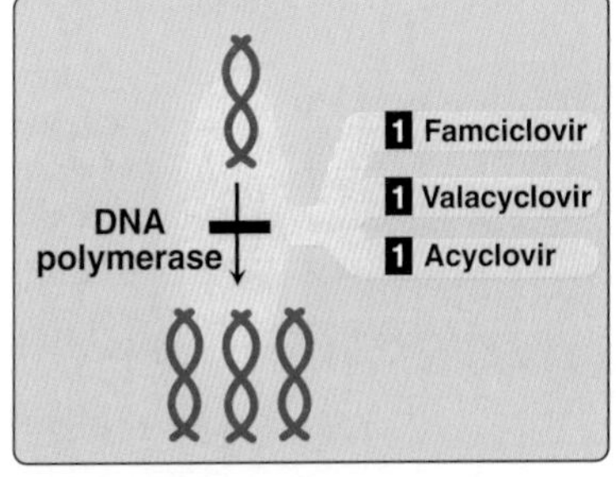

Figure 25.13
Drug therapy for varicella virus.
1 Indicates first-line drugs.

A. Epidemiology and pathogenesis

Initial infection with HCMV commonly occurs during childhood. Depending on geographic location and socioeconomic group, 35 to 90 percent of the population have antibody against the virus by adulthood.

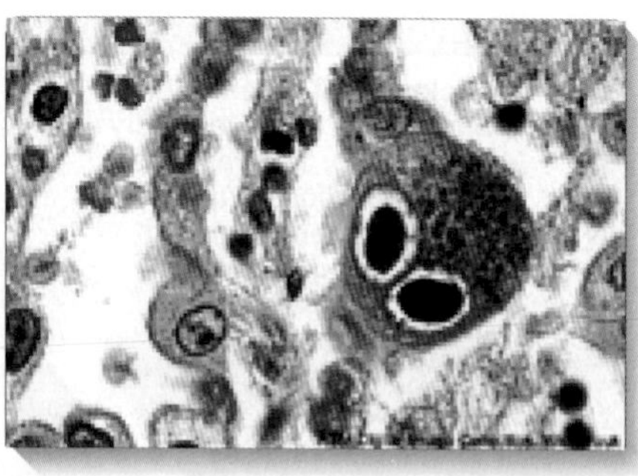

Figure 25.14
Cytomegalovirus infection. Lung section showing typical owl-eye inclusions.

1. **Transmission:** Infection in children is usually asymptomatic, and these children continue to shed virus for months in virtually all body fluids, including tears, urine, and saliva. Transmission is by intimate contact with these fluids, although saliva may be the most common source. In adults, the virus can also be transmitted by: 1) sexual means because it is present in semen and vaginal secretions, 2) organ transplants, and 3) blood transfusions. Similarly, virus is present in breast milk, and neonates can be infected by this route. HCMV can also cross the placenta and infect a fetus *in utero*. Initial replication of the virus in epithelial cells of the respiratory and gastrointestinal (GI) tracts is followed by viremia and infection of all organs of the body. In symptomatic cases, kidney tubule epithelium, liver, and CNS, in addition to the respiratory and GI tracts, are most commonly affected.

2. **Latency and reactivation:** A distinctive feature of HCMV latency is the phenomenon of repeated episodes of asymptomatic virus shedding over prolonged periods. Latency is probably established in monocytes and macrophages, but other cell types, such as those of the kidney, are also involved.

B. Clinical significance

In healthy individuals, primary HCMV infection is usually subclinical (no apparent symptoms). Although most infections occur in childhood, primary infection as an adult may result in a mononucleosis syndrome clinically identical to that caused by EBV (see p. 268). It is estimated that about 8 percent of infectious mononucleosis (IM) cases are caused by HCMV. Persistent fever, muscle pain, and lymphadenopathy are characteristic IM symptoms, as are elevated levels of abnormal lymphocytes and liver enzymes. The major distinguishing feature of HCMV IM is the absence of the heterophile antibodies that characterize IM caused by EBV (see p. 268). Two specific situations have greater clinical significance, namely, congenital infections and infection of immunocompromised patients.

1. **Congenital infections:** HCMV is the most common intrauterine viral infection. However, there is a great disparity in incidence of fetal infection and severity of outcome, depending on whether the mother is experiencing a primary or recurrent infection. In women experiencing their first HCMV infection during pregnancy (who, therefore, have not yet produced antibodies against HCMV), 35 to 50 percent of fetuses will be infected, and 10 percent of these will be symptomatic (Figure 25.15). It is known as cytomegalic inclusion disease, and the severity of the symptoms is most pronounced when infection occurs during the first trimester. Results of the infection range from varying degrees of damage to liver, spleen, blood-forming organs, and components of the nervous system to fetal death. Damage to the nervous system is a common cause of hearing loss and mental retardation. Even in infants who are asymptomatic at birth, hearing deficits and ocular damage (for example, chorioretinitis) may appear later and continue to progress during the first few years of life. Congenitally and perinatally infected infants may continue to excrete virus for years after birth, serving as an important virus reservoir.

2. **Infections of immunosuppressed and immunodeficient patients:** Immunosuppressed transplant recipients are multiply at risk from: 1) HCMV present in the tissue being transplanted, 2) virus carried in leukocytes in the associated blood transfusions, and 3) reactivation of their own endogenous latent virus. Immune suppression for the transplant can negate any protective advantage of a seropositive recipient. Destruction of GI tract tissue, hepatitis, and pneumonia are common, the latter being a major cause of death in bone marrow transplant recipients. HCMV infection is also associated with decreased survival of solid tissue grafts (i.e., heart, liver, kidney). HCMV coinfection of patients with HIV infection occurs frequently, probably because of their similar modes of transmission (see p. 364). As a common opportunistic infection in AIDS patients, invasive HCMV infections arising from reactivation of latent virus become increasingly important as CD4+ lymphocyte counts and immune competence decline (see p. 300). Although any organ system can be affected, pneumonia and blindness caused by HCMV retinitis are especially common. Encephalitis, dementia, esophagitis, enterocolitis, and gastritis are other significant problems. In addition, coinfection with HCMV may accelerate the progression of the pathology of AIDS (Figure 25.16).

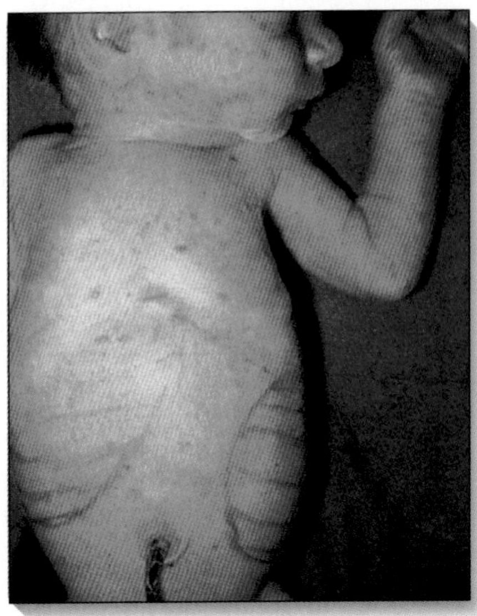

Figure 25.15
Newborn with congenital cytomegalovirus disease, showing hepatosplenomegaly and rash.

C. Laboratory identification

Because the incidence of HCMV infection in the population is so high, and periodic inapparent recurrent infections occur frequently, simple detection of virus or anti-HCMV antibody is not generally useful. Recovery of virus is not usually done. Serologic diagnosis using ELISA (or, enzyme-linked immunosorbent assay) techniques can distinguish primary from recurrent infection by demonstrating IgG seroconversion or the presence of HCMV-specific IgM. Direct determination of the presence and amount of viral DNA or proteins in white blood cells is useful as an indicator of invasive disease, whereas extracellular virus in urine or saliva may simply result from asymptomatic recurrence. Any of these techniques can also be used to screen transplant donors and recipients to determine HCMV status.

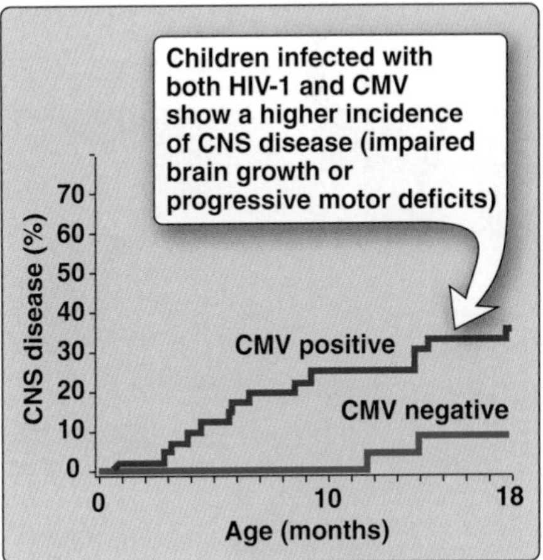

Figure 25.16
Incidence of central nervous system (CNS) disease in HIV-1-infected children, with or without cytomegalovirus (CMV) infection.

D. Treatment and prevention

Treatment of HCMV infection is indicated primarily in immunocompromised patients (Figure 25.17). Acyclovir is ineffective because HCMV lacks its own thymidine kinase. However, two inhibitors of HCMV DNA polymerase are available: ganciclovir, a guanine analog that is phosphorylated by a virus-coded protein kinase, and cidofovir, a deoxycytidine analog. A third inhibitor of DNA polymerase, unrelated to the two just described, is phosphonoformic acid (foscarnet). Ganciclovir is used for invasive infections of transplant recipients and AIDS patients, but it has considerable toxicity. For retinitis in AIDS patients, toxic adverse effects can be avoided by direct intraocular placement of a ganciclovir-impregnated implant. Following organ transplants, patients are treated prophylactically with gancyclovir or anti-HCMV Ig. Alternatively, patients are monitored for the first sign of HCMV replication and then treated preemptively with antivirals. A vaccine for active immunization is not available.

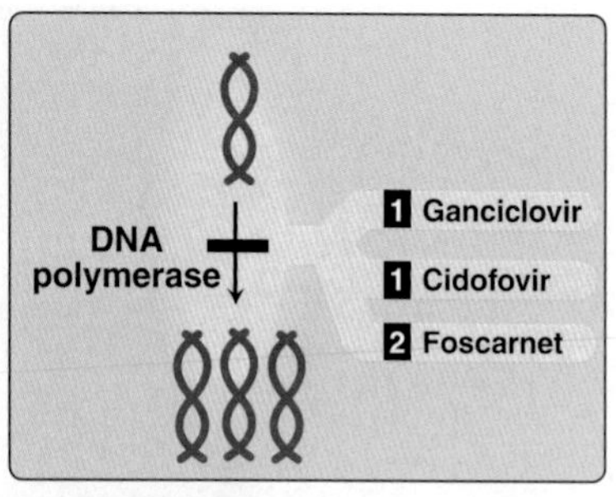

Figure 25.17
Drug therapy for cytomegalovirus.
1 Indicates first-line drugs;
2 indicates alternative drug.

VI. HUMAN HERPESVIRUS TYPES 6 AND 7

HHV-6 and HHV-7, classified as members of the Betaherpesvirinae, have marked similarities to HCMV in biologic and genome characteristics. Both HHV-6 and HHV-7 are causative agents of roseola infantum (exanthem subitum), although infection with HHV-7 is more frequently asymptomatic. Two variants of HHV-6 have been recognized: HHV-6A and HHV-6B. HHV-6B is virtually ubiquitous and is the causative agent of roseola infantum. HHV-6A has been implicated in the progression of HIV disease to full-blown AIDS.

A. Epidemiology and pathogenesis

Most infections with HHV-6 and HHV-7 occur during the first 3 years of life, with overall incidence of antibody approaching 90 percent of the population by age 3. Transmission is thought to be via oral secretions because the viruses replicate in the oropharynx as well as in B and T lymphocytes. HHV-7, in particular, is commonly recovered from healthy individuals' saliva. These viruses also infect peripheral blood lymphocytes and the cells of various solid organs. HHV-6A infection of lymphoid cells induces a number of significant cell responses, including the synthesis of CD4 glycoprotein, interferon-α, tumor necrosis factor-α, and interleukin-1-β. The ability of HHV-6A to induce expression of CD4 in cells not normally expressing it extends the range of cells that can be infected by HIV. In addition, HHV-6A transactivates transcription of HIV, accelerating the rate of cell death in coinfected cells. Latently infected cells are found among the peripheral blood lymphocyte population. HHV-6A was shown to accelerate AIDS progression in an animal model of the disease.

B. Clinical significance

HHV-6 infections resulting in disease are most common in infants and individuals who are immunocompromised.

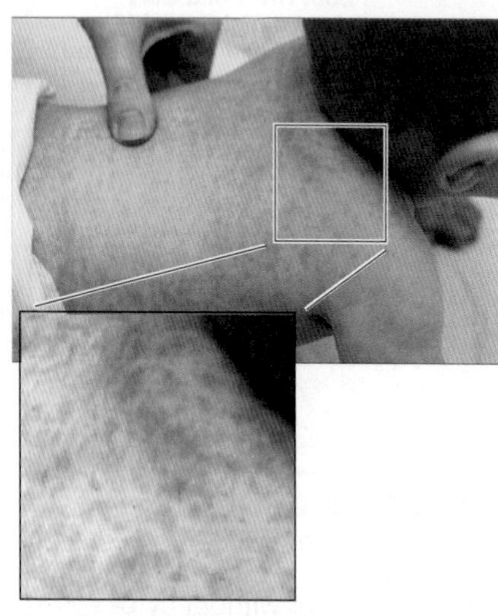

Figure 25.18
Roseola infantum.

1. **Primary infections:** Symptomatic roseola infantum (exanthem subitum) occurs in roughly one third to one half of infants with a primary HHV-6 infection. It is characterized by a high fever of 3 to 5 days' duration, after which a characteristic erythematous macular rash appears on the neck and trunk, resolving after several more days without sequelae (Figure 25.18). HHV-7 infection has been shown to produce an identical clinical picture. Of greater clinical significance is that primary HHV-6 infection of infants is the cause of many acute febrile illnesses and febrile seizures in the absence of the characteristic rash. In some of these cases, HHV-7 has been shown to be the causative agent, whereas, in others, the patient was coinfected with both HHV-6 and HHV-7. Over 20 percent of emergency room visits for febrile illness in infants and one third of febrile seizures are caused by primary infection with HHV-6 and/or HHV-7 (Figure 25.19).

2. **Recurrent infections:** Following immunosuppression for organ transplantation or immunocompromise related to HIV infection, reactivation of latent HHV-6, frequently together with HCMV, has

been associated with sometimes-fatal interstitial pneumonitis, fever, hepatitis, and encephalitis as well as with transplant rejection. The relationship of HHV-6A to AIDS has not been completely elucidated. Three factors may accelerate the progression from early HIV infection to terminal AIDS: 1) HHV-6A broadens the range of cell types infected by HIV by inducing CD4, 2) coinfected cells are killed more rapidly, and 3) extensively disseminated HHV-6A infection frequently occurs in terminal AIDS patients. The most common clinical syndrome associated with HHV-6 in AIDS patients is encephalitis (Figure 25.20).

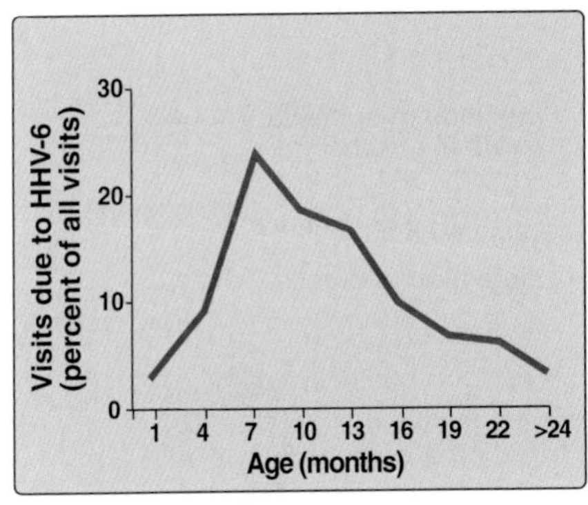

Figure 25.19
Percentage of visits to the emergency department for febrile illness associated with human herpesvirus type 6 (HHV-6).

C. Laboratory identification

A simple diagnostic test for primary infection with HHV-6 or HHV-7 is not available. PCR amplification has been used to demonstrate HHV-6 DNA in the CSF of patients with neurologic disease and in the serum of patients undergoing posttransplant reactivation of a latent infection.

D. Treatment and prevention

Because of its genetic relationship to HCMV, HHV-6 is generally inhibited by the same drugs (ganciclovir, cidofovir, and foscarnet), but extensive clinical trials have not yet been done. In AIDS patients, treatment of the HIV infection appears to reduce the amount of HHV-6 as well. No vaccine is currently available for these viruses.

VII. HUMAN HERPESVIRUS TYPE 8

HHV-8 infection appears not to occur as frequently as the other human herpesviruses in the normal, healthy population. Yet the virus genome and/or viral proteins have been detected in more than 90 percent of patients with KS, but in less than 1 percent of non-KS tissues. The primary method for detection of HHV-8 is PCR amplification.

VIII. EPSTEIN-BARR VIRUS

EBV is most commonly known as the causative agent of IM in young adults. Its initial discovery in association with the childhood disease Burkitt lymphoma (BL) led to its recognition as the first human virus clearly related to a malignancy. More recently, EBV has been associated with several additional human neoplastic diseases.

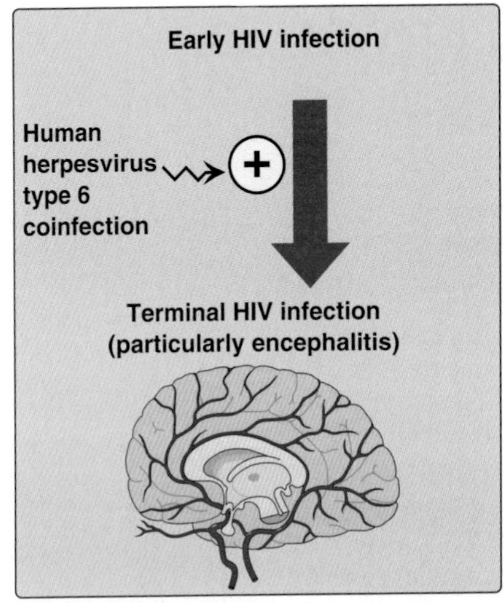

Figure 25.20
Coinfection with human herpesvirus type 6 accelerates the progression of HIV symptoms.

A. Epidemiology and pathogenesis

Most transmission of EBV occurs by intimate contact with saliva that contains virus during both primary infection and in repeated episodes of asymptomatic shedding. The initial site of virus replication appears to be the oropharyngeal epithelium, following which some of the progeny viruses infect B lymphocytes (Figure 25.21). The B-cell receptor for EBV is the complement component C3b receptor. During B-cell infection, only a limited number of early proteins are synthesized. Expression of these gene products results in latency and immortalization of the B cell. The EBV genome is main-

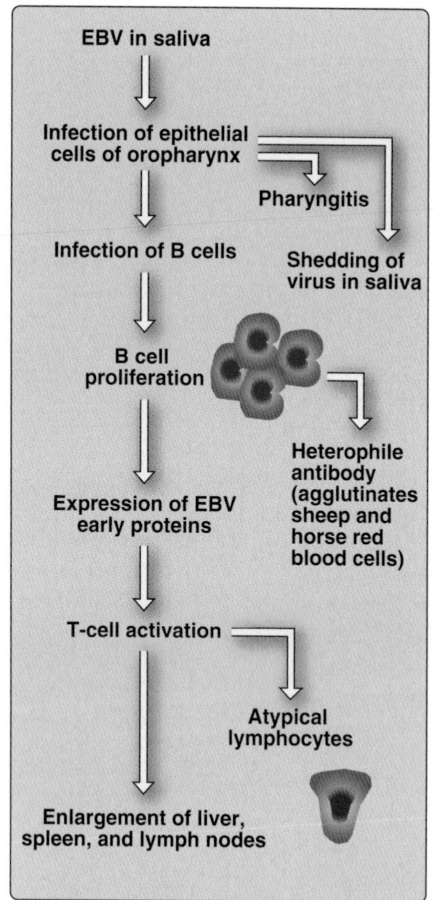

Figure 25.21
Pathogenesis of infectious mononucleosis caused by Epstein-Barr virus (EBV).

tained as a circular plasmid-like form called an episome during latency. One protein that is expressed during latency is called EBNA1, and one of its key functions is to segregate the episomes into daughter cells following cell division. EBV infection of B cells also causes the induction of a number of cellular lymphokines, including B-cell growth factors. In contrast to other herpesviruses, the early genes of EBV induce cell multiplication and immortalization, rather than cell death. Thus, infection induces a polyclonal B-cell proliferation and an accompanying nonspecific increase in total IgM, IgG, and IgA. The IgM class contains heterophile antibodies that agglutinate sheep and horse red blood cells. These antibodies are the basis for the classic diagnostic test for EBV-associated IM (see p. 269).

B. Clinical significance

As stated earlier, primary infection in infancy or childhood is usually asymptomatic, but as many as 50 percent of those infected later in life develop IM. Although B cells are the primary targets of infection as a result of the presence of the EBV-receptor molecule, EBV has more recently been found to be associated with a small number of T-cell malignancies as well. In patients who are immunodeficient or immunosuppressed, the lack of cell-mediated immune control increases the likelihood of lymphoproliferative disorders of various kinds. Throughout life, healthy EBV carriers continue to have episodes of asymptomatic virus shedding. The source of this virus seems to be the productively infected oropharyngeal cells that acquire the virus from latently infected B cells in which the lytic cycle has been activated.

1. **Infectious mononucleosis:** The manifestations and severity of primary EBV infection vary greatly, but the typical IM syndrome appears after an incubation period of 4 to 7 weeks and includes pharyngitis, lymphadenopathy, fever, splenomegaly, and increased levels of liver enzymes in the blood (Figure 25.22). Headache and malaise often precede and accompany the disease, which may last several weeks. Complete recovery may take much longer.

2. **EBV and malignancies:** Following the initial discovery of EBV in association with BL, it has been shown to be associated with a number of other human neoplastic diseases.

   a. **Burkitt lymphoma:** BL was first described in 1958 as a rather unique malignancy of the jaw, found in an unusually high frequency in children in regions of equatorial Africa. BL cells all contain one of three characteristic chromosome translocations. The breakpoints of these translocations are such that the c-myc proto-oncogene on chromosome 8 is constitutively activated. Malarial infection and HIV infection are known risk factors for development of BL.

   b. **Epstein-Barr–associated nasopharyngeal carcinoma:** Nasopharyngeal carcinoma (NPC) is one of the most common cancers in southeast Asia and North Africa and in the Inuit population, but it is less common elsewhere. NPC differs from BL in that there is no characteristic chromosomal alteration, and the cells involved are epithelial in origin. A role for EBV is suggested because all cells of the tumor contain cytoplasmic viral DNA molecules (episomes).

c. **Epstein-Barr virus infections in immunocompromised and immunosuppressed patients:** In BL and NPC, EBV infection appears to be only one step in a multistep, disease-causing process, and its specific role is still not well defined. In contrast, EBV alone appears to be sufficient for induction of B-cell lymphomas in immunocompromised patients, such as transplant recipients and individuals with AIDS, who cannot control the cell multiplication induced by the early proteins. For example, many AIDS patients develop a B-cell malignancy of some type: BL of the sporadic type occurs with high frequency in earlier stages of AIDS progression, whereas non–BL-type lymphoblastic lymphomas are more characteristic in late-stage AIDS patients. Not all of the HIV-associated BL cases contain the EBV genome. AIDS patients infected with EBV may exhibit nonmalignant, white-gray lesions on the tongue ("hairy leukoplakia") as shown in Figure 25.23.

C. Laboratory identification

Atypical lymphocytes (cytotoxic T cells) can be observed in the blood smear of a patient with IM (Figure 25.24). The classic test for IM, the Paul-Bunnell test, is based upon the nonspecific elevation of all Igs, including heterophile antibodies that specifically agglutinate horse and sheep red blood cells, during polyclonal stimulation of B cells by EBV infection. These heterophile antibodies are diagnostic for EBV-related IM, although they are not present in all cases of EBV IM. Antibodies specific for EBV are also produced during infection. IgM and IgG antibodies specific for EBNA1 and capsid proteins can be detected by serological techniques.

D. Treatment and prevention

Although acyclovir inhibits EBV replication, none of the antiherpes drugs have been effective in modifying the course or severity of IM due to EBV or in preventing development of EBV-related B-cell malignancies. Acyclovir has been successful in treating oral hairy leukoplakia, in which the virus is actively replicating in the epithelial cells of the tongue. No vaccine for prevention of EBV infections is currently available. Some properties of the common herpesvirus infections are summarized in Figure 25.25.

IX. POXVIRIDAE

Poxviruses belong to a family of large, genetically complex viruses having no obvious symmetry. Members of this family are widely distributed in nature. The agent of previous medical importance to humans, variola virus, was the cause of smallpox, the first infectious disease to be declared eradicated from the Earth. Among the factors that led to this

A Classic clinical triad of infectious mononucleosis:

- Fever
- Pharyngitis
- Lymphadenopathy
  (usually enlargement of anterior and posterior cervical lymph nodes)

Note: Acute infection is often asymptomatic in children, whereas adolescents and young adults show the typical symptoms of infectious mononucleosis.

B Transmission:

- Exposure to oropharyngeal secretions

C Clinical manifestations of Epstein-Barr–associated infectious mononucleosis by age-group:

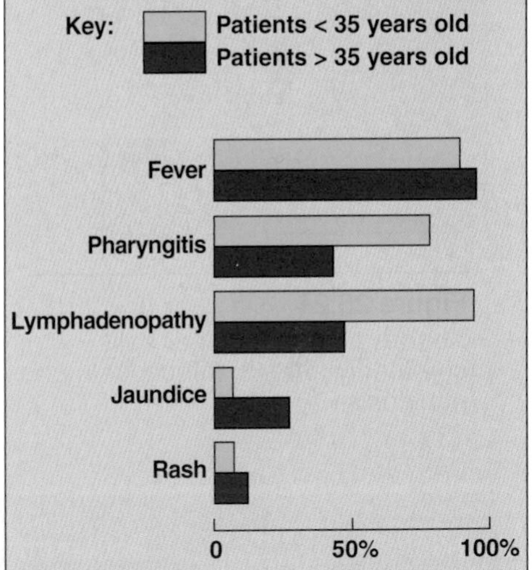

D Incidence of Epstein-Barr–associated infectious mononucleosis:

- Peak incidence occurs between ages 15 and 19 years.
- Incidence is 30 times higher in blacks than whites in the United States.
- No difference in incidence between sexes.
- Ninety percent of the general population shows evidence of previous infection with Epstein-Barr virus.

Figure 25.22
Characteristics of infectious mononucleosis.

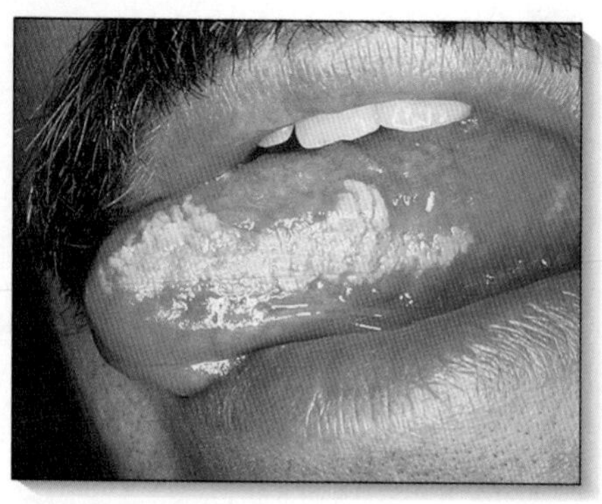

Figure 25.23
Hairy leukoplakia caused by Epstein-Barr virus infection.

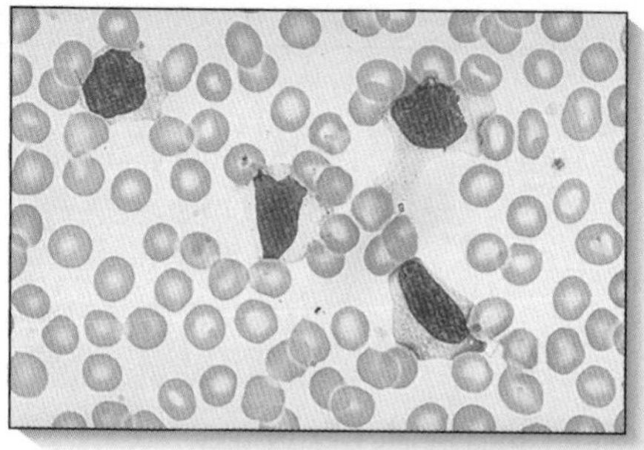

Figure 25.24
Abnormal mononuclear cells commonly seen in infectious mononucleosis.

success are: 1) the availability of an effective, attenuated vaccine; 2) variola's antigenic stability (that is, only a single antigenic type existed); 3) the absence of asymptomatic cases or persistent carriers; 4) the absence of an animal reservoir; and 5) the emotional effect of this highly lethal, disfiguring disease, which helped to galvanize public support of and cooperation in the eradication efforts. The highly effective poxvirus vaccine contains live vaccinia virus (which causes cowpox), and the viral genome is currently being used in attempts to construct vectors carrying immunizing genes from other infectious agents. Finally, the poxvirus, molluscum contagiosum virus (MCV), causes small, wart-like tumors (not to be confused with true warts caused by papilloma virus, see p. 245).

A. Structure and classification of the family

The genome is a single linear molecule of double-stranded DNA, with a coding capacity for more than 200 polypeptides. The virion contains enzymes that are involved in early steps of replication. The vertebrate poxviruses are related by a common nucleoprotein antigen but are otherwise quite distinct. Humans are the natural host for variola and MCV, but monkeypox, cowpox, and several other animal poxviruses can also cause human disease.

B. Replication of the poxviruses

Poxviruses follow the basic replication pattern for DNA viruses (see p. 238), with a few notable exceptions. The most striking of these is that the entire replication cycle takes place in the cytoplasm, the virus providing all of the enzymes (including a viral DNA-dependent RNA polymerase) necessary for DNA replication and gene expression. Final maturation by acquisition of a lipoprotein envelope occurs as the virus buds from the cell. The replication cycle is rapid and results in early shut-off of all cell macromolecular syntheses, causing the death of the cell.

VIRUS	VIRUS SUBFAMILY	CLINICAL MANIFESTATIONS OF PRIMARY INFECTION	CLINICAL MANIFESTATIONS OF RECURRENT INFECTION	SITE OF INITIAL INFECTION	SITE OF LATENCY
Herpes simplex-1	α	**Keratoconjunctivitis, gingivostomatitis, pharyngitis, tonsilitis**	**Herpes labialis ("cold sores")**	**Mucoepithelial**	**Trigeminal sensory ganglia**
Herpes simplex-2	α	**Genital herpes, perinatal disseminated disease**	**Genital herpes**	**Mucoepithelial**	**Lumbar or sacral sensory ganglia**
Varicella-zoster virus	α	**Varicella ("chickenpox")**	**Herpes-Zoster ("shingles")**	**Mucoepithelial**	**Trigeminal and dorsal root ganglia**
Cytomegalovirus	β	**Congenital infection (in utero), mononucleosis-like syndrome**	**Asymptomatic shedding of virus**	**Monocytes, lymphocytes, and epithelial cells**	**Monocytes, lymphocytes**
Epstein-Barr virus	γ	**Infectious mononucleosis, Burkitt lymphoma**	**Asymptomatic shedding of virus**	**Mucosal epithelium, B lymphocytes**	**B lymphocytes**

Figure 25.25
Properties of common herpesvirus infections.

C. Epidemiology and clinical significance

The stages of smallpox are illustrated in Figure 25.26. Although naturally occurring smallpox is no longer a threat, the mutation of one of the animal poxviruses to a form more virulent for humans has continued to be of concern. Human infections with monkeypox are clinically similar to smallpox and, although somewhat less severe, nevertheless have a mortality rate of about 11 percent. Such infections have only been observed where the human population comes into close contact with infected animals. In its natural state, monkeypox is not readily transmitted among humans. MCV infection occurs only in humans, causing benign wartlike tumors on various body surfaces. Usually spread by direct contact, the virus can be spread among adults via sexual contact.

D. Laboratory identification

The unique cellular localization of poxvirus replication has enabled rapid diagnosis by observation of DNA-containing intracytoplasmic inclusion bodies in cells scraped from skin lesions.

E. Treatment and prevention

Although immunization with vaccinia is no longer done routinely, it is still carried out in certain groups, such as the military and laboratory workers. Although one of the safest vaccines in healthy recipients, individuals with eczema may develop a generalized vaccinia rash covering the surface of the body. Immunocompromised patients are likely to develop progressive vaccinia, which has a high mortality rate. Postvaccinal encephalitis, with a mortality of 40 percent, is a rare secondary hazard accompanying vaccination.

F. Smallpox as a biologic weapon

Smallpox is potentially a devastating biologic weapon because it is highly contagious and has a high case fatality rate—more than 30 percent among unvaccinated persons. In 1972, the United States stopped routine vaccination of civilians against smallpox. As a result, more than 40 percent of the population is now susceptible to smallpox infection, with the percentage increasing each year. As a result of Project Bioshield, the United States supported the development of a new-generation smallpox vaccine that would be administered in the event of a bioterrorism attack. The new vaccine (called MVA for modified vaccinia Ankara) contains a mutant form of the vaccinia virus, which cannot replicate in humans. The vaccine is safe, even in immunocompromized individuals, and protective against monkeypox in a primate infection model.

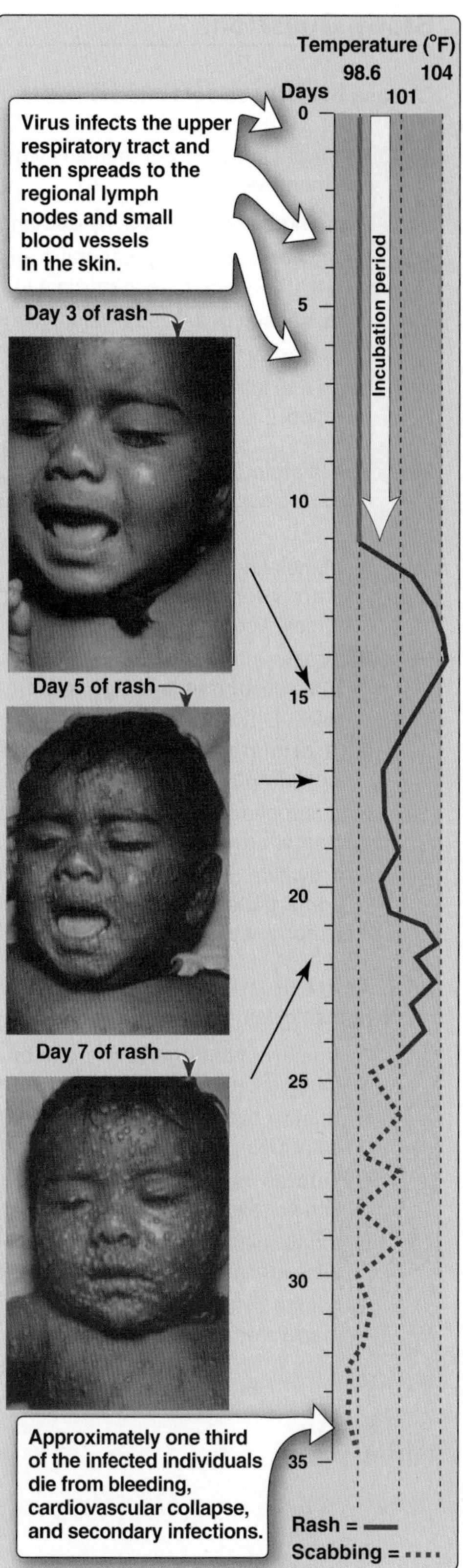

Figure 25.26
Time course of smallpox.

Study Questions

Choose the ONE correct answer.

25.1 The initial infection with human cytomegalovirus most commonly occurs:

A. during early childhood, by exchange of body fluids.
B. *in utero*, by transplacental transmission from a latently infected pregnant woman.
C. by transfer of saliva between young adults.
D. by sexual intercourse.
E. as a result of blood transfusion or organ transplantation.

Correct answer = A. Depending on the population, up to 90 percent have antibody by adulthood. B: The most serious complications of infection are those resulting from transplacental transmission, but this is not the common mode of transmission. C and D: Transmission by kissing or sexual intercourse can occur, but most individuals would have already been infected. E: This mode of transmission has serious consequences in antibody-negative recipients, but most recipients had been infected at an earlier age. More common is reactivation of latent HCMV in recipients who have been immunosuppressed for purposes of transplantation.

25.2 The histological presentation typical of infectious mononucleosis caused by Epstein-Barr virus is due to:

A. stimulation of B-cell proliferation by the Epstein-Barr virus early proteins synthesized in the infected cells.
B. proliferation of cytotoxic T cells responding to Epstein-Barr virus antigens expressed on the surface of infected B cells.
C. a primary humoral immune response to the Epstein-Barr virus infection.
D. macrophages responding to the death of Epstein-Barr virus–infected cells.
E. activation of an oncogene resulting from a chromosome translocation in Epstein-Barr virus–infected lymphocytes.

Correct answer = B. The proliferation of cytotoxic T cells results in the increased numbers of atypical lymphocytes detected in blood smears of Epstein-Barr virus (EBV)-infected patients. A: Polyclonal stimulation of B cells by EBV infection occurs and results in the appearance of the characteristic heterophile antibodies, but it is the cytotoxic T-lymphocyte response that results in atypical lymphocytosis of infectious mononucleosis. C: EBV-specific humoral immune response is not related to lymphocytosis. D: B cells are not killed by infection with EBV. E: Although this is the process that results in EBV-associated Burkitt lymphoma, it occurs only years after the initial virus infection.

25.3 Acyclovir is largely ineffective in the treatment of human cytomegalovirus infections because:

A. human cytomegalovirus exhibits a high rate of mutation in the target enzyme.
B. human cytomegalovirus depends upon the host cell's DNA polymerase for replication of its DNA.
C. human cytomegalovirus lacks the thymidine kinase required for activation of acyclovir.
D. the tissues in which human cytomegalovirus multiplies are largely inaccessible to the drug.
E. human cytomegalovirus codes for an enzyme that inactivates the drug.

Correct answer = C. The specificity of acyclovir derives from its necessary phosphorylation by the herpes simplex virus or varicella-zoster virus thymidine kinase in order to be an active inhibitor of viral DNA synthesis. Human cytomegalovirus (HCMV) does not have a corresponding enzyme. A: HCMV develops resistance to those drugs that are effective, such as ganciclovir and cidofovir, after long-term therapy, but because their mechanisms of action are different, mutants resistant to one are usually not resistant to the other. B: All herpesviruses code for their own DNA polymerase. D: In those cases where access is a problem for treatment of herpesvirus infections, direct inoculation of the drug has been done. E: Resistance to antiherpesvirus drugs has generally involved mutation of the enzyme interacting with the drug, not inactivation of the drug.

Hepatitis B and Hepatitis D (Delta) Viruses

26

I. OVERVIEW

Hepatitis (inflammation of the liver) can be caused by a variety of organisms and toxins. For example, there are many viral diseases that involve some degree of liver damage as a secondary effect (such as infectious mononucleosis caused by the Epstein-Barr virus, see p. 268). However, the viruses referred to as "hepatitis viruses" are those whose pathogenesis specifically involves replication in and destruction of hepatocytes. This chapter describes the only human hepatitis virus that has a DNA genome, hepatitis B virus (HBV) as shown in Figure 26.1. This chapter also discusses the defective agent that sometimes accompanies HBV during infections: the "delta agent," or hepatitis D virus (HDV). With the exception of HBV, hepatitis viruses thus far identified (hepatitis A, C, D, and E viruses) contain RNA and belong to several different families (see Figure 26.1), but the acute disease produced by each is similar. (See pp. 291 and 378 for summaries of hepatitis). Outcome of infection and mode of transmission, however, differ significantly from virus to virus (Figure 26.2). Worldwide, chronic HBV infection affects almost 300 million people, three quarters of whom are in Asia. HBV is a leading cause of chronic hepatitis, cirrhosis, and hepatocellular carcinoma, accounting for 1 million deaths annually.

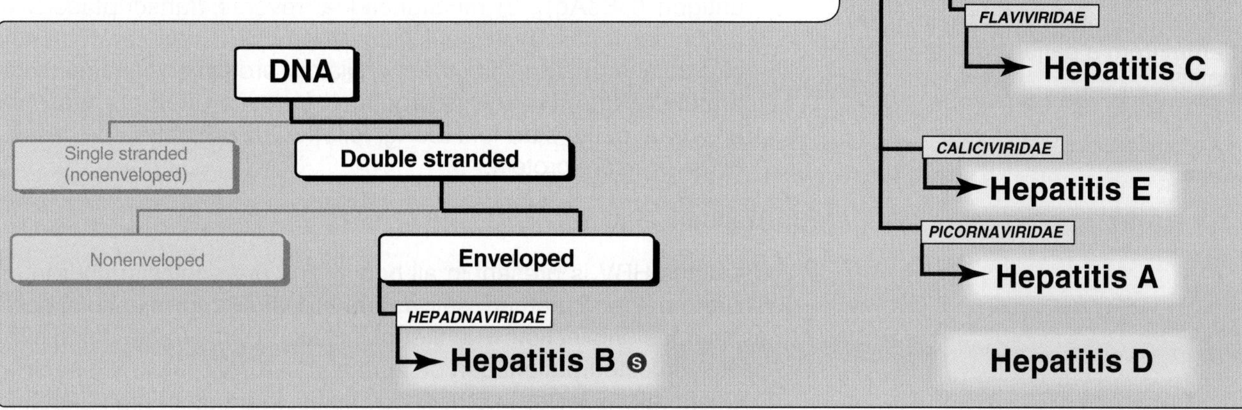

Figure 26.1
Classification of major viral agents causing hepatitis. [Note: Hepatitis D is a defective virus and is classified in its own "floating" genus. Hepatitis A, C, and E are discussed in Chapter 27.] See p. 355 for a summary of this virus.

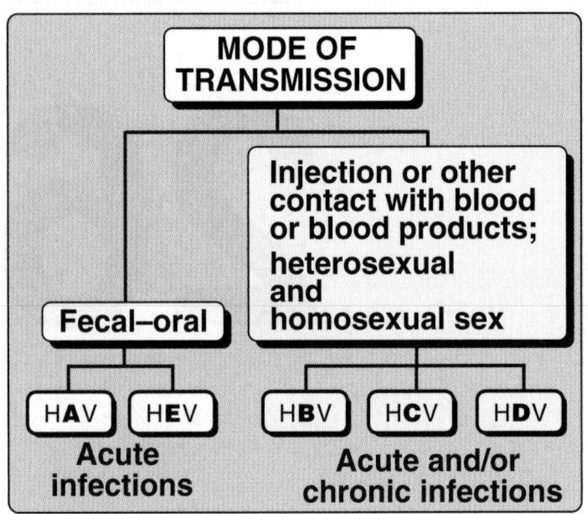

Figure 26.2
Classification of hepatitis viruses based on mode of transmission. HAV, HEV, HBV, HCV, and HDV each refer to the specific hepatitis virus.

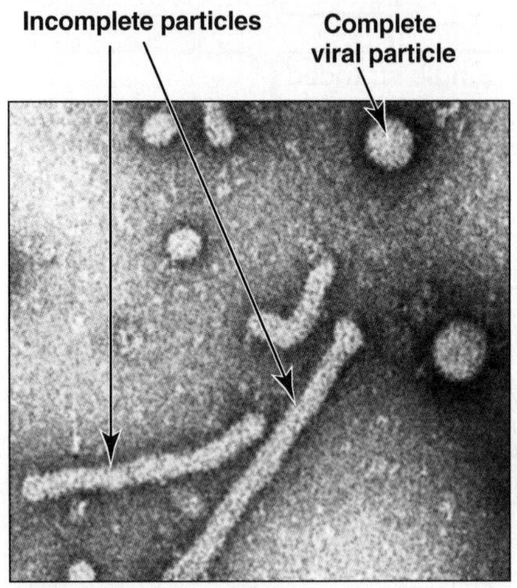

Figure 26.3
Electron micrograph of a fraction of serum from a patient with severe hepatitis.

II. HEPADNAVIRIDAE

The family Hepadnaviridae (hepatotropic DNA viruses) consists of hepatitis-causing viruses with DNA genomes. Each hepadnavirus has a narrow host range in which it produces both acute and chronic, persistent infections, but HBV is the only member of this family that infects humans. Because highly infectious virus is present in the blood of both symptomatic and asymptomatic patients, chronically infected individuals pose a serious threat to all healthcare workers, immunization of whom is generally required. A highly effective vaccine produced in genetically engineered yeast cells is available and included among routine childhood immunizations (see p. 39). Biologically, HBV is unique among human disease agents in that replication of the DNA genome proceeds via an RNA intermediate, which, in turn, is "reverse transcribed" by a viral enzyme homologous to the retrovirus reverse transcriptase (see p. 296). However, although retroviruses package an RNA genome, Hepadnaviridae package a DNA genome.

A. Structure and replication of hepatitis B virus

The HBV virion, historically referred to as the "Dane particle," consists of an icosahedral nucleocapsid enclosed in an envelope (Figure 26.3).

1. **Organization of the hepatitis B virus genome:** The short HBV DNA genome is unusual in that it is a partly single-stranded, partly double-stranded, noncovalently closed, circular DNA molecule (that is, one strand is longer than the other) as shown in Figure 26.4. The short "plus" strand, which can vary in length, is only 50 to 80 percent as long as its complementary strand, the "minus" strand. The circular structure of the genome is maintained by base-pairing the strands at one end. A summary of HBV replication is shown in Figure 26.4.

2. **Viral proteins:** The four proteins encoded by viral DNA are: 1) the core protein [hepatitis B nucleocapsid core antigen (HBcAg)]; 2) envelope protein [a glycoprotein referred to as hepatitis B surface antigen (HBsAg)]; 3) multifunctional reverse transcriptase/DNA polymerase, which is complexed with the DNA genome within the capsid; and 4) a nonstructural regulatory protein designated the "X protein." [Note: HBeAg is produced from an alternate start site upstream of the start for HBcAg, followed by proteolytic processing of the pre-core protein.]

B. Transmission

Infectious HBV is present in all body fluids of an infected individual. Therefore, blood, semen, saliva, and breastmilk, for example, serve as sources of infection. The titer of infectious virus in the blood of an acutely infected patient can be as high as 10^8 virus particles per ml but generally is lower in other body fluids. In areas of high endemicity (for example, Southeast Asia, Africa, and the Middle East), the majority of the population becomes infected at or shortly after birth from a chronically infected mother or from infected siblings. Individuals infected at this young age have a significant chance of becoming chronic carriers, maintaining the high prevalence of virus in the population. Individuals infected at an early age also have an increased risk of developing hepatocellular carcinoma later in life. In the United States and other Western countries, the carrier rate is much lower, and primary infection rarely occurs in newborns. Hepatitis B is primarily a disease of infants in developing nations, and, in Western countries, it is mostly confined to adults who usually contract HBV infection through sexual intercourse or blood exposure from shared needles during injecting drug use.

C. Pathogenesis

Fully differentiated hepatocytes are the primary cell type infected by HBV. The primary cause of hepatic cell destruction appears to be the cell-mediated immune response, which results in inflammation and necrosis. The cells involved are cytotoxic T cells, which react specifically with the fragments of nucleocapsid proteins (HBcAg and HBeAg), expressed on the surface of infected hepatocytes. This response also contributes to control of the infection by eliminating virus-producing cells. Enhanced natural killer cell activity, as well as production of interferon-γ also contributes to limiting the extent of infection. Anti-HBsAg antibody, which is the neutralizing antibody, does not appear until well into the convalescence period, when it may aid in clearing any remaining circulating free virus. More importantly, this antibody provides protection against reinfection. However, it is this same humoral antibody that is considered the source of extrahepatic damage seen in 10 to 20 percent of patients, through the formation and deposition of HBsAg/anti-HBsAg antibody immune complexes and the consequent activation of complement.

D. Clinical significance: acute disease

HBV is important medically and in public health, not only as the cause of acute liver disease but also as the cause of chronic, persistent infections that can result in the eventual death of infected individuals from cirrhosis and liver cancer. Chronically infected people serve as the reservoir of transmissible virus in the population. In most individuals, the primary infection is asymptomatic and resolves as a result of an effective cell-mediated immune response (Figure 26.5).

1. **Phases in acute hepatitis B virus infections:** Following infection, HBV has a long but variable incubation period of between 45 and 120 days. Following this period, a pre-icteric (prejaundice) phase occurs, lasting several days to a week. This is characterized by mild fever, malaise, anorexia, myalgia, and nausea. The acute, icteric phase then follows and lasts for 1 to 2 months. During this phase, dark urine, due to bilirubinuria, and jaundice (a yellowish coloration of mucous membranes, conjunctivae, and skin) are evident. There usually is an enlarged and tender liver as well. In 80 to 90 percent of adults, a convalescent period of several more months is followed by complete recovery (Figure 26.6).

2. **Monitoring the course of acute hepatitis B virus infection:** Whereas liver-specific enzymes are important clinical determinants of all of

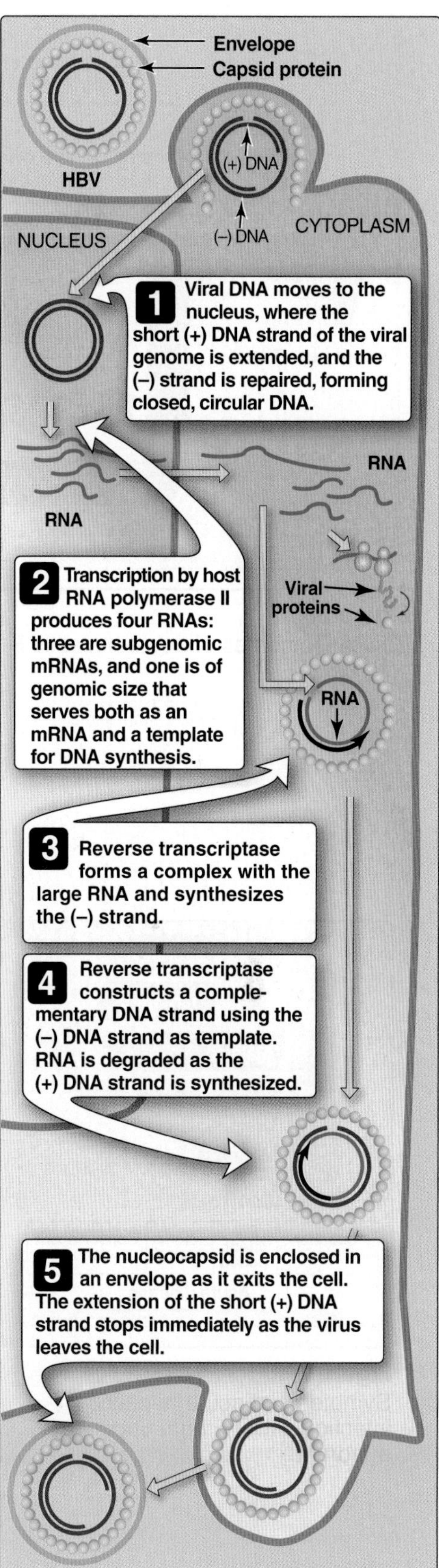

Figure 26.4
Replication of hepatitis B virus (HBV).

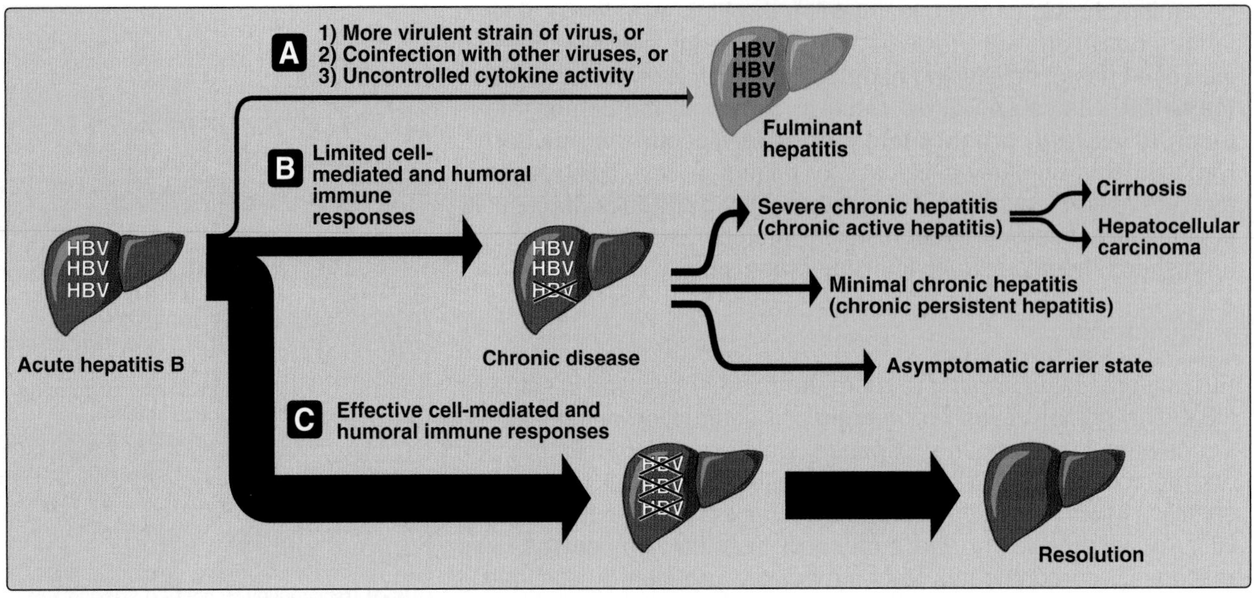

Figure 26.5
Clinical outcomes of acute hepatitis B virus (HBV) infection.

the viral hepatitides, HBV infection is unusual in that the quantities of virions and virion components in the blood are so great that the time course of their appearance and clearance, along with that of the antibodies directed against them, serve as convenient markers of the stage of the disease and the likely future course.

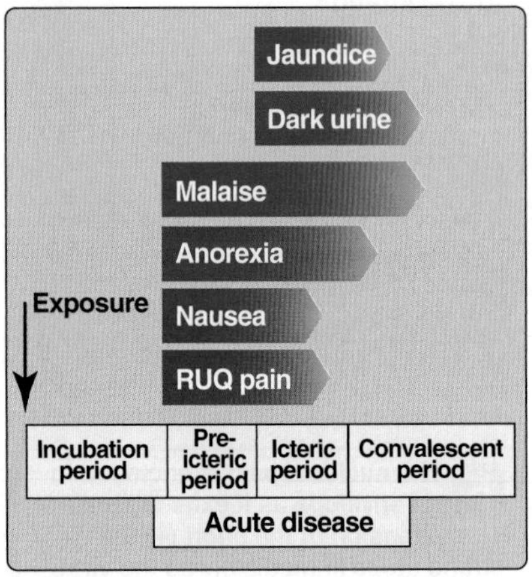

a. **Appearance of viral antigens:** During the incubation period, HBsAg and hepatitis B e antigen (HBeAg) are the first indicators of HBV infection to appear in the blood (Figure 26.7). Their presence indicates an active infection but does not distinguish between acute and chronic infections. Next, viral DNA, viral DNA polymerase, and complete virions become detectable. These continue to increase during the acute disease phase, when a patient's blood has the highest titer of infectious virus.

Jaundice
Dark urine
Malaise
Anorexia
Exposure
Nausea
RUQ pain
Incubation period
Pre-icteric period
Icteric period
Convalescent period
Acute disease

Figure 26.6
Symptoms of acute hepatitis B infection. RUQ = right upper quadrant.

b. **Appearance of antiviral antibodies:** Antibodies to HBcAg rise concurrently with liver enzymes in the serum, whereas anti-HBeAg antibodies and, still later, anti-HBsAg antibodies do not appear until the beginning of convalescence (generally after the respective antigens have disappeared from the blood, see Figure 26.7). In those patients in whom the infection resolves completely, anti-HBcAg and anti-HBsAg antibodies remain present for life, providing immunity to reinfection. Continued presence of HBsAg beyond 6 months and absence of anti-HBsAg indicates that the infection has become chronic (Figure 26.8). A patient suffering chronic HBV infection is capable of eliciting an immune response against HBsAg but the anti-HBs antibody levels are too low to be detectable. All of the antibody that develops is complexed with circulating HBsAg.

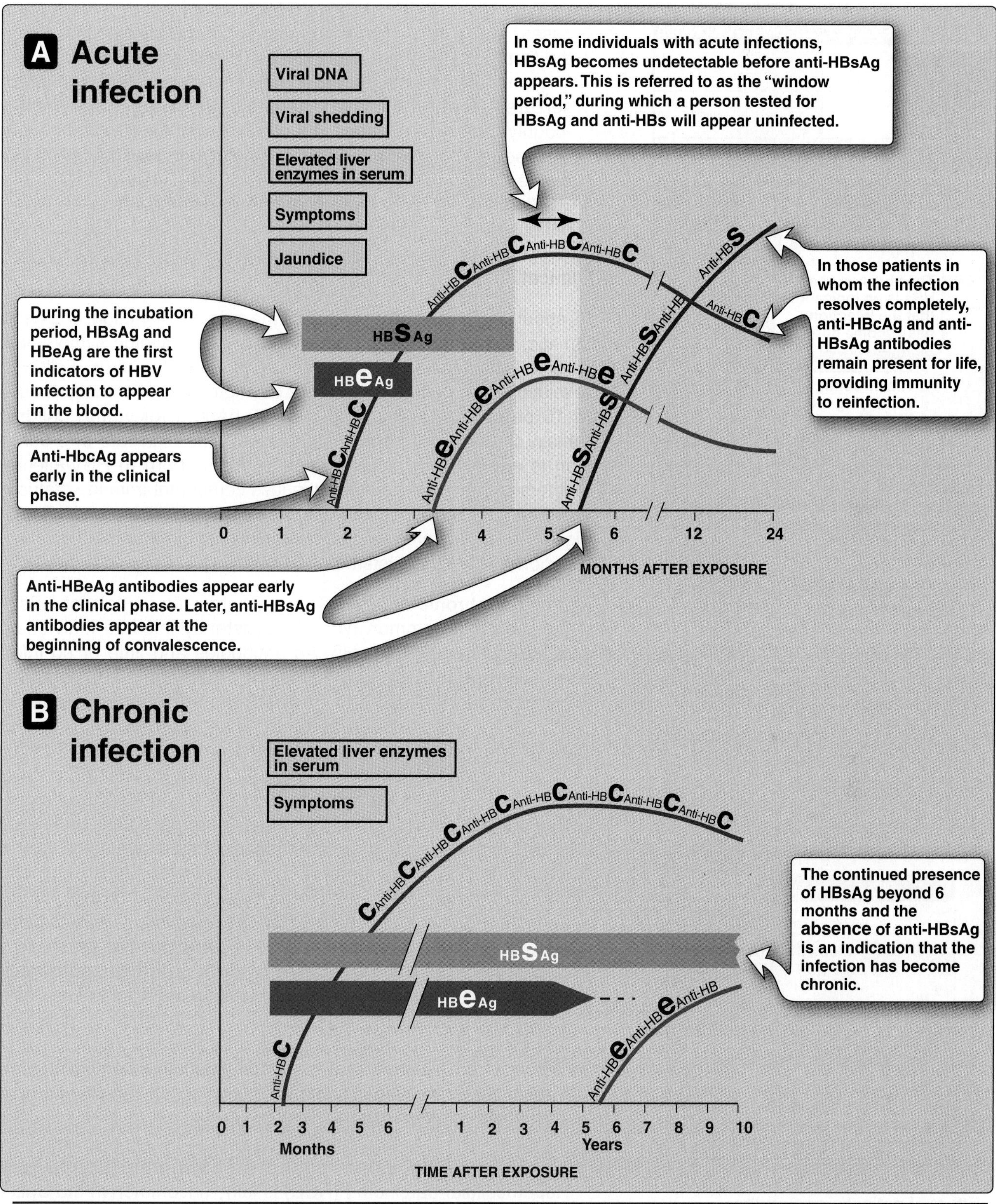

Figure 26.7
Typical course of hepatitis B virus infection. A. Acute infection. B. Chronic infection. HBsAg = hepatitis B surface antigen; HBeAg = hepatitis B e antigen; HBcAg = hepatitis B nucleocapsid core antigen; anti-HBsAg, anti-HBeAg, and anti-HBcAg each refer to antibodies to the corresponding antigen.

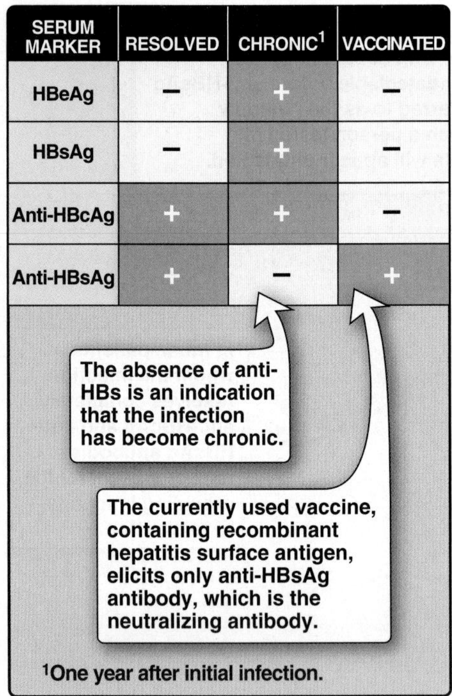

SERUM MARKER
RESOLVED
CHRONIC¹
VACCINATED
HBeAg
HBsAg
Anti-HBcAg
Anti-HBsAg
The absence of anti-HBs is an indication that the infection has become chronic.
The currently used vaccine, containing recombinant hepatitis surface antigen, elicits only anti-HBsAg antibody, which is the neutralizing antibody.
¹One year after initial infection.

Figure 26.8
Interpretation of serologic markers of hepatitis B infection. HBeAg = hepatitis B e antigen; HBsAg = hepatitis B surface antigen; anti-HBcAg, and anti-HBsAg each refer to antibodies to the corresponding antigen.

3. **Fulminant hepatitis:** In 1 to 2 percent of acute symptomatic cases, much more extensive necrosis of the liver occurs during the first 8 weeks of the acute illness. This is accompanied by high fever; abdominal pain; and eventual renal dysfunction, coma, and seizures. Termed fulminant hepatitis, this condition is fatal in roughly 8 percent of cases. Although it is not clear why the acute disease takes this course, a more highly virulent strain of HBV, coinfection with HDV or another hepatitis virus (for example, HCV), and/or perhaps an uncontrolled immune response by the patient, are thought to play a role.

E. Clinical significance: chronic disease

In about two thirds of individuals, the primary infection is asymptomatic, even though such patients may later develop symptomatic chronic liver disease, indicating persistence of the virus. Following resolution of the acute disease (or asymptomatic infection), about 2 to 10 percent of adults and over 25 percent of young children remain chronically infected (Figure 26.9). The high rate of progression to chronic liver disease seen in infants born to HBV-infected mothers is thought to relate to the less competent immune status of newborns. Adults with immune deficiencies also have a considerably higher probability of developing chronic infection than do individuals with normal immune systems.

1. **Types of chronic carriers:** The asymptomatic carriers of HBsAg are the most common type of persistently infected individuals. They usually have anti-HBeAg antibodies and little or no infectious virus in their blood (see Figures 26.7B and 26.8). Later progression of liver damage or recurrence of acute episodes of hepatitis is rare in such patients. Those carriers with minimal chronic hepatitis (formerly, "chronic persistent hepatitis") are asymptomatic most of the time but have a higher risk of reactivation of disease, and a small fraction does progress to cirrhosis. Severe chronic hepatitis (formerly, "chronic active hepatitis") results in more frequent exacerbations of acute symptoms, including progressive liver damage, potentially leading to cirrhosis and/or hepatocellular carcinoma (see below), chronic fatigue, anorexia, malaise, and anxiety. These symptoms are accompanied by active virus replication and the corresponding presence of HBeAg in the blood. Serum levels of liver enzymes and bilirubin are increased to varying degrees, reflecting the extent of necrosis. The risk of developing cirrhosis is highest in those carriers with more frequent recurrences of acute disease and those in whom HBeAg is not cleared from the blood, indicating continuing virus replication. Overall life expectancy is significantly shorter in those individuals with cirrhosis.

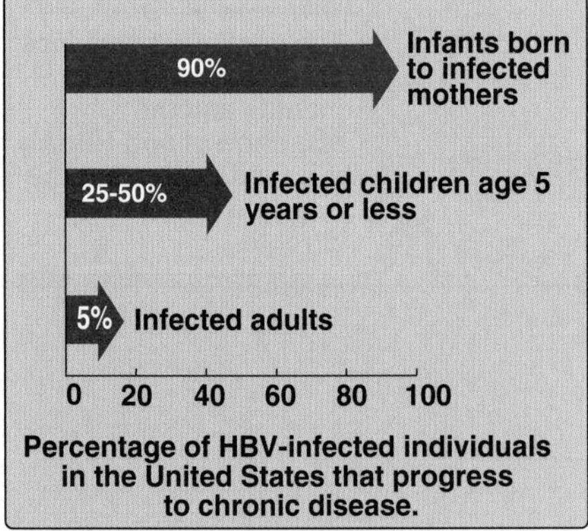

Figure 26.9
Effect of patient's age on the tendency of acute hepatitis B virus (HBV) infection to progress to chronic disease.

2. **Development of hepatocellular carcinoma (hepatoma):** Hepatocellular carcinoma (HCC) is fairly uncommon in the United States, whereas it is 10 to 100 times more frequent in areas of high HBV endemicity. In all populations, males experience a higher rate of chronic HBV infections; a higher rate of progression to cirrhosis; and, ultimately, a higher rate of HCC, for which the male-to-female ratio is 6:1. HCC typically appears many years

after the primary HBV infection, and the tumor itself is rather slow growing and only occasionally metastasizes. Clinically, a patient with HCC exhibits weight loss, right-upper-quadrant pain, fever, and intestinal bleeding. Although there is no doubt that chronic HBV infection greatly increases the risk of HCC, the mechanisms relating HBV and HCC are not completely understood. By causing continuing liver necrosis, followed by regeneration of the damaged tissue, chronic HBV infection provides the opportunity for chromosomal rearrangements and mutations. Because HBV is a DNA virus, integration of the viral genome into the host's chromosome can also result in mutation and insertion, with concomitant changes in cell growth control. In fact, recent evidence suggests that the HBV gene product X is actively involved in tumor formation, following integration of the gene into the host's chromosome. HCC is a major cause of death due to malignancy worldwide, and its distribution parallels HBV incidence (approximately 80 percent of primary HCCs occur in HBV-infected individuals).

F. Laboratory identification

The purpose of diagnostic laboratory studies of patients with clinical hepatitis is to, first, determine which hepatitis virus is the cause of the illness and, second (for HBV), to distinguish acute from chronic infections. The diagnosis of hepatitis is made on clinical grounds, coupled with biochemical tests that evaluate liver damage. Elevations of aminotransferases, bilirubin, and prothrombin time all contribute to the initial evaluation of hepatitis. Commonly known as ELISA, enzyme-linked immunosorbent assay (see p. 27), and other immunologic techniques for detection of viral antigens and antibodies are the primary means to distinguish among HAV, HBV, HCV, and HDV. In addition, identification of the presence or absence of specific antiviral antibodies and viral antigens permits differentiating between acute and chronic HBV infections (see Figure 26.7).

G. Treatment

1. **Acute hepatitis:** Specific treatment for acute hepatitis B is usually not needed, because, in about 95 percent of adults, the immune system controls the infection and eliminates the virus within about 6 months. Although drug therapy is usually only required in chronic hepatitis, it may also be required with the acute severe liver impairment that accompanies fulminant hepatitis.

2. **Chronic hepatitis:** The goal for treatment in patients with chronic hepatitis is to reduce the risk of progressive chronic liver disease and other long-term complications from chronic HBV, such as cirrhosis and hepatocellular carcinoma. The most commonly used drugs include interferon-α or one of a large number of nucleoside/nucleotide antiviral agents (Figure 26.10). The drug of choice depends on multiple factors, including the antibody and antigen status of the patient. Pegylated interferon-α (if the patient does not have cirrhosis), entecavir, or tenofovir are often preferred for initial treatment. The two most commonly used markers to monitor the efficacy of therapy are seroconversion to anti-HBeAg and sustained suppression of HBV DNA.

Interferon and pegylated interferon

- Many side effects
- No drug resistance
- Administered subcutaneously
- High cost
- Pegylated interferon, a long acting interferon taken once a week, is given for one year.[1]

[1]This is in contrast to the other hepatitis treatments, which are given by mouth for many years until a desired response is achieved.

Lamivudine

- High rate of drug resistance
- Low cost
- Many years of experience confirm its safety, including its use during pregnancy

Adefovir

- Potential nephrotoxicity
- Activity against lamivudine-resistant HBV

Entecavir

- High cost
- Has potent antiviral activity and a low rate of drug resistance

Telbivudine

- High rate of drug resistance
- Role as primary therapy is limited

Tenofovir

- Potential nephrotoxicity
- First line treatment in treatment-naïve patients, and in patients with lamivudine, telbivudine, or entecavir resistance, preferably as additional treatment in these patients

Figure 26.10
Drugs used in the treatment of hepatitis B. HBV = hepatitis B virus.

Routine immunization
- All infants and previously unvaccinated children by age 11 years

Increased risk of hepatitis B
- People with multiple sexual partners
- Sexual partner or household contacts of HBsAg-positive people
- Men who have sex with men
- Users of illicit injection drugs
- Travelers to regions of endemic disease
- People occupationally exposed to blood or body fluids
- Hemodialysis patients
- Patients receiving clotting-factor concentrates

Figure 26.11
Candidates for hepatitis B virus immunization. HBsAg = hepatitis B surface antigen.

H. Prevention

The purpose of controlling the spread of HBV infection is to prevent cases of acute hepatitis. An additional goal is to decrease the pool of chronically infected individuals who serve as reservoirs for infectious virus in the population and who are at greatly increased risk for developing cirrhosis and liver cancer. The availability of a highly effective vaccine has led to a several-pronged approach: 1) protection of those adults who are at risk because of lifestyle or occupation, 2) protection of newborns from infection by transmission from HBV-positive mothers (important because of the high rate of resulting chronic infections, see p. 274), and 3) protection of siblings and other children from infection by chronically infected family members.

1. **Active immunization:** HBsAg is used to prepare vaccines conferring protection because antibody to the virion component neutralizes infectivity. HBV vaccination is now recommended as a routine infant immunization, as is the immunization of adolescents who were not given the vaccine as infants. An unusual feature of the recommended vaccination schedule is to initiate an HBV vaccine series at birth. This is possible because infants have adequate antibody response to neonatal vaccination with the HBV vaccine. Other individuals who are candidates for HBV vaccine are shown in Figure 26.11.

2. **Passive immunization:** Hepatitis B immunoglobulin (HBIG) is prepared from the blood of donors having a high titer of anti-HBsAg antibody. Immediate administration of HBIG is recommended as the initial step in preventing infection of individuals accidentally exposed to HBV-contaminated blood by needlestick or other means and of those exposed to infection by sexual contact with an HBV-positive partner. In such cases, this should be accompanied by a course of active immunization with the hepatitis B vaccine. It is also strongly recommended that pregnant women should be screened for HBsAg. Infants born to mothers who are HBV positive are given HBIG plus hepatitis B vaccine at birth, followed by additional doses of vaccine at 1 and 6 months.

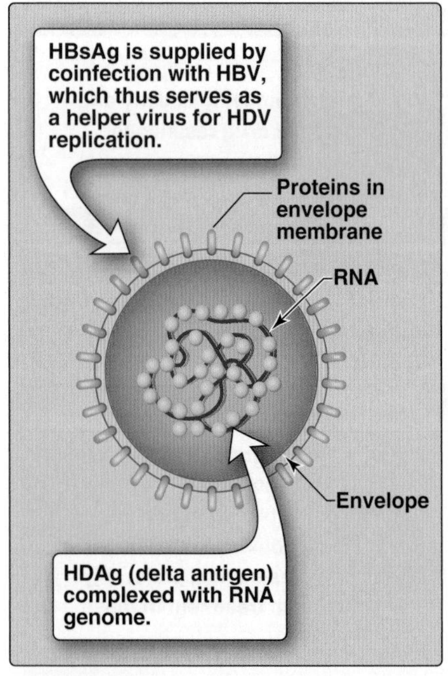

Figure 26.12
Structure of hepatitis D virus. HBsAg = hepatitis B surface antigen.

III. HEPATITIS D VIRUS (DELTA AGENT)

HDV is found in nature only as a coinfection with HBV. It is significant because its presence results in more severe acute disease, with a greater risk of fulminant hepatitis and, in chronically infected patients, a greater risk of cirrhosis and liver cancer.

A. Structure and replication

HDV does not fall into any known group of animal viruses. It has a circular, single-stranded RNA genome with negative polarity that codes for one protein (delta antigen), with which the genome is complexed in the virion (Figure 26.12). In the infectious particle, the nucleoprotein complex is enclosed within an envelope containing

HBV-coded HBsAg. Thus, HDV requires HBV to serve as a helper virus for infectious HDV production. The HDV RNA genome is replicated and transcribed in the nucleus by cellular enzymes, whose specificity is probably modified by complexing with the delta protein. [Note: This phase of HDV replication is independent of HBV, whose only helper function is to supply HBsAg for the envelope.]

B. Transmission and pathogenesis

Because HDV exists only in association with HBV, it can be transmitted by the same routes. However, it does not appear to be transmitted sexually as frequently as HBV or HIV (human immunodeficiency virus). Pathologically, liver damage is essentially the same as in other viral hepatitides, but the presence of HDV usually results in more extensive and severe damage.

C. Clinical significance

HDV disease can occur in one of three variations (Figure 26.13). First, simultaneous primary coinfection with both HBV and HDV can cause an acute disease that is similar to that caused by HBV alone, except that, depending on the relative concentrations of the two agents, two successive episodes of acute hepatitis may occur. The risk of fatal fulminant hepatitis caused by the presence of HDV is also considerably higher than with HBV alone. The likelihood of progression to the second variation of HDV disease (chronic coinfection with HBV) is greatly increased as well. In this case, cirrhosis and HCC or death due to liver failure also develop more frequently than with HBV infection alone. The third variation, primary HDV infection of a chronically HBV-infected individual, leads to an episode of severe acute hepatitis after a short incubation period and develops into chronic HDV infection in more than 70 percent of cases. Again in this situation, the risk of acute hepatitis becoming fulminant is greatly increased, and the persistent infection is often the severe chronic type (see p. 276).

D. Laboratory identification

The immunologically based methods used to diagnosis HBV are also applied to HDV. The delta (D) antigen and immunoglobulin M antibodies against it can be detected in serum. The presence of HDV RNA in serum or liver tissue, as detected by hybridization with or without the use of reverse transcriptase and polymerase chain reaction amplification, is an indicator of active infection.

E. Treatment and prevention

No treatment specific for HDV infection is available. Because HDV depends on coinfection with HBV, the approaches for preventing HBV infection are also effective in preventing HDV infection. There is no vaccine specifically for HDV. Therefore, those who are chronically infected with HBV can only be protected from HDV infection by limiting chances for exposure. Those who are protected against HBV infection through vaccination will not be affected by HDV.

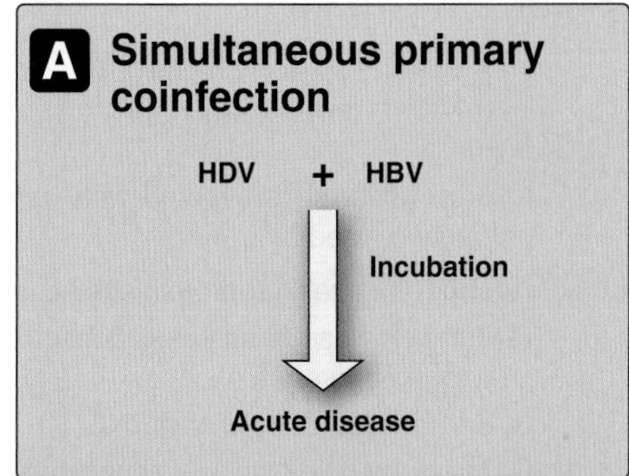

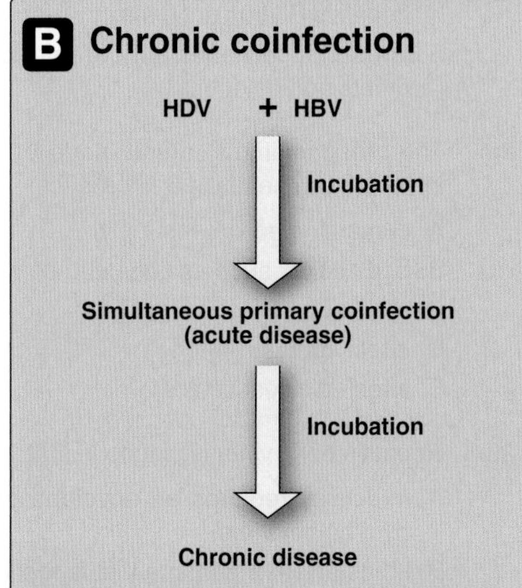

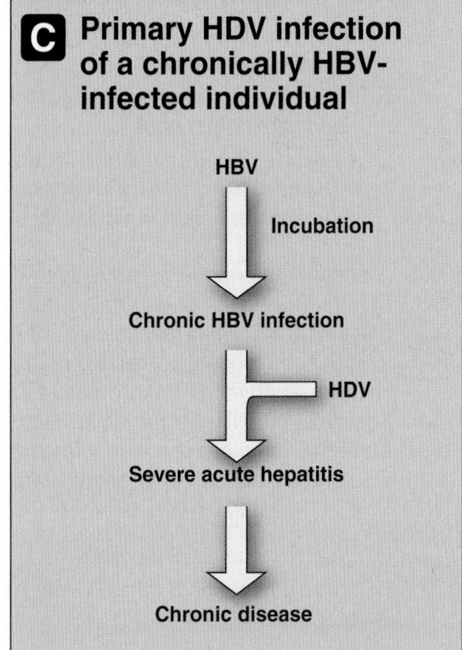

Figure 26.13
Consequences of hepatitis D virus (HDV) infection. HBV = hepatitis B virus.

Study Questions

Choose the ONE correct answer.

26.1 Killing of liver cells infected with hepatitis B virus is primarily caused by:

A. shut-off of cellular protein synthesis.
B. intracytoplasmic accumulation of hepatitis B virus antigen aggregates.
C. degradation of cellular mRNA.
D. attack by cytotoxic T lymphocytes directed against hepatitis B virus antigens.
E. virus-induced aberrant chromosome rearrangements and deletions.

Correct answer = D. There is no evidence that hepatitis B virus (HBV) infection is cytocidal. Protein synthesis is not shut off, and mRNA is not degraded in infected cells. Accumulation of HBV proteins is not seen, rather, they are actively exported. Although chromosome damage is observed in cells of primary hepatocellular carcinoma, it is not characteristic of nonmalignant infected liver cells.

26.2 The most common natural mode of transmission of infection with hepatitis B virus is via:

A. contaminated water supply.
B. body fluids, such as urine and semen.
C. respiratory droplets.
D. direct contact.
E. infected insect vectors.

Correct answer = B. Hepatitis B virus is found at high levels in all body fluids, which results in transmission from mother to newborn, from sibling to sibling, and through sexual intercourse as well as by infection by virus-containing blood. Contaminated water or food is the typical source of hepatitis A and E infection.

26.3 Hepatitis delta virus is unique in that:

A. infectivity requires an envelope protein provided by a helper virus.
B. it has an RNA genome that is replicated by a replicase supplied by a coinfecting helper virus.
C. its mRNA is transcribed by a transcriptase supplied by a helper virus.
D. the virion contains a reverse transcriptase provided by a helper virus.
E. it encodes a protein delta antigen (HDAg) that replaces helper virus glycoproteins in the envelopes of helper virus particles.

Correct answer = A. The only function of the hepatitis B virus (HBV) helper is to supply the envelope. B: Genome replication requires a cell RNA polymerase, presumably modified by the hepatitis D virus (HDV) delta protein such that it can use the HDV RNA as a template. C: Transcription likewise depends on cell enzymes. D: The virion contains only the delta protein. E: HDAg is complexed with the RNA genome in the HDV virion and is not found in the HBV virion.

26.4 A patient suffering from hepatitis underwent a battery of laboratory tests to determine the cause of the disease. The following results were obtained from serological and biochemical testing of the patients serum: HBsAg positive, HBeAg positive, anti-HBcAg IgM positive, anti-HBsAg negative, HDV RNA negative, elevated liver enzymes. From these results, how would you diagnose this patient's infection?

A. Acute hepatitis B disease
B. Chronic hepatitis B disease
C. Chronic hepatitis B disease with hepatitis D superinfection
D. Acute hepatitis D disease
E. Chronic hepatitis D disease

Correct answer = A. The presence of HBs (surface) and HBe antigens is consistent with early or acute hepatitis B virus (HBV) disease. Antibodies against HBsAg have not yet developed, and immunoglobulin (Ig) M against HBcAg (nucleocapsid core) occurs early in the course of infection. The IgM isotype subsequently switches to IgG during convalescence. The absence of hepatitis D virus (HDV) RNA indicates that this person is not superinfected with HDV. D and E are incorrect because HDV does not infect alone but requires HBV as a helper virus. Thus, a person who has infection caused by HDV must be simultaneously infected with HBV.

Positive-strand RNA Viruses

27

I. OVERVIEW

Viruses with a positive-strand RNA genome (that is, one that can serve as a messenger RNA in the infected cell) include the viral families *Picornaviridae*, *Togaviridae*, *Flaviviridae*, *Caliciviridae*, and *Coronaviridae*. The viruses in these families cause a broad spectrum of diseases but share the following features: 1) they replicate in the cytoplasm; 2) genomic RNAs serve as messenger RNAs and are infectious; 3) genomic RNAs are nonsegmented; 4) virions do not contain any enzymes; and 5) virus-specified proteins are synthesized as polyproteins that are processed by viral and cellular proteases, giving rise to individual viral proteins. Some positive-strand RNA viruses are enveloped, whereas others are not. Figure 27.1 summarizes the positive-strand RNA viruses discussed in this chapter.

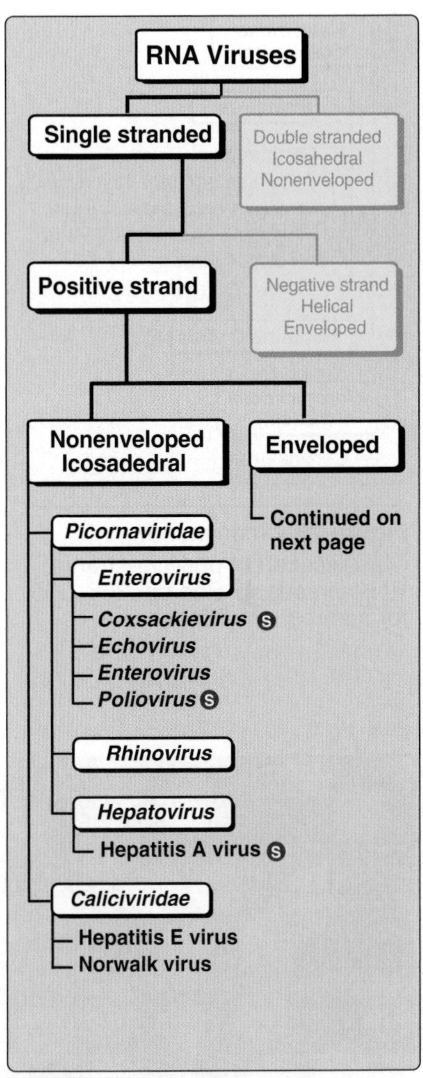

Figure 27.1
Classification of positive-strand RNA viruses (continued on next page). See p. 363 for summaries of these viruses.

II. PICORNAVIRIDAE

Picornaviruses are small, naked (nonenveloped), icosahedral viruses (Figure 27.2), which contain a single-stranded, nonsegmented RNA genome and four structural proteins. *Picornaviridae* are divided into five genera: enteroviruses, rhinoviruses, cardioviruses, aphthoviruses, and hepatoviruses. *Cardiovirus* species cause encephalitis and myocarditis in mice, whereas *Aphthovirus* species is represented by "foot-and-mouth" disease virus, which infects cattle. *Enterovirus*, *Rhinovirus*, and *Hepatovirus* species cause a wide variety of clinical syndromes in humans. Although the most intensively studied picornavirus is poliovirus, what has been learned about the structure and replication of poliovirus also applies in large measure to the other viruses in this family.

A. *Enterovirus*

More than seventy enteroviruses have been identified. Currently, as new enteroviruses are identified, they are not assigned to one of these groups but are simply given numerical designations (for example, enterovirus 68, enterovirus 69, and so forth).

1. **Epidemiology:** Individuals are infected with enteroviruses by ingestion of contaminated food or water. Enteroviruses are stable at the low pH of the stomach, replicate in the gastrointestinal (GI) tract, and are excreted in the stool. Thus, these viruses are said to be transmitted by the fecal–oral route. The virus can replicate in a

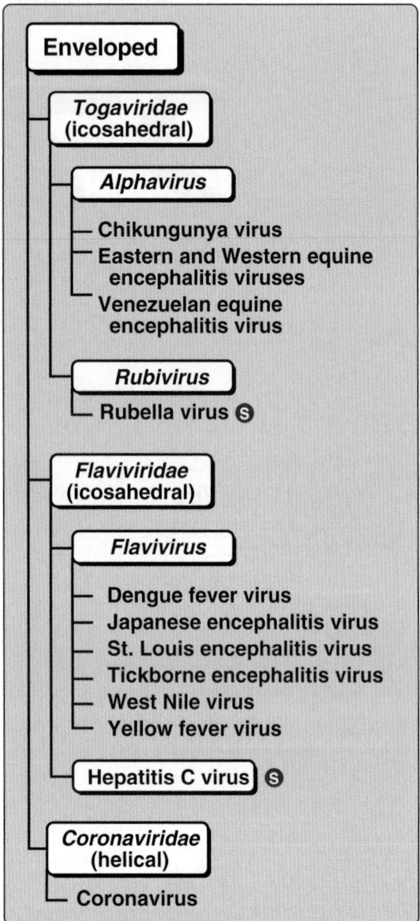

Figure 27.1 (continued)
Classification of positive-strand RNA viruses. Ⓢ See pp. 366, 355 for summaries of these viruses.

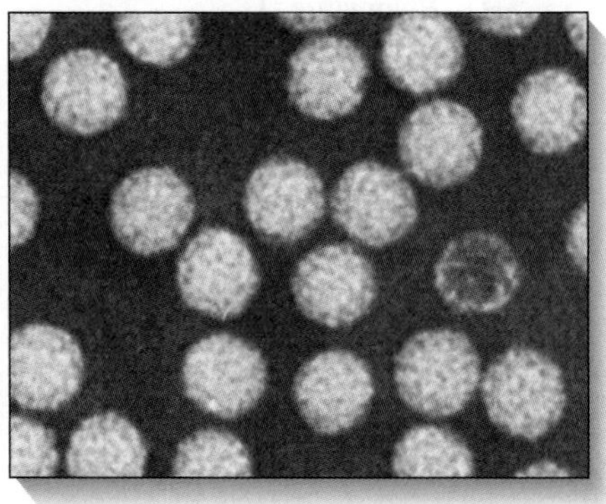

Figure 27.2
Poliovirus, a type of *Picornavirus*, is one of the simplest and smallest viruses.

variety of tissues. For example, after replicating in the oropharynx and intestinal tract lymphoid tissue, enteroviruses can enter the bloodstream and, thereby, spread to various target organs (for example, poliovirus spreads to the central nervous system [CNS]). Although the great majority of infections are asymptomatic, infection, whether clinical or subclinical, usually results in protective immunity. Enteroviruses account for an estimated 10 to 15 million symptomatic infections per year in the United States.

2. **Viral replication:** Enteroviruses bind to specific receptors on host cell surfaces. For example, poliovirus binds to a receptor that is a member of the immunoglobulin (Ig) supergene family of proteins. Cells lacking these specific receptors are not susceptible to infection.

   a. **Mechanism of genome replication:** This is the same process as described for Type I RNA viruses (see p. 239): Namely, the incoming parental RNA serves as the template for a genome-size, negative-strand RNA, and this, in turn, serves as a template for multiple copies of progeny positive-strand RNA.

   b. **Translation:** *Enterovirus* RNA contains a single, long, open reading frame. Translation of this message results in the synthesis of a single, long polyprotein, which is processed by viral proteases into structural proteins and nonstructural proteins, including the viral RNA polymerase needed to synthesize additional copies of the viral genome.

3. **General clinical significance of enterovirus infections:** All enteroviruses can cause CNS disease. For example, enteroviruses are currently the major recognizable cause of acute aseptic meningitis syndrome, which refers to any meningitis (infectious or noninfectious) for which the cause is not clear after initial examination plus routine stains and cultures of the cerebrospinal fluid (CSF). Viral meningitis is a common infection in the United States, with an estimated 75,000 cases each year. Viral meningitis can usually be distinguished from bacterial meningitis because: 1) the viral disease is milder; 2) there is an elevation of lymphocytes in the CSF, rather than the elevated neutrophils seen in bacterial meningitis; and 3) the glucose concentration in the CSF is not decreased. Viral meningitis occurs mainly in the summer and fall, affecting both children and adults. The treatment is symptomatic, and the course of the illness is usually benign. Viruses can be isolated from the stool or from various target organs (CNS in meningitis cases and from conjunctival fluid in conjunctivitis cases). Evidence of infection can also be obtained by demonstration of a rise in antibody titer against a specific enterovirus. No antiviral drugs are available for treatment of infections caused by *Enterovirus* species.

4. **Clinical significance of poliovirus infection:** Poliomyelitis is an acute illness in which the poliovirus selectively destroys the lower motor neurons of the spinal cord and brainstem, resulting in flaccid, asymmetric weakness or paralysis. In the United States, no cases of paralytic poliomyelitis caused by wild-type poliovirus

have occurred in more than 20 years. The few cases of polio that occur (less than 10 per year) are all caused by the reversion to virulence of the virus in the live-attenuated Sabin polio vaccine (see below). In countries with low immunization rates, paralytic polio continues to occur. There are only three countries that remain polio endemic: Afganistan, Pakistan, and Nigeria. The number of countries is down significantly from 125 in 1988. Notably, India was polio free for the first time in 2011. Although this represents significant progress toward the goal of eradicating polio from the world, in 2009–2010, 23 previously polio-free countries were reinfected due to importation of the virus.

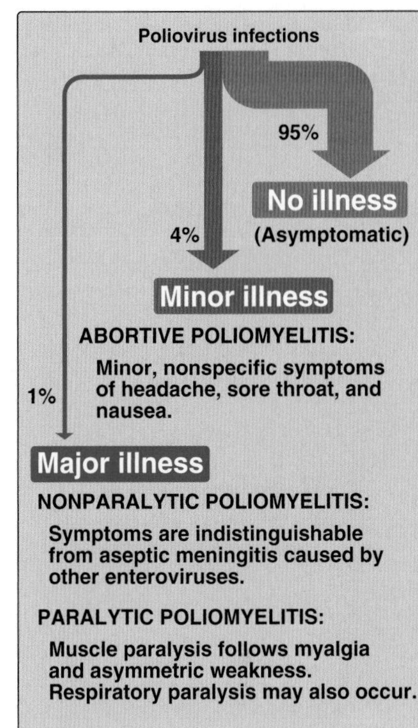

Figure 27.3
Clinical outcomes of infection with poliovirus.

a. **Transmission and pathogenesis:** Poliovirus infections may follow one of several courses: 1) asymptomatic infection, which occurs in 90 to 95 percent of cases and causes no disease and no sequelae; 2) abortive infection; 3) nonparalytic infection; or 4) paralytic poliomyelitis (Figure 27.3). The classic presentation of paralytic poliomyelitis is flaccid paralysis, most often affecting the lower limbs. This is a result of viral replication in, and destruction of, the lower motor neurons in the anterior horn of the spinal cord (Figure 27.4). Respiratory paralysis may also occur, following infection of the brainstem. Poliomyelitis should be considered in any unimmunized person with the combination of fever, headache, neck and back pain, asymmetric flaccid paralysis without sensory loss, and lymphocytic pleocytosis (an increase in the number of lymphocytes in the spinal fluid).

b. **Prognosis:** Permanent weakness is observed in approximately two thirds of patients with paralytic poliomyelitis. Complete recovery is less likely when acute paralysis is severe, and patients requiring mechanical ventilation because of respiratory paralysis rarely recover without some permanent disability.

c. **Postpoliomyelitis syndrome:** Approximately 20 to 30 percent of patients who partially or fully recover from paralytic poliomyelitis experience a new onset of muscle weakness, pain, atrophy, and fatigue 25 to 35 years after the acute illness.

d. **Treatment and prevention:** Specific antiviral agents for the treatment of poliomyelitis are not available. Management, therefore, is supportive and symptomatic. Vaccination is the only effective method of preventing poliomyelitis (see p. 40). Poliomyelitis can be prevented by either live-attenuated (Sabin) or killed (Salk) polio vaccines. These vaccines have led to the elimination of wild-type polio from Western Europe, Japan, and the Americas. Killed polio vaccine has no adverse effects, whereas live polio vaccine may undergo reversion to a virulent form while it multiplies in the human intestinal tract and cause vaccine-associated paralytic poliomyelitis in those receiving the vaccine. Because the small numbers of cases of paralytic poliomyelitis in the United States since 1979 were due to vaccine-derived strains, the CDC changed its recommendation for routine polio vaccination to killed (inactivated) polio vaccine (IPV) in 2000.

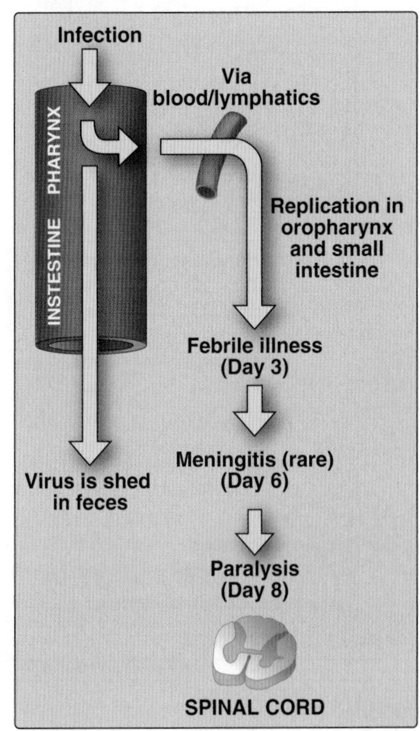

Figure 27.4
Central nervous system invasion by poliovirus.

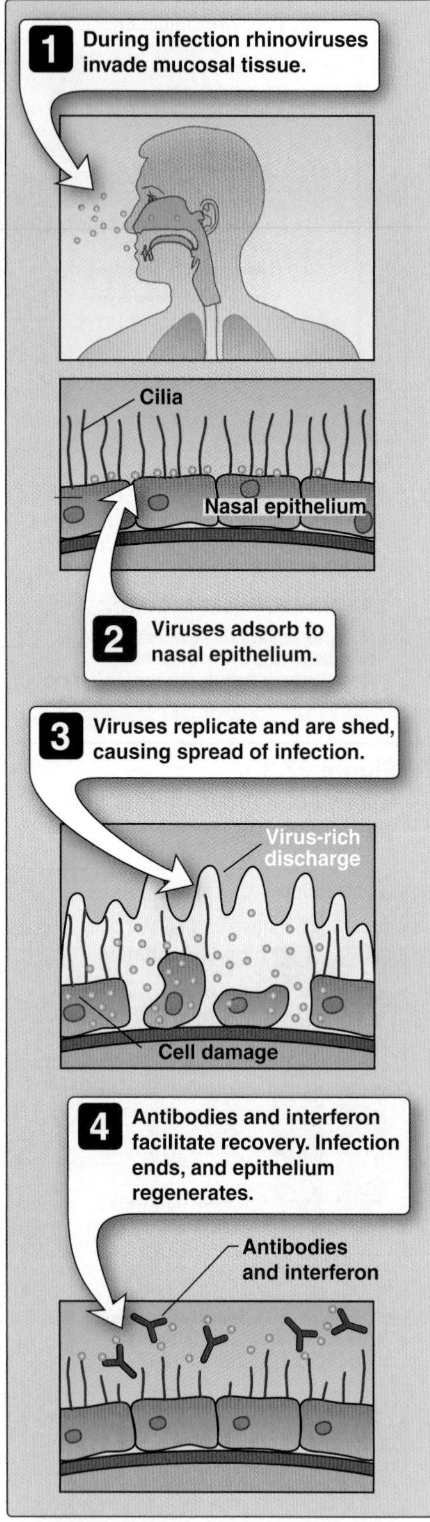

Figure 27.5
Pathogenesis of the common cold showing stages from infection to recovery.

5. **Clinical significance of coxsackievirus and echovirus infections:** These give rise to a large variety of clinical syndromes, including meningitis, upper respiratory infections, gastroenteritis, herpangina (severe sore throat with vesiculoulcerative lesions), pleurisy, pericarditis, myocarditis, and myositis.

6. **Clinical significance of enteroviruses 70 and 71 infections:** These have been associated with severe CNS disease. A particularly acute form of extremely contagious hemorrhagic conjunctivitis has also been associated with enterovirus 70.

B. *Rhinovirus*

Rhinoviruses cause the common-cold syndrome (Figure 27.5). They differ in two important respects from enteroviruses. First, whereas enteroviruses are acid stable (they must survive the acid environment of the stomach), rhinoviruses are acid labile. Second, rhinoviruses, which replicate in the nasal passages, have an optimal temperature for replication that is lower than that of enteroviruses. This permits rhinoviruses to replicate efficiently at temperatures several degrees below body temperature. Rhinovirus replication is similar to that of the poliovirus (see p. 284). Because there are more than 100 serotypes of rhinoviruses, development of a vaccine is impractical. Studies have shown that in addition to being spread by respiratory droplets, rhinoviruses can also be spread by hand-to-hand contact. Therefore, hand washing at appropriate intervals can be a useful preventive measure.

C. *Hepatovirus*

The sole member of this genus is hepatitis A virus (HAV). Although at one time HAV was also known as enterovirus 72, sufficient differences have been found between HAV and the enteroviruses to warrant placing HAV in a genus by itself. HAV, of which there is only one serotype, causes viral hepatitis. As with the enteroviruses, transmission is by the fecal–oral route, and the virus is shed in the feces. For example, a common mode of transmission of the virus is through eating uncooked shellfish harvested from sewage-contaminated water. The main site of replication is the hepatocyte. Viral replication results in severe cytopathology, and liver function is significantly impaired (Figure 27.6). In contrast to most other picornaviruses, HAV grows poorly in tissue culture. The prognosis for patients with acute hepatitis A is generally favorable, and the development of persistent infection and chronic hepatitis is uncommon. HAV infection is most common in developing countries with poor sanitation (Figure 27.7). Prevention depends on taking measures to avoid fecal contamination of food and water. Immune globulin has been used for many years, mainly as postexposure prophylaxis. Vaccines prepared from whole virus inactivated with formalin are now available. HAV vaccination is recommended for children over age 1 year and for persons traveling to developing countries. A combination vaccine (Twinrix) is available to protect against both hepatitis A and hepatitis B virus infection.

III. CALICIVIRIDAE

Caliciviruses are small, nonenveloped, spherical particles. Each contains a single-stranded, nonsegmented RNA genome, and a single species of capsid protein. In contrast to the picornaviruses, the caliciviruses genome contains three open reading frames. Norovirus is the prototype human calicivirus. There are at least four strains of human caliciviruses.

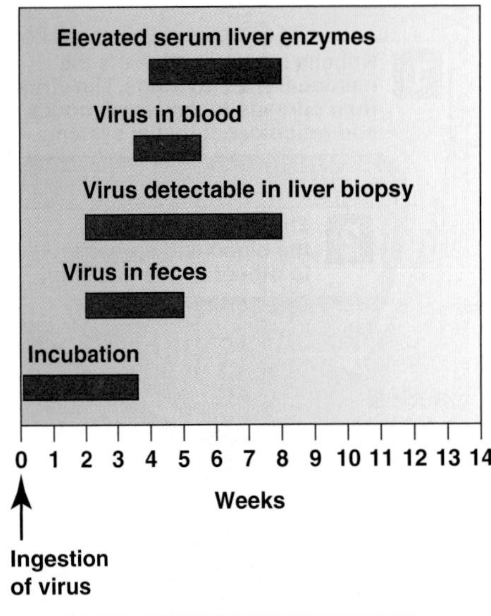

Figure 27.6
Time course of hepatitis A infection.

A. Caliciviruses

Norovirus (formerly known as Norwalk-like virus) replicates in the GI tract and is shed in the stool. Infection by the Norovirus is by the fecal–oral route, following ingestion of contaminated food or water, by person-to-person contact, or by contact with contaminated surfaces. Norovirus is a major cause of epidemic acute gastroenteritis, particularly at schools, camps, military bases, prisons, and other closed environments such as cruise ships. It affects primarily adults and school-age children but not infants. The clinical presentation is characterized by nausea, vomiting, and diarrhea. Symptoms last 24 to 48 hours, and the disease is self-limited. Radioimmunoassays and ELISA (enzyme-linked immunosorbent assay) tests are available for the detection of antiviral antibodies (see p. 27). No specific antiviral treatment is available. Careful attention to hand washing and measures to prevent contamination of food and water supplies should reduce the incidence of these infections.

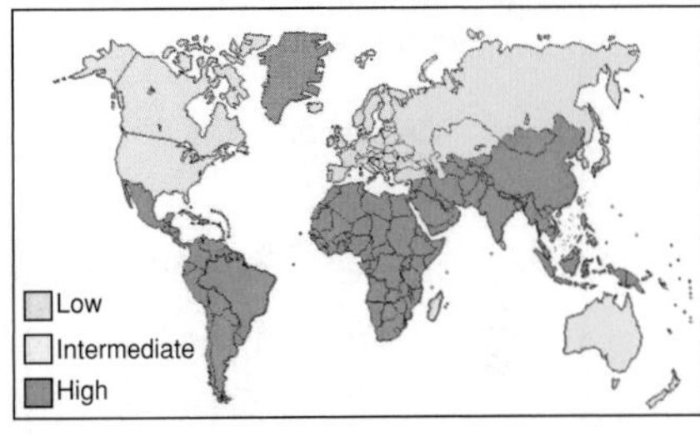

Figure 27.7
Distribution of hepatitis A virus infection worldwide.

B. Hepatitis E virus (HEV)

HEV is a nonenveloped, single-stranded RNA virus. It is a major cause of enterically transmitted, waterborne hepatitis in developing countries. The peak incidence is in young adults, and the disease is especially severe in pregnant women, in whom death can result from HEV infection. Viral RNA can be detected in the feces of infected individuals by RT-PCR (see p. 29), and nearly all serologically confirmed epidemics of HEV can be attributed to fecally contaminated water. Apart from epidemic situations, the diagnosis of HEV cannot be made in an infected individual solely on clinical grounds. However, specific tests are available to detect antibodies to HEV. The signs and symptoms are similar to those seen with other forms of acute viral hepatitis, but, as with hepatitis A, progression to chronic hepatitis is not seen. Interestingly, in regions of the world where HEV is rarely, if ever, diagnosed, antibodies to HEV can still be found. Neither antiviral treatment nor vaccine is currently available.

IV. TOGAVIRIDAE

The togaviruses are enveloped, icosahedral viruses that contain a positive-sense, single-stranded RNA genome and generally three structural proteins. The capsid (C) protein encloses the viral RNA, forming the nucleocapsid, and the two other proteins (E1 and E2) are glycoproteins that form the hemagglutinin-containing viral spikes that project from the lipid bilayer. The family *Togaviridae* is divided into two genera: *Alphavirus* and *Rubivirus*.

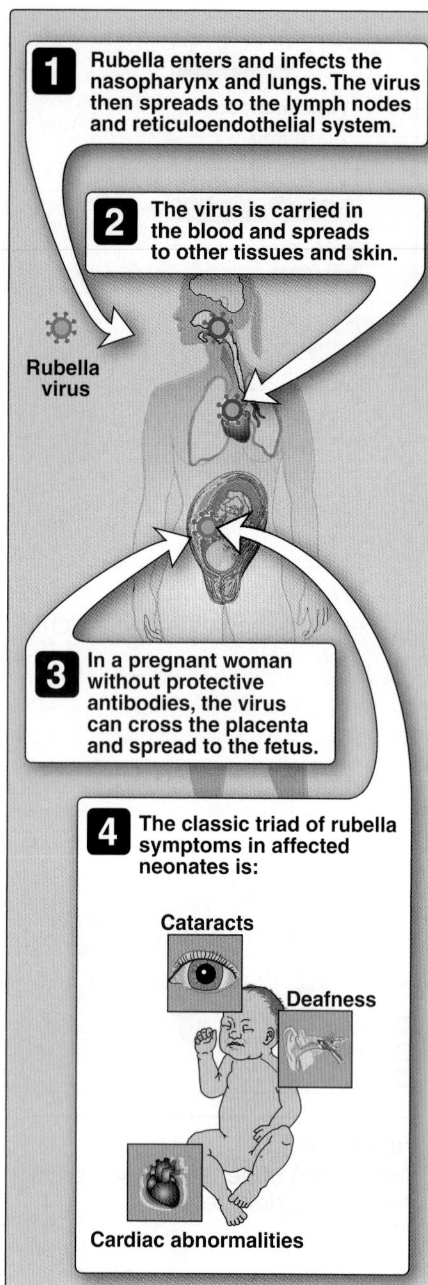

1 Rubella enters and infects the nasopharynx and lungs. The virus then spreads to the lymph nodes and reticuloendothelial system.
2 The virus is carried in the blood and spreads to other tissues and skin.
Rubella virus
3 In a pregnant woman without protective antibodies, the virus can cross the placenta and spread to the fetus.
4 The classic triad of rubella symptoms in affected neonates is:
Cataracts
Deafness
Cardiac abnormalities

Figure 27.8
Pathology of rubella virus infection.

A. *Alphavirus*

The alphaviruses, of which there are approximately 26, are arthropod-borne viruses (arboviruses), which are transmitted to humans and domestic animals by mosquitoes. All alphaviruses share a common group antigen. Some arboviruses were initially isolated from horses, hence, the word "equine" in their names (see below).

1. **Epidemiology and pathogenesis:** Alphaviruses have a broad host range, being able to replicate in organisms that are widely separated phylogenetically, such as mosquitoes and humans. Following inoculation of an *Alphavirus* by a mosquito, the patient is observed to have a viremia, following which the virus may be seeded in various target organs (for example, the CNS in the encephalitis viruses).

2. **Viral replication:** Following attachment to the cell surface, the virus is internalized by receptor-mediated endocytosis. Like the picornaviruses, genome replication is as described for Type I RNA viruses (see p. 239).

3. **Clinical significance:** Several different clinical syndromes are associated with *Alphavirus* infections of humans. These include: 1) acute encephalitis (Eastern and Western equine encephalitis viruses), 2) acute arthropathy (Chikungunya virus), and 3) a febrile illness with a flulike syndrome (Venezuelan equine encephalitis virus). However, the majority of infections are subclinical and can be diagnosed only by the demonstration of an immune response.

4. **Laboratory identification:** This is generally accomplished by the demonstration of a rise in antibody titer (that is, comparing acute and convalescent sera). The virus can also be isolated from CSF, blood, or tissue. IgM antibody specific for the pathogen can be detected in the CSF of patients suffering from acute infection.

5. **Prevention:** The most important measure for prevention of infections caused by *Alphavirus* is control of the mosquito vector population. A Venezuelan equine encephalitis vaccine is available.

B. *Rubivirus*

The sole member of the *Rubivirus* genus is rubella virus. The structure and replication of rubella virus are basically as described for the alphaviruses (see p. 287). Respiratory secretions of an infected person are the primary vehicles for rubella virus transmission. Rubella causes a mild clinical syndrome that is characterized by a generalized maculopapular rash and occipital lymphadenopathy. [Note: This is known as "German measles," not to be confused with "measles" (rubeola), caused by the measles virus (see p. 313).] In most cases, these symptoms may be hardly noticeable, and the infection remains subclinical. For this reason, the only reliable evidence for a prior infection with rubella virus is the demonstration of antirubella antibodies. The clinical significance of rubella lies not in the primary infection described above but, rather, in the severe damage possible to the developing fetus (especially in the first trimester) when a woman is infected during pregnancy (congenital rubella). This damage can include congenital heart disease; cataracts; hepatitis; and abnormalities related to the CNS, such as mental retardation, motor dysfunction, and deafness (Figure 27.8). Fetal damage resulting from rubella infection is preventable by use of the live attenuated rubella vaccine (see p. 41) that is included with the routine childhood vaccinations. This vaccine, which has few complications, is effective in preventing congenital rubella because it reduces the reservoir of the virus in the childhood populations and also ensures that women reaching childbearing age are immune to rubella infection. The vaccine should not be given to women who are already pregnant or to immunocompromised patients, including babies. In the United States, rubella outbreaks often begin among infected persons from countries where rubella is not included in routine immunizations.

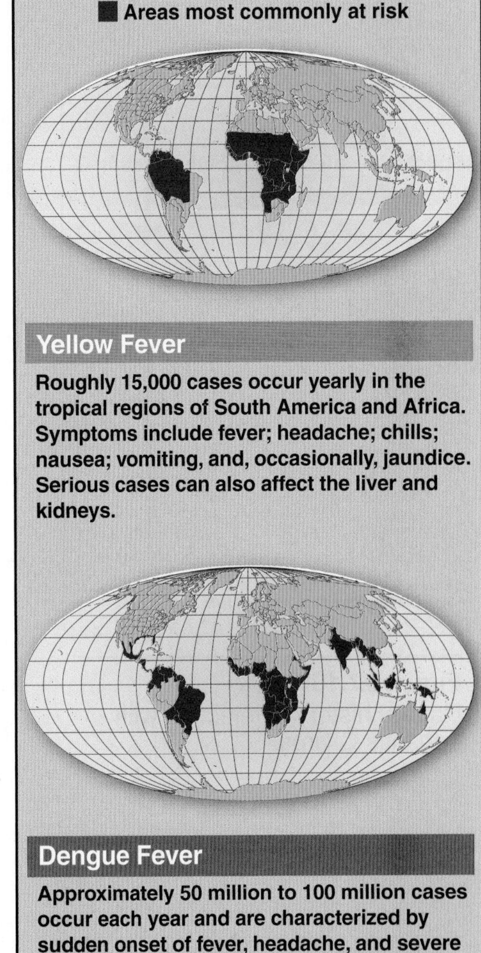

Areas most commonly at risk
Yellow Fever
Roughly 15,000 cases occur yearly in the tropical regions of South America and Africa. Symptoms include fever; headache; chills; nausea; vomiting, and, occasionally, jaundice. Serious cases can also affect the liver and kidneys.
Dengue Fever
Approximately 50 million to 100 million cases occur each year and are characterized by sudden onset of fever, headache, and severe myalgia. Severe dengue may lead to shock, hemorrhaging, and death.

Figure 27.9
Global distribution of yellow fever and dengue fever.

V. FLAVIVIRIDAE

The members of this family are enveloped viruses that contain a single-stranded RNA genome and three structural proteins. The capsid (C) protein and the viral RNA form the icosahedral nucleocapsid, and the other two proteins are envelope associated. Currently, the family *Flaviviridae* is divided into three genera: *Flavivirus*, Hepatitis C virus, and *Pestivirus*. However, the viruses in the genus *Pestivirus* (classical swine fever virus and bovine viral diarrhea virus) are only of veterinary interest.

A. *Flavivirus*

The genus Flavivirus comprises more than sixty viruses. These include many viruses of medical importance, such as yellow fever, St. Louis encephalitis, Japanese encephalitis, dengue fever viruses, and West Nile virus, all of which are mosquito transmitted. Tickborne encephalitis virus is, of course, transmitted by ticks. [Note: Like the viruses in the *Alphavirus* genus of the family *Togaviridae* (see p. 287), most of the viruses in this genus are, therefore, arboviruses.] All of the viruses in the genus *Flavivirus* share a common group antigen.

1. **Epidemiology and pathogenesis:** As arboviruses, the medically important members of this genus are transmitted to humans by the bite of an infected mosquito or tick. These viruses are maintained in nature by replicating alternately in an arthropod vector and a vertebrate host. Figure 27.9 shows the global distributions of yellow fever and dengue fever.

2. **Replication:** Following attachment to the cell surface, the virus is taken up by receptor-mediated endocytosis (see Figure 23.9). Replication of the viral RNA is as described for Type I RNA viruses (see p. 239). Only one species of viral mRNA, the genomic RNA, is found in infected cells. It is translated into a single, long polyprotein, which is processed by virus-coded and cellular proteases, giving rise to three structural and seven nonstructural proteins. Nucleocapsids are formed in the cyto-

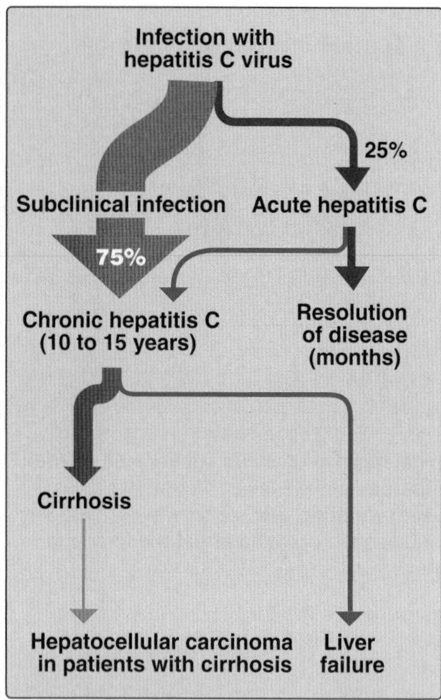

Figure 27.10
Natural history of infection with hepatitis C virus.

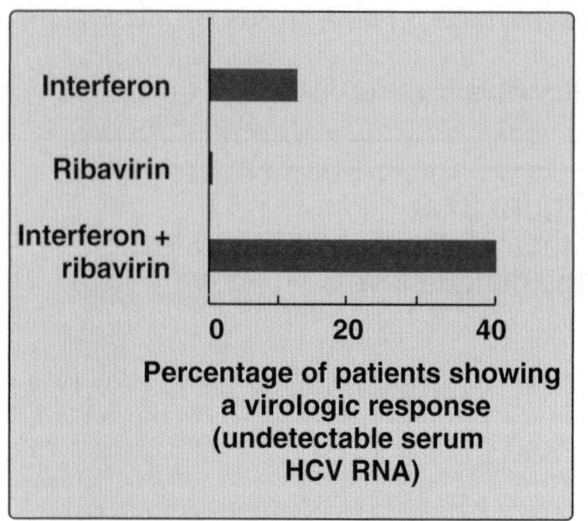

Figure 27.11
Combination treatment with interferon and ribavirin for chronic hepatitis C. [Note: Patients receiving ribavirin alone showed a biologic and histologic response, but no decrease in circulating hepatitis C virus.]

plasm, and maturation of the viral particle occurs by envelopment of the nucleocapsid, not at the plasma membrane as with viruses in the family *Togaviridae*, but, instead, at cytoplasmic Golgi membranes. Virus particles then accumulate in vesicles and are extruded when the vesicles move to the cell surface.

3. **Clinical significance:** Viruses in the genus *Flavivirus* are associated with several different clinical syndromes. These include: encephalitis (St. Louis encephalitis, Japanese encephalitis, and tickborne encephalitis viruses); hemorrhagic fever (yellow fever virus); and fever, myalgia, and rash (dengue viruses). Although there is little mortality associated with classic dengue fever, in certain parts of the world, such as Southeast Asia, a severe form of dengue infection occurs, particularly in infants and young children. Called dengue hemorrhagic fever or dengue shock syndrome, it is associated with a significant mortality (10 percent or higher) if untreated. Like dengue fever, West Nile fever is a mosquito-transmitted, acute, usually self-limited illness that presents chiefly with fever, malaise, lymphadenopathy, and rash. Infection may also result in aseptic meningitis or meningoencephalitis, especially in older adults. The first outbreak of West Nile encephalitis in the United States occurred in the New York City area in the summer of 1999. The outbreak was preceded by a significant die-off of wild crows and exotic birds at the Bronx zoo. The West Nile virus, following bird migration, has now spread to all 48 contiguous states in the United States.

4. **Laboratory identification:** A specific diagnosis is most often made by serologic means (that is, by demonstrating at least a fourfold rise in antibody titer, when comparing acute and convalescent sera). In some cases, virus isolation or demonstration of specific viral antigens is also feasible.

5. **Prevention:** A safe, highly effective, live attenuated vaccine for yellow fever has been available for many years. In China and Japan, a formalin-inactivated Japanese encephalitis virus vaccine is used, whereas, in central Europe, a formalin-inactivated vaccine is widely used to prevent tickborne encephalitis. Another important method of prevention is vector control. In urban areas, elimination of breeding sites can dramatically reduce the population of *Aedes aegypti* mosquitoes, which serve as the vector for both yellow fever and dengue viruses.

B. Hepatitis C viruses

Hepatitis C virus (HCV) was discovered in 1988 in the course of searching for the cause of non-A, non-B, transfusion-associated hepatitis. At that time, HCV accounted for 90 percent of the cases of non-A, non-B hepatitis. The hepatitis C viruses are heterogeneous and can be divided into six types on the basis of their nucleotide sequences.

1. **Transmission and pathogenesis:** Although HCV was initially identified as a major cause of posttransfusion hepatitis, intravenous

drug users and patients on hemodialysis are also at high risk for infection with HCV. Tattooing is also a leading cause of HCV infection. In addition, there is evidence for sexual transmission of HCV as well as for transmission from mother to infant. In the infected individual, viral replication occurs in the hepatocyte and, probably, also in mononuclear cells (lymphocytes and macrophages). Destruction of liver cells may result both from a direct effect of the activities of viral gene products and from the host immune response, including cytotoxic T cells. Although DNA viruses are associated with chronic infection and cancer development, this is not generally the case for RNA viruses. Nonetheless, certain strains of HCV have been associated with hepatocellular carcinoma development, even in the absence of cirrhosis. Particular alleles of the core gene of HCV have been strongly associated with development of hepatocellular carcinoma. Variant core gene alleles have also been associated with interferon-γ (IFN-γ) treatment failures.

2. **Clinical significance:** The majority of infections with HCV are subclinical, but about 25 percent of infected individuals present with acute hepatitis, including jaundice (Figure 27.10). More importantly, a significant proportion of infections progress to chronic hepatitis and cirrhosis. Finally, some of these individuals go on to develop hepatocellular carcinoma many years after the primary infection.

3. **Laboratory identification:** A specific diagnosis can be made by demonstration of antibodies that react with a combination of recombinant viral proteins. Sensitive tests are also now available for detection of the viral nucleic acid by RT-PCR (reverse transcription of the viral RNA followed by polymerase chain reaction to amplify the DNA copy, see p. 29).

4. **Treatment and prevention:** Tests to screen blood for HCV have been available for several years, so that HCV as a cause of transfusion-associated hepatitis is now unusual. Treatment of patients with chronic hepatitis by IFN-γ is sometimes beneficial but, in most cases, only for the period during which the patient is receiving the IFN-γ. Treatment with IFN-γ plus ribavirin provides a significantly improved response, and combination therapy is the treatment of choice (Figure 27.11). Chronic hepatitis resulting in severe liver damage may be an indication for a liver transplant. Figure 27.12 summarizes hepatitis A, B, and C.

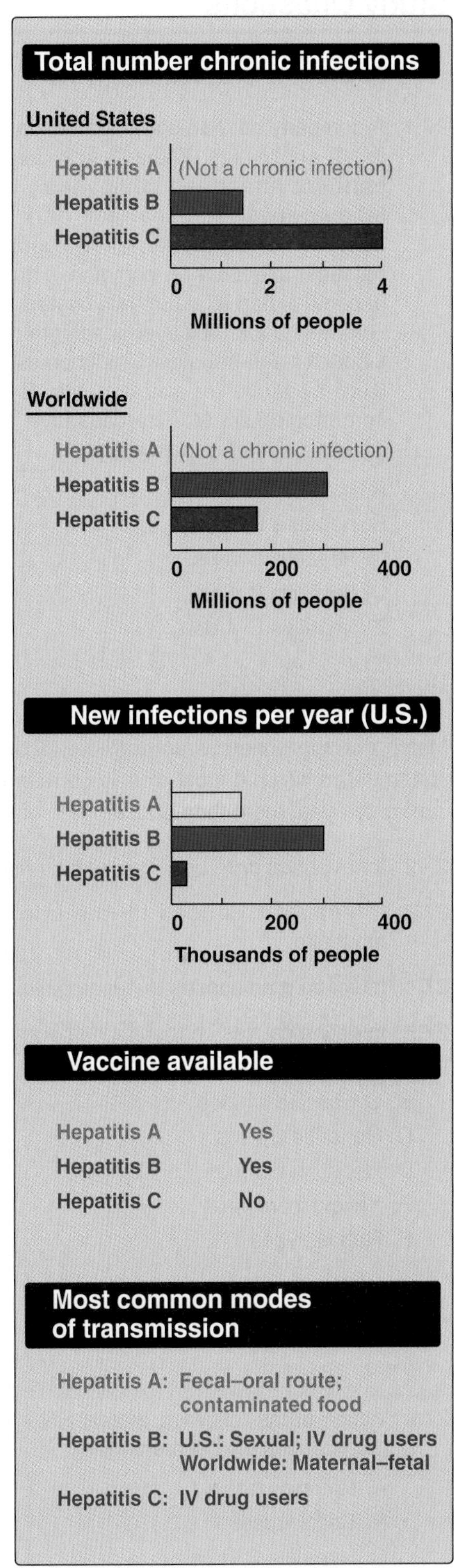

Figure 27.12
Summary of hepatitis A, B, and C.

VI. CORONAVIRIDAE

Coronaviruses are large, enveloped, pleomorphic particles, with a distinctive arrangement of spikes (peplomers) projecting from their surfaces. [Note: These projections have the appearance of a solar corona, which gives the virus its name.] The *Coronavirus* genome is the largest described for any RNA virus thus far. Human coronaviruses have been most commonly implicated in upper respiratory infections, causing 10 percent to 30 percent of cases of the common cold.

Study Questions

Choose the ONE correct answer.

27.1 A company held an elaborate holiday dinner party for its 42 employees. Within 3 to 4 weeks, many of the banquet attendees complained of experiencing fatigue, fever, nausea, and dark urine and were observed to be jaundiced. The group exhibited no bacterial infections in common. The employees who became ill had all eaten raw oysters at the party. The company doctor assayed a sample of the employees' blood for anti-hepatitis B antibodies, but all samples were negative for anti-hepatitis B surface antigen immunoglobulin M. The causative agent consistent with this history is most likely:

A. hepatitis A virus.
B. hepatitis B virus.
C. hepatitis C virus.
D. hepatitis D virus.
E. hepatitis E virus.

Correct answer = A. Hepatitis A is transmitted by the fecal–oral route and is most frequently acquired by eating contaminated shellfish or by contact with a carrier. The symptoms that were exhibited by the partygoers are consistent with liver damage caused by, for example, hepatitis. Hepatitis B infection is excluded because of the negative test for antibodies. Hepatitis C infection is acquired most commonly by intravenous drug users, patients on dialysis, and tattoo recipients. Hepatitis D infection occurs only in combination with hepatitis B infection. Hepatitis E is a major cause of enterically transmitted, waterborne hepatitis in developing countries.

Questions 27.2 to 27.5:

Match the appropriate virus from the following list with the statement to which it most closely corresponds. Each virus can match one, more than one, or none of the statements.

27.2 Intravenous drug users are at high risk for the virus.

27.3 Infection is caused by the bite of an infected mosquito.

27.4 Infection predisposes to hepatocellular carcinoma.

27.5 Infection causes congenital malformations.

A. Hepatitis A virus
B. Coxsackie viruses
C. Hepatitis C virus
D. Hepatitis E virus
E. Yellow fever virus
F. Rubella virus

Correct answer = C. Until the recent development of tests for the presence of hepatitis C virus (HCV) in blood, HCV was an important cause of transfusion-associated hepatitis. Intravenous drug users are one of several groups still at high risk for infection with this virus.

Correct answer = E. Yellow fever virus is an arthropod-borne virus, which is transmitted by the bite of an infected *Aedes aegypti* mosquito. The virus does not spread from person to person.

Correct answer = C. Unlike hepatitis A virus, hepatitis C virus infection has a strong tendency to lead to chronic hepatitis and cirrhosis, often resulting after many years in hepatocellular carcinoma.

Correct answer = F. Infection with rubella virus is generally of little consequence to the adult. The exception is the pregnant woman, in whom rubella virus infection can result in congenital malformations in the fetus. The risk is highest in the first trimester. These malformations can affect the central nervous system, the liver, the heart, and the eye.

27.6 Which of the following groups RNA viruses are common causes of viral meningitis?

A. Rhinoviruses
B. Caliciviruses
C. Hepatitis C virus
D. Flaviviruses
E. Enteroviruses

Correct answer = E. All of the enteroviruses can cause CNS disease. The enteroviruses are the major cause of aseptic meningitis. Rhinoviruses cause the common cold whereas the Caliciviruses cause gastrointestinal diseases. Hepatitis virus C causes hepatitis and cirrhosis. Flaviviruses cause encephalitis and hemorrhagic fever. While West Nile virus can cause meningitis, this manifestation is not typical of the entire Flavivirus group.

Retroviruses and AIDS

28

I. OVERVIEW

The family *Retroviridae* includes a large number of disease-producing animal viruses, several of which are of clinical importance to humans (Figure 28.1). Retroviridae are distinguished from all other RNA viruses by the presence of an unusual enzyme, reverse transcriptase, which converts a single-stranded RNA viral genome into double-stranded viral DNA. Because these viruses reverse the order of information transfer (RNA serving as a template for DNA synthesis, rather than DNA serving almost universally as a template for RNA synthesis), they are termed retroviruses. [Note: "Retro" is Latin for backward.] Retroviridae contain two genera that are of human interest: 1) *Lentivirus*, which includes human immunodeficiency viruses 1 and 2 (HIV-1 and -2) and 2) the human T-cell lymphotropic virus–bovine leukemia virus group (HTLV-BLV group), which contains human T-cell lymphotropic viruses 1 and 2 (HTLV-1 and -2). The lentiviruses cause neurologic and immunologic diseases but do not have the oncogenic properties of the HTLV-BLV group. In this chapter, a consideration of the features common to all retroviruses is presented, following which HIV and HTLV are discussed in detail.

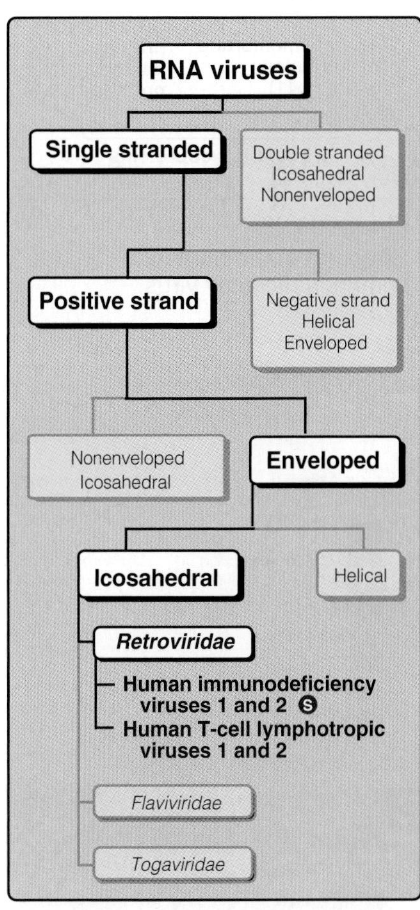

Figure 28.1
Classification of retroviruses that cause disease in humans. See p. 364 for a summary of these viruses.

II. RETROVIRUS STRUCTURE

Despite their wide range of disease manifestations, all retroviruses are similar in structure, genome organization, and mode of replication. Retroviruses are enveloped particles (Figure 28.2). The viral envelope, formed from the host cell membrane, contains a complex HIV protein that protrudes through the surface of the virus particle and appears as spiked knobs on electron micrographs of the virus. The full-length protein, called gp160, is cleaved into two peptides by a viral protease. [Note: The designation "gp" indicates that the protein is glycosylated.] The resulting transmembrane protein is called gp41, or TM, whereas the surface exposed portion of the protein is called gp120, or SU. Host cell proteins, including the major histocompatibility complex class II proteins, are also found in the envelope. The virion has a cone-shaped, icosahedral core containing the major capsid protein called p24, or CA. Between the capsid and the envelope is an outer matrix protein (p17, or MA), which directs entry of the double-stranded DNA provirus into the nucleus and is later essential for the process of virus assembly. There are two identical copies of the positive-sense, single-stranded RNA

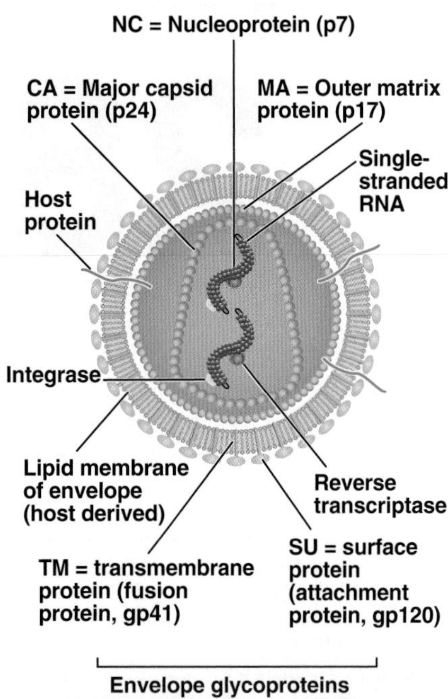

Figure 28.2
Structure of the human immunodeficiency virus.

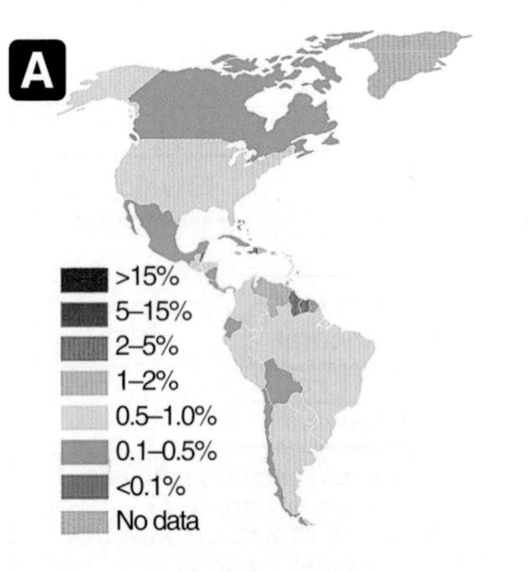

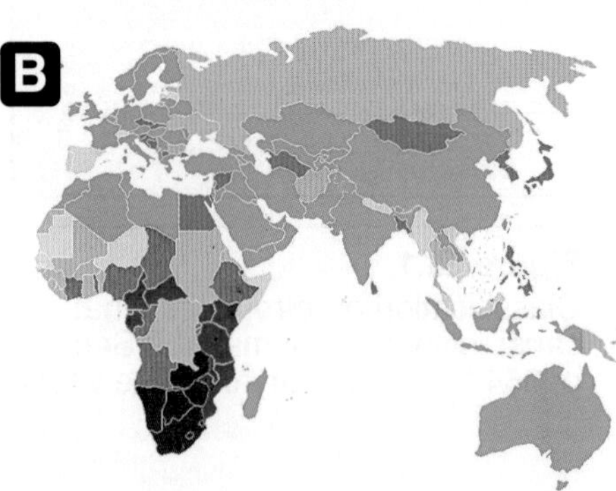

Figure 28.3
Estimated population prevalence of worldwide HIV infections (2008). A. The Americas. B. Europe, Africa, Asia and Australia.

genome in the capsid (that is, unlike other viruses, retroviruses are diploid). The RNA is tightly complexed with a basic protein (p7, or NC) in a nucleocapsid structure that differs in morphology among the different retrovirus genera. Also found within the capsid are the enzymes reverse transcriptase and integrase (which are required for viral DNA synthesis and integration into the host cell chromosome) and protease (essential for virus maturation).

III. HUMAN IMMUNODEFICIENCY VIRUS

Acquired immune deficiency syndrome (AIDS) was first reported in the United States in 1981. The earliest cases of AIDS were seen in large urban centers, such as Los Angeles, San Francisco, and New York City. Clusters of young men who have sex with men (MSM) exhibited a puzzling collection of symptoms, including severe pneumonia caused by *Pneumocystis jiroveci* (ordinarily a harmless eukaryotic organism), Kaposi sarcoma ([KS] ordinarily an extremely rare form of cancer), sudden weight loss, swollen lymph nodes, and general suppression of immune function. This constellation of signs and symptoms associated with illness came to be known as AIDS. Early attempts at understanding the disease focused on the possibility of immune suppression induced by chronic injectable drug use (IDU) or infection. Soon, however, cases were reported in MSM and non-IDU patients who had received blood or blood products by transfusion. By 1984, AIDS was recognized as an infectious disease caused by a virus, and, eventually, HIV was isolated from AIDS patients. In the decade after this initial recognition, AIDS killed more U.S. citizens than the Korean and Vietnam wars combined. According to World Health Organization estimates, more than 33 million people worldwide were living with HIV in 2009 (more than 1.1 million in the United States). There were estimated to be about 2.5 million new infections worldwide and 1.8 million deaths due to AIDS in 2009. Worldwide, new infections are almost equally distributed between men and women, with heterosexual activity accounting for the majority of cases. Although the United States and other developed countries have identified combinations of drugs that significantly slow the progression of AIDS, 95 percent of HIV-infected people live in developing countries (Figure 28.3), where, for logistic and financial reasons, few have access to these drugs. Figure 28.4 shows the incidence and deaths due to AIDS in the United States. The two types of HIV, HIV-1 and HIV-2, are similar but have different pathogenic potentials and geographic distributions. HIV-1 is more virulent, more infective, and more widespread geographically, whereas HIV-2 is not as virulent and is localized exclusively to West Africa.

A. Organization of the HIV genome

The HIV RNA genome contains three major genes: *gag*, *pol*, and *env* (Figure 28.5). The *gag* gene encodes p17 (MA), p24 (CA), and p7 (NC) (core and matrix proteins). The *pol* gene encodes reverse transcriptase, protease, integrase, and ribonuclease. Finally, the *env* gene encodes gp41 (TM) and gp120 (SU) (transmembrane and surface proteins). Genes for additional regulatory and accessory proteins of diverse function are located between the *pol* and *env* genes. The 5' end of the viral RNA contains a unique sequence, U5, which houses part of the site required for viral integration into the host cell chromosome and also the tRNA primer-binding site for initiation of reverse transcription. The 3' end of the viral RNA contains the nucleotide sequence U3, which houses sequences that are important in the control of transcription of the DNA provirus. As with cellular mRNAs synthesized by RNA polymerase II, the 5' end of the viral RNA synthesized from proviral DNA has a methylated cap, and the 3' end has a poly-A tail.[1] At both ends of the viral genome is a repeated sequence, R, which is involved in reverse transcription. Synthesis of the double-stranded DNA provirus results in duplication of the R and U sequences, producing two identical repeat units designated long terminal repeats (LTRs). The genomic organization of the DNA provirus is illustrated in Figure 28.5. A brief overview of retrovirus replication is presented in Chapter 23 (see Figure 23.15), and additional details of some steps in the cycle are discussed below.

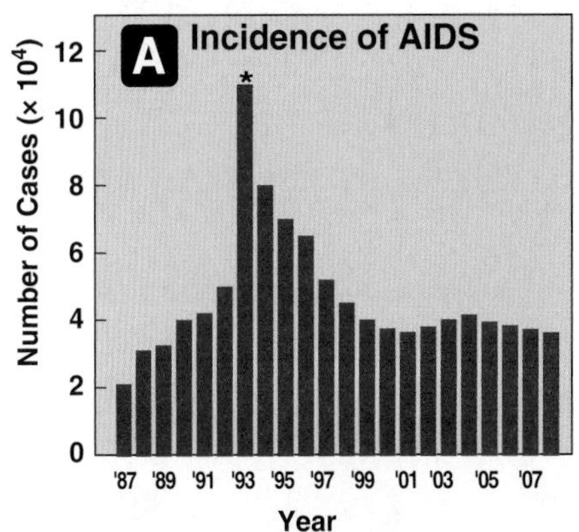

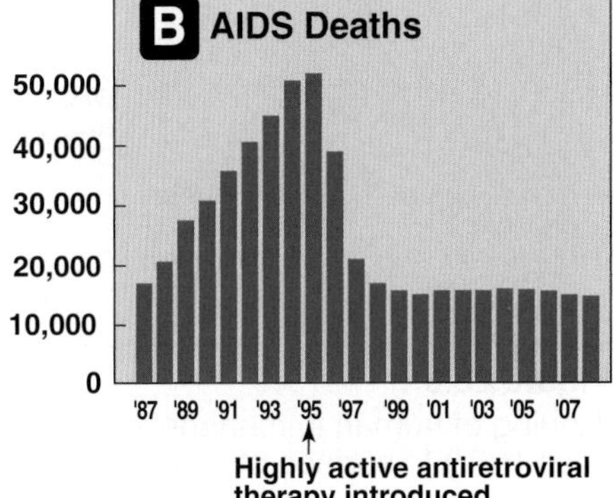

Figure 28.4
A. Incidence of AIDS in the United States. *Increase in 1993 resulted from several changes introduced in January 1993 in the case definition of AIDS. B. Deaths due to AIDS in the United States.

B. HIV replication

The first phase of HIV replication, which includes viral entry, reverse transcription, and integration of the virus into the host genome, is accomplished by proteins provided by the virus. The second phase of replication, which includes the synthesis and processing of viral genomes, mRNAs, and structural proteins, uses the host cell machinery for transcription and protein synthesis. The end result of HIV replication in most cell types is cell death.

1. **Attachment to a specific cell surface receptor:** Attachment is accomplished via the gp120 fragment of the *env* gene product on the HIV surface, which preferentially binds to a CD4 receptor molecule (Figure 28.6). Thus, the virus infects helper T cells, lymphocytes, monocytes, and dendritic cells, which contain this protein in their cell membranes (Figure 28.7).

2. **Entry of virus into the cell:** An additional coreceptor, a chemokine receptor, is required for entry of the viral core into the cell (see Figure 28.6). [Note: A chemokine is a cytokine with chemotactic properties, produced by lymphocytes and macrophages.]

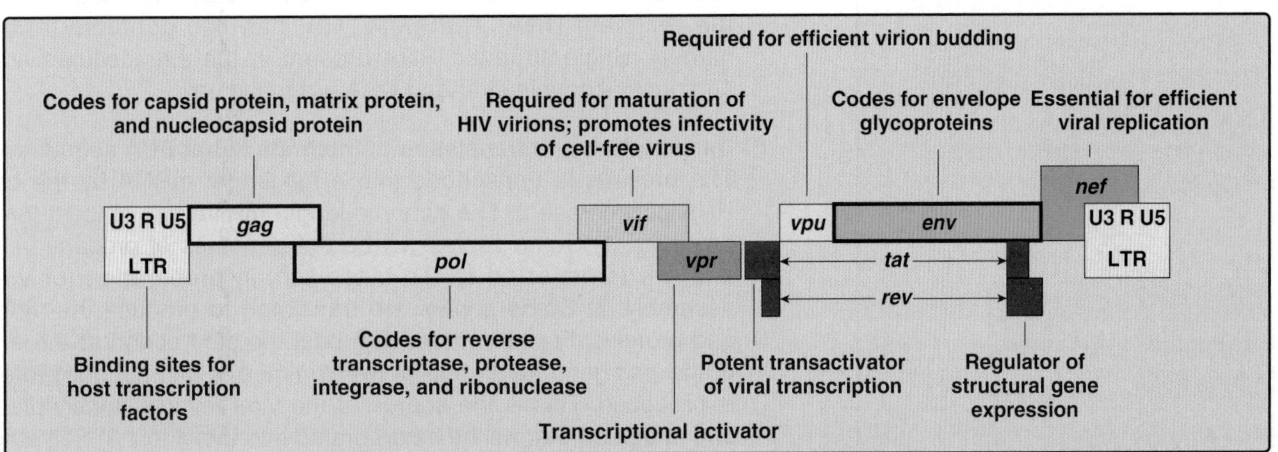

Figure 28.5
Human immunodeficiency virus (HIV) proviral genome. The *rev* and *tat* genes are divided into noncontiguous pieces, and the gene segments are spliced together in the RNA transcript. LTR = long terminal repeat.

[1]See Chapter 30 in ***Lippincott's Illustrated Reviews: Biochemistry*** for a discussion of the cap and poly-A tail of mRNA.

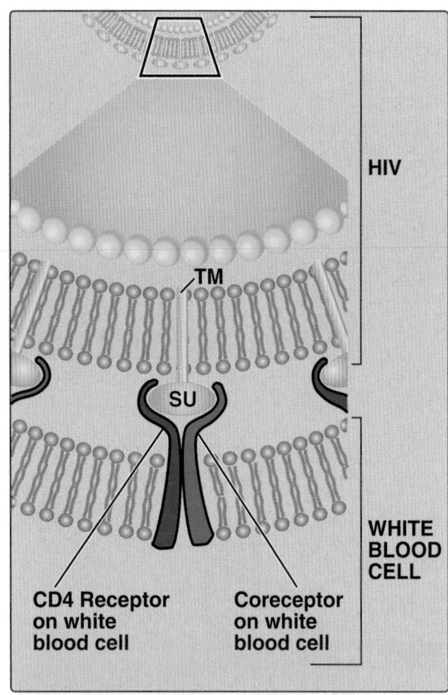

Figure 28.6
Binding of human immunodeficiency virus (HIV) to surface of lymphocyte.

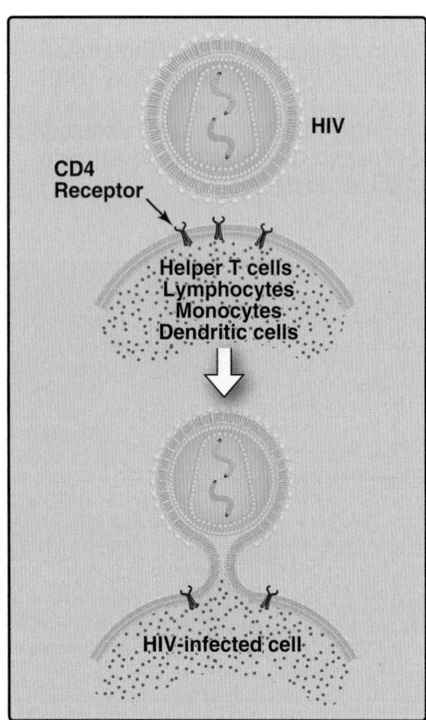

Figure 28.7
Attachment and entry of human immunodeficiency virus (HIV).

Macrophages and T cells express different chemokine receptors that fulfill this function. Two chemokine receptors that are employed by HIV as coreceptors are CCR5 and CXCR4, which are expressed differentially on different cell types. The tropism of particular variants of HIV is determined, in part, by which coreceptor is present. Binding to a coreceptor activates the viral gp41 gene product, triggering fusion between the viral envelope and the cell membrane (Figure 28.8).

3. **Reverse transcription of viral RNA:** After entering the host cell, the HIV RNA is not translated. Instead, it is transcribed into DNA by reverse transcriptase, an RNA-directed DNA polymerase that enters host cells as part of the viral nucleocapsid (see Figure 28.8). A host cellular transfer RNA (tRNA) is hydrogen-bonded to a specific site on each viral RNA molecule, where it functions as a primer for initiation of reverse transcription. This process takes place in the cytoplasm. The viral reverse transcriptase first synthesizes a DNA-RNA hybrid molecule, and then its RNase activity degrades the parental RNA molecule while synthesizing the second strand of DNA. This process results in duplication of the ends to form the LTRs. The resulting linear molecule of double-stranded DNA is the provirus. LTRs at either end of the provirus contain promoter and enhancer sequences[2] that control expression of the viral DNA. Because the reverse transcriptase enzyme has no proofreading capacity, errors often occur during the conversion of genomic RNA into the DNA provirus. This error-prone process gives rise to 1 to 3 mutations per newly synthesized virus particle.

4. **Integration of the provirus into host cell DNA:** The provirus, still associated with virion core components, is transported to the nucleus with the aid of p17 (MA). In the nucleus, viral integrase cleaves the chromosomal DNA and covalently inserts the provirus. The integrated provirus, thus, becomes a stable part of the cell genome and can never be eliminated (see Figure 28.8). The insertion is random with respect to the site of integration in the recipient DNA. Therefore, HIV has two genomic forms: namely, single-stranded RNA present in the extracellular virus and proviral double-stranded DNA within the cell.

5. **Transcription and translation of integrated viral DNA sequences:** The provirus is transcribed into a full-length mRNA by the cell RNA polymerase II. The genome-length mRNA has at least three functions: 1) Some copies will be the genomes of progeny virus and are transported to the cytoplasm in preparation for viral assembly. 2) Some copies are translated to produce the virion gag proteins. Further, by reading past the stop codon at the end of the *gag* gene about one of twenty times, a gag-pol polyprotein is produced. This is the source of the viral reverse transcriptase and integrase that will be incorporated into the virion. 3) Still other copies of viral RNA are spliced, creating new translatable sequences (see Figure 28.8). In all retroviruses, one of the spliced mRNAs is translated into the envelope proteins. In the complex viruses, such as HIV and HTLV, additional spliced

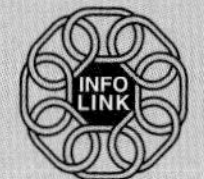

[2]See Chapter 30 in ***Lippincott's Illustrated Reviews: Biochemistry*** for a discussion of the role of promoters and enhancers in gene regulation.

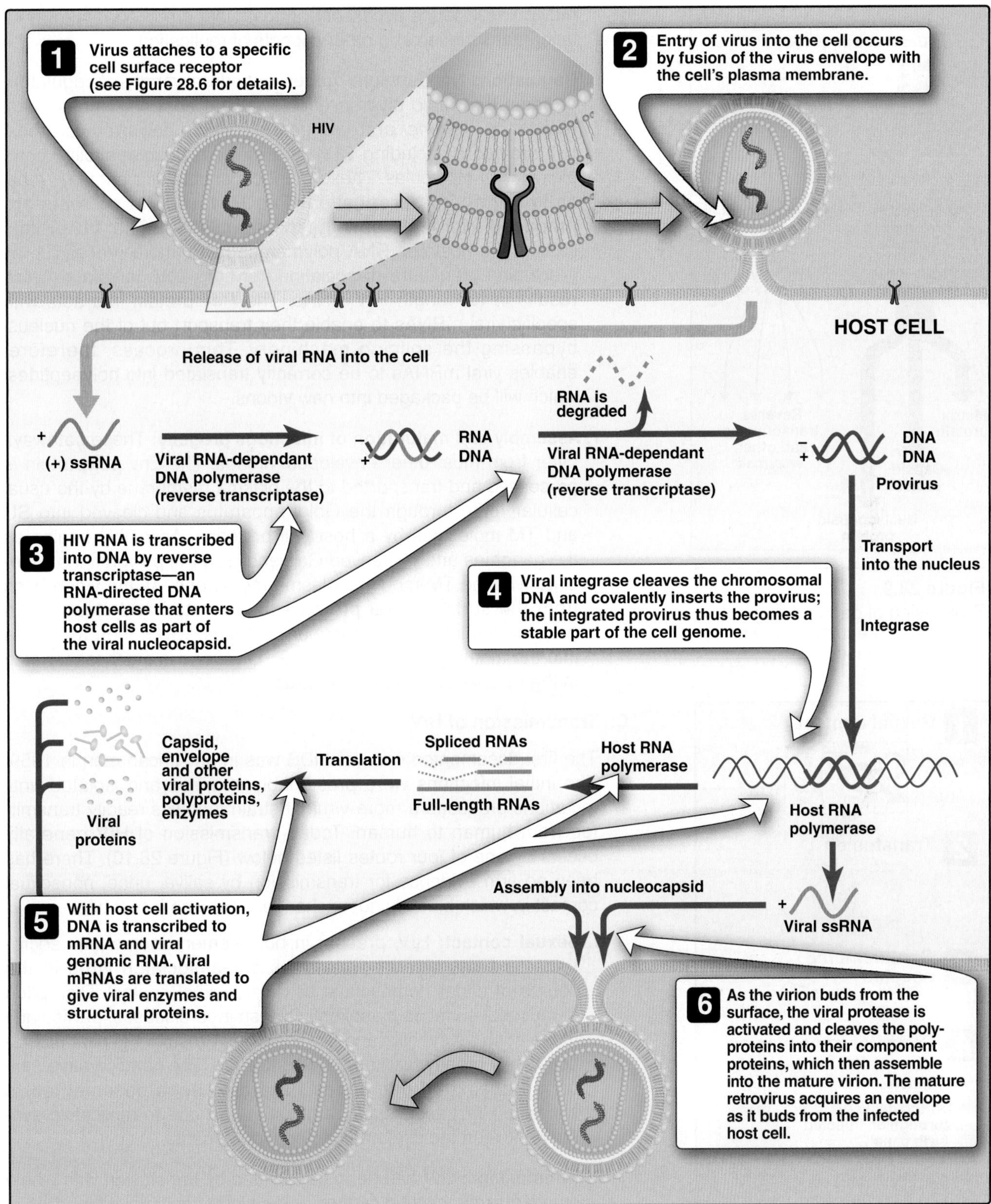

Figure 28.8
The human immunodeficiency virus (HIV) replication cycle. ssRNA = single strand RNA.

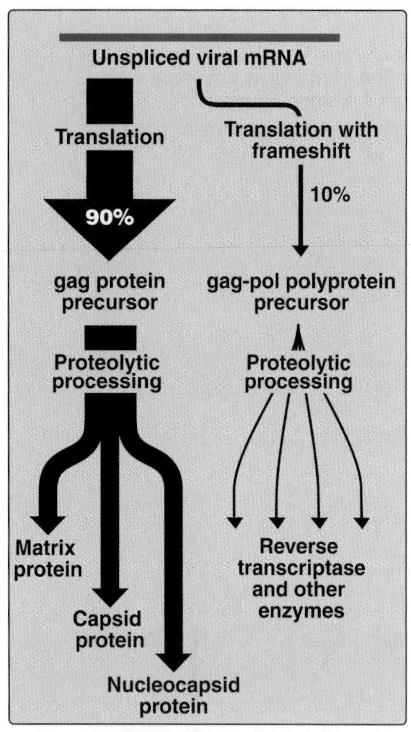

Figure 28.9
Processing of gag and gag-pol polyprotein precursor proteins by the viral protease.

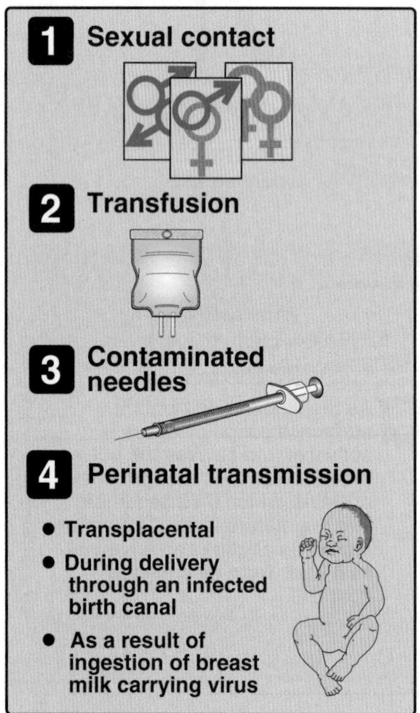

Figure 28.10
Common modes of transmission of human immunodeficiency virus (HIV).

molecules produce accessory proteins that are important in regulating transcription and other aspects of replication.

6. **Regulation:** Nonstructural genes encode a variety of regulatory proteins that have diverse effects on the host cell and on viral replication. The *nef* and *vpu* gene products down-regulate host cell receptors, including CD4 and major histocompatibility complex class I molecules. These products enable efficient virus replication and viron production. The Rev and Tat proteins are produced from differentially spliced mRNAs. The Tat protein causes the host cell RNA polymerase to be more processive by preventing premature dissociation from the DNA template, which results in full-length HIV RNAs. The Rev protein interacts with specific viral mRNAs to enable their transport out of the nucleus, bypassing the splicing machinery. This process, therefore, enables viral mRNAs to be correctly translated into polypeptides, which will be packaged into new virions.

7. **Assembly and maturation of infectious progeny:** These pathways differ from most other enveloped viruses. The Env polyprotein is processed and transported to the plasma membrane by the usual cellular route through the Golgi apparatus and cleaved into SU and TM molecules by a host cell protease. Assembly begins as the genomes and uncleaved Gag and Gag-Pol polyproteins associate with the TM-modified plasma membrane. As the virion buds from the surface, viral protease is activated and cleaves the polyproteins into their component proteins, which then assemble into the mature virion (Figure 28.9). Cleavage is a necessary step in the maturation of infectious virus.

C. Transmission of HIV

The first documented case of AIDS was in an African man in 1959. The initial infections were presumably sporadic and isolated until mutations produced a more virulent strain that was readily transmitted from human to human. Today, transmission of HIV generally occurs by one of four routes listed below (Figure 28.10). There has been no firm evidence for transmission by saliva, urine, nonsexual contact in which blood is not exchanged, or by an insect bite.

1. **Sexual contact:** HIV, present in both semen and vaginal secretions, is transmitted primarily as cell-associated virus in the course of either homosexual or heterosexual contact. Disruption of mucosal surfaces by sexually transmitted diseases, particularly those such as syphilis and chancroid that result in genital ulcerations, may greatly facilitate HIV-1 infection. The nonulcerative sexually transmitted pathogens have also been documented to enhance HIV transmission, at least in part due to replicative synergy between the viral and bacterial pathogens.

2. **Transfusions:** HIV has been transmitted by transfusion with whole blood, plasma, clotting factors, and cellular fractions of blood.

3. **Contaminated needles:** Transmission can occur by inoculation with HIV-contaminated needles or syringes among drug users or accidentally if a contaminated needle punctures the skin of a health care worker.

4. **Perinatal transmission:** An HIV-infected woman has a 15 to 40 percent chance of transmitting the infection to her newborn, either transplacentally, during passage of the baby through the birth canal, or via breastfeeding. Because of the high rates of HIV-1 infection in women of childbearing age in developing countries, perinatally acquired HIV-1 infection is responsible for approximately 20 percent of all AIDS cases in these areas. Figure 28.11 compares the modes of transmission worldwide with those occurring in the United States.

D. Pathogenesis and clinical significance of HIV infection

The pathology of HIV disease results from either tissue destruction by the virus itself or the host's response to virus-infected cells. In addition, HIV can induce an immunodeficient state that leads to opportunistic diseases that are rare in the absence of HIV infection. The progression from HIV infection to AIDS develops in 50 percent of HIV-infected individuals in an average of 10 years, and, if untreated, it is uniformly fatal, generally within 2 years of diagnosis. However, there is a significant fraction (about 10 percent) of HIV-infected individuals who have not developed AIDS after 20 years. Development from HIV infection to end-stage AIDS progresses through several phases (Figure 28.12).

1. **Initial infection:** After the acquisition of HIV, the initially infected cells are generally macrophages within the genital tract. From this initial localized infection, HIV disseminates via the blood, and virus may then localize in dendritic cells throughout the lymphoid tissue. From the surface of follicular dendritic cells, HIV can then infect CD4+ lymphocytes moving through the germinal centers of lymph nodes. This process creates a reservoir of chronically HIV-infected cells within the lymphatic tissue throughout the body. Some individuals are resistant to some variants of HIV-1 due to a deletion in the gene that encodes the coreceptor (C-C chemokine receptor type 5, or CCR5) for the virus.

2. **Acute phase viremia:** Several weeks after the initial infection with HIV, one-third to two-thirds of individuals experience an acute disease syndrome (also referred to as the primary infection) similar to infectious mononucleosis. During this period, there is a high level of virus replication occurring in CD4+ cells. Large amounts of virus and capsid protein (CA antigen) are present in the blood, but circulating antibody does not appear until 1 to 10 weeks after the initial infection (seroconversion). During this window of time, antibody tests will not identify HIV-infected people. Lymph nodes also become infected during this time and later serve as the sites of virus persistence during the asymptomatic period.

3. **Latent period:** The acute phase viremia is eventually reduced significantly with the appearance of a HIV-specific cytotoxic T-lymphocyte response, followed by a humoral antibody response. A clinically asymptomatic or "latent" period lasting from months to many years follows the acute infection. During this latent period, the majority (90 percent) of HIV proviruses are transcriptionally silent, so that only 10 percent of the cells containing integrated HIV DNA also contain viral mRNA or viral proteins. A constant

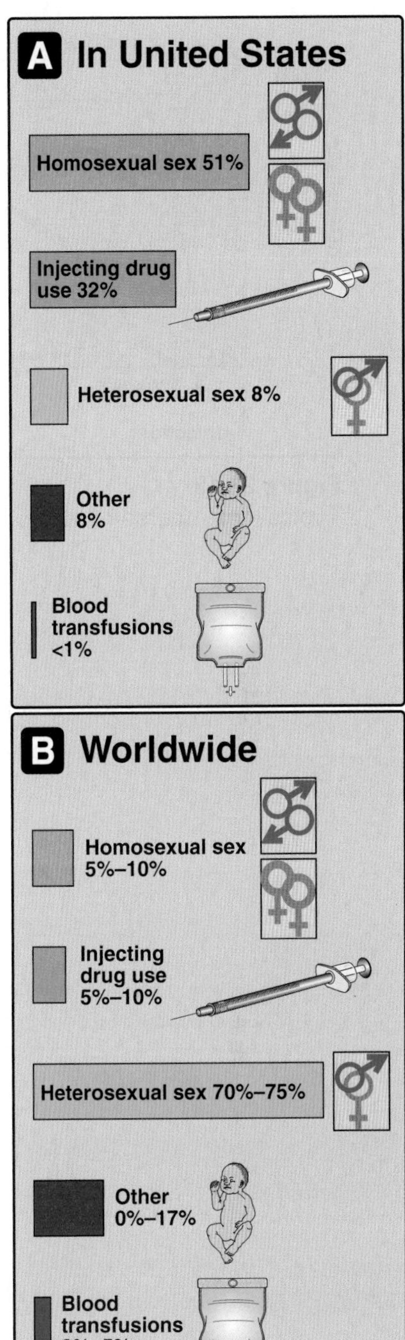

Figure 28.11
Modes of HIV transmission in the United States compared with those worldwide. (A) In the United States, the primary mode of HIV transmission is homosexual sex. Transmission in western Europe is similar to that in the United States. (B) In most of the world, transmissior is primarily by heterosexual sex. [Note: Segment labeled "Other" includes perinatal transmission.]

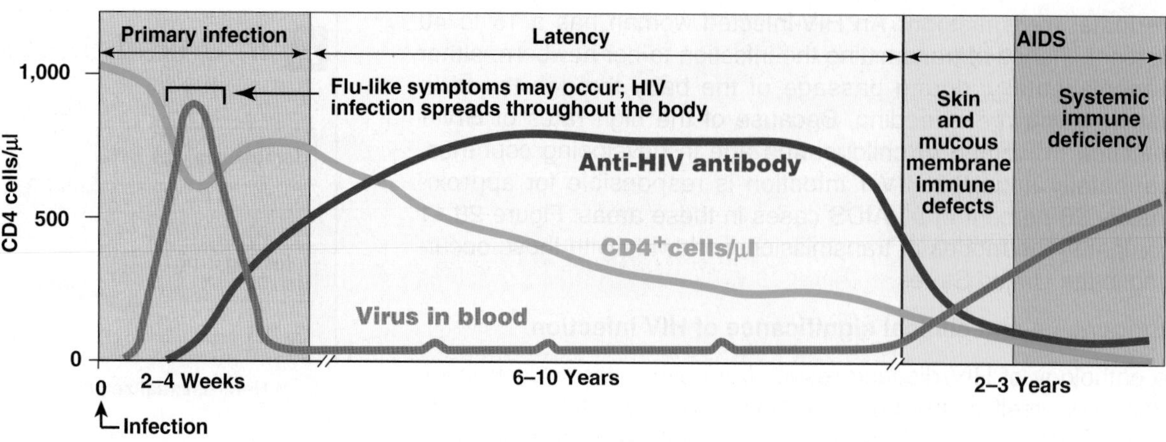

Figure 28.12
Typical time course of human immunodeficiency virus (HIV) infection.

level of virus and virus-infected cells is maintained by a combination of replacement of the CD4+ cells killed by HIV infection with cells newly produced in lymphoid organs and the subsequent infection of these new cells with progeny virus. There are transient peaks of viremia that are often correlated with stimulation of the immune system by infection with other pathogens or by immunization. Although there is continuous loss of those CD4+ cells in which HIV is replicating, active replacement through stem cell multiplication compensates for this loss, and the CD4+ count declines only slowly over a period of years. In addition, the host immune response is still sufficiently effective to maintain a relatively stable, low level of virus production. It has been estimated that 10^{11} virions and 10^{9} CD4 T cells are produced each day. Virus isolated during this period is also less cytopathic for CD4+ cells and replicates more slowly than does virus isolated later during symptomatic AIDS. Despite the nearly normal levels of CD4+ cells, however, impairment of T-cell responses to specific antigens is evident. The infection remains relatively clinically asymptomatic as long as the immune system is functional. The actual level of virus replication in peripheral blood cells varies greatly among patients, and those with a higher steady-state viral load progress more rapidly to symptomatic AIDS and death.

4. **Clinical complications of HIV infection during the latent period:** During this period (of variable length but lasting on average about 10 years), there are multiple, nonspecific conditions, such as persistent, generalized lymphadenopathy (swollen lymph nodes); diarrhea; chronic fevers; night sweats; and weight loss. The more common opportunistic infections, such as herpes zoster and candidiasis, may occur repeatedly during this period as well as when patients progress to AIDS.

5. **Progression to AIDS:** The progression from asymptomatic infection to AIDS is not sudden but, in fact, occurs as a continuum of clinical states. A number of virologic and immunologic changes occur that affect the rate of this progression. For example, coinfection with a number of the herpesviruses, such as human herpesvirus type 6 (see p. 255), can transactivate transcription from

the silent HIV provirus, increasing HIV replication. Any stimulation of an immune response causing activation of resting T cells also activates HIV replication. Not only does this increase the number of infected CD4+ cells, but it also increases the opportunity to create generations of virus mutants. Eventually, a more highly cytocidal, more rapidly multiplying variant appears. This transition is also often accompanied by the appearance of a CXCR4-tropic virus variant, whereas the infecting variants tend to be CCR5-tropic. [Note: The CXCR4 receptor is one of several chemokine receptors that HIV isolates can use to infect CD4+ T cells.] In addition, these variants are often highly syncytium-inducing, promoting fusion between infected and previously uninfected cells. T-cell precursors in the lymphoid organs are also infected and killed, so the capacity to generate new CD4+ cells is gradually lost. The capacity to contain the infection is further compromised by the appearance of HIV mutants with altered antigenic specificity, which are not recognized by the existing humoral antibody or cytotoxic T lymphocytes. The eventual result of these accumulating, interacting factors is an increasingly rapid decline in CD4+ count, accompanied by loss of immune capacity. With the CD4+ count falling below 200/μl and the appearance of increasingly frequent and serious diseases and opportunistic infections ("AIDS-defining illnesses"), the patient is said to have AIDS.

6. **End-stage AIDS:** Nearly all systems of the body can be affected as a result of HIV infection, either by HIV itself or by opportunistic organisms. The weakening immune system leads to many complications, including malignancies.

   a. **Spread of HIV to additional body sites:** Cell types other than CD4+ lymphocytes can be infected by HIV. Infection of these cells produces some of the additional manifestations of end-stage disease. Chief among these are infected cells of the monocyte-macrophage lineage, which are not killed as rapidly as CD4+ T cells and can transport the virus into other organs (Figure 28.13). For example, microglia are the HIV-infected cells present in brains of patients with AIDS encephalopathy, which typically evolves over a period of 1 year, with gradual deterioration resulting in severe dementia. This appears to be unrelated to CD4+ depletion but, rather, to an expanded tropism of variant HIV. The basis for damage to neuronal cells is not known, however. Similarly, the wasting syndrome seen in late stages of AIDS probably relates to HIV-infected macrophages being induced to produce various cytokines, especially tumor necrosis factor. HIV infection of blood cell progenitors in the bone marrow leads to the anemia seen in most AIDS patients.

   b. **Opportunistic infections in AIDS:** Multiple recurrent bouts of infections with fungi, bacteria, and viruses occur as the CD4+ cell count declines (Figure 28.14). For example, the nervous system can be the site of opportunistic infections with *Toxoplasma*, *Cryptococcus*, JC virus, and mycobacteria. The eye can be infected with HIV, but also with opportunistic agents, the most prominent of which is cytomegalovirus (CMV), a cause of retinal destruction. The lungs are also pri-

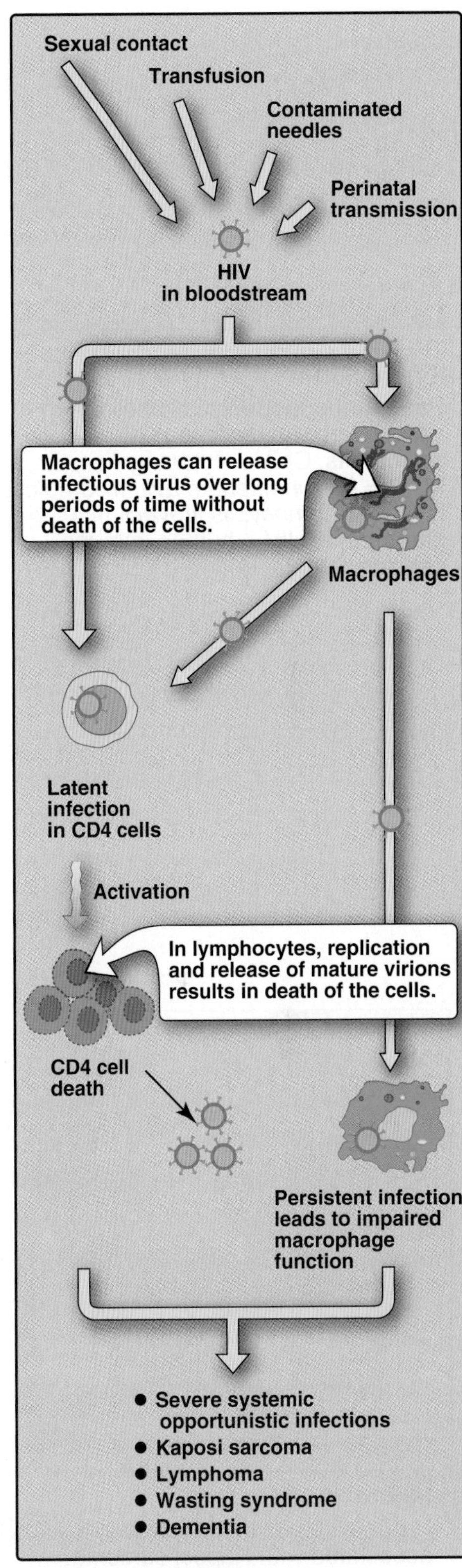

Figure 28.13
Pathogenesis of human immunodeficiency virus (HIV).

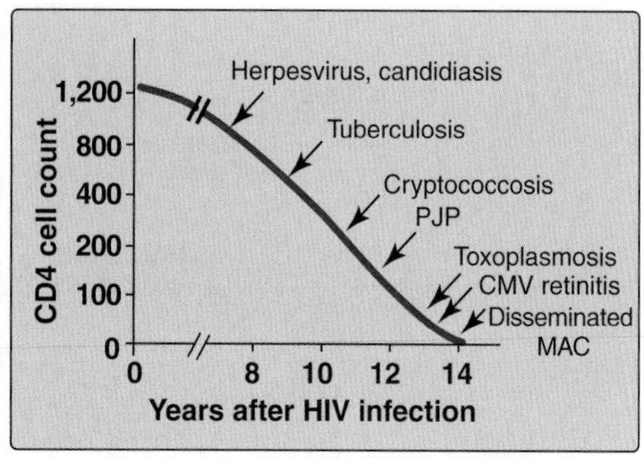

Figure 28.14
Pattern of opportunistic infections associated with declining CD4+ cell counts. CMV = cytomegalovirus; MAC = *Mycobacterium avium* complex; PJP = *Pneumocystis jiroveci* pneumonia; HIV = human immunodeficiency virus.

marily affected by opportunistic infections, *P. jirovecci* pneumonia being one of the most common. Mycobacterial infections are also a common problem in the lung. For example, currently, 30 percent of AIDS patients die from tuberculosis (see p. 186). Serious gastrointestinal (GI) tract illnesses are due to opportunistic pathogens, but these may be in concert with HIV infection. CMV colitis is a common problem, but HIV is often present as well. Protozoal parasitic diseases, as well as infections with gram-negative enteric bacteria are other sources of GI disorders. The immune deficiency also provides the opportunity for latent infections to recur repeatedly or to become chronic and spread extensively. Recurrent infections by Epstein-Barr virus (EBV), varicella zoster virus, human papillomavirus, and herpes simplex virus are common. Mucocutaneous candidiasis (for example, oral, esophageal, or vaginal) is an ongoing problem in AIDS patients as well. In fact, vaginal candidiasis is the most frequent reason HIV-infected females seek medical attention. See Figure 28.14 for a summary of common AIDS-defining opportunistic infections.

c. **Malignancies associated with AIDS:** A number of malignancies commonly arise in HIV-infected patients. The most characteristic neoplasm present in AIDS patients is KS, which involves skin, mucous membranes, and deep viscera. Various lymphomas, including those of the central nervous system (CNS), are also common. These are probably the result of the immune compromise and not HIV itself. KS has been associated with human herpesvirus, type 8 (HHV-8) as shown in Figure 28.15. In AIDS patients, body cavity lymphomas are also usually associated with HHV-8 infection, whereas many other lymphomas are EBV associated (see p. 268).

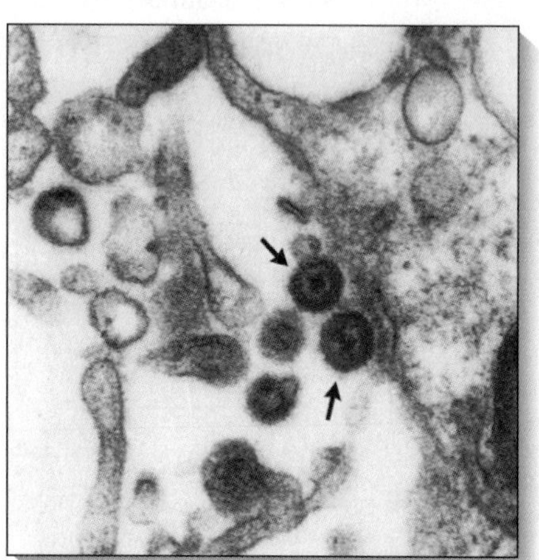

Figure 28.15
Herpesvirus 8 virions (arrows) associated with Kaposi sarcoma.

E. Laboratory identification

1. **Demonstration of virus or virus components:** Amplification of viral RNA or DNA proviruses by the polymerase chain reaction (PCR) technique (see p. 30) is the most sensitive method for early detection of virus in blood or tissue specimens. Recent adaptation of the technique to obtain quantitative estimates of viral load (measured, for example, as the amount of viral RNA per milliliter of blood plasma) now permit evaluation of the stage of the disease, effectiveness of a drug regimen, and prognosis. In addition, the circulating virus can be genotyped by sequencing, allowing physicians to determine the most appropriate initial therapy or to establish whether drug-resistant virus has emerged. For purposes of initial screening of the blood supply, ELISA (for enzyme-linked immunosorbent assay) testing (see p. 27) for the CA (p24) antigen in serum can detect otherwise undetectable infection in individuals who are infectious by screening for anti-HIV antibodies.

2. **Demonstration of immune response:** The usual screening procedure for HIV infection is a two-step process, used both for purposes of diagnosing individuals who may be infected and for protection of the blood supply. The first step in screening is an

ELISA procedure (see p. 27) in which the serum sample is reacted with whole virus lysates or synthetic HIV peptides. The latter can detect antibody much earlier than the former and is now standard. At its most sensitive, there is still a 25-day window between the time that virus is first present in the blood and when antibody can be detected. Although the ELISA test is highly specific, there are false-positives, so any positive result is confirmed using the Western blot technique.[3] Antigen (p24) and antibody tests have been combined into a fourth generation test, which allows detection of infected samples during the window of time before antibodies develop.

F. Treatment

Because of the progressive nature of the disease, it is the HIV infection that is treated as the clinical problem, rather than focusing on the end stage (that is, AIDS) alone. Virtually every step in the HIV replication cycle is a potential target for an antiviral drug, but only those directed against reverse transcriptase, viral protease, viral fusion and integration have so far been used successfully (Figure 28.16). Used early in the infection, a combination of three different drugs administered together can reduce the plasma viral load to undetectable levels, at least temporarily.

1. **Strategy for multiple-drug therapy in treating HIV infections:** Unlike DNA polymerase, which makes few mistakes in the replication of DNA because of its proofreading activity, reverse transcriptase has no ability to proofread. Therefore, DNA synthesis by the viral reverse transcriptase produces many errors (about one per cycle of synthesis). This results in mutations in all of the HIV genes and accumulation of a pool of mutant viruses in any individual patient. In the presence of an antiviral drug, there is strong selection for mutations that confer resistance to that drug, and the high mutation rate ensures that such mutations will occur. The answer to this therapeutic dilemma has been to simultaneously use multiple drugs that act on different steps in the viral replication cycle because the probability of several different mutations occurring concurrently in the targeted genes in the same genome is low. In addition, certain drug combinations are synergistic, the effect on reducing viral load being considerably greater than merely the sum of the individual drug effects. The use of potent combination regimens can limit viral replication and dissemination to lymphoid tissue, creating a smaller reservoir of chronically infected cells, and limiting the potential for viral mutations (acquired during the replicative process) that could lead to acquisition of drug resistance. However, even this approach is not entirely effective because HIV also exhibits a relatively high rate of recombination, enabling mutations from two different genomes to be combined into one virus particle.

2. **Early therapy:** Approaches to therapy are evolving as more is learned about the nature of the disease. For example, it has been determined that the steady-state level of replicating virus in the plasma (that is, the "viral load") is a prognostic indicator of the

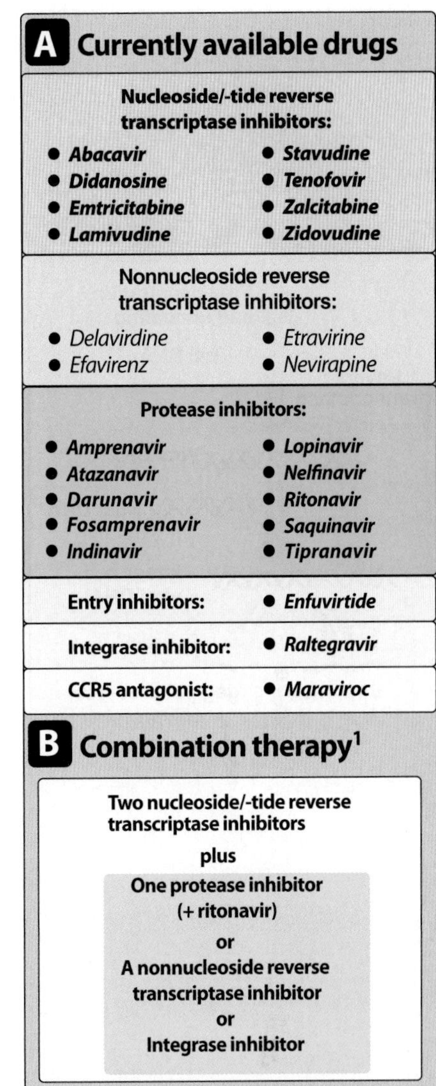

A Currently available drugs
Nucleoside/-tide reverse transcriptase inhibitors:
• Abacavir
• Didanosine
• Emtricitabine
• Lamivudine
• Stavudine
• Tenofovir
• Zalcitabine
• Zidovudine
Nonnucleoside reverse transcriptase inhibitors:
• Delavirdine
• Efavirenz
• Etravirine
• Nevirapine
Protease inhibitors:
• Amprenavir
• Atazanavir
• Darunavir
• Fosamprenavir
• Indinavir
• Lopinavir
• Nelfinavir
• Ritonavir
• Saquinavir
• Tipranavir
Entry inhibitors: • Enfuvirtide
Integrase inhibitor: • Raltegravir
CCR5 antagonist: • Maraviroc
B Combination therapy¹
Two nucleoside/-tide reverse transcriptase inhibitors
plus
One protease inhibitor (+ ritonavir)
or
A nonnucleoside reverse transcriptase inhibitor
or
Integrase inhibitor

Figure 28.16
Highly active antiretroviral therapy (HAART). [1]Choice of a drug regimen is individualized based on criteria such as tolerability, drug–drug interactions, convenience/adherence, and possible baseline resistance. The availability of well-tolerated combination antiretroviral tablets that can be dosed once daily has greatly simplified early treatment of human immunodeficiency virus infection. CCR5 = C-C chemokine receptor type 5 that can function as viral coreceptor.

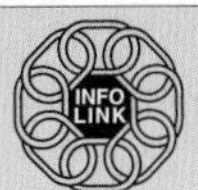

[3]See Chapter 33 in ***Lippincott's Illustrated Reviews: Biochemistry*** for a discussion of the use of ELISA assay and Western blots in testing for HIV exposure.

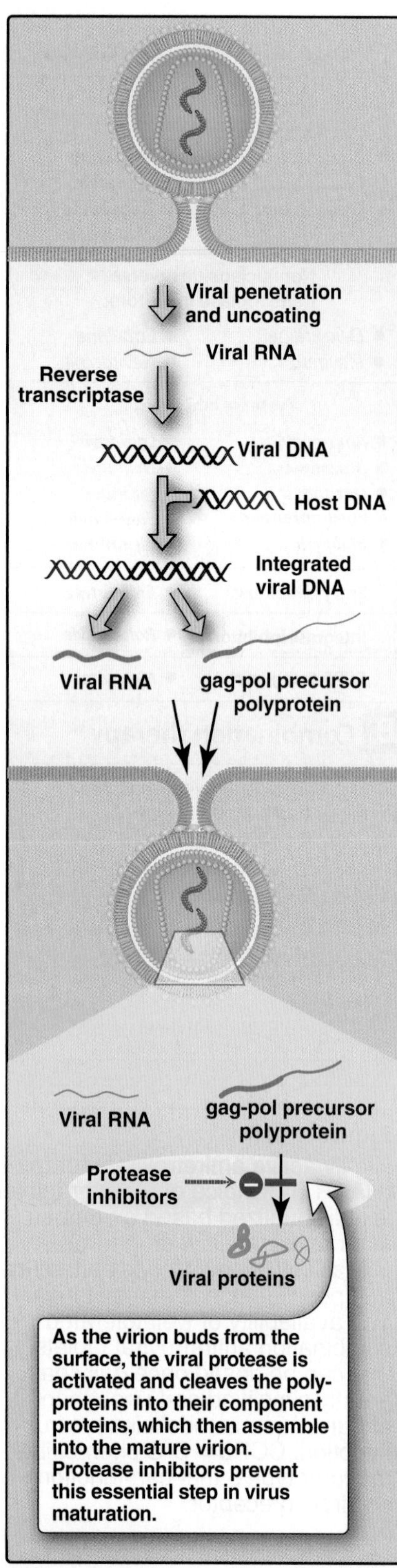

Figure 28.17
Role of human immunodeficiency virus protease in viral replication.

rate of progression to AIDS. This has led to the principle that HIV infection should be treated as aggressively and as early as possible, minimizing the initial spread of the virus. Not only does this approach yield a lower steady-state level of virus, but it has the additional advantage of increased drug efficacy insofar as drugs are administered at a time when mutants are still rare.

3. **Highly active antiretroviral therapy:** Currently, combinations of various drugs described below that are given three at a time are being evaluated for efficacy, both in short-term reduction of viral load and/or increase in CD4+ cell count and in long-term survival. Choice of a drug regimen is individualized based on criteria such as tolerability, drug–drug interactions, convenience/adherence, and possible baseline resistance. [Note: All such multiple-drug therapies are commonly referred to as "highly active antiretroviral therapy," or HAART (see Figure 28.16).] Unfortunately, although multidrug therapies can lower the viral load to undetectable levels, virus reemerges if HAART is stopped, indicating that the HIV has not been eradicated. Therefore, with current drug therapy, HIV continues to exist in sanctuaries, such as the CNS, testes, lymphoid tissue, and nonreplicating T-lymphocyte reservoirs. Thus, HIV infection is currently both chronic and incurable.

   a. **Nucleoside and nucleotide analog reverse transcriptase inhibitors:** Reverse transcriptase inhibitors prevent the copying of the HIV RNA genome into a proviral DNA genome. There are both nucleoside analogs and nonnucleoside inhibitors of the viral reverse transcriptase.[4] Nucleoside and nucleotide analogs inhibit primarily by serving as chain terminators after insertion into the growing DNA chain by the reverse transcriptase. Resistant mutants inevitably arise after long-term treatment with any one of these drugs. However, because cross-resistance is incomplete, zidovudine (AZT) in combination with one of the other drugs has been successful in minimizing the effect of mutation. Significant adverse effects accompany use of these drugs. The use of combined therapy in some cases permits less toxic doses to be administered.

   b. **The nonnucleoside reverse transcriptase inhibitors:** These drugs act by targeting the reverse transcriptase itself. They bind in a noncompetitive, reversible manner to a unique site on the enzyme, altering its ability to function. Their major advantage is their lack of effect on the host's blood-forming elements and lack of cross-resistance with nucleoside analog reverse transcriptase inhibitors.

   c. **Protease inhibitors:** The products of the *gag* and *pol* genes are translated initially into large polyprotein precursors that must be cleaved by the viral protease to yield the mature proteins. Protease inhibitors, which include ritonavir, nelfinavir, saquinavir, amprenavir, indinavir, and lopinavir interfere with the processing of the polyproteins in the budding virion and result in noninfectious particles (Figure 28.17). However, viral resis-

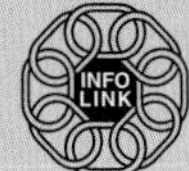

[4]See Chapter 29 in ***Lippincott's Illustrated Reviews: Biochemistry*** for a discussion of reverse transcriptase.

tance develops if protease inhibitors are used alone. Further, lipodystrophy (redistribution of fat, so that the limbs become skinny, and fat is deposited along the abdomen and the upper back) and hyperglycemia can occur with these drugs.

d. **Fusion inhibitor:** Enfuvirtide is a 36 amino acid peptide that binds to gp41 and inhibits the fusion of HIV with the membrane of the host cell.

e. **Integrase inhibitor:** Raltegravir targets the viral enzyme that catalyses the integration of the proviral DNA into the host's genome. Only one drug of this class is currently approved, although others are in clinical trials. This potent drug has few side effects or negative drug interactions.

f. **Coreceptor blockers:** Maraviroc is a CCR5 antagonist that interferes with binding and entry of the virus into susceptible cells. Circulating virus must be genotyped before the drug is utilized to determine whether the inhibitor will block virus entry, because not all variants are CCR5-tropic.

4. **Effect of HAART on the incidence of opportunistic infections:** The incidence of opportunistic infections in AIDS patients is decreasing in response to widespread use of aggressive multidrug treatment. This is true for virtually all opportunistic infections (Figure 28.18).

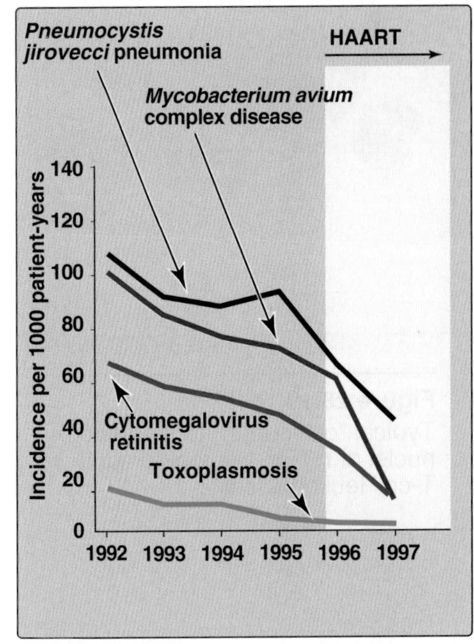

Figure 31.18
Incidence of selected opportunistic infections in patients with HIV infection. [Note: The shaded area labeled "HAART" indicates the period of wide availability of highly active antiretroviral therapy (HAART). The decline in opportunistic infections after 1995 largely reflects the effect of HAART.]

5. **Perinatal treatment:** Zidovudine when administered to HIV-1–infected pregnant women during the second and third trimesters of pregnancy, followed by administration to the infants during the first 6 weeks of life, reduces risk of maternal–infant transmission of HIV-1 from approximately 23 percent to 8 percent. The availability of this effective intervention, which decreases perinatal transmission of HIV-1, has led to increased efforts to screen all pregnant women (with their consent) for the presence of HIV-1 infection. Postnatal transmission of HIV via breast milk can, however, occur.

6. **Pre-exposure prophylaxis:** Three trials have investigated different populations: heterosexual couples in East Africa in which one person was HIV positive, and the other was not; sexually active young adults in Botswana; and, in the United States and other countries, MSM. In each trial, Truvada, a once-daily tablet containing tenofovir and emtricitabine, significantly reduced the risk of acquiring HIV infection. The drug is already approved to treat HIV infection but must be used in combination with other drugs to prevent the emergence of resistant HIV strains. The drug is useful for people at high risk of infection, like MSM with multiple sex partners, and individuals who are in relationships with someone who is HIV positive.

G. Prevention

Due to lower availability of antiretroviral drugs in developing countries and lack of a vaccine, education concerning methods for pre-

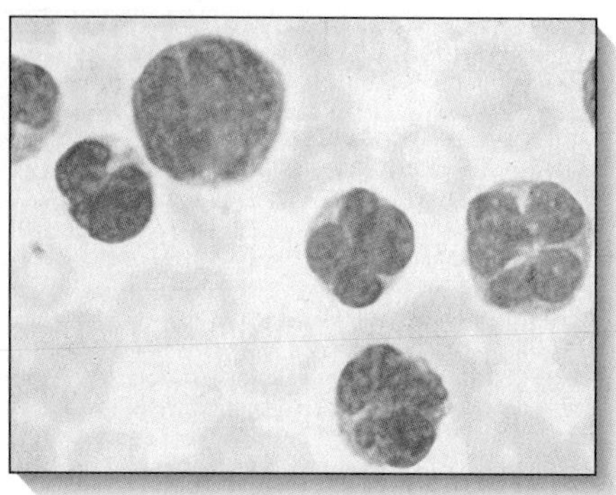

Figure 28.19
Typical "cloverleaf" appearance of nuclei of HTLV-1–infected adult T-cell leukemic cells.

venting transmission of HIV is currently the primary means of preventing spread of the virus.

1. Attempts to produce a vaccine: An effective vaccine is not yet available despite intensive efforts to produce one. HIV has a high mutation rate, and antigenically distinct strains exist worldwide.

2. Other measures: Screening of the blood supply has nearly eliminated transmission by that route. Strict adherence to standard precautions by healthcare workers can minimize risk in that setting. It is recommended that physicians screen for HIV infection in all adolescents and adults at increased risk of HIV infection. The Centers for Disease Control and Prevention has more recently recommended an "opt-out" strategy in which everyone between ages 13 and 64 years should be tested for HIV, regardless of perceived risk factors, unless he/she opts out of this testing.

IV. HUMAN T-CELL LYMPHOTROPIC VIRUSES, TYPES 1 AND 2

Human T-cell lymphotropic viruses, types 1 and 2 (HTLV-1 and -2) are genetically and biologically similar. However, their worldwide distribution differs. HTLV-1 has definitively been associated with a human malignant disease, adult T-cell leukemia (ATL), and a less common neurologic condition, HTLV-associated myelopathy/tropical spastic paraparesis (HAM/TSP). There are six subclasses of HTLV-1, each of which is endemic to different regions of the world. No conclusive evidence links HTLV-2 to any known disease.

A. Transmission of HTLV

The distribution of HTLV infection varies greatly with geographic area and socioeconomic group. HTLV transmission occurs primarily by cell-associated virus, via one of three routes. First, in highly endemic regions, mother to fetus or newborn is the most common mode of transmission. This is accomplished via infected lymphocytes either transplacentally or in breast milk. Second, infection can be transmitted sexually by infected lymphocytes contained in semen. Third, any blood products containing intact cells are also a potential source of infection. There is little evidence for transmission by cell-free fluids.

B. Pathogenesis and clinical significance of adult T-cell leukemia

Both HTLV-1 and HTLV-2 infect lymphocytes: HTLV-1 has a tropism for CD4 lymphocytes, whereas HTLV-2 preferentially infects CD8 lymphocytes. HTLV-1 infection both stimulates mitosis and immortalizes T lymphocytes, which acquire an "antigen-activated" phenotype. Following infection, the virus becomes integrated in the host cell as a provirus and transforms a polyclonal population of T cells. Although these cells all have an integrated provirus, there is no common integration site in different tumors. No HTLV mRNA is transcribed, and no recognized oncogene is activated. Continued multiplication of T lymphocytes over a period of many years results in the accumulation of many chromosomal aberrations. Peripheral blood smears show lymphoid cells with hyperlobulated nuclei (Figure 28.19). Selection of monoclonal populations leads to cells that have an increasingly malignant phenotype. HTLV-I seroprevalence rates are strongly age- and sex-dependent, with higher rates associated with older age and with female sex (Figure 28.20) The majority of infected individuals are asymptomatic carriers who have an estimated 2 to 4 percent chance of developing ATL within their lifetime. ATL typically appears 20 to 30 years after initial infection, when an increasingly larger population of monoclonal malignant ATL cells develops, and infiltration of various visceral organs by these cells occurs. There are accompanying serum chemistry abnormalities, and impairment of the immune system leads to opportunistic infections. Median survival after appearance of acute ATL is about 6 months.

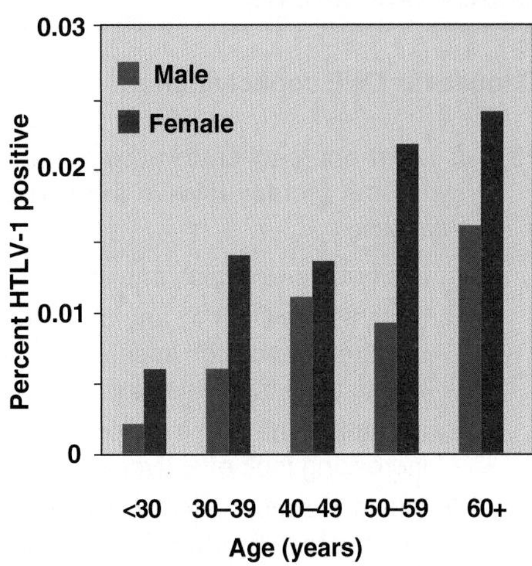

Figure 28.20
Age- and sex-specific seroprevalence of human T-cell lymphotropic virus type I in U.S. blood donors.

C. Pathogenesis and clinical significance of HTLV-associated myelopathy/tropical spastic paraparesis

About 1 to 2 percent of HTLV-1–infected individuals will go on to develop HAM/TSP. HAM/TSP is distinctly different from ATL in that it usually appears only a few years after infection. CNS involvement is indicated by: 1) the presence of anti-HTLV-1 antibody in the cerebrospinal fluid, 2) lymphocytic infiltration and demyelination of the thoracic spinal cord, and 3) brain lesions. The lymphocyte count is normal, although there is a polyclonal nonmalignant fraction with integrated HTLV. HAM occurs with lower frequency than ATL among HTLV-infected populations. It is characterized by progressive spasticity and weakness of the extremities, urinary and fecal incontinence, hyperreflexia, and some peripheral sensory loss.

D. Other manifestions of HTLV-1 infection.

HTLV-1 infections have also been associated with uveitis and retinal vasculitis. In addition, a chronic, severe form of infectious dermatitis can result from vertical transmission of the HTLV-1 virus and has been linked with an earlier onset of HAM/TSP.

E. Laboratory identification

Screening of blood donors for HTLV is done by ELISA or agglutination tests (see p. 27), but the existence of false-positives necessitates confirmatory testing by Western blotting. Test sensitivity is also a problem caused by the low and variable antibody titers in infected individuals. PCR amplification can be used to distinguish between HTLV-1 and HTLV-2 infections and to quantify viral load, which is a marker for the progression to HAM/TSP.

F. Treatment and prevention

The usual agents used in cancer chemotherapy have proven to be ineffective in treating ATL, and attempts to treat HAM/TSP, for the most part, have been equally unsuccessful. Treatment of both diseases is symptomatic. An estimated 15 to 20 million people worldwide are infected with HTLV-1 or -2, and 5 percent of these will eventually develop either ATL or HAM/TSP.

Study Questions

Choose the ONE correct answer.

28.1 Current approaches to acquired immune deficiency syndrome therapy involve the use of multiple drugs because:

A. it is not known which one will be effective.
B. mutants resistant to any one drug appear rapidly, but the chance for appearance of mutants resistant to all of them is small.
C. all inhibit the same step in replication, thereby increasing their effectiveness.
D. this is the most effective means of curing cells of integrated human immunodeficiency virus genomes.
E. each tends to neutralize the toxicity of the others.

Correct answer = B. The major problem with chemotherapy of acquired immune deficiency syndrome is the high mutation rate of the virus, leading to rapid appearance of mutants resistant to any single drug. By choosing drugs that act at different steps in the replication cycle or with different mechanisms of action, mutations in each of the affected proteins would have to occur in the same virus genome. The chance for this to occur is considerably lower than for either one individually. D: There is no way known to cure cells of their integrated genomes. E: Although these drugs do not neutralize each other's toxicity, it is possible in some cases to use a lower dose of each of the drugs, decreasing the toxic adverse effects.

28.2 The "asymptomatic period" following the initial acute disease caused by human immunodeficiency virus infection is characterized by:

A. high levels of human immunodeficiency virus replication in lymphoid tissue.
B. high levels of human immunodeficiency virus replication in circulating T lymphocytes.
C. inability of the immune system to respond to antigenic stimuli.
D. absence of detectable human immunodeficiency virus genomes or mRNA in circulating lymphocytes.
E. high titers of free virus in the blood.

Correct answer = A. During this period, a relatively large fraction of circulating lymphocytes can be shown to contain integrated human immunodeficiency virus (HIV) genomes, but a considerably smaller fraction have HIV mRNA, and virus replication occurs in relatively few cells. Infectious virus is largely confined to the lymphoid organs, although occasional bursts of viremia do occur, usually as the result of antigenic stimulation. The immune system retains its ability to respond to mitogenic stimuli generally, but there is some impairment of responses to specific antigens.

28.3 After infection of a cell by a retrovirus, synthesis of progeny genomes is carried out by:

A. the DNA-dependent RNA polymerase activity of viral reverse transcriptase.
B. the retrovirus RNA-dependent RNA polymerase.
C. the host cell DNA polymerase.
D. a host cell RNA polymerase.
E. a complex of reverse transcriptase and a second virus protein that enables it to synthesize RNA rather than DNA.

Correct answer = D. Progeny virus RNA is synthesized by the same transcription process as that of cellular genes. A and E: Reverse transcriptase is involved only in the initial step, converting the infecting parental RNA genome into double-stranded DNA. B: Unlike other RNA viruses, retroviruses do not encode an RNA-dependent RNA polymerase. C: The host cell DNA polymerase replicates the integrated provirus but plays no role in synthesis of progeny.

28.4 Which one of the following correctly describes human T-cell lymphotropic virus, type 1 (HTLV-1)?

A. The majority of infected individuals develop adult T-cell leukemia (ATL)
B. HTLV-1 causes myelopathy more frequently than ATL.
C. ALT typically appears 2 to 3 years after initial infection.
D. Virion entry into lymphocytes occurs most efficiently by direct cell-to-cell contact, rather than from virions free in plasma.
E. HTLV-1 induces death of infected lymphocytes.

Correct answer = D. Transmission rarely occurs by virons free in the plasma. The majority of infected individuals are asymptomatic carriers who have an estimated 2 to 4 percent chance of developing ATL within their lifetime. ATL typically appears 20 to 30 years after initial infection. ATL is more common than HTLV-associated myelopathy. Adult ALT typically appears 20 to 30 years after initial infection. HTLV-1 does not induce death of lymphocytes, but rather causes cell proliferation and transformation.

Negative-strand RNA Viruses

29

I. OVERVIEW

Medically important negative-strand RNA viruses are shown in Figure 29.1. They have several things in common: 1) they are all enveloped; 2) their virions contain an RNA-dependent RNA transcriptase that synthesizes viral mRNAs using the genomic negative-strand RNA as a template; 3) the genomic negative-strand viral RNAs are not infectious, in contrast to the genomic RNAs of positive-strand viruses (see p. 283); and 4) following entry and penetration, the first step in the replication of negative-strand RNA viruses is the synthesis of mRNAs, whereas with positive-strand RNA viruses, the first step in replication is translation of the incoming genomic RNA (see p. 239). Some negative-strand RNA viruses have segmented genomes, whereas others have nonsegmented genomes. Although most of these viruses replicate in the cytosol, the replication of influenza virus RNA (an orthomyxovirus) occurs in the nucleus.

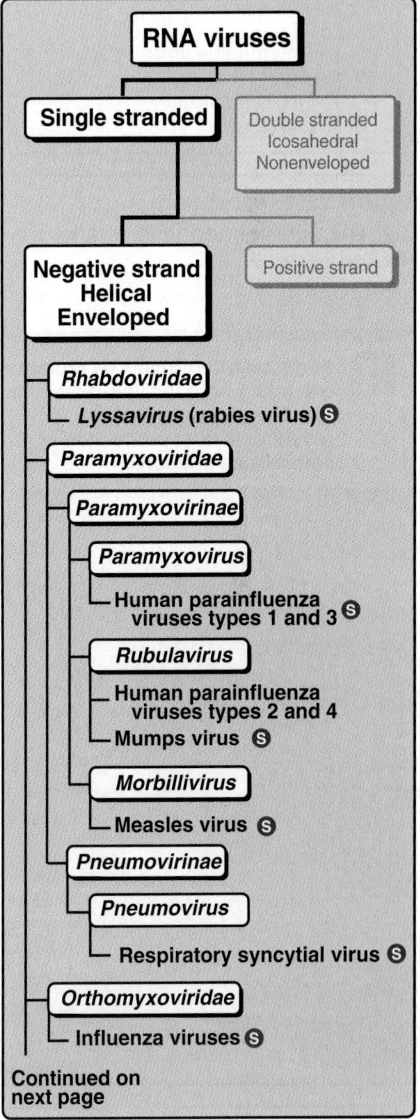

Figure 29.1
Classification of negative-strand RNA viruses (continued on next page). Ⓢ See pp. 365, 361, 360 for summaries of these viruses.

II. RHABDOVIRIDAE

Rhabdoviruses are enveloped, bullet-shaped viruses (Figure 29.2). Each contains a helical nucleocapsid (see p. 235). The viruses in the family *Rhabdoviridae* known to infect mammals are divided into two genera: *Lyssavirus* (rabies virus, the rhabdovirus of greatest medical importance to humans), and *Vesiculovirus* [vesicular stomatitis virus (VSV), a virus of horses and cattle, and the best-studied virus in this family]. Other rhabdoviruses infect invertebrates, plants, or other vertebrates.

A. Epidemiology

A wide variety of wildlife, such as raccoons, skunks, squirrels, foxes, and bats, provide reservoirs for the rabies virus (Figure 29.3B). In developing countries, domestic dogs and cats also constitute important reservoirs for rabies. Cases of human rabies are rare in the United States. However, in developing areas, such as rural Africa and Asia, rabies causes approximately 55,000 deaths a year. Humans are usually infected by the bite of an animal, but, in some cases, infection is via inhalation (for example, of droppings from infected bats). Sequence analysis of the viral RNA has shown that most human cases in the United States are from a bat strain of rabies virus.

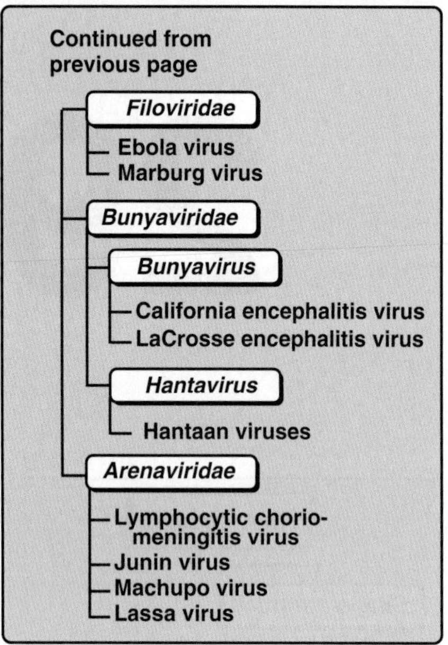

Figure 29.1 (continued)
Classification of negative-strand RNA viruses.

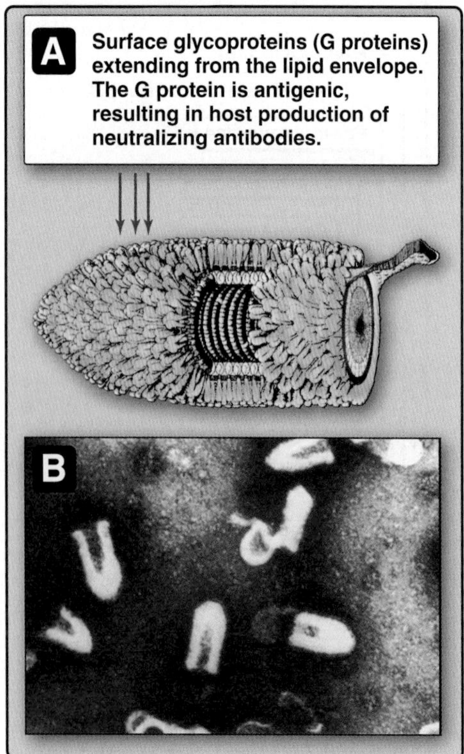

A
Surface glycoproteins (G proteins) extending from the lipid envelope. The G protein is antigenic, resulting in host production of neutralizing antibodies.
B

Figure 29.2
Rabies virus. A. Schematic drawing. B. Electron micrograph.

B. Viral replication

The genomic negative-strand RNA is nonsegmented. The virion contains five proteins, one of which, the G (for "glyco-") protein, is an envelope protein composed of viral spikes (see Figure 29.2). The rabies virion attaches via its glycoprotein spikes to cell-surface receptors. It enters the cell via receptor-mediated endocytosis, following which the viral envelope fuses with the endocytotic vesicle's membrane, releasing the viral nucleocapsid into the cytosol, where replication occurs. Five different mRNAs are transcribed from the genomic RNA template by the virion's RNA-dependent RNA polymerase (transcriptase function), each of which encodes one viral protein. The polymerase that produces the mRNA also synthesizes positive-strand copies of the viral RNA template (replicase function), from which new negative-strand RNA genomic molecules can be transcribed. This process is an example of the Type II virus genome replication described on p. 240. Viral structural proteins plus the negative-strand viral RNA form new helical nucleocapsids, which move to the cell surface. There, each nucleocapsid acquires its envelope by budding through a region of virus-modified plasma membrane (see Figure 23.16).

C. Pathology

Following inoculation, the virus may replicate locally but then travels via retrograde transport within peripheral neurons to the brain, where it replicates primarily in the gray matter (Figure 29.3A). From the brain, the rabies virus can travel along autonomic nerves, leading to infection of the lungs, kidney, adrenal medulla, and salivary glands. [Note: Contamination of saliva potentially leads to further transmission of the disease (for example, through a bite from an infected animal).] The extremely variable incubation period depends on the host's resistance, amount of virus transferred, and distance of the site of initial infection from the central nervous system (CNS). Incubation generally lasts 1 to 8 weeks but may range up to several months or, in unusual cases, as long as several years following exposure. Clinical illness may begin with an abnormal sensation at the site of the bite, then progress to a fatal encephalitis, with neuronal degeneration of the brain and spinal cord. Symptoms include hallucinations; seizures; weakness; mental dysfunction; paralysis; coma; and, finally, death. Many, but not all, patients show the classic rabid sign of hydrophobia. In this case, "hydrophobia" refers to the infected individual's painful inability to swallow liquids (due to pharyngeal spasms), leading to avoidance. Once symptoms begin, death is almost always inevitable.

D. Laboratory identification

Clinically, diagnosis rests on a history of exposure and signs and symptoms characteristic of rabies. However, a reliable history of exposure is often not obtainable, and the clinical presentation, especially in the initial stages, may not be characteristic. Therefore, a clinical diagnosis may be difficult. Postmortem, in approximately 80 percent of cases, characteristic eosinophilic cytoplasmic inclusions

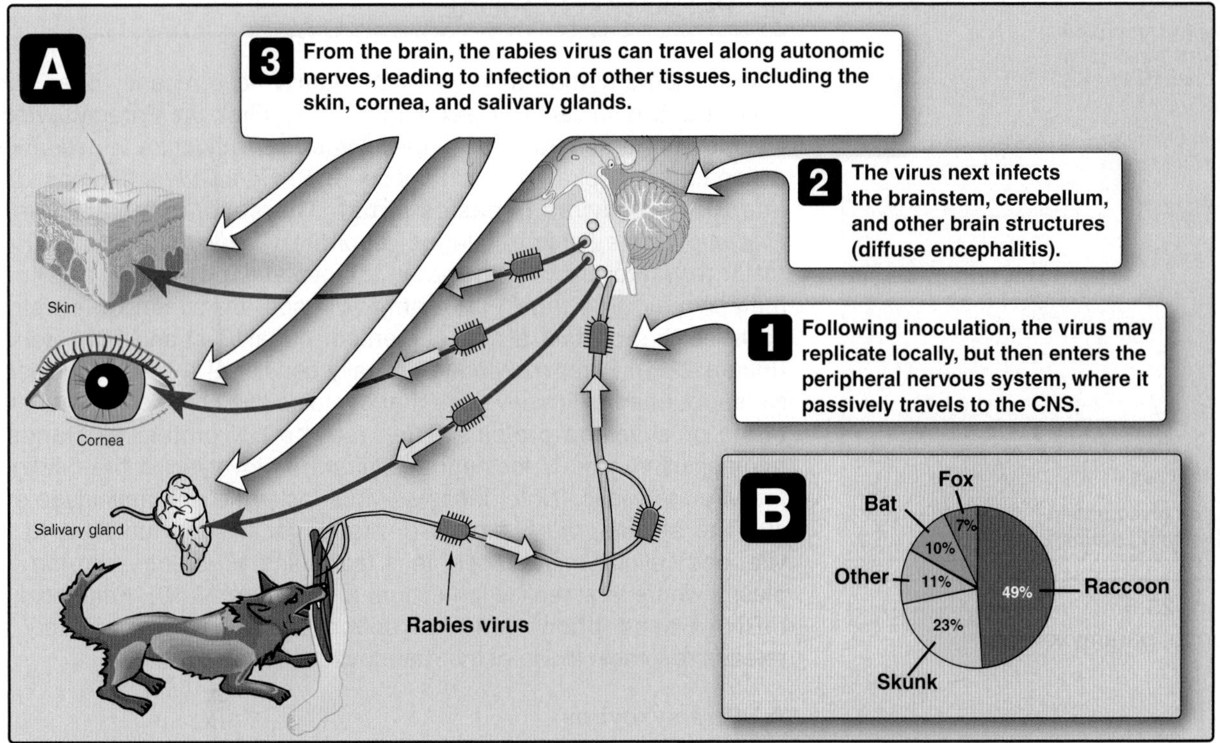

Figure 29.3
A. Schematic representation of pathogenesis of rabies infection. B. Wildlife rabies in the United States.

(Negri bodies) may be identified in certain regions of the brain such as the hippocampus. These cytoplasmic inclusion bodies are virus production foci and diagnostic of rabies (Figure 29.4). Prior to death, the diagnosis can be made by identification of viral antigens in biopsies of skin from the back of the neck or from corneal cells or by demonstration of the viral nucleic acid by reverse transcription polymerase chain reaction (RT-PCR) in infected saliva (see p. 30).

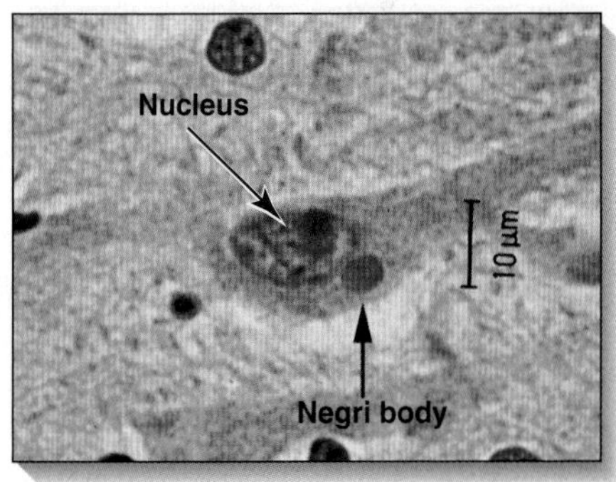

Figure 29.4
An oval Negri body in a brain cell from a human rabies case.

E. Treatment and prevention

Once an individual has clinical symptoms of rabies, there is no effective treatment. However, a killed rabies virus vaccine is available for prophylaxis. In the United States, two vaccine formulations are approved by the Food and Drug Administration. Both contain inactivated virus grown in cultured cells (chick embryo cells or human diploid cells). Preexposure prophylaxis is indicated for individuals at high risk because of the work they do (for example, for veterinarians). Postexposure prophylaxis refers to treatment instituted after an animal bite or exposure to an animal (or human) suspected of being rabid, and consists of thorough cleaning of the wound, passive immunization with antirabies immunoglobulin, and active immunization with the rabies vaccine (HDCV, the human diploid cell vaccine). Prevention of initial exposure is, however, clearly the most important mechanism for controlling human rabies.

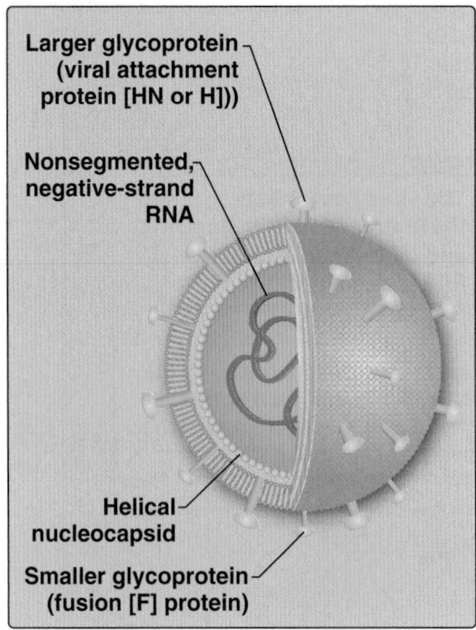

Figure 29.5
Model of paramyxovirus.

III. PARAMYXOVIRIDAE

The members of the *Paramyxoviridae* family have recently been subdivided into two subfamilies (see Figure 29.1). First, the Paramyxovirinae, includes three genera: 1) *Paramyxovirus* (parainfluenza viruses, which cause upper respiratory tract infections); 2) *Rubulavirus* (mumps virus); and 3) *Morbillivirus* (measles virus). The second subfamily is the *Pneumovirinae*, which includes respiratory syncytial virus (RCV), a major respiratory tract pathogen in the pediatric population, and human metapneumovirus (hMPV). Paramyxoviruses are spherical, enveloped particles that contain a nonsegmented, negative-strand RNA genome (Figure 29.5). Paramyxoviridae typically consist of a helical nucleocapsid surrounded by an envelope that contains two types of integral membrane or envelope proteins. The first, the HN protein (H stands for hemagglutinin and N for neuraminidase), is involved in the binding of the virus to a cell. [Note: Measles virus lacks the neuraminidase activity.] The second, the F protein (F stands for fusion), functions to fuse viral and cellular membranes, thus facilitating virus entry into the cytoplasm, where viral replication occurs (see Figure 23.10). *Paramyxovirus* mRNA transcription, genome replication, and viral assembly and release resemble those of the rhabdoviruses (see p. 309).

A. *Paramyxovirus*

The clinically important viruses in this genus are types 1 and 3 human parainfluenza viruses (hPIV). They cause croup, pneumonia, and bronchiolitis, mainly in infants and children. The term "parainfluenza" was first coined because infected individuals may present with influenza-like symptoms, and, like influenza virus, these viruses have both hemagglutinating and neuraminidase activities.

B. *Rubulavirus*

This genus contains hPIV types 2 and 4 and mumps virus.

1. **Types 2 and 4 human parainfluenza viruses:** The clinical features of infection with parainfluenza virus type 2 are similar to those of types 1 and 3 viruses. Type 4 hPIV has been associated only with a mild upper respiratory tract illness, affecting both children and adults.

2. **Mumps virus:** Mumps used to be one of the commonly acquired childhood infections. Adults who escape the disease in childhood could also be infected. In the prevaccine period, mumps was the most common cause of viral encephalitis. Complete recovery, however, was almost always achieved. The virus spreads by respiratory droplets. Although about one third of infections are subclinical, the classic clinical presentation and diagnosis center on infection and swelling of the salivary glands, primarily the parotid glands (Figure 29.6). However, infection is widespread in the body and may involve not only the salivary glands but also the pancreas, CNS, and testes. Orchitis (inflammation of the testis) caused by mumps virus may cause sterility. A live, attenuated vaccine has been available for many year and has resulted in a dramatic drop in the number of cases of mumps. [Note: Individuals who have had the disease develop lifelong immunity.]

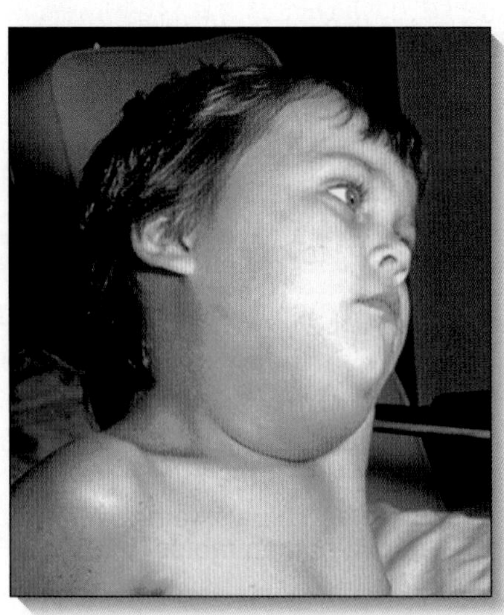

Figure 29.6
Child with mumps showing swollen parotid gland.

C. *Morbillivirus*

Measles virus is the only virus in this genus that causes disease in humans. Other viruses in the genus *Morbillivirus* are responsible for diseases in animals (for example, canine distemper virus). Measles virus differs in several ways from the other viruses in the family Paramyxoviridae.

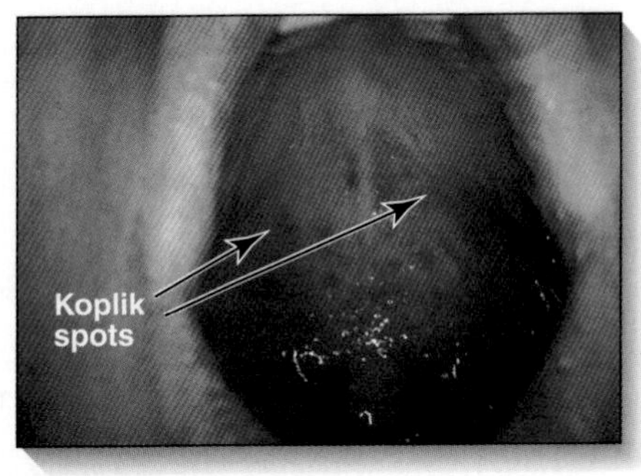

Figure 29.7
Koplik spots in the mouth caused by measles virus.

1. **Viral replication:** The cellular receptor for measles virus is the CD46 molecule, a protein whose normal function is to bind certain components of complement. Although the viral attachment protein has hemagglutinating activity, it lacks neuraminidase activity. Hence, it is referred to as the H protein, rather than HN protein. An F protein facilitates uptake of the virion. Measles virus replication in tissue culture and certain organs of the intact organism is characterized by the formation of giant multinucleate cells (syncytium formation), resulting from the action of the viral spike F protein.

2. **Pathology:** Measles virus is transmitted by sneeze- or cough-produced respiratory droplets. The virus is extremely infectious, and almost all infected individuals develop a clinical illness. Measles virus replicates initially in the respiratory epithelium and then in various lymphoid organs. Classically, measles (previously referred to as rubeola) begins with a prodromal period of fever, cough, coryza (runny nose), and conjunctivitis (often referred to as the "3 C"s). Two to three days later, specific diagnostic signs develop. First, Koplik spots (small white spots on bright red mucous membranes of the mouth and throat) appear (Figure 29.7), followed by a generalized macular rash, beginning at the head and traveling slowly to the lower extremities (Figure 29.8). Soon after the rash appears, the patient is no longer infectious. The major morbidity and mortality caused by measles are associated with various complications of infection, especially those affecting the lower respiratory tract and the CNS. The most important of these is postinfectious encephalomyelitis, which is estimated to affect 1 of 1,000 cases of measles, usually occurring within 2 weeks after the onset of the rash. This is an autoimmune disease associated with an immune response to myelin basic protein. Figure 29.9 shows the time course of measles virus infection. Children are particularly susceptible, especially those weakened by other diseases or malnutrition. Measles is, therefore, an important cause of childhood mortality in developing countries.

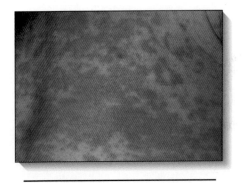

Figure 29.8
The measles rash consists of large, slightly raised lesions called maculopapules. These run into each other to form irregular blotches.

3. **Diagnosis:** In most cases, there is little difficulty in making a diagnosis of measles on clinical grounds, especially in an epidemic situation. The presence of Koplik spots provides a definitive diagnosis. If a laboratory diagnosis is necessary, it is usually made by demonstrating an increase in the titer of antiviral antibodies.

4. **Prevention:** Measles is usually a disease of childhood and is followed by lifelong immunity. A live, attenuated measles vaccine, which has been available for many years, has greatly reduced the incidence of the disease. Nevertheless, occasional outbreaks of measles continue to occur, especially in older children and young

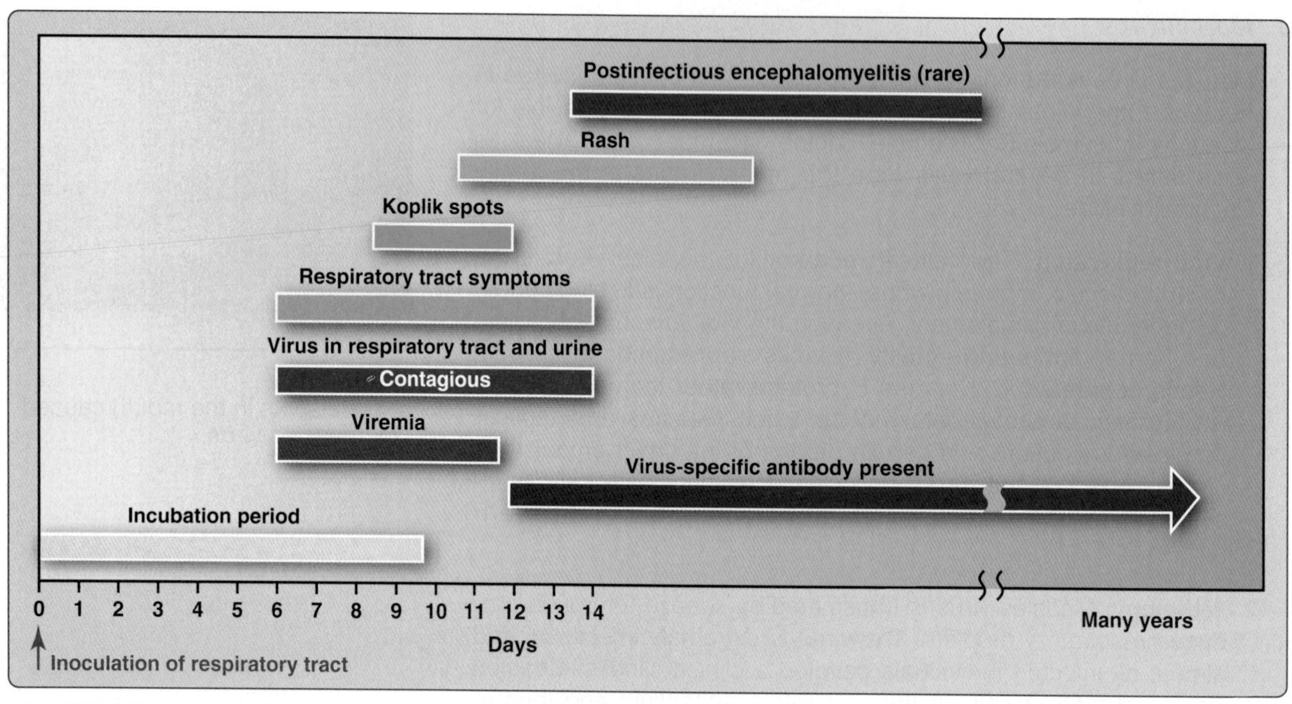

Figure 29.9
Time course of measles virus infection.

adults, possibly due to waning immunity. Thus, two doses of the vaccine, in the form of the measles-mumps-rubella (MMR) vaccine (see p. 39), are now recommended, the first at 12 to 18 months, the second at 4 to 6 years. Parental resistance to the MMR vaccine has led to populations of children who are susceptible to measles. Importation of the virus by returning international travelers has led to recent outbreaks in the United States among unvaccinated children.

D. *Pneumovirus*

There are two viruses in this genus that are of medical importance: RSV and hMPV. RSV is the major viral respiratory tract pathogen in the pediatric population and the most important cause of bronchiolitis in infants. hMPV is the second leading cause of bronchiolitis in infants but can also cause pneumonia and croup in children. RSV may also cause pneumonia in young children, an influenza-like syndrome in adults, and severe bronchitis with pneumonia in older adults and organ transplant recipients. The viruses in the subfamily *Pneumovirinae*, genus *Pneumovirus*, are set apart from those in the other three genera in the Paromyxovirus family by a somewhat more complex genome and a larger number of virus-specific proteins. Nevertheless, the basic strategy of replication is as described for the other viruses in this family (see p. 312). RSV has one envelope protein that functions as an attachment protein and another that functions as a fusion protein, but, like measles virus, RSV lacks neuraminidase activity. RSV is transmitted by respiratory droplets or by contaminated hands carrying the virus to the nose or mouth. Repeated infections are common. Definitive diagnoses of RSV or hMPV infection can be made only on the basis of laboratory findings, including culture of virus from nasopharyngeal secretions, detection of viral RNA by RT-PCR or detection of viral antigen by enzyme-linked immunosorbent assay (ELISA) techniques. The only specific treatment for RSV is ribavirin, administered by aerosol, and this is only of moderate benefit. Handwashing and avoiding others with the infection are the major preventive measures, because no vaccine is available to prevent infection with either virus.

IV. ORTHOMYXOVIRIDAE

Orthomyxoviruses are spherical, enveloped viruses containing a segmented, negative strand RNA genome. Viruses in this family infect humans, horses, and pigs, as well as nondomestic waterfowl, and are the cause of influenza. Orthomyxoviruses are divided into three types: influenzae A, B, and C. Only influenza virus types A and B are of medical importance. Type A influenza viruses differ from type B viruses in that they have an animal reservoir and are divided into subtypes. Influenza virus C is not a significant human pathogen.

A. Structure

Influenza virions are spherical, enveloped, pleomorphic particles (Figure 29.10). Two types of spikes project from the surface: One is composed of H protein and the second of N protein. [Note: This is in contrast to the paramyxoviruses, in which H and N activities reside in the same spike protein.] Both the H and N influenza proteins are integral membrane proteins. The M (matrix) proteins underlie the viral lipid membrane. The RNA genome, located in a helical nucleocapsid, is composed of eight distinct segments of RNA, each of which encodes one or more viral proteins. Each nucleocapsid segment contains not only the viral RNA but also four proteins (NP, the major nucleocapsid protein, and three P (polymerase) proteins that are present in much smaller amounts than NP and are involved in synthesis and replication of viral RNA).

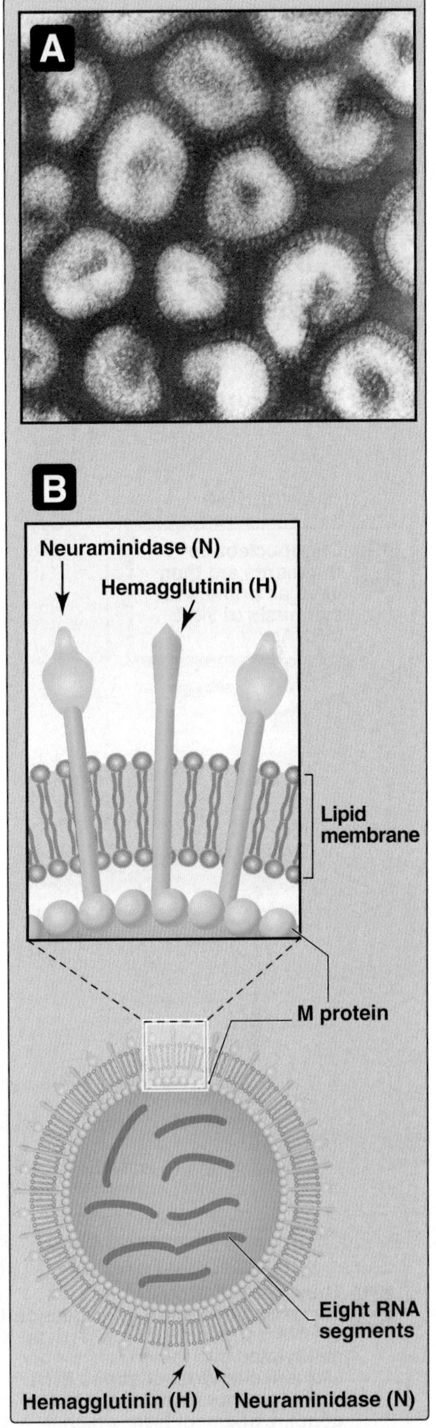

Figure 29.10
Influenza virus. A. Electron micrograph. B. Schematic drawing showing envelope proteins—called H and N spikes—that protrude from the surface. M protein = matrix protein.

B. Viral replication

There are two unusual features associated with synthesis and replication of influenza viral RNAs that distinguish the influenza viruses from the other RNA viruses discussed up to this point. First, the synthesis of influenza virus mRNAs and the replication of the viral genome occur in the nucleus. This is in contrast to the replication of other RNA viruses, which occurs completely in the cytoplasm. [Note: The retroviruses are an exception to this generalization (see p. 295).] Second, compounds such as actinomycin D and α-amanitin, which inhibit mRNA transcription by eukaryotic RNA polymerase II (Pol II), also inhibit the replication of influenza virus.

1. **Viral entry into the cell:** Influenza virus attaches to sialic acid residues on host cell glycoproteins or glycolipids. Entry then occurs via receptor-mediated endocytosis (see Figure 23.10). Both the attachment and the fusion functions are associated with the H protein.

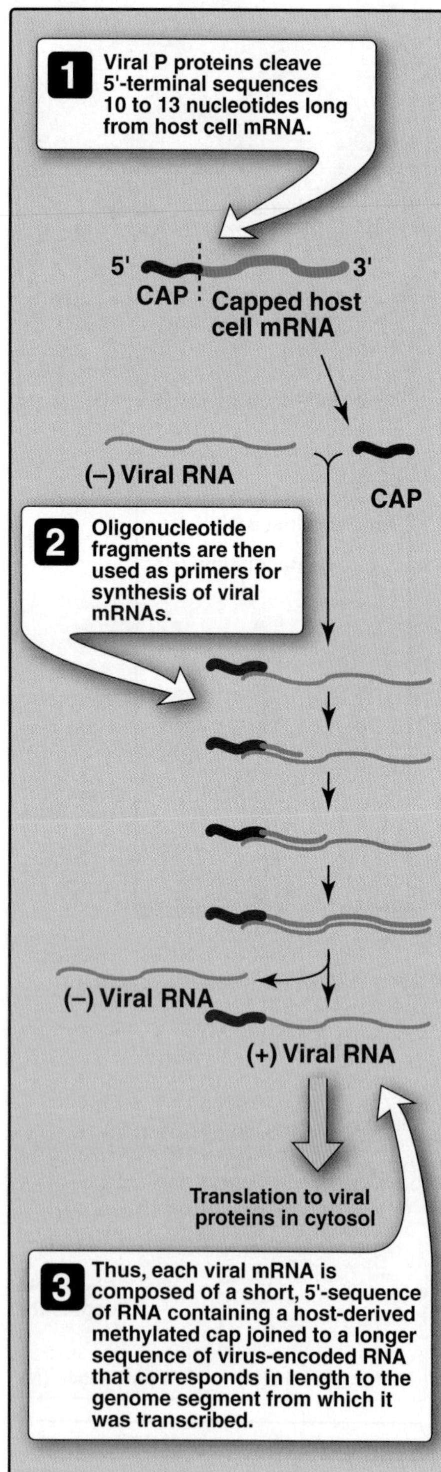
1
Viral P proteins cleave 5'-terminal sequences 10 to 13 nucleotides long from host cell mRNA.
5'
3'
CAP
Capped host cell mRNA
(–) Viral RNA
CAP
2
Oligonucleotide fragments are then used as primers for synthesis of viral mRNAs.
(–) Viral RNA
(+) Viral RNA
Translation to viral proteins in cytosol
3
Thus, each viral mRNA is composed of a short, 5'-sequence of RNA containing a host-derived methylated cap joined to a longer sequence of virus-encoded RNA that corresponds in length to the genome segment from which it was transcribed.

Figure 29.11
"Cap snatching" by influenza virus prior to viral mRNA translation.

2. **Synthesis and translation of viral mRNAs:** The nucleocapsid segments are released into the cytosol, and, as with the other negative-strand RNA viruses, the viral genomic RNA serves as the template for synthesis of viral mRNAs. Each of the eight genome segments directs the synthesis of one positive-strand mRNA. However, influenza virus is distinguished from the other negative-strand viruses in that, although the virions contain proteins that can transcribe mRNAs, these enzymes lack the ability to cap and methylate viral mRNAs. The synthesis of influenza virus mRNA, therefore, begins with "cap snatching," in which the viral P proteins cleave 5'-terminal sequences (10 to 13 nucleotides long) from nascent host cellular Pol II transcripts that had been previously synthesized, capped, and methylated in the nucleus. The oligonucleotide fragments are then used as primers for the synthesis of the viral mRNAs (Figure 29.11). Thus, each viral mRNA is composed of a short, 5'-sequence of RNA containing a host-derived methylated cap joined to a longer sequence of virus-encoded RNA that corresponds in length to the genome segment from which it was transcribed.

3. **Assembly and release of influenza virus particles:** Once the viral mRNAs are made and translated, the NP and the three P proteins move into the nucleus, whereupon replication of the eight genomic segments begins, and progeny nucleocapsids are assembled. Meanwhile, certain regions of the plasma membrane are virus modified by insertion of H and N proteins and alignment of the M protein on the inner side of the plasma membrane. The nucleocapsids move from the nucleus to the cytosol and, finally, to virus-modified regions of the plasma membrane, through which they bud, giving rise to extracellular viral particles (Figure 29.12). Viral release is facilitated by the N protein, which cleaves neuraminic acid on the cell surface.

C. Pathology and clinical significance

In humans, influenza is spread by respiratory droplets and is an infection solely of the respiratory tract (Figure 29.13). There is rarely viremia or spread to other organ systems. Destruction of respiratory epithelial cells is attributed to the host immune response, specifically cytotoxic T cells. Typically, influenza has an acute onset, with symptoms including a nonproductive cough and chills, followed by high fever, muscle aches (caused by circulating cytokines), and extreme drowsiness. Runny nose is unusual, differentiating influenza virus infection from the common cold. The disease runs its course in 4 to 5 days, after which recovery is gradual. The most serious problems, such as development of pneumonia, occur in the very young, older adults, and people with chronic cardiac or pulmonary disease or those who are immunodeficient. Reye syndrome is a rare and serious complication of viral infections in children, especially in those who have had chickenpox or influenza B. Aspirin, used to lower virus-induced fever, contributes to the appearance of this syndrome. Therefore, acetaminophen is usually recommended for fevers of unknown origin in children.

D. Epidemiology

Influenza virus infections are seasonal, with peaks in incidence from October through May. Between 5 and 20 percent of the U.S. population contracts the flu each year, resulting in over 200,000 hospitalizations and more than 36,000 deaths.

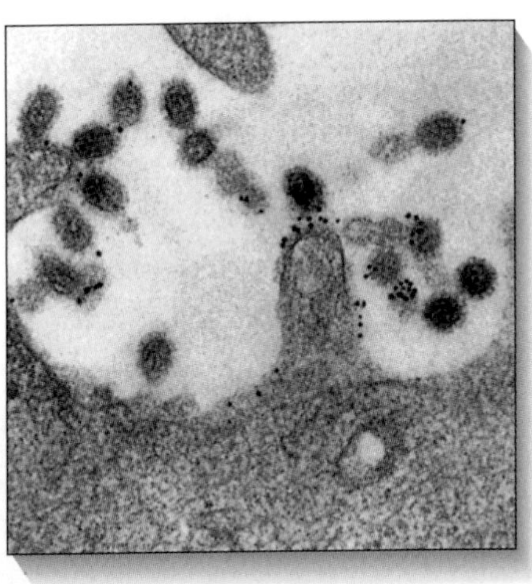

Figure 29.12
Influenza virus budding from the surface of an infected cell (electron micrograph).

E. Influenza virus immunology

When individuals are infected with influenza virus, antibodies are made against the various viral proteins. However, it is the antibodies made against the H protein that are neutralizing and the best index of protection. The antigenic properties of the influenza virus proteins are also important because they serve as the basis for the classification of influenza viruses.

1. **Types and subtypes:** Influenza viruses are classified as types A, B, and C, depending on their inner proteins, mainly the M and NP proteins. Thus, all type A viruses share common internal antigens that are distinct from those shared by all type B viruses. Only the type A viruses are broken down into subtypes. The classification into subtypes depends on antigens associated with the outer viral proteins, H and N. Taking into consideration animal as well as human influenza viruses, 16 H and 9 N subtypes have been described. Subtypes of influenza viruses are, therefore, designated by the unique combinations of H and N antigens, for example: H1N1, H2N2, and H3N2.

2. **Antigenic variability of influenza viruses:** In contrast to viruses such as polio or measles virus that have maintained antigenic stability since they were first isolated, influenza viruses have shown marked variation over the years in antigenic properties, specifically H and N proteins. Two distinct phenomena account for this observation: antigenic drift and antigenic shift.

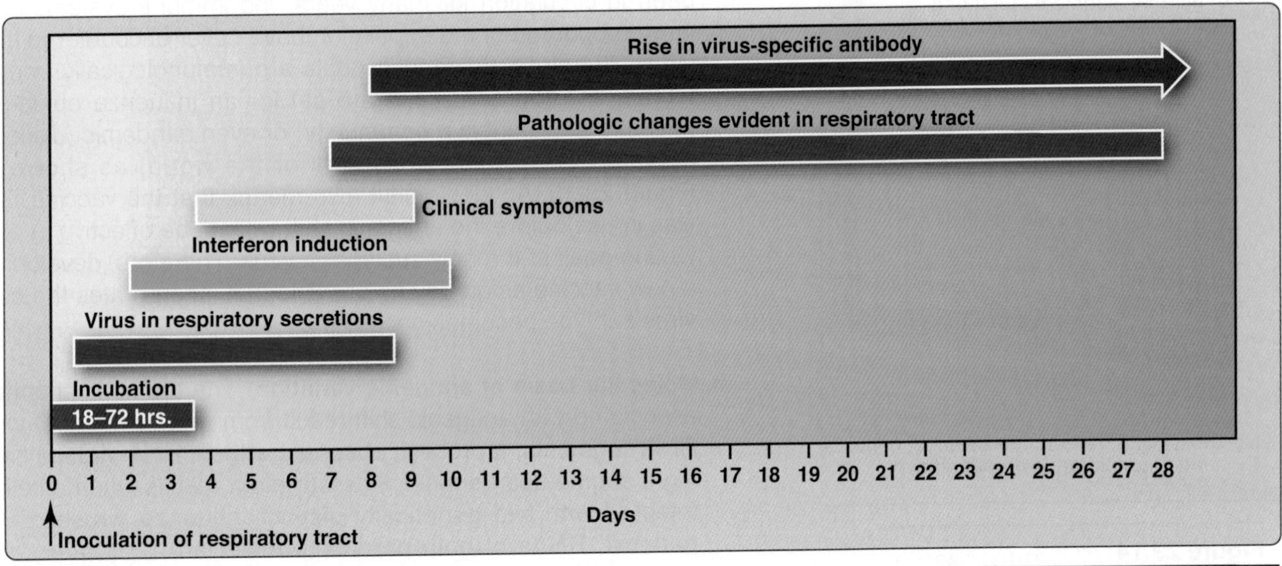

Figure 29.13
Time course of influenza A virus infection. The classic "flu syndrome" occurs early. Later, pneumonia may result from secondary bacterial infection.

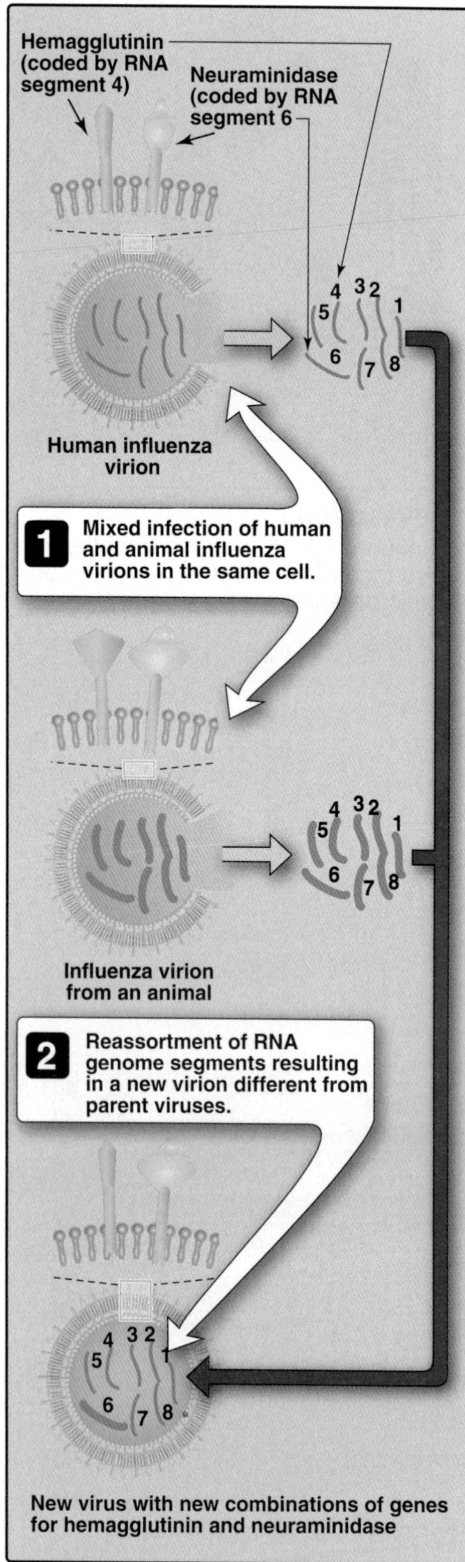
Hemagglutinin (coded by RNA segment 4)
Neuraminidase (coded by RNA segment 6
Human influenza virion
1 Mixed infection of human and animal influenza virions in the same cell.
Influenza virion from an animal
2 Reassortment of RNA genome segments resulting in a new virion different from parent viruses.
New virus with new combinations of genes for hemagglutinin and neuraminidase

Figure 29.14
Mechanism of antigenic shift in influenza virus.

a. **Antigenic drift:** This refers to minor antigenic changes in H and N proteins that occur each year. Antigenic drift does not involve a change in the viral subtype. This phenomenon can be easily explained by random mutations in viral RNA and single or a small number of amino acid substitutions in H and N proteins.

b. **Antigenic shift:** This phenomenon involves a much more dramatic change in the antigenic properties of the H and/or N proteins (Figure 29.14), and a change in subtype, for example, from H1N1 to H3N2. Antigenic shift occurs only infrequently, perhaps every 10 or 20 years. For example, the appearance of a new, extremely virulent H1N1 virus, due presumably to antigenic shift, probably accounted for the pandemic of 1918–1919 that resulted in the death of an estimated 20 million people worldwide, including more than 500,000 in the United States (Figure 29.15). In 1957, antigenic shift again occurred, and H1N1 virus was replaced by subtype H2N2. In 1968, H2N2 was replaced by H3N2. Since 1977, multiple subtypes of influenza A have been circulating around the world. In most years, both type A and type B influenza viruses can be isolated from patients. Both type A and B viruses undergo antigenic drift, but only type A viruses show antigenic shift. H5N1 (an avian flu subtype) was first isolated in 1997 from a human. The virus affects individuals who live closely with domestic birds such as chickens. Passage from human to human has not been seen, but rather from bird to bird, including wild birds that migrate. The primary infections have been in Asia and the Middle East. Over 50 percent of reported cases have been fatal.

c. **Consequences of antigenic variation:** When antigenic shift occurs, giving rise to a subtype of virus appears that has not been in circulation for many years, the immune systems of a large proportion of the population have never encountered that virus. Therefore, these individuals are immunologically unprotected, and the conditions are set for an influenza epidemic (disease prevalent in a community) or even pandemic (disease prevalent over a whole country or the world) as shown in Figure 29.15. Antigenic shift also means that the vaccine that was in use before the antigenic shift will not be effective in protecting against the new subtype of virus. Therefore, developing a new vaccine as quickly as possible that incorporates the new virus subtype becomes necessary.

d. **Molecular basis of antigenic variation:** The dramatic changes associated with antigenic shift result from reassortment of viral RNA segments, a process observed with all RNA viruses having a segmented genome. Reassortment results when a cell is infected with two genetically distinct influenza viruses: The genomic RNAs of both parental viruses are replicated, and progeny viruses are assembled that contain genomic RNA segments from one of the parental viruses and other genomic segments from the second parent (see Figure 29.14). In this

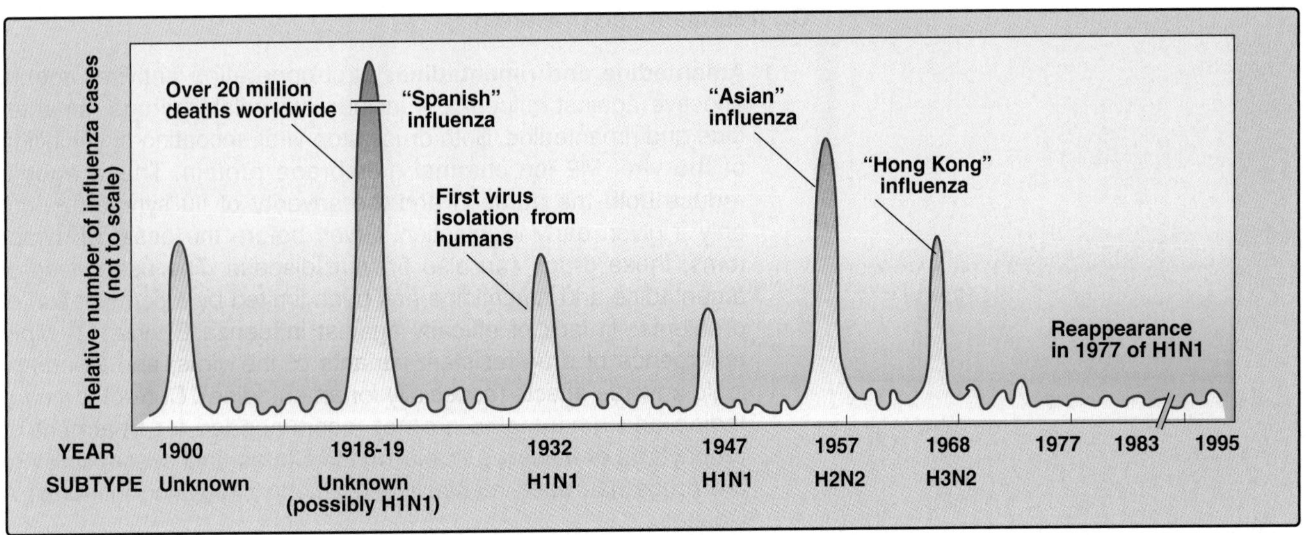

Figure 29.15
Time line showing the occurrence of some of the major outbreaks and antigenic shifts associated with type A influenza during the 1900s.

way, new viruses can be generated that differ from both parents. Although all eight of the influenza virus RNA genome segments undergo reassortment, for antigenic shift to occur, it is the reassortment of the RNA segments that specify the mRNAs for H and N proteins (the proteins that define the antigenic subtypes) that is most critical. How does this reassortment occur? We know that influenza type A viruses are found in many different animals, including horses, pigs, and wild migrating waterfowl. Furthermore, it has been demonstrated that reassortment can occur between influenza A viruses that infect different animal and avian species. For example, pigs can be infected by human- and avian-specific influenza viruses. In environments where pigs, birds and humans coexist, it is possible for a pig to be simultaneously infected with multiple influenza subtypes. "Reassortants" can, therefore, be produced within one host animal (the pig), in which the mRNAs encoding the H and N antigens have been reassorted into unique combinations. The reassortant virus then has the potential to spread among humans, birds, and pigs.

F. Diagnosis

The collection of influenza-like symptoms described above can also be caused by other viruses such as RSV (see p. 314). Therefore, a definitive diagnosis cannot be made on clinical grounds except in an epidemic situation. In most cases, it is not practical to make a specific laboratory diagnosis. Isolation of virus from nasopharyngeal washings in culture is the gold standard, but is difficult and time consuming. Detection of viral RNA by RT-PCR is sensitive and specific. Rapid tests are also available in which viral antigens (neuraminidase or nucleoprotein) can be detected in nasopharyngeal swab specimens.

G. Treatment and prevention

1. **Amantadine and rimantadine:** First-generation antiviral agents effective against influenza A include two related drugs, amantadine and rimantadine. Both drugs stop viral uncoating by inhibition of the viral M2 ion channel membrane protein. These agents reduce both the duration and the severity of flu symptoms, but only if given early in infection. Given before the onset of symptoms, these drugs can also prevent disease. The usefulness of amantadine and rimantidine has been limited by a combination of problems: 1) lack of efficacy against influenza B virus, 2) rapid emergence of drug-resistant variants of the virus, and 3) neurologic adverse effects (especially for amantadine). Currently, amantadine and rimantadine are not recommended for treatment or prophylaxis of influenza in the United States until susceptibility to the drugs has been reestablished among circulating influenza A isolates.

2. **Zanamivir and oseltamivir:** Second-generation antiviral agents effective against influenza A and B include zanamivir and oseltamivir. They inhibit viral neuraminidase, which is present in both influenza A and B viruses. Neuraminidase is an enzyme that is essential for the production progeny virus. The enzyme cleaves terminal sialic acid residues from glycoconjugates to allow the release of the virus from infected cells. The neuraminidase inhibitors are indicated for uncomplicated acute illness in individuals ages 7 years and older who have been symptomatic for no more than 2 days. Zanamivir must be taken by inhalation. In contrast, oseltamivir is well absorbed when administered orally and has proven to be effective for symptomatic patients over age 1 year as well as for prophylaxis (for example, to prevent the spread of influenza long-term care facilities and hospitals). For maximum benefit, therapy should begin within 2 days of symptom onset. For example, oseltamivir taken within 24 hours of symptom onset shortens the duration of illness by about 2 days, with patients reporting feeling better within 1 day of starting treatment.

3. **Vaccine:** As useful as new therapies are, they are not a substitute for the vaccine. A vaccine consisting of formalin-inactivated influenza virus has been available for many years. The vaccine is administered intramuscularly and is approved for use in anyone over age 6 months. It is recommended for all persons who might contract the influenza virus, particularly older adults and children, in addition to health care workers. It is of critical importance that the vaccine contains the specific subtypes of influenza virus that are in circulation at any given time. The circulating strains worldwide are monitored each season, and the following year's vaccine includes the principal strains recovered during the previous year (usually, one type B influenza and two type A influenza strains). A live, attenuated influenza virus vaccine has also been approved for use in persons between ages 2 and 49 years. The virus is temperature sensitive, capable of replication only at the lower temperatures found in the nose but not at higher temperatures typical of the lower respiratory tract. The vaccine, consisting of H1N1 and H2N3 subtypes and administered intranasally, elicits very good

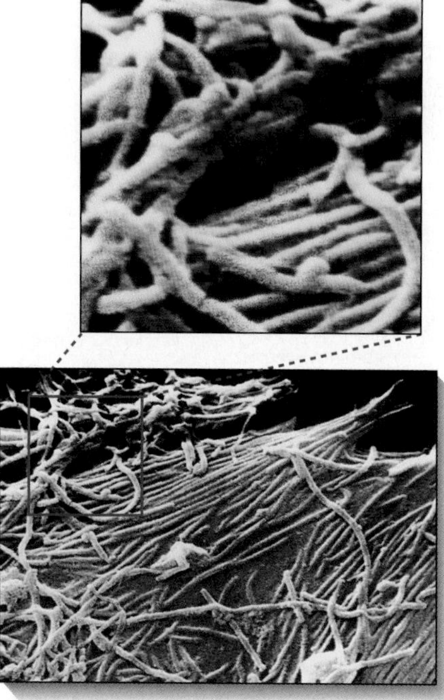

Figure 29.16
Electron micrograph of Ebola virus.

protective immunity, including mucosal immunoglobulin A, particularly in children.

V. FILOVIRIDAE

Filoviruses are pleomorphic viruses with unusual morphologies (Figure 29.16) that cause rare zoonotic infections. They are generally seen as long, filamentous, enveloped particles that may be branched. Marburg virus was initially isolated in Germany and Yugoslavia (now Serbia) from laboratory workers who became severely ill while preparing primary cell cultures from African green monkeys. Since this outbreak, only a few sporadic cases have been reported, all in Africa. Ebola virus was first isolated from patients with hemorrhagic fever in Zaire and the Sudan. Ebola and Marburg viruses are not related antigenically but both cause severe hemorrhagic fever, characterized by widespread bleeding into the skin, mucous membranes, visceral organs, and the gastrointestinal tract. The mortality rate is high, often greater than 50 percent. Death is thought to be due to visceral organ necrosis. Although the natural reservoir for these viruses is unknown, they can be transmitted to humans from infected monkeys and probably other animals or by exposure to blood or other body fluids from an infected patient. Outbreaks of hemorrhagic fever caused by these viruses continue to occur in research facilities and in Africa. Laboratory identification is made by the demonstration of antiviral antibodies, for example, by ELISA assays (see p. 27). If virus can be recovered, the morphology of the particles is quite characteristic. There is no specific treatment for infections caused by these viruses. Strict barrier techniques are essential when caring for infected individuals or handling infected specimens. Because of the hazards of working with filoviruses, they are studied in only a few reference laboratories around the world.

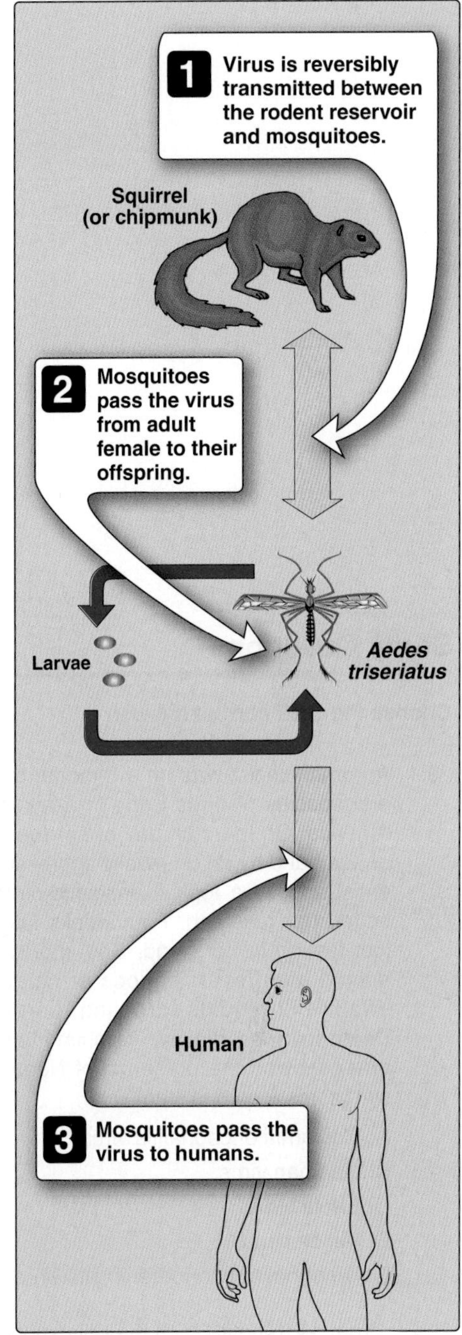
1 Virus is reversibly transmitted between the rodent reservoir and mosquitoes.
Squirrel (or chipmunk)
2 Mosquitoes pass the virus from adult female to their offspring.
Larvae
Aedes triseriatus
Human
3 Mosquitoes pass the virus to humans.

Figure 29.17
Transmission of California encephalitis virus.

VI. BUNYAVIRIDAE

In the United States, the most clinically important viruses in this family are LaCrosse virus (genus, *Bunyavirus*), which cause meningitis and encephalitis, and the Hantaan viruses (genus, *Hantavirus*), which are associated with hemorrhagic fever, and hantavirus pulmonary syndrome, a condition associated with high mortality. The viruses in this family are spherical, enveloped particles, with spikes projecting from the surface of the virions. Because the RNA genome is divided into three segments, reassortment of RNA segments between closely related viruses is possible. Arthropods serve as vectors for most viruses in the family *Bunyaviridae* that are transmitted to humans (Figure 29.17). However, because viruses in the genus *Hantavirus* do not have an arthropod vector, they are transmitted to humans by rodents via aerosols formed from their dried excretions. No effective antiviral agent is currently available.

VII. ARENAVIRIDAE

Arenaviruses are enveloped, spherical particles with a bipartite (two-segment) RNA genome that exists in virions as helical nucleocapsids.

Both RNAs have an ambisense organization, which means that coding information is contained in both the genomic and antigenomic viral RNAs. Viral particles mature by budding from the plasma membrane. Viruses in this family are associated with chronic infections of rodents, and humans are infected by inhaling contaminated aerosols, eating food containing viral particles, or by exposure of open wounds to infected soil. Lymphocytic choriomeningitis virus, a cause of viral meningitis, is a relatively benign infection with little mortality. In Latin America, Junin and Machupo viruses are associated with Argentine and Bolivian hemorrhagic fevers, respectively. These are diseases with mortality rates of 25 to 30 percent. In Africa, Lassa virus infection can be asymptomatic, or it can cause Lassa fever, which is a severe infection that is associated with shock, hemorrhage, and bleeding from mucosal membranes. Only 20 percent of cases are multisystemic, but, among this group, mortality reaches 15 percent. Ribavirin appears to be of benefit both in Lassa fever and hemorrhagic fever. The most important measure in prevention, however, is rodent control.

Study Questions

Choose the ONE correct answer.

29.1 An ornithologist was on a 3-month trip to study several species of birds living in a rain forest in South America. On the 10th day of her trip, she was bitten on the hand by an unusually aggressive bat. The scientist applied a topical antibiotic ointment and continued her research. Four weeks later, the scientist lost feeling in her hand. She shortly began experiencing high fever, periods of rigidity, difficulty in swallowing liquids, drooling, and disorientation. Death followed rapidly. A postmortem biopsy of her brain showed the presence of Negri bodies. These symptoms are consistent with:

A. California encephalitis virus.
B. Hantaan virus.
C. Ebola virus.
D. rabies virus.
E. lymphocytic choriomeningitis virus.

Correct answer = D. Rabies virus is usually transmitted via the bite of an infected animal, and the woman's symptoms are consistent with those of rabies. California encephalitis virus, transmitted by arthropods, causes meningitis and encephalitis. Hantaan virus is transmitted through aerosols formed from dried rodent excretions. This virus causes hemorrhagic fever and severe pulmonary infections. Ebola virus can be transmitted by an animal, but infection causes severe hemorrhagic fever. Lymphocytic choriomeningitis virus is a cause of viral meningitis and a relatively benign infection with little mortality. Humans are infected by inhaling contaminated aerosols, by eating food containing viral particles, or by exposure of open wounds to infected soil.

29.2 From 1918 until 1956, the only subtype of influenza observed in humans was H1N1. In 1957, H1N1 was replaced by H2N2. This is an example of:

A. viral interference.
B. phenotypic mixing.
C. antigenic shift.
D. antigenic drift.
E. viral transformation.

Correct answer = C. A marked antigenic change in the N (neuraminidase) protein, the H (hemagglutinin) protein, or both is termed antigenic shift. In antigenic drift, there is also an antigenic change in one or both of these proteins, but the change is much less significant. With antigenic drift, although the H protein does change antigenically, H1 remains H1, for example.

Double-stranded RNA Viruses: Reoviridae

30

I. OVERVIEW

The single genus of medical importance in this family is *Rotavirus*, which causes severe viral gastroenteritis, primarily in infants and young children (Figure 30.1). Viruses in the family *Reoviridae* are spherical, nonenveloped particles that have an icosahedral structure. The viral genome consists of 10 to 12 segments of double-stranded (ds) RNA. The virions contain all the enzymes needed to make positive-strand RNA transcripts, which are capped and methylated. Reoviruses replicate completely in the cytoplasm. The name "reovirus" stands for respiratory and enteric orphan virus. Although an orphan virus is typically one that is not known to cause any disease, this is no longer the case for reoviruses. Echoviruses (p. 283) were also initially considered orphan viruses but were soon discovered to cause a large number of clinical syndromes. Therefore, for viruses, being an orphan may be only a temporary state.

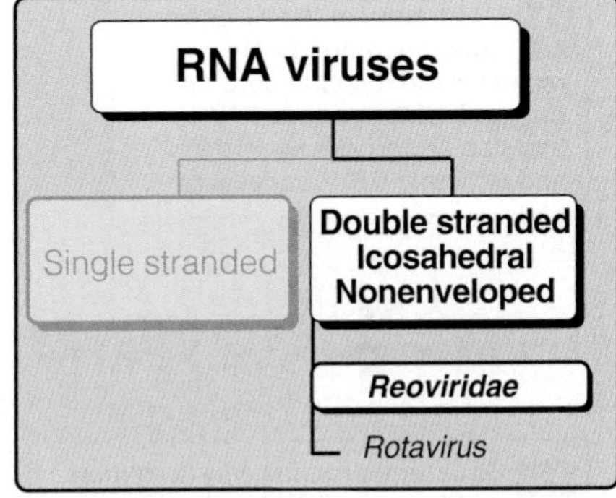

Figure 30.1
Classification of double-stranded, nonenveloped RNA viruses.

II. ROTAVIRUS

Rotaviruses, found in many mammalian species, often have a fairly broad host range. Rotaviruses have a characteristic morphology that distinguishes them from other reoviruses: Namely, they have the appearance of wheels with spokes radiating from the center and a smooth outer rim (Figure 30.2). The particles also have a large number of channels connecting the outer surface of the virion to the inner core. It has been postulated that these channels are involved in the import of substrates needed for RNA transcription and the extrusion of newly synthesized RNA transcripts. These channels are necessary because viral replication in the cytoplasm occurs without complete uncoating of the virion particle.

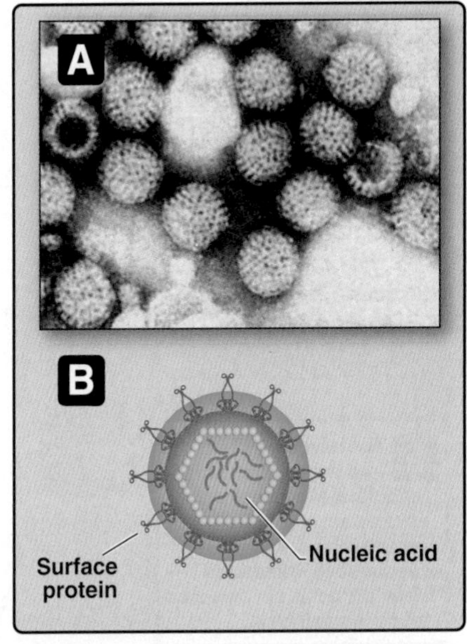

Figure 30.2
Structure of rotavirus. A. Electron micrograph. B. Schematic drawing.

A. Epidemiology

Rotaviruses are divided into seven serogroups (A through G) of which group A is the most important cause of outbreaks of disease in humans. Transmission of rotaviruses is via the fecal–oral route. Marked seasonal incidence is associated with rotavirus infections, with the peak months in the United States being January through

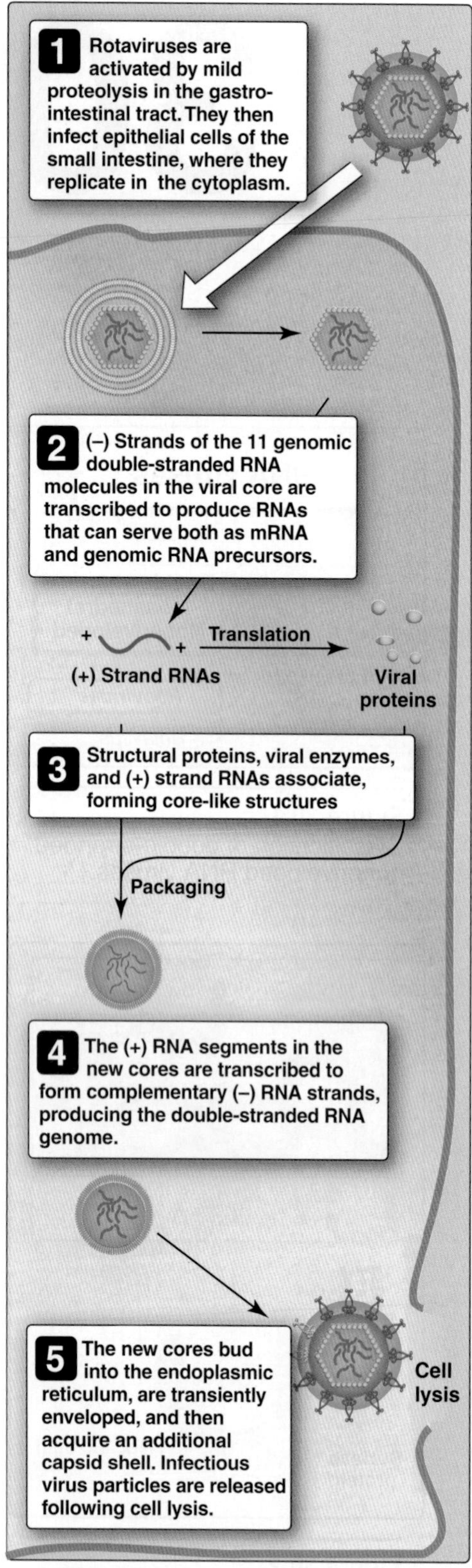

1 Rotaviruses are activated by mild proteolysis in the gastrointestinal tract. They then infect epithelial cells of the small intestine, where they replicate in the cytoplasm.
2 (–) Strands of the 11 genomic double-stranded RNA molecules in the viral core are transcribed to produce RNAs that can serve both as mRNA and genomic RNA precursors.
Translation
(+) Strand RNAs
Viral proteins
3 Structural proteins, viral enzymes, and (+) strand RNAs associate, forming core-like structures
Packaging
4 The (+) RNA segments in the new cores are transcribed to form complementary (–) RNA strands, producing the double-stranded RNA genome.
5 The new cores bud into the endoplasmic reticulum, are transiently enveloped, and then acquire an additional capsid shell. Infectious virus particles are released following cell lysis.
Cell lysis

Figure 30.3
Replication of rotavirus.

March. Because infectious particles are relatively stable, they can survive for extended periods on various surfaces. Rotavirus infections account for about 50 percent of cases of severe diarrhea in infants and young children (up to age 2 years).

B. Viral replication

After attachment to and uptake by the host cell, rotaviruses become partially uncoated in a lysosome. The rotavirus genome has 11 segments of linear, dsRNA, each of which codes for a single protein. Reassortment of the RNA segments (see p. 318) can occur when a cell is infected with two different rotaviruses. The viral particles contain enzymes (such as RNA-dependent RNA polymerase) that are needed to synthesize positive-sense RNA transcripts with a 5' cap. These positive RNA strands function not only as mRNA but also as templates for the synthesis of negative-strand RNA (see Figure 23.14). After the negative-strand RNA is made, it stays associated with its positive-strand template, giving rise to a dsRNA segment that is packaged in the virion. Rotaviruses are released following cell lysis rather than by budding through the membrane, thus accounting for the lack of a viral envelope. Figure 30.3 illustrates additional details of rotavirus replication.

C. Clinical significance

Following ingestion, rotaviruses infect the epithelial cells of the small intestine, primarily the jejunum (Figure 30.4). Rotaviruses are able to reach the small intestine because they are resistant to the acid pH of the stomach. The incubation period is usually 48 hours or less. Infection can be subclinical or may result in symptoms ranging from mild diarrhea and vomiting to severe, nonbloody, watery diarrhea with dehydration and loss of electrolytes. Although rotavirus infections are probably equally widespread around the world, the outcomes of infection vary significantly in different regions, and malnutrition dramatically increases the severity of the infection. For example, more than 90 percent of children in the United States may have antibodies to rotaviruses by age 3 or 4 years, and mortality in younger children is low because patients who are severely ill are generally hospitalized, with fluid and electrolyte losses rapidly corrected. Infection results in some degree of lifelong immunity with reinfected adults suffering a much milder illness. Infants who are breastfed also suffer milder disease manifestations. However, in developing countries and areas where medical facilities or personnel may be lacking, the mortality is significant: An estimated 1 million deaths per year worldwide result from rotavirus infection.

D. Laboratory identification

Severe diarrhea, dehydration, and electrolyte loss can be due to a variety of causes. Accordingly, a definitive diagnosis cannot be made on clinical grounds alone. As with many other viral infections, identification can be made by detection of viral capsid anti-

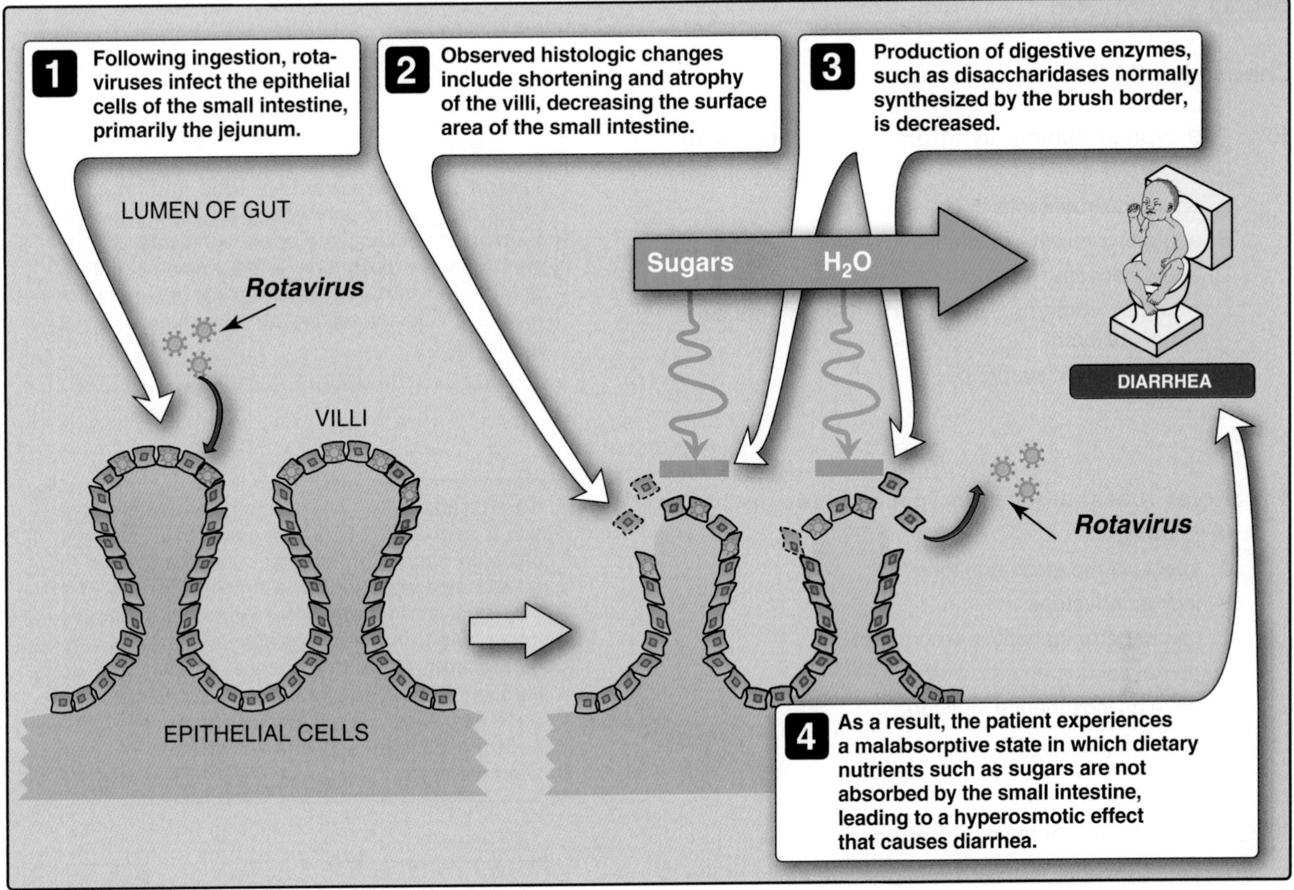

Figure 30.4
Mechanism of rotavirus diarrhea.

gens in stool samples using enzyme-linked immunosorbent assay (see p. 27). An increase in the titer of antiviral antibody in a patient's serum can also be diagnostic. Electron microscopy of stool specimens, although not a routine diagnostic measure, can aid in the identification of the virus because rotaviruses have a distinctive appearance (see Figure 30.2).

E. Treatment and prevention

There is no specific antiviral drug appropriate for treatment of rotavirus infections. The most important clinical intervention is the rapid and efficient replacement of fluids and electrolytes, usually intravenously. Formulations are also being produced that can be used in developing countries so that fluids and electrolytes can be replaced orally. Two oral vaccines using weakened live virus have been shown to be highly efficacious in protecting infants against severe rotavirus gastroenteritis and not associated with increased risk of intussusception (telescoping of one portion of the intestine into another). Prevention of rotavirus infections requires improved sanitation measures.

Study Questions

Choose the ONE correct answer.

30.1 The typical clinical syndrome associated with rotavirus infection is:

A. acute gastroenteritis of young adults.
B. acute bronchiolitis of infants.
C. acute hepatitis.
D. nausea, vomiting, and diarrhea in infants and young children.
E. acute paralytic syndrome.

Correct answer = D. Rotaviruses infect and replicate in the gastrointestinal tract and typically affect infants and very young children. Although rotavirus infections are seen worldwide, significant mortality exists only in developing countries or in situations where good medical treatment (for example, fluid and electrolyte replacement), is not available.

30.2 Rotaviruses differ from polioviruses in that rotaviruses:

A. infect via the fecal–oral route.
B. lack an envelope.
C. can undergo genetic reassortment.
D. do not contain any enzymes.
E. have an icosahedral structure.

Correct answer = C. Because rotaviruses contain a segmented genome, infection of a single cell with two different rotaviruses can result in genetic reassortment and the emergence of a new viral strain with some genomic segments from one parent and the remaining genomic segments from the other parent. Rotaviruses do contain the enzymes required to synthesize viral mRNAs. A, B, D, E: No differences exist between polioviruses and rotaviruses in these characteristics.

30.3 The diagnosis of a rotavirus infection:

A. can be made, in most cases, on the basis of the clinical presentation.
B. can be made based upon the detection of viral capsid antigens in stool samples.
C. is routinely made by electron microscopy of suitably treated stool samples.
D. can only be made on epidemiologic grounds (for example, if there is an epidemic).
E. must be made rapidly so that specific antiviral therapy is initiated as soon as possible.

Correct answer = B. The diagnosis of rotavirus infection is readily made by detection of viral antigens in the stool by enzyme-linked immunosorbent assay. Although the diagnosis can be made by electron microscopy, it is not a routine procedure. The clinical presentation is not sufficiently distinctive to make the diagnosis, and there is no specific antiviral treatment for rotavirus infections

30.4 Appropriate treatment of rotavirus infection includes which of the following?

A. Fluid and electrolyte replacement
B. Antiviral drugs targeting membrane fusion
C. Metronidazole
D. Antiviral drugs targeting reverse transcriptase
E. Antiviral drugs targeting proteolytic processing

Answer: A. There are no specific antiviral treatments for rotavirus infection. The most effective treatment simply involves fluid and electrolyte replacement. The virus is non-enveloped and therefore membrane fusion does not occur. Metronidazole is used to treat infections with anaerobic bacteria and some parasitic infections. Unlike HIV, rotavirus does not have reverse transcriptase or proteases that are required for virus maturation.

Unconventional Infectious Agents

31

I. OVERVIEW

The designation "unconventional infectious agent" refers to a distinctive, transmissible, infectious agent that, although having some properties in common with viruses, does not fit the classic definition of a virus (Figure 31.1). One such highly unconventional infectious agent, the prion, has been implicated as the causative agent of transmissible spongiform encephalopathies (TSEs). These infections are transmissible to uninfected animals and humans. The primary disease manifestation, encephalopathy, should be distinguished from encephalitis. TSEs are characterized by their distinct absence of inflammatory signs, whereas encephalitis is distinguished by inflammation and the infiltration of white cells. TSEs occurring in humans are designated as kuru, Creutzfeldt-Jakob disease (CJD), Gerstmann-Straussler syndrome (GSS), and fatal familial insomnia (FFI). Important TSEs of animals include scrapie in sheep, bovine spongiform encephalopathy (BSE) in cattle (popularly called "mad cow disease"), and chronic wasting disease (found in deer and elk). Histologically, these diseases are characterized by spongiform vacuolation of neuronal processes and gray matter; accumulation of a unique protein (prion protein, or PrP, as shown in Figure 31.2); and, in certain cases, deposition in the brain of extracellular amyloid plaques composed of PrP. Such diseases are sometimes referred to as transmissible amyloidoses.

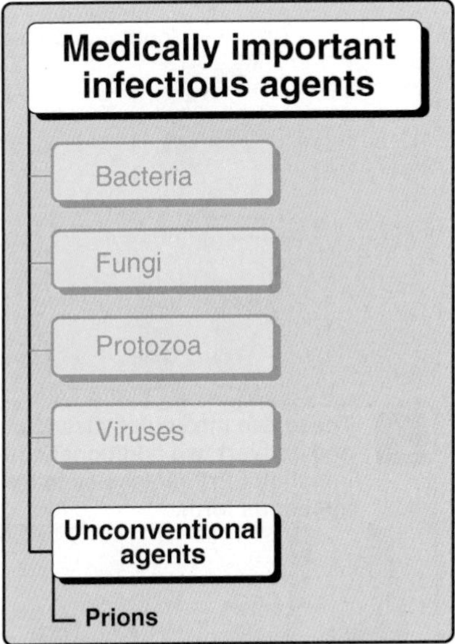

Figure 31.1
Classification of unconventional infectious agents.

II. PRIONS

After an extensive series of purification procedures, scientists were astonished to find that the infectivity of the agent causing scrapie in sheep was associated with a single protein species, with no detectable associated nucleic acid. This infectious protein is designated the prion protein. It is relatively resistant to proteolytic degradation and, when infectious, tends to form insoluble aggregates of fibrils, similar to the amyloid found in other diseases of the brain.

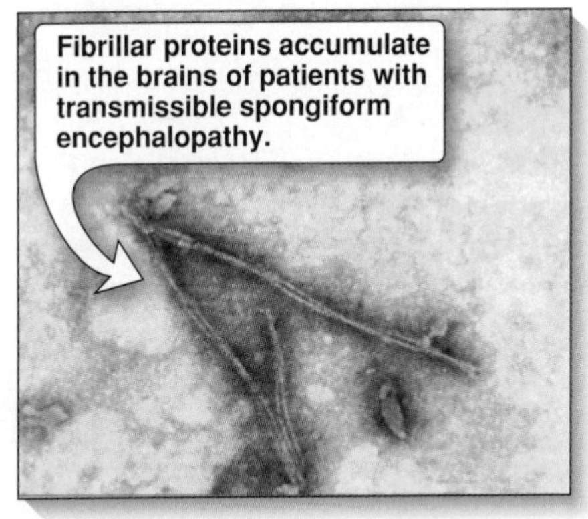

Fibrillar proteins accumulate in the brains of patients with transmissible spongiform encephalopathy.

Figure 31.2
Electron micrograph of fibrillar prion proteins.

A. Presence of prion protein in normal mammalian brain

A noninfectious form of PrP, having the same amino acid and gene sequences as the infectious agent, is present in normal mammalian brains on the surface of neurons and glial cells. It is referred to as PrP^C (cellular prion protein). Although the function of noninfectious PrP^C is unknown, it is highly conserved in nature, with the amino acid and gene sequences differing little among divergent mam-

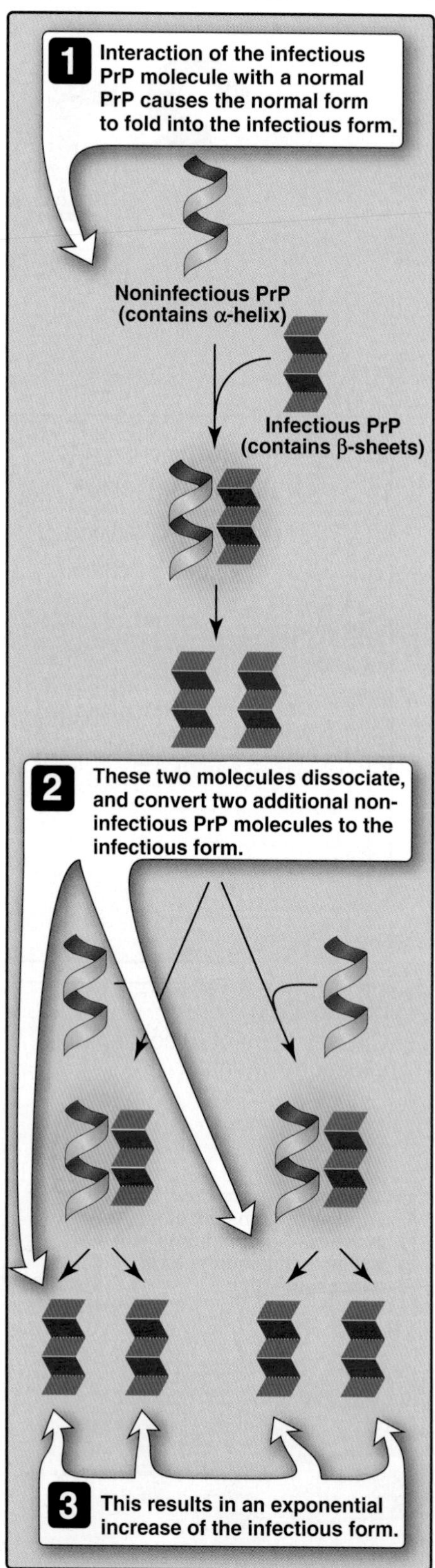

1
Interaction of the infectious PrP molecule with a normal PrP causes the normal form to fold into the infectious form.
Noninfectious PrP (contains α-helix)
Infectious PrP (contains β-sheets)
2
These two molecules dissociate, and convert two additional non-infectious PrP molecules to the infectious form.
3
This results in an exponential increase of the infectious form.

Figure 31.3
One proposed mechanism for "reproduction" of the infectious prion protein (PrP).

malian species. Recent evidence suggests that the wild-type protein participates in signal transduction and/or metal homeostasis. The primary structure and posttranslational modifications of the normal and the infectious forms of the protein are closely related or identical. However, specific mutational changes of single amino acids at a few sites appear to be determinants of susceptibility to exogenous infection and the probability for spontaneous conversion of the normal PrP^{C} to the infectious form (PrP^{Sc}). The key to becoming infectious apparently lies in the three-dimensional conformation of the PrP. It has been observed that several α-helices present in noninfectious PrP^{C} are replaced by β-sheets in the infectious form. Presumably, this conformational difference confers relative resistance to proteolytic degradation on infectious prions, thereby distinguishing them from normal PrP^{C} in infected tissue. A model for "reproduction" of the agent is shown in Figure 31.3.

B. Epidemiology

The normal mode of transmission among animals (for example, among sheep in a flock infected with scrapie) has not been elucidated. It is clear, however, that several diseases of domestic animals have been transmitted via feed prepared from other diseased animals.

1. **Bovine spongiform encephalopathy:** BSE, commonly called mad cow disease, arose in British cattle presumably caused by their feed processed with animal parts prepared from diseased sheep and cattle. The obvious question raised by this occurrence is whether the BSE from infected cattle can be transmitted to humans. Although such a risk was originally considered negligible, a study of infectious material from a cluster of histologically distinctive British CJD cases in unusually young patients (now referred to as "variant," or vCJD) indicated that animal-to-human transmission very likely did take place. Because the incubation time for symptoms to appear varies from 4 to 40 years, the likelihood of a potential epidemic caused by BSE is unknown.

2. **Kuru:** An example of human-to-human transmission of a TSE is found in kuru, a disease in which the infectious agent is acquired by an individual's exposure to diseased brain tissue in the course of ritualistic cannibalism among members of a tribe in New Guinea. Infection occurs by consuming contaminated brain tissue or via inoculation through breaks in the skin following the handling of diseased tissue. With cannibalism cessation in the late 1950s, the disease is disappearing.

3. **Creutzfeldt-Jakob disease:** Of more general significance are the documented cases of iatrogenic (unintentionally introduced by medical procedures) transmission of CJD, for example, by use of prion-contaminated human pituitary–derived growth hormone prepared from individuals who died from CJD. In addition, corneal transplants, implantation of contaminated brain electrodes, and blood transfusions have resulted in documented cases of disease transmission. Thus far, there has been no evidence of transplacental transmission or transmission by person-to-person contact. In about 15 percent of CJD cases, the condition is inherited as a mutation in the PrP gene. However, most CJD cases are

sporadic and have an unknown etiology (that is, they occur with no known exposure or mutational change). The incidence of sporadic CJD is low (about 1 to 2 per million population) but in those families with a PrP mutation, an attack rate of 50 to 100 percent is seen in those carrying the mutation. In contrast to CJD, all cases classified as GSS or FFI have involved inheritance of specific PrP mutations. Despite the inherited nature of the disease, brain tissues from these patients are nevertheless infectious. Knockout mice lacking the gene that encodes PrP^C appear normal but are immune to infection with prions.

C. Pathology

Ingestion or other extracerebral exposure to prions results in significant multiplication of prion agents in the follicular dendritic cells within lymphoid tissues and in the spleen, but it is invasion of the central nervous system that results in the typical clinical effects. The basis for the pathogenic consequences of abnormal PrP^{Sc} deposition has not been clarified. Diseased brain tissue is characterized by accumulation of abnormal PrP^{Sc} in the form of amyloid fibrils in neuron cytoplasmic vesicles (see Figure 31.2) and in the form of extracellular amyloid plaques. There is, in addition, extensive vacuolation within neurons, neuronal loss, and astroglial proliferation. The extensive destruction results in the characteristic spongiform appearance of gray matter in histologic sections. Whereas TSE amyloid plaques are morphologically similar to those of Alzheimer disease, the PrP gene is located on a different chromosome than the gene for the Alzheimer amyloid-β-protein precursor, and there is no nucleotide or amino acid homology between the two. Recent evidence suggests that these two proteins may physically interact with one another and participate in the same signaling or transport pathways in neurons.

D. Clinical significance

TSEs are a group of progressive, ultimately fatal, neurodegenerative diseases affecting humans and a number of animal species. The disease process is fundamentally the same in all TSEs, but their clinical manifestations and histopathologies differ. TSEs also share some similarities with conventional infectious diseases, but their differences are striking (Figure 31.4).

1. **Molecular basis of inherited TSEs:** In each inherited TSE, specific, single amino acid substitutions or insertions of nucleotide repeat sequences are found in the PrP gene. These are thought to increase greatly (10^6-fold) the probability of transition to the infectious conformation. In the spontaneously occurring, sporadic disease (that is, with no known exposure to infectious material and no inheritance of a mutated PrP gene), it is proposed that the altered folding occurs randomly with low probability. Importantly, once formed, the abnormal PrP^{Sc} acquires both the ability to "multiply," as well as the properties of an infectious agent. It has been recognized, however, that certain amino acid substitutions at one specific site increase susceptibility to infection.

2. **Major symptoms:** All TSEs involve deposition of the PrP^{Sc} protein. In the inherited forms, each PrP^{Sc} mutation is associated with a

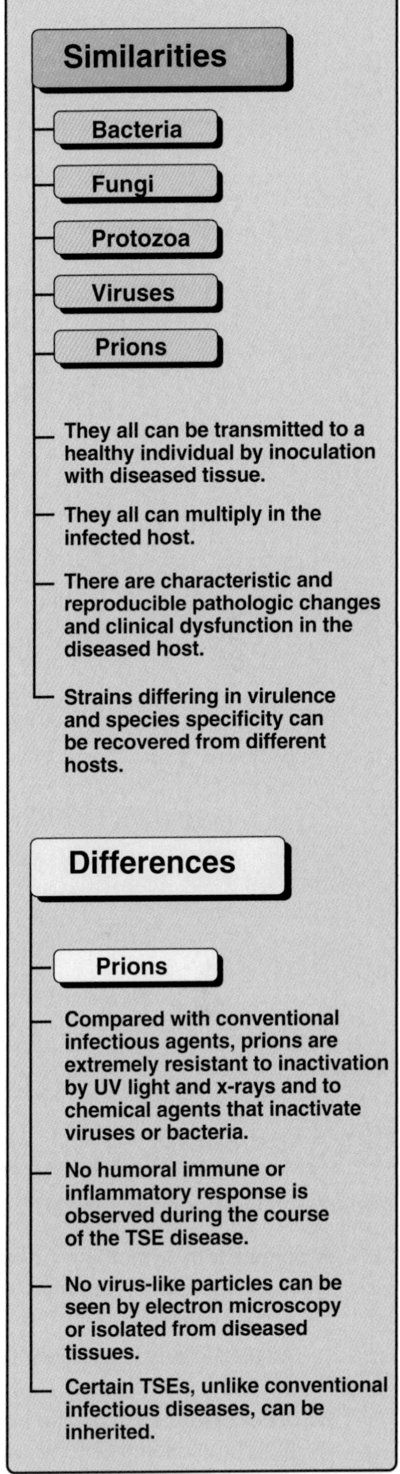

Similarities
Bacteria
Fungi
Protozoa
Viruses
Prions
They all can be transmitted to a healthy individual by inoculation with diseased tissue.
They all can multiply in the infected host.
There are characteristic and reproducible pathologic changes and clinical dysfunction in the diseased host.
Strains differing in virulence and species specificity can be recovered from different hosts.
Differences
Prions
Compared with conventional infectious agents, prions are extremely resistant to inactivation by UV light and x-rays and to chemical agents that inactivate viruses or bacteria.
No humoral immune or inflammatory response is observed during the course of the TSE disease.
No virus-like particles can be seen by electron microscopy or isolated from diseased tissues.
Certain TSEs, unlike conventional infectious diseases, can be inherited.

Figure 31.4
Similarities and differences between conventional and unconventional agents. TSE = Transmissible spongiform encephalopathies. UV = ultraviolet.

characteristic clinical phenotype. For example, the most prominent features of CJD are rapidly progressive dementia and behavioral disturbances, ending in death within 1 year. In GSS, ataxia is the more prominent feature, with death resulting in 2 to 6 years. FFI, also fatal within 1 year, has the additional symptom of uncontrollable insomnia. Although there is some difference in age of onset, all human TSEs (with the exception of BSE-associated vCJD) occur relatively late in life, typically between ages 40 and 60 years.

E. Laboratory identification

A presumptive diagnosis can be made on clinical grounds, but there is some overlap with other dementing illnesses. Routine laboratory tests of serum and cerebrospinal fluid are generally normal. The presence of infectious PrP^{Sc} in peripheral lymphatic tissue provides specimens for analysis without the need for brain biopsy. Currently, however, definitive diagnosis of these diseases is made by postmortem histopathologic examination of brain sections. Conversion from the wild-type PrP^{C} protein to the abnormal PrP^{Sc} is associated with changes in iron homeostasis within the host, leading to the hypothesis that iron-binding proteins could be used as a biomarker for TSE diseases.

F. Treatment and prevention

TSEs are invariably fatal, and no treatment is currently available that can alter this outcome. The unusually high resistance of the infectivity to most disinfecting agents makes transmission prevention by the usual infection control procedures ineffective. Current recommendations for decontamination of a CJD brain specimen are autoclaving at 132°C, plus immersion in either undiluted sodium hypochlorite or 1N sodium hydroxide. With respect to preventing possible transfer of BSE to humans, all animals showing signs of illness are destroyed, and preparation of animal feed from internal organs of potentially infected animals has ceased.

Study Questions

Choose the ONE correct answer.

31.1 A patient with symptoms of variant Creutzfeldt-Jacob disease caused by eating contaminated beef would most likely exhibit which of the following?

A. Circulating antibodies specific for bovine central nervous system antigens

B. DNA copies of the bovine infectious agent integrated into chromosomes of the patient's diseased central nervous system tissue

C. Cytotoxic T lymphocytes directed against central nervous system–specific antigens found in both cattle and humans

D. Amyloid deposits that have bovine rather than the human amino acid sequences

E. Lack of any bovine-specific protein or nucleic acid or an immune response

Correct answer = E. Histologically, varient Creutzfeldt-Jacob disease is characterized by spongiform vacuolation of neuronal processes and gray matter and accumulation of prion protein. Unlike encephalitis, transmissable spongiform encephalopathies do not provoke an inflammatory response. A and C: An important characteristic of the prion diseases is that there is no unique immune response to either the prion or to central nervous system antigens. B: A second distinguishing feature of these agents is the absence of a detectable nucleic acid genome. D: The amyloid deposits found in these diseases are composed of the diseased host's proteins, not of proteins from the source of the infection.

UNIT V:
Clinical Microbiology Review

Quick Review of Clinically Important Microorganisms

32

I. OVERVIEW

Although all of the microorganisms presented in this volume have clinical significance, some play a more critical role than do others in the pathology of disease in the United States. This chapter presents a summary of these particularly important microorganisms, organized alphabetically, but continuing the use of icons and color coding to aid the reader in retaining the morphology and classification of the microorganisms. At the top of each box in which a new organism is introduced in this summary chapter, a color-coded entry indicates the general group of bacteria or viruses to which the organism belongs, according to the definitions in Figure 32.1A or B. The name in large type above the arrow in the **bacteria** section is the name of the **genus** to which the organism(s) listed below the arrow belong (exceptions will be noted in the text). In the **virus** section, the names in large type above the arrow refer to the **family** of which the individual viruses listed below the arrow are members. [Note: Only the bacteria and viruses that are summarized in this chapter are listed below the arrows. Additional organisms belonging to the same genus or family are described in the body of the text.] The order of the microorganisms in this chapter is presented in Figure 32.2.

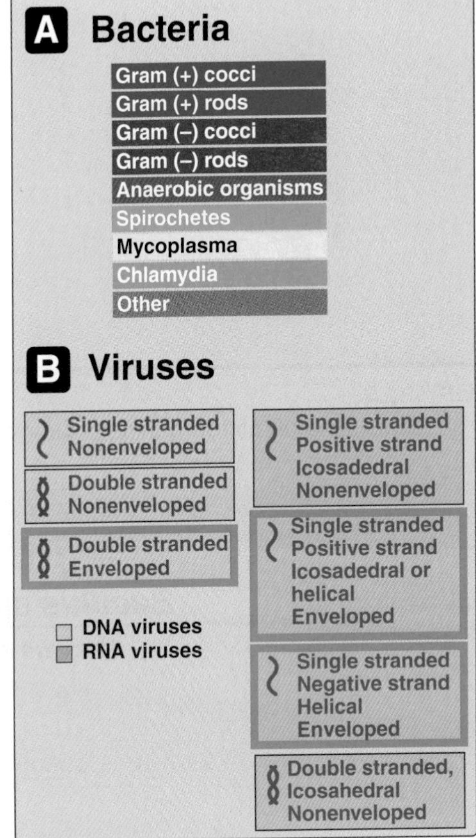

Figure 32.1
Representations of medically important bacteria and viruses.

BACTERIA

VIRUSES

FIGURE 32.2
Alphabetical listing of microorganisms summarized in this chapter. Page numbers refer to location in this chapter.

BACTERIA

Gram (+) rods

Bacillus species

Bacillus anthracis

Common characteristics

- **Gram-positive**
- **Blunt-ended bacilli that occur singly, in pairs, or frequently in long chains**
- **Form oval, centrally located endospores**
- **Nonmotile; has antiphagocytic capsule**
- **Culture on blood agar**

[*B. anthracis* is is continued on the next page.]

Bacillus anthracis (continued)

Pathogenesis/Clinical Significance

B. anthracis infects primarily domestic herbivores, such as sheep, goats, and horses. Human infection usually occurs through contact with infected animal products or spore-contaminated dust that is inoculated through incidental skin abrasions or is inhaled. *B. anthracis* spores are highly resistant to physical and chemical agents, and may remain viable for many years in contaminated pastures or animal materials. *B. anthracis* produces two plasmid-coded exotoxins: edema factor, which causes elevation of intracellular cyclic adenosine monophopshate, leading to severe edema, and lethal factor, which disrupts cellular signalling and induces cytokines. The *B. anthracis* capsule is essential for full virulence.

- **Cutaneous anthrax**

  Upon introduction of organisms or spores that germinate, a papule develops. It rapidly evolves into a painless, black, severely swollen "malignant pustule", which eventually crusts over (an eschar). The organisms may invade regional lymph nodes, and then the general circulation, leading to a fatal septicemia. The overall mortality rate in untreated cutaneous anthrax is about 20 percent.

- **Pulmonary anthrax ("wool-sorter's disease")**

  Caused by inhalation of spores, this disease is characterized by progressive hemorrhagic pneumonia and lymphadenitis (inflammation of the lymph nodes), and has a mortality rate approaching 100 percent if untreated.

- **Gastrointestinal form of anthrax**

  This unusual form of anthrax is caused by ingestion of spores, for example, by eating raw or inadequately cooked meat containing *B. anthracis* spores. This is the portal of entry commonly seen in animals.

Treatment and Prevention

- **Treatment:** *B. anthracis* is sensitive to ciprofloxacin. However, antibiotics are effective in cutaneous anthrax only when administered early in the course of the infection. Multidrug therapy is recommended in pulmonary anthrax.
- **Prevention:** Because of the resistance of endospores to chemical disinfectants, autoclaving is the only reliable means of decontamination. A cell-free vaccine is available for workers in high-risk occupations.

Laboratory Identification

- Cultured on blood agar, *B. anthracis* forms large, grayish, nonhemolytic colonies with irregular borders.
- A direct immunofluorescence assay aids in the identification of the organism.

Gram (–) rods ←

Bordetella species

Bordetella pertussis

Common characteristics

- **Gram-negative**
- **Small coccobacilli that grow singly or in pairs**
- **Encapsulated**
- **Aerobic**
- **Culture on Regan-Lowe agar**

Pathogenesis/Clinical Significance

B. pertussis is transmitted primarily by droplets spread by coughing. The organism survives only briefly in the environment. *B. pertussis* binds to ciliated epithelium in the upper respiratory tract. There, the bacteria produce a variety of toxins and other virulence factors that interfere with ciliary activity, eventually causing the death of these cells.

- **Pertussis ("whooping cough")**

  The incubation period for this disease ranges from 1 to 3 weeks. The disease can be divided into two phases: 1) the **catarrhal phase**, which begins with relatively nonspecific symptoms, and then progresses to include a dry, nonproductive cough; and 2) the **paroxysmal phase**, in which the cough worsens, causing paroxysms of coughing followed by a "whoop" as the patient inspires rapidly. Large amounts of mucus are typically produced. During the 3–4 week convalescent period, secondary complications, such as encephalopathy, seizures, and/or pneumonia, may occur.

Treatment and Prevention

- **Treatment:** Erythromycin is the drug of choice for *B. pertussis* infections, both as chemotherapy and as chemoprophylaxis for household contacts. Trimethoprim-sulfamethoxazole is an alternative choice for erythromycin treatment failures.
- **Prevention:** Two forms of vaccine are currently available (one of killed whole cells, and one that is acellular, containing purified *B. pertussis* proteins). Both are formulated in combination with diphtheria and tetanus toxoids.

Laboratory Identification

- *B. pertussis* from nasopharyngeal samples can be cultured on selective agar such as Regan-Lowe medium, where the organism produces pinpoint, hemolytic colonies.
- More rapid diagnosis may be accomplished using a direct fluorescent antibody test to detect *B. pertussis* in smears of nasopharyngeal specimens.

Spirochetes

Borrelia species

Borrelia burgdorferi

Common characteristics

- **Gram-negative, but stain poorly and need to be visualized by other means**
- **Long, slender, flexible, spiral- or corkscrew-shaped rods**
- **Highly motile**
- **Difficult and time consuming to culture**

Pathogenesis/Clinical Significance

B. burgdorferi is transmitted to humans by the bite of a small tick (genus *Ixodes*), which must feed for at least 24 hours to deliver an infectious dose. Deer, mice, other rodents, and birds serve as reservoirs for the spirochete. The organism is not spread from human to human.

- **Lyme disease**

  The first stage of the disease begins 3 to 22 days after a tick bite, with a characteristic red, circular rash with a clear center (erythema migrans) appearing at the site of the bite. Flu-like symptoms can accompany the rash. The organism spreads via the lymph or blood to musculoskeletal sites, the skin, central nervous system (CNS), heart, and other organs. Weeks to months after the initial symptoms, the second stage of the disease begins with symptoms such as arthritis, arthralgia, cardiac complications, and neurologic complications such as meningitis. The third stage begins months to years later, with chronic arthritis and progressive CNS disease.

Treatment and Prevention

- **Treatment:** Cephalosporins, amoxicillin, or doxycycline are useful in treating the early stages of Lyme disease. If arthritic symptoms have already appeared, longer courses of antibiotics are used.
- **Prevention:** A previously licensed vaccine was withdrawn and is no longer available. The best prevention is wearing clothing that limits skin exposure to ticks, and using insect repellent.

Laboratory Identification

- The polymerase chain reaction used to assist in detection of *B. burgdorferi* in body fluids provides the most definitive test.
- *B. burgdorferi* infection can be diagnosed serologically, but the number of false positives can outnumber the true positives.

Gram (–) rods

Brucella species

Brucella abortus
Brucella canis
Brucella melitensis
Brucella suis

Common characteristics

- **Gram-negative**
- **Small coccobacilli, arranged singly or in pairs**
- **Unencapsulated**
- **Aerobic, intracellular parasites**
- **Culture on blood agar**

Pathogenesis/Clinical Significance

Brucellosis is a chronic, lifelong infection in animals. Organisms localize in reproductive organs (male and female), and are shed in large numbers, for example, in milk and urine. Transmission to humans usually occurs either through direct contact with infected animal tissues or ingestion of unpasteurized milk or milk products. Human-to-human transmission is rare.

Brucellae typically enter the body through cuts in the skin or through the gastrointestinal (GI) tract. They are transported via the lymphatic system to the regional lymph nodes, where they survive and multiply within host phagocytes. They are then carried by the blood to organs that are involved in the reticuloendothelial system, including the liver, spleen, kidneys, bone marrow, and other lymph nodes. Lipopolysaccharide is the major virulence factor.

- **Brucellosis (undulant fever)**

  Symptoms of brucellosis are nonspecific and flu-like (malaise, fever, sweats, anorexia and GI symptoms, headache, and back pains), and may also include depression. Untreated patients may develop an undulating pattern of fever. Brucellosis may involve any of a variety of organ systems, including the GI tract, and the skeletal, neurologic, cardiovascular, and pulmonary systems.

Treatment and Prevention

- **Treatment:** Combination therapy involving rifampin plus a tetracycline is generally recommended for brucellosis. Prolonged treatment (for example, 6 weeks) is generally necessary to prevent relapse and to reduce the incidence of complications.

Laboratory Identification

- A detailed history is often crucial because of the nonspecific symptoms.
- The organism can be cultured from blood and other body fluids, or from tissue specimens, but isolation of the organism is difficult and time consuming.
- Serologic tests for agglutinating antibodies are diagnostically useful. Titers greater than 1:160 and rising are considered indicative of brucella infection.

Gram (–) rods

Campylobacter species

Campylobacter jejuni

Common characteristics

- **Gram-negative**
- **Curved, spiral, or S-shaped rods**
- **Single, polar flagellum results in characteristic darting motion**
- **Microaerophilic**
- **Do not ferment carbohydrates**
- **Culture on selective medium (blood agar containing antibiotics to inhibit growth of other fecal flora)**

Pathogenesis/Clinical Significance

C. jejuni is widely distributed in nature, existing as part of the normal flora of many vertebrate species, including both mammals and fowl, wild and domestic. Transmission is via the fecal-oral route through direct contact, or exposure to contaminated meat (especially poultry) or to contaminated water.

C. jejuni infects the intestine, where it can cause ulcerative, inflammatory lesions in the jejunum, ileum, or colon. An enterotoxin related to cholera toxin and a cytotoxin are important virulence factors.

- **Acute enteritis**

  C. jejuni is the leading cause of food-borne disease in the United States. Symptoms may be both systemic (fever, headache, myalgia) and intestinal (abdominal cramping and diarrhea, which may or may not be bloody). *C. jejuni* is a cause of both traveler's diarrhea and pseudoappendicitis. Rare complications include septic abortion, reactive arthritis, and Guillain-Barré syndrome.

Treatment and Prevention

- **Treatment:** Diarrhea should be treated symptomatically (fluid and electrolyte replacement). If disease is severe, ciprofloxacin is the drug of choice.
- **Prevention:** No vaccine or preventive drug is available. Good hygiene, avoiding contaminated water, pasteurizing milk and milk products, and thoroughly cooking potentially contaminated food (for example, poultry) is important in prevention of infection.

Laboratory Identification

- Presumptive diagnosis can be made on the basis of finding curved organisms with rapid, darting motility in a wet mount of feces.

Chlamydia

Chlamydia species

Chlamydia pneumoniae
Chlamydia psittaci
Chlamydia trachomatis

Common characteristics

- **Not routinely stained with Gram stain**
- **Small, round to ovoid**
- **Obligate intracellular parasites, the organisms replicate in endocytic vacuoles, creating characteristic cytoplasmic inclusion bodies**

Chlamydia pneumoniae

Pathogenesis/Clinical Significance

C. pneumoniae is generally transmitted by respiratory droplets. *Chlamydia* are energy parasites, and require exogenous ATP and NAD^+ for growth. They acquire these compounds by replicating inside host cells.

- **Community-acquired respiratory infection**

  C. pneumoniae is a significant cause of respiratory infections worldwide, causing pharyngitis, laryngitis, bronchitis, and interstitial pneumonia. Epidemic outbreaks have been reported.

[*CHLAMYDIA* SPECIES ARE CONTINUED ON THE NEXT PAGE]

Treatment and Prevention

- **Treatment:** Doxycycline and erythromycin are the drugs of choice.
- **Prevention:** No vaccine or preventive drug is available.

Laboratory Identification

- Neither serologic tests nor recovery by culturing is routinely available.

Chlamydia psittaci

Pathogenesis/Clinical Significance

- **Psittacosis (ornithosis)**
  This is a zoonotic disease transmitted to humans by inhalation of dust contaminated with respiratory secretions or feces of infected birds (such as parrots). *C. psittaci* infection of humans targets the respiratory tract, causing a dry cough, flu-like symptoms, and pulmonary infiltrates. Enlargement of the liver and spleen frequently occurs.

Treatment and Prevention

- **Treatment:** Tetracycline and doxycycline are the drugs of choice.

Laboratory Identification

- Demonstration of a rise in antibody titer, using either complement fixation or indirect immunofluorescence tests, can aid in diagnosis.

Chlamydia trachomatis

Pathogenesis/Clinical Significance

- **Nongonococcal urethritis (NGU)**
  C. trachomatis is the major causative agent of NGU, which is the most common sexually transmitted bacterial disease in the United States. It is transmitted by personal contact, and affects both sexes. Repeated or chronic exposure to *C. trachomatis* can lead to sterility and ectopic pregnancy. Women may develop **pelvic inflammatory disease (PID).**
- **Trachoma**
  C. trachomatis causes eye infections (**chronic keratoconjunctivitis**) with symptoms that range from simple irritation of the eye to blindness. This disease is widely prevalent in developing countries. It is transmitted by personal contact with infected humans or contaminated surfaces, and by flies.
- **Inclusion conjunctivitis of the newborn (ICN)**
  Infants born to mothers infected with *C. trachomatis* can become infected during passage through the birth canal. This can lead to an acute, purulent conjunctivitis.
- **Lymphogranuloma venereum (LGV)**
  C. trachomatis causes LGV, an invasive, sexually transmitted disease that is uncommon in the United States, but is endemic in Asia, Africa, and South America. LGV is characterized by transient papules on the external genitalia, followed in 1 to 2 months by painful swelling of inguinal and perirectal lymph nodes. Regional lymphatic drainage can become blocked.

Treatment and Prevention

- **Treatment:** Azithromycin, erythromycin, and tetracyclines such as doxycycline are useful in treating chlamydial infections. [Note: Erythromycin is used for young children and pregnant women.]
- **Prevention:** No vaccine is available. Erythromycin or silver nitrate in ointment or eyedrops is applied prophylactically to newborns' eyes, especially those at risk. Proper precautions should be taken during sexual contact to prevent transmission of NGU.

Laboratory Identification

- Microscopic examination of infected cells stained with direct fluorescent antibodies reveals characteristic cellular cytoplasmic inclusions.
- Nucleic acid amplification tests can detect *C. trachomatis* with a high degree of sensitivity.

Anaerobic organisms ←

Clostridia species

Clostridium botulinum
Clostridium difficile
Clostridium perfringens
Clostridium tetani

Common characteristics

- **Gram-positive**
- **Large, blunt-ended rods that produce endospores**
- **Most species are motile**
- **Obligate anaerobe**
- **Culture anaerobically on blood agar**

Clostridium botulinum

Pathogenesis/Clinical Significance

C. botulinum is found in soil and aquatic sediments. Its spores contaminate vegetables, meat, and fish. *C. botulinum* exotoxin inhibits the release of acetylcholine at the neuromuscular junctions, preventing contraction and causing flaccid paralysis.

- **Botulism (food poisoning) and floppy baby syndrome**
  These diseases are caused by ingestion of exotoxin, leading to flaccid paralysis, vomiting, and diarrhea. Death can occur due to respiratory paralysis. In infants, *C. botulinum* spores germinate in the large intestine, producing exotoxin that is slowly absorbed. Lethargy, poor muscle tone, and constipation result.

Treatment and Prevention

- **Treatment:** Antitoxin (horse antiserum) that neutralizes unbound botulinum toxin should be administered as soon as possible in suspected botulinum intoxication.
- **Prevention:** Proper food preservation techniques prevent the production of the clostridial exotoxin.

Laboratory Identification

- *C. botulinum* toxin can be detected in food, intestinal contents, and serum.
- The organism can be cultured and identified by standard anaerobic methods.

[*CLOSTRIDIA* SPECIES ARE CONTINUED ON THE NEXT PAGE.]

Clostridium difficile

Pathogenesis/Clinical Significance

C. difficile is found as a normal but minor component of the flora of the large intestine. Its spores can contaminate indoor as well as outdoor environments. *C. difficile* can overgrow in the colon of an individual on antibiotics that deplete the normal flora.

C. difficile exotoxins A and B catalyze the glucosylation of host guanosine triphosphate–binding proteins leading to cytoskeleton rearrangement, interference with signalling cascades, and cell death.

- **Pseudomembranous colitis**
  Caused by toxins A and B, this condition is characterized by watery, explosive diarrhea and pseudomembrane formation in the colon.

Treatment and Prevention

- **Treatment:** Discontinue the predisposing drug, and replace fluids and electrolytes. *C. difficile* is resistant to many antibiotics. Oral administration of vancomycin or metronidazole may be added in severe cases.
- **Prevention:** No vaccine or preventive drug is available.

Laboratory Identification

- The enterotoxin can be detected in stool samples using the enzyme-linked immunosorbent assay (ELISA) test for exotoxins A and B.
- The presence of a pseudomembrane in the colon can be detected by endoscopy.

Clostridium perfringens

Pathogenesis/Clinical Significance

C. perfringens is part of the normal flora of the vagina and gastrointestinal tract. Its spores are found in soil. *C. perfringens* α toxin is a phospholipase C (lecithinase) that causes lysis of endothelial and blood cells. The bacterium produces at least 11 additional exotoxins that have hemolytic or other cytotoxic and necrotic effects.

- **Myonecrosis (gas gangrene)**
  Spores germinate in open wounds, such as those caused by GI tract surgery, burns, puncture wounds, and war wounds, and produce cytotoxic factors. Fermentation of organic compounds in host tissues causes formation of gas bubbles. As the disease progresses, increased capillary permeability leads to exotoxins being carried by the circulation from the damaged tissues to other organs, resulting in systemic effects, such as shock, renal failure, and intravascular hemolysis. Untreated myonecrosis is uniformly fatal.
- **Acute food poisoning**
  This condition is caused by the germination of spores in improperly cooked food. The resulting vegetative bacteria produce an enterotoxin that disrupts ion transport in the lower portion of the small intestine. This causes loss of fluid and intracellular proteins.
- **Anaerobic cellulitis**
  This is a clostridial infection of connective tissue in which bacterial growth spreads rapidly along fascial planes.

Treatment and Prevention

- **Treatment of gas gangrene:** Immediate treatment and wound debridement or amputation and exposure of the wound to hyperbaric oxygen are important mechanisms for treating the infection. High doses of penicillin G or doxycycline should be administered.
- **Treatment of food poisoning:** Clostridial food poisoning is usually self-limiting and requires only supportive care.
- **Prevention:** No vaccine or preventive drug is available. Prevention of food poisoning is a matter of appropriate food handling practices.

Laboratory Identification

- When specimens from diseased tissue are Gram stained, large, gram-positive rods are observed.
- When cultured anaerobically on blood agar, *C. perfringens* produces a unique double zone of β-hemolysis.
- Other diagnostic biochemical tests are available that measure such characteristics as sugar fermentation and organic acid production.

Clostridium tetani

Pathogenesis/Clinical Significance

C. tetani spores are common in soil. *C. tetani* exotoxin, tetanospasmin, binds irreversibly, penetrating neurons and blocking neurotransmitter release at inhibitory synapses. This causes severe, prolonged muscle spasms.

- **Tetanus**
  Caused by *C. tetani* spores infecting a puncture wound, a severe burn or postsurgical incision. In the early stages, the jaw muscles are affected, so that the mouth cannot open (**trismus**, or "lockjaw"). Gradually, other voluntary muscles become involved. Death is usually the result of paralysis of the chest muscles, leading to respiratory failure.

Treatment and Prevention

- **Treatment:** Preferred treatment is with human hyperimmune (tetanus immune) globulin. Sedatives and muscle relaxants are administered, and proper ventilation should be maintained. *C. tetani* is sensitive to penicillin or metronidazole.
- **Prevention:** Inactivated tetanus toxoid (formalin-inactivated toxin) is given as part of the DPT vaccine (D = diphtheria toxoid; P = pertussis antigen).

Laboratory Identification

- Diagnosis is based on clinical findings, because laboratory identification is difficult (*C. tetani* is difficult to culture, and, frequently, few organisms can be isolated from infected tissue).

Gram (+) rods

Corynebacterium species

Corynebacterium diphtheriae

Common characteristics

- **Gram-positive; stain unevenly**
- **Small, slender, pleomorphic rods that form characteristic clumps that look like Chinese characters or a picket fence (palisade arrangement)**
- **Nonmotile and unencapsulated**
- **Most species are facultative anaerobes**
- **Culture aerobically on selective medium such as Tinsdale agar**

Pathogenesis/Clinical Significance

C. diphtheriae is found on the skin, and in the nose, throat, and nasopharynx of carriers and patients with diphtheria. The organism is spread primarily by respiratory droplets.

Diphtheria is caused by the local and systemic effects of a single exotoxin that inhibits eukaryotic protein synthesis. This toxin inactivates eukaryotic polypeptide chain elongation factor EF-2 by ADP-ribosylation, thus terminating protein synthesis. [Note: The structural gene for the toxin is coded for by a bacteriophage. Only those strains of *C. diphtheriae* that are lysogenic for this phage can produce toxin and are, therefore, virulent.]

- **Diphtheria**

  This life-threatening disease begins as a local infection, usually of the throat. The infection produces a distinctive thick, grayish, adherent exudate (called a pseudomembrane) that is composed of cell debris from the mucosa, and inflammatory products. The exudate coats the throat and may extend into the nasal passages or respiratory tract where it sometimes obstructs the airways, leading to suffocation. Generalized symptoms are due to dissemination of the toxin. Although all human cells are sensitive to diphtheria toxin, major clinical effects involve the heart (myocarditis may lead to congestive heart failure and permanent heart damage) and peripheral nerves (neuritis of cranial nerves and paralysis of muscle groups such as those that control movement of the palate or the eye).

Treatment and Prevention

- **Treatment:** A single dose of horse serum antitoxin inactivates any circulating toxin, although it does not affect toxin that is already bound to a cell-surface receptor. [Note: Serum sickness caused by a reaction to the horse protein may cause complications.] Eradication of the organism is accomplished with any of several antibiotics, such as erythromycin or penicillin.
- **Prevention:** Immunization with toxoid, usually administered in the DPT triple vaccine (together with tetanus toxoid and pertussis antigens) should be started in infancy. Booster injections of diphtheria toxoid (with tetanus toxoid) should be given at approximately 10 year intervals throughout life.

Laboratory Identification

- The initial diagnosis and decision to treat for diphtheria must be made based on clinical observation, because no reliable, rapid laboratory test is available.
- *C. diphtheriae* can be cultured on selective media such as Tinsdale agar, which contains potassium tellurite, an inhibitor of other respiratory flora. The organism can then be tested for toxin production using an immunologic precipitin reaction.

Gram (+) cocci

Enterococcus species

Enterococcus faecalis

Enterococcus faecium

Common characteristics

- **Gram-positive**
- **Round-to-ovoid in shape, occurring in pairs or chains**
- **α-Hemolytic or nonhemolytic**
- **Catalase negative**
- **Grow in 6.5 percent NaCl; culture on bile-esculin agar**

Pathogenesis/Clinical Significance

Enterococcus faecalis and *Enterococcus faecium* are part of the normal fecal flora.

- **Nosocomial infections:** Enterococci are frequent causes of such infections, especially in intensive care units. Under conditions where host resistance is lowered, or where the integrity of the gastrointestinal or genitourinary tract has been disrupted, enterococci can spread to normally sterile sites, causing urinary tract infections, bacteremia/sepsis, subacute bacterial endocarditis, biliary tract infection, and intra-abdominal abscesses.

Treatment and Prevention

- **Treatment:** A combination of a penicillin and an aminoglycoside, or the glycopeptide vancomycin is used to treat enterococcal infections. Newer antibiotics, such as the combination of quinupristin and dalfopristin, are used to treat vancomycin-resistant infections.
- **Prevention:** No vaccine is available against enterococci. Careful attention to handwashing and other cleanliness measures among hospital personnel can significantly decrease the incidence of nosocomial infections.

Laboratory Identification

- Enterococci are distinguished from the non–Group D streptococci by their ability to survive in 6.5 percent sodium chloride. They can also hydrolyze the polysaccharide esculin in the presence of bile.

Gram (–) rods

Escherichia species

Escherichia coli

Common characteristics

- **Gram-negative**
- **Short rods**
- **Facultative anaerobe**
- **Ferments glucose and a wide range of carbohydrates**
- **Catalase positive, oxidase negative**
- **Culture on MacConkey agar**

Pathogenesis/Clinical Significance

E. coli is part of the normal flora in the colon of humans and other animals, but can be pathogenic both within and outside the gastrointestinal tract. *E. coli* species possess three types of antigens: O, K, and H. Pili facilitate the attachment of the bacterium to human epithelial surfaces. Pathogenic *E. coli* "virotypes" differ from the normal flora *E. coli* by the acquisition of genes that encode new virulence factors allowing for toxin production and attachment to or invasion of host cells.

- **Urinary tract infections (UTI)**

  E. coli is the most common cause of UTIs, especially in women. Symptoms include dysuria, urinary frequency, hematuria, and pyuria.

- **Diarrhea**

  Several categories of diarrhea are caused by different strains of *E. coli*. Among the most prevalent are the following:

  Enterotoxigenic *E. coli* (ETEC): This organism is a common cause of "**traveler's diarrhea**" in developing countries. It infects only humans, with transmission occurring through food and water contaminated with human waste, or by person-to-person contact. ETEC colonizes the small intestine and in a process mediated by an enterotoxin that stimulates increased cAMP production, causes prolonged hypersecretion of chloride ions and water while inhibiting the reabsorption of sodium. ETEC strains produce a heat labile toxin that is very similar to cholera toxin, in addition to a heat stable toxin that also invokes diarrhea.

  Enteropathogenic *E. coli* (EPEC): This organism is an important cause of diarrhea in infants, especially in developing countries. The newborn becomes infected during birth or *in utero*. EPEC attaches to mucosal cells in the small intestine, causing destruction of microvilli and development of characteristic lesions. Watery diarrhea results, which may become chronic.

  Enterohemorrhagic *E. coli* (EHEC): EHEC binds to cells in the large intestine, and produces one of two different Shiga-like toxins that destroy microvilli, causing a severe form of copious, bloody diarrhea (**hemorrhagic colitis**) and acute renal failure (**hemolytic uremic syndrome**). Serotype O157:H7 is the most common strain of *E. coli* that produces Shiga-like toxin. The primary reservoir of EHEC is cattle. Therefore, the possibility of infection can be greatly decreased by thoroughly cooking ground beef and pasteurizing milk.

- **Meningitis in infants**

  E. coli and group B streptococci are the leading causes of neonatal meningitis. Newborns lack IgM, and therefore, are particularly susceptible to *E. coli* sepsis, which can result in the organism's being carried to the brain. *E. coli* strains that cause meningitis express the K1 capsule, which is chemically identical to the capsule produced by serogroup B meningococci.

Treatment and Prevention

- **Treatment for UTIs:** Trimethoprim-sulfamethoxazole or a fluoroquinolone, such as ciprofloxacin, are the drugs of choice. [Note: Isolated microorganisms must be tested for antibiotic sensitivity because multiple drug resistance, carried by transmissible plasmids, is common.]
- **Treatment for meningitis:** The combination of a cephalosporin, such as cefotaxime, plus gentamicin is usually recommended.
- **Treatment for diarrhea:** Antibiotics cited above shorten the duration of the disease. Patients with diarrhea must be rehydrated and have their electrolytes replaced. Antibacterial treatment of hemolytic uremic syndrome caused by EHEC is not recommended because bacterial cell death can lead to increased toxin circulation and worse outcomes.
- **Prevention:** No vaccine or preventive drug is available. Diarrhea can be prevented by taking precautions in food and water consumption. Spread of infection between people can be controlled by handwashing and disinfection.

Laboratory Identification

- *E. coli* can be cultured on differential medium such as MacConkey agar.
- Carbohydrate fermentation patterns are observed. For example, most strains of *E. coli* ferment lactose, produce gas during glucose fermentation, and show a positive test for mannitol fermentation.

Gram (–) rods

Francisella species

Francisella tularensis

Common characteristics

- **Gram-negative**
- **Small, pleomorphic coccobacillus with a lipid-rich capsule**
- **Facultative intracellular parasite**
- **Strict aerobe**
- **Primarily pathogen of animals**
- **Rarely cultured**

Pathogenesis/Clinical Significance

The host range of *F. tularensis* is broad, and includes wild and domestic mammals, birds, and house pets. A number of biting or blood-sucking arthropods serve as vectors. Transmission is, thus, by contact with infected animal tissues, contaminated water, or an arthropod bite. Tularemia is an occupational risk for veterinarians, hunters and trappers, domestic livestock workers, and meat handlers.

F. tularensis is an intracellular parasite that can survive and multiply within host macrophages as well as in other cells. After cutaneous inoculation, *F. tularensis* multiplies locally, producing a papule that ulcerates after several days. Organisms spread from the local lesion to the regional lymph nodes, where they cause enlarged, tender nodes that may suppurate. From the lymph nodes, the organisms spread via the lymphatic system to various organs and tissues, including lungs, liver, spleen, kidneys, and the central nervous system.

- **Tularemia**

  Tularemia varies in severity from mild to fulminant and fatal. Onset of symptoms is usually abrupt. The most common symptoms are flu-like (chills, fever, headache, malaise, anorexia, and fatigue), although respiratory and gastrointestinal symptoms may also occur. Ulcers may result from contact with animal products or from insect bites (ulceroglandular tularemia). Lymphadenopathy is characteristic.

Treatment and Prevention

- **Treatment:** The drug of choice for treatment of tularemia is streptomycin or gentamicin plus a tetracycline such as doxycycline.
- **Prevention:** Avoiding insect vectors and taking precautions when handling wild animals or animal products are the best means of prevention of *F. tularensis* infection.

Laboratory Identification

- Clinical presentation and history consistent with possible exposure is of primary importance in the diagnosis of tularemia. Confirmation of the clinical diagnosis is most commonly made serologically.
- The organism is rarely cultured.

Gram (–) rods

Haemophilus species

Haemophilus influenzae

Common characteristics

- **Gram-negative**
- **Pleomorphic in shape, ranging from small coccobacilli to long, slender filaments**
- **Obligate parasite, requiring hemin and NAD^+ for growth**
- **Culture on chocolate agar containing hemin and NAD^+**

Pathogenesis/Clinical Significance

H. influenzae is a normal resident of the human upper respiratory tract, and may also colonize the conjunctiva and genital tract. Transmission is by respiratory droplets.

H. influenzae may be unencapsulated, or may produce a capsule (capsular type b is associated with the most serious, invasive disease). After attaching to and colonizing the respiratory mucosa, the infection can become systemic, with bacteria spreading via the blood to the central nervous system.

- **Bacterial meningitis**

  H. influenzae can cause bacterial meningitis, especially in infants and very young children.

[*H. INFLUENZAE* IS CONTINUED ON THE NEXT PAGE.]

Treatment and Prevention

- **Treatment:** Antibiotic sensitivity testing should be done to determine appropriate antibiotic. Generally, a third-generation cephalosporin, such as cefotaxime or ceftriaxone, is effective in the treatment of meningitis. Sinusitis, otitis media, and other upper respiratory tract infections are treated with trimethoprim-sulfamethoxazole or ampicillin plus clavulanate.

Laboratory Identification

- *H. influenzae* can be cultured on chocolate agar containing hemin (factor X) and NAD^+ (factor V).
- Capsular swelling (quellung reaction) can be observed, and the capsule can be identified by immunofluorescent staining.
- Capsular antigen can also be detected in CSF or other body fluids using immunologic techniques.

Haemophilus influenzae (continued)

Pathogenesis/Clinical Significance

- **Upper respiratory tract infections**

  H. influenzae is a major cause of otitis media, sinusitis, and epiglottitis, primarily in children.

- **Pneumonia**

  This organism causes pneumonia, particularly in older adults or immunocompromised individuals.

Treatment and Prevention

- **Prevention:** A conjugated vaccine against *H. influenzae* capsular polysaccharide type b is administered to infants. Rifampin is given prophylactically.

Laboratory Identification

Gram (–) rods ←

Helicobacter species

Helicobacter pylori

Common characteristics

- **Gram-negative**
- **Curved or spiral rods**
- **Multiple polar flagella give the organism rapid, corkscrew motility**
- **Urease-positive**
- **Culture on selective medium containing antibiotics to inhibit growth of other fecal flora**

Pathogenesis/Clinical Significance

H. pylori is unusual in its ability to colonize the stomach, where low pH normally protects against bacterial infection. Transmission is thought to be from person to person (the organism has not been isolated from food or water). Untreated, infections tend to be chronic and life-long.

H. pylori colonizes gastric mucosal cells in the stomach, surviving in the mucous layer that coats the epithelium. The organism is noninvasive, but recruits and activates inflammatory cells, thus causing a chronic inflammation of the mucosa. *H. pylori* secretes urease, producing ammonium ions that neutralize stomach acid in the vicinity of the organism, thus favoring bacterial multiplication. Ammonia can damage the gastric mucosa, and may also potentiate the effects of a cytotoxin produced by *H. pylori*.

- **Acute gastritis**

  Initial infection with *H. pylori* results in decreased mucous production, and leads to acute gastritis. Both **duodenal ulcers** and **gastric ulcers** are closely correlated with infection by *H. pylori*. The organism appears to be a risk factor for development of **gastric carcinoma** and **gastric B-cell lymphoma**.

Treatment and Prevention

- **Treatment:** Elimination of *H. pylori* requires combination therapy with two or more antimicrobials due to rapid appearance of resistant strains. A typical regimen includes tetracycline plus metronidazole plus a proton pump inhibitor such as omeprazole.
- **Prevention:** No vaccine or preventive drug is available.

Laboratory Identification

- Characteristic corkscrew movement can be seen in smears of biopsied gastric mucosa.
- Urease-positivity can be measured by a breath test (radioactively labeled urea is cleaved by bacterial enzyme, releasing radioactive CO_2 in expired breath).
- Serologic tests are available, including enzyme-linked immunosorbent assay (ELISA) for serum antibodies to *H. pylori*.

Gram (–) rods

Legionella species

Legionella pneumophila

Common characteristics

- **Gram-negative (faintly staining)**
- **Slender rod in nature; coccobacillary in clinical material**
- **Facultative, intracellular parasite**
- **Organisms are unencapsulated with monotrichous flagella**
- **Culture on specialized medium**

Pathogenesis/Clinical Significance

L. pneumophila's normal habitats are free living ameba found in water and soil, and the organism within its ameba host resides in cooling towers, humidifiers, air conditioners, and water distribution systems. The organism is chlorine tolerant and, thus, survives water treatment procedures.

Infections generally result from inhalation of aerosolized organisms. The resulting pathology is, therefore, initially confined primarily to the respiratory tract. Macrophages phagocytose the *L. pneumophila*, but the phagosome fails to fuse with a lysosome. Instead, the organisms multiply within this protected environment until the cell ruptures, releasing increased numbers of infectious bacteria.

- **Legionnaires' disease**

  This is an acute lobar pneumonia with multisystem symptoms. Predisposing factors include immunocompromise, pulmonary compromise (due, for example, to heavy smoking or chronic lung disease), and debilitation brought on by excessive alcohol consumption, age, or surgery. Pneumonia (associated with a cough that is only slightly productive) is the predominant symptom. Watery, nonbloody diarrhea occurs in 25 to 50 percent of cases. Nausea, vomiting, and neurologic symptoms may also occur.

- **Pontiac fever**

  This is an influenza-like illness that characteristically infects otherwise healthy individuals. Recovery is usually complete within 1 week.

Treatment and Prevention

- **Treatment:** Macrolides, such as erythromycin or azithromycin, are the drugs of choice for Legionnaire's disease. Fluoroquinolones are also effective. No specific therapy is required for Pontiac fever.
- **Prevention:** No vaccine or preventive drug is available. Measures such as flushing the water supply with extremely hot water decrease the chance of contamination.

Laboratory Identification

- Culture *L. pneumophila* from respiratory secretions using buffered charcoal yeast extract enriched with L-cysteine, iron, and α-ketoglutarate.
- Serologic tests include a direct fluorescent antibody test and a radioimmunoassay for *L. pneumophila* antigen in the urine.
- Hybridization with a *L. pneumophila*-specific DNA probe is also available.

Spirochetes

Leptospira species

Leptospira interrogans

Common characteristics

- **Gram-negative, but stains poorly, and needs to be visualized by other means**
- **Long, very slender, flexible, spiral- or corkscrew-shaped rods**
- **Highly motile**
- **Culture on specialized medium**

Pathogenesis/Clinical Significance

A number of wild and domestic animals serve as reservoirs for *L. interrogans*. Transmission to humans occurs following ingestion of food or water contaminated, for example, by animal urine containing the spirochete. These organisms can survive for several weeks in stagnant water, but are sensitive to drying.

- **Leptospirosis**

  Different strains of *L. interrogans* are found worldwide, and cause leptospirosis, known under various local names such as **infectious jaundice**, **marsh fever**, **Weil's disease**, and **swineherd's disease**. Fever occurs about 1 to 2 weeks after infection, and *L. interrogans* is present in the blood. The organisms next infect various organs, particularly the liver and kidneys, resulting in jaundice, hemorrhage, and tissue necrosis. Large numbers of leptospira are shed into the urine by the diseased kidneys. The second phase of the disease involves a rise in IgM antibody titer accompanied by aseptic meningitis. Hepatitis frequently occurs.

Treatment and Prevention

- **Treatment:** Penicillin G or a tetracycline such as doxycycline are used during early stages of the infection.
- **Prevention:** No vaccine is available. Doxycycline is effective prophylactically. Prevention of exposure to contaminated water, and rodent control, can both help decrease the chance of infection.

Laboratory Identification

- *L. interrogans* does not stain well. However, the organisms can sometimes be observed in a fresh blood smear by dark-field microscopy.
- *L. interrogans* can be detected by serologic agglutination tests.

Gram (+) rods

Listeria species

Listeria monocytogenes

Common characteristics

- **Gram-positive, staining darkly**
- **Slender, short rods, sometimes occurring as diplobacilli or in short chains**
- **Facultative intracellular parasites**
- **Catalase positive**
- **Distinctive tumbling motility in liquid medium**
- **Grow facultatively on a variety of enriched media**

Pathogenesis/Clinical Significance

Listeria species are widespread among animals in nature. Infections with the pathogenic *L. monocytogenes* may occur as sporadic cases or in small epidemics, which are usually food-borne (dairy products, ground meats, and poultry).

L. monocytogenes is a facultative, intracellular parasite. It attaches to and enters a variety of mammalian cells by phagocytosis. Once inside the cell, it escapes from the phagocytic vacuole by producing a membrane-damaging toxin, **listeriolysin**. *Listeria* grows in the cytosol, and utilizes actin-based motility and the protein ActA to facilitate its direct passage from cell to cell.

- **Listeriosis**

  Septicemia and meningitis are the most commonly reported forms of listeria infection. The organism can be transmitted from an infected mother to her newborn (*Listeria* is a relatively common cause of newborn meningitis), or to the fetus, initiating abortion. Immunocompromised individuals, especially those with defects in cellular immunity, are susceptible to serious, generalized infections.

Treatment and Prevention

- **Treatment:** A variety of antibiotics have been successfully used to treat *L. monocytogenes* infections, including ampicillin or trimethoprim plus sulfamethoxazole.
- **Prevention:** No vaccine is available against *L. monocytogenes.* Prevention of *Listeria* infections can be accomplished by proper food preparation and handling.

Laboratory Identification

- *L. monocytogenes* can be isolated from blood, cerebrospinal fluid, and other clinical specimens.
- On blood agar, the organism produces a small colony surrounded by a narrow zone of β-hemolysis.
- *Listeria* species can be distinguished by morphology, positive motility, and the production of catalase.

Other

Mycobacterium species

Mycobacterium leprae

Mycobacterium tuberculosis

Common characteristics

- **Not stained by Gram stain due to lipid-rich cell walls**
- **Long, slender, nonmotile rods**
- **Aerobic**
- **Resistant to drying**
- **Culture *M. tuberculosis* on specialized medium such as Lowenstein-Jensen agar; *M. leprae* does not grow in culture**

Mycobacterium leprae

Pathogenesis/Clinical Significance

M. leprae has low infectivity. It is transmitted from human to human through prolonged contact, for example between exudates of a leprosy patient's skin lesions, and the abraded skin of another individual. Some cases in the United States have been linked to contact with or ingestion of armaidillos, a known reservoir of the pathogen. No *M. leprae* toxins or virulence factors are known.

- **Hansen disease (leprosy)**

  Leprosy is a chronic granulomatous condition of peripheral nerves and skin. There are two clinical forms: **tuberculoid leprosy**, in which destructive lesions due to the host's cell-mediated immune response occur as large macular plaques in cooler body tissues such as skin (especially nose and outer ears), testicles, and in superficial nerve endings, and **lepromatous leprosy**, in which the cell-mediated immune response is severely depressed, and the disease becomes slow but progressive, with large numbers of organisms in the lesions and blood.

[*MYCOBACTERIUM* SPECIES ARE CONTINUED ON THE NEXT PAGE.]

Treatment and Prevention

- **Treatment for tuberculoid form:** Treatment of leprosy consists of multiple drug treatment with dapsone, rifampicin, and, for lepromatous disease, clofazimine. Both tuberculoid and lepromatous forms require long-term antibiotic treatment.
- **Prevention:** No preventive drug is available. Vaccination with bacillus Calmette-Guerin shows some protective effects against leprosy.

Laboratory Identification

- **Tuberculous leprosy:** Organisms in clinical samples are very rare, and diagnosis relies on clinical findings and the histology of biopsy material.
- **Lepromatous leprosy:** Acid-fast stains of skin scrapings from nasal mucosa or other infected areas can show the presence of *M. leprae.*

Mycobacterium tuberculosis

Pathogenesis/Clinical Significance

M. tuberculosis survives and grows in host macrophages, where it can remain viable but quiescent for decades. Immunosuppression can lead to reactivation. *M. tuberculosis* produces no demonstrable endo- or exotoxins.

Tuberculosis is the principal chronic bacterial disease in humans, and is the leading cause of death from infection worldwide. Transmission is by aerosol droplets produced by coughing, and depends on crowded conditions and poor ventilation.

- **Tuberculosis:**

  Tubercles (productive granulomatous lesions) form in the lung following infection by *M. tuberculosis.* Their formation is mediated by the host immune response. The lesion may arrest and become fibrotic and calcified, or it can break down, resulting in spread of the infection via the lymph and bloodstream. *M. tuberculosis* can seed different tissues, causing, for example, chronic pneumonitis, tuberculous osteomyelitis, or tuberculous meningitis. If active tubercles develop throughout the body, this serious condition is known as miliary (disseminated) tuberculosis.

Treatment and Prevention

- **Treatment:** A long course of combined antibiotic treatment (6 months or more) with isoniazid, rifampin, pyrazinamide, and ethambutol is required for a cure.
- **Prevention:** Bacille Calmette-Guerin vaccine is available, and is used for tuberculin-negative individuals under sustained heavy risk of infection. Isoniazid is used prophylactically, for example, for tuberculin-positive, asymptomatic individuals, who need immunosuppressive therapy for other illnesses.

Laboratory Identification

- Acid-fast bacteria can be observed in clinical specimens treated with Ziehl-Neelsen stain.
- Nucleic acid probes can be used to detect *M. tuberculosis* DNA that has been amplified by polymerase chain reaction.
- The organism can be cultured on specialized media such as Lowenstein-Jensen agar.

Mycoplasma ←

Mycoplasma species

Mycoplasma pneumoniae

Common characteristics

- **Not seen with Gram stain because it lacks peptidoglycan cell walls**
- **Plastic, pleomorphic shape (neither rods nor cocci)**
- **Three-layer (trilaminar) cell membrane contains sterols**
- **Rarely cultured for diagnostic purposes**

Pathogenesis/Clinical Significance

M. pneumoniae is found as part of the normal flora of the human mouth and and genitourinary tract. It is transmitted person to person by respiratory droplets.

M. pneumoniae has a membrane-associated cytoadhesin (P1) that binds to ciliated bronchial epithelial cells, and inhibits ciliary action. This results in an inflammatory response in bronchial tissues. *M. pneumoniae* produces an exotoxin that is similar to pertussis toxin.

- **Primary atypical pneumonia:**

  This disease of the lower respiratory tract is the best-known form of *M. pneumoniae* infection. It is also referred to as "walking pneumonia" because the signs and symptoms may be minimal, and the patient usually remains ambulatory throughout the illness. *M. pneumoniae* infection also causes bronchitis, pharyngitis, and nonpurulent otitis media. The highest incidence of disease occurs in older children and young adults (6 to 20 years old).

[*M. PNEUMONIASE* IS CONTINUED ON THE NEXT PAGE.]

Treatment and Prevention

- **Treatment:** Doxycycline, azithromycin, erythromycin or levofloxacin are the drugs of choice.

Laboratory Identification

- Serologic tests such as complement fixing antibodies to *M. pneumoniae* are the most widely used procedures for establishing an identification of primary atypical pneumonia.
- *M. pneumoniae* is difficult and expensive to culture.
- Commercially available DNA probes can be used to detect *M. pneumoniae* in sputum specimens.

Mycoplasma pneumoniae (continued)

Pathogenesis/Clinical Significance	Treatment and Prevention	Laboratory Identification
		• Cold agglutinins are detectable after *M. pneumoniae* infection. These RBC-specific antibodies agglutinate RBCs in the cold.

Gram (–) cocci ←

Neisseria species

Neisseria gonorrhoeae
Neisseria meningitidis

Common characteristics

- **Gram-negative**
- **Kidney bean–shaped diplococci**
- **Piliated**
- **Oxidase-positive**
- **Aerobic**

Neisseria gonorrhoeae

Pathogenesis/Clinical Significance

The normal habitat of *N. gonorrhoeae* is the human genital tract. It is usually transmitted during sexual contact, but can also be transmitted during the passage of a baby through an infected birth canal.

N. gonorrhoeae is highly sensitive to dessication, and is unencapsulated. Bacterial proteins (pili and outer membrane proteins) enhance the attachment of the bacterium to host epithelial and mucosal cell surfaces, such as those of the urethra, rectum, cervix, pharynx, and conjunctiva, followed by colonization. Pilin antigenic variation contributes to immune evasion and an IgA protease allows gonococci to evade mucosal IgA.

- **Gonorrhea**

  Gonorrhea is the second most commonly reported infectious disease in the United States. In males, symptoms include urethritis, purulent discharge, and pain during urination. In females, infection is usually localized to the endocervix, sometimes causing a purulent vaginal discharge. If the woman's disease progresses to the fallopian tubes, **gonococcal salpingitis** (which may lead to tubal scarring and infertility), **pelvic inflammatory disease**, and fibrosis can occur. Alternatively, the infection may be asymptomatic.

- **Ophthalmia neonatorum**

  This is a purulent conjunctivitis acquired by a newborn during passage through the birth canal of a mother infected with the gonococcus. If untreated, acute conjunctivitis can lead to blindness.

- **Septic arthritis**

  Blood-borne (disseminated) *N. gonorrhoeae* infection is the most common cause of infectious arthritis in sexually active adults.

Treatment and Prevention

- **Treatment for uncomplicated gonorrhea:** Ceftriaxone is currently the antibiotic of choice. A tetracycline, such as doxycycline, is added when *Chlamydia* is a suspected co-pathogen.
- **Treatment for ophthalmia neonatorum:** A single dose of ceftriaxone is given systemically. Neonatal prophylaxis: Erythromycin is instilled into newborns' eyes to eradicate both *N. gonorrhoeae* and *Chlamydia trachomatis.*
- **Prevention:** No vaccine or preventive drug is available. Newborns whose eyes are at risk for infection with *N. gonorrhoeae* are treated prophylactically with erythromycin. Taking precautions during sex (that is, using condoms) can prevent transmission of the disease.

Laboratory Identification

- Gram-negative diplococci are visible within neutrophils in urethral exudates.
- Oxidase-positive cultures grow on Thayer-Martin agar with additional CO_2.
- *N. gonorrhoeae* utilizes glucose but not maltose.

Neisseria meningitidis

Pathogenesis/Clinical Significance

N. meningitidis is one of the most frequent causes of meningitis. Transmission is via respiratory droplets, and pili allow the attachment of *N. meningitidis* to the nasopharyngeal mucosa. The meningococcal polysaccharide capsule is antiphagocytic, and is, therefore, the most important virulence factor aiding in maintenance of the infection. *N. meningitidis* also makes IgA protease (see *N. gonorrhoeae*). A truncated endotoxin called LOS is responsible for most of the tissue damage in meningococcal disease.

[*N. MENINGITIDIS* IS CONTINUED ON THE NEXT PAGE.]

Treatment and Prevention

- **Treatment:** Penicillin G, cefotaxime, and ceftriaxone are the drugs of choice.

Laboratory Identification

- Under the light microscope, *N. meningitidis* obtained from cerebrospinal fluid appear as gram-negative diplococci, often inside of and in association with polymorphonuclear leukocytes.

Neisseria meningitidis (continued)

Pathogenesis/Clinical Significance

- **Meningitis**

  The epithelial lining of the nasopharynx normally serves as a barrier to bacteria. If meningococci penetrate that barrier and enter the blood stream they rapidly multiply, causing **meningococcemia**. This septicemia can result in intravascular coagulation, circulatory collapse, and potentially fatal shock (for which the bacterial endotoxin is largely responsible). If *N. meningitidis* crosses the blood–brain barrier, it can infect the meninges, causing an acute inflammatory response that results in a purulent **meningitis**. The initial fever and malaise can rapidly evolve into severe headache, rigid neck, vomiting, and sensitivity to bright light. Coma can occur within a few hours.

- **Waterhouse-Friderichsen syndrome**

  This syndrome is an acute, fulminating meningococcal septicemia seen mainly in young children. It is associated with adrenal hemorrhage.

Treatment and Prevention

- **Prevention:** A conjugate vaccine comprised of capsular material from serogroups A, C, Y and W-135 is now recommended for adolescents and young adults. Unfortunately, the polysaccharide of serogroup B does not elicit an effective immune response.
- **Prophylaxis:** Rifampin can be used to treat family members and other close associates of an infected individual.

Laboratory Identification

- *N. meningitidis* can be cultured on chocolate agar.
- The organism is oxidase-positive, and utilizes both glucose and maltose in an atmosphere of 5 percent CO_2.

Gram (–) rods

Pseudomonas species

Pseudomonas aeruginosa

Common characteristics

- **Gram-negative**
- **Motile rods (polar flagella) with alginate capsule**
- **Aerobic or facultative**
- **Oxidase-positive**
- **Produces diffusible green and blue pigments**
- **Oxidizes but does not ferment carbohydrates such as lactose**
- **Culture on MacConkey agar**

Pathogenesis/Clinical Significance

P. aeruginosa is widely distributed in nature (soil, water, plants, animals). It may colonize healthy humans without causing disease but is also a significant opportunistic pathogen and a major cause of nosocomial infections. *P. aeruginosa* is regularly a cause of nosocomial pneumonia; nosocomial infections of the urinary tract, surgical sites, and severe burns; and of infections of patients with cystic fibrosis, and those who are undergoing either chemotherapy for neoplastic diseases or antibiotic therapy for other infections. *P. aeruginosa* can grow in distilled water, laboratory hot water baths, hot tubs, wet intravenous tubing, and other water-containing vessels. This explains why the organism is responsible for so many nosocomial infections.

P. aeruginosa disease begins with attachment and colonization of host tissue. Virtually any tissue/organ may be affected. Pili mediate adherence, and extracellular proteases, cytotoxin, hemolysins, and pyocyanin promote tissue damage and local invasion and dissemination of the organism. Systemic disease is promoted by an antiphagocytic capsule, and endo- and exotoxins.

- **Localized infections:**

  Localized *P. aeruginosa* infections may occur in the eye, ear, skin, urinary tract, respiratory tract, gastrointestinal tract (GI), and central nervous system (CNS). In most cases, localized infections have the potential to lead to disseminated infection.

- **Systemic infection**

  The GI tract is a particularly common site for penetration. The resulting systemic infections may include bacteremia, secondary pneumonia, bone and joint infections, endocarditis, and infections of the skin/soft tissue and CNS.

Treatment and Prevention

- **Treatment:** Because resistance to a variety of antibiotics is common in this species, antimicrobial therapy often requires a combination of bactericidal antibiotics, such as an aminoglycoside and an antipseudomonal β-lactam.
- **Prevention:** No vaccine or preventive drug is available. Prevention of burn wound infection requires the use of topical silver sulfadizine.

Laboratory Identification

- *P. aeruginosa* does not ferment lactose, and is oxidase positive.
- *P. aeruginosa* produces colorless colonies on MacConkey agar. Cultured organisms produce blue (pyocyanin) and fluorescent green (pyoverdin) pigments.

Other

Rickettsia species

Rickettsia rickettsii

Common characteristics

- **Gram-negative, but stain poorly**
- **Small, rod-like or coccobacillary in shape**
- **Grow only inside living host cells**
- **Transmitted by infected tick**
- **Not routinely cultured because of obligate intracellularity**

Pathogenesis/Clinical Significance

R. rickettsii is transmitted to humans by the bite of an infected wood or dog tick. It parasitizes endothelial cells lining the capillaries throughout the circulatory system, ultimately killing the host cell. This results in the formation of focal thrombi in various organs including the skin. A variety of small hemorrhages and hemodynamic disturbances create the symptoms of illness.

- **Rocky Mountain spotted fever**

  This disease is characterized by high fever, malaise, and a prominent rash that begins on the palms and soles, and then spreads to cover the body. The rash can progress from macular to petechial or frankly hemorrhagic. Untreated, infection can lead to myocardial or renal failure. The disease occurs most frequently in children and teenagers, but mortality rates are highest (5 to 30 percent) among individuals older than 40 years of age.

Treatment and Prevention

- **Treatment:** Doxycycline is the drug of choice for *R. rickettsii* infections, provided it is administered early in the illness. Because the principal diagnostic methods await the demonstration of seroconversion, a decision to treat must be made on clinical grounds, together with a history or suspicion of contact with a tick.
- **Prevention:** No antirickettsial vaccine is licensed in the United States, and no preventive drug is available. Prevention depends on vector control, wearing proper clothing that minimizes bare skin, and immediate removal of attached ticks.

Laboratory Identification

- Serologic procedures rely on the demonstration of a rickettsia-specific antibody response during the course of infection.
- Indirect fluorescent antibody tests using rickettsia-specific antibodies are available, primarily in reference laboratories.

Gram (–) rods

Salmonella species

Salmonella enterica serovar Typhi

Salmonella enterica serovar Typhimurium

Common characteristics

- **Gram-negative rods**
- **Facultative anaerobes**
- **Ferment glucose and a wide range of carbohydrates, but most species of *Salmonella* do not ferment lactose**
- **Catalase positive, oxidase negative**
- **Culture on MacConkey agar**

Salmonella enterica serovar Typhi

Pathogenesis/Clinical Significance

S. enterica serovar Typhi is transmitted between humans, without animal or fowl reservoirs. Infection is via the oral–fecal route, generally through food or water contaminated by human feces. Young children and older adults are particularly susceptible to *Salmonella* infections, as are individuals in crowded institutions or living conditions.

S. enterica serovar Typhi causes disease by attaching to and invading macrophages of the intestinal lymphoid tissue (Peyer's patches). The bacteria replicate rapidly within these cells, and eventually spread to the reticuloendothelial system (including both liver and spleen, which become enlarged) and potentially to the gallbladder.

- **Enteric (typhoid) fever**

  This is a severe, life-threatening systemic illness, characterized by fever and, frequently, by abdominal symptoms. About 30 percent of patients have a faint, maculopapular rash on the trunk (termed "rose spots"). After 1 to 3 weeks of incubation, *S.* serovar Typhi can enter the blood, with the resulting bacteremia causing fever, headache, malaise, and bloody diarrhea. Bacterial endotoxin can cause encephalopathy, myocarditis, and intravascular coagulation. Perforations of the intestine can lead to hemorrhage. Some infected individuals may become chronic carriers for periods as long as years due to persistent residual infection of the gallbladder. Public food handlers and health care deliverers who are carriers can present a serious public health problem (remember "Typhoid Mary"!).

[*SALMONELLA* SPECIES ARE CONTINUED ON THE NEXT PAGE.]

Treatment and Prevention

- **Treatment:** Ceftriaxone and fluoroquinolones such as ciprofloxacin are the first-line drugs of choice.
- **Prevention:** Two vaccines are available. One consists of a live attenuated strain of *S. enterica* serovar Typhi and is administered orally. The other vaccine contains capsular material and is delivered parenterally. Prevention requires maintaining proper hygiene and cooking food thoroughly.

Laboratory Identification

- Serovar Typhi can be isolated from blood, feces, bone marrow, urine, or tissue from rose spots.
- Serovar Typhi can be cultured on MacConkey agar, where it produces colorless, non–lactose-fermenting colonies.
- Serologic tests for antibodies against O antigen in patient's serum also aid in the diagnosis.

Salmonella enterica serovar Typhimurium

Pathogenesis/Clinical Significance

S. enterica serovar Typhimurium (and other *Salmonella* species that cause enterocolitis) reside in the gastrointestinal tracts of humans, other animals, and fowl. They are transmitted through contaminated food products, or via the oral/fecal route.

- **Enterocolitis (gastroenteritis, foodborne infection)**
  Contaminated poultry products including eggs are the primary vehicles for infection of humans by serovar Typhimurium, although raw milk and pets such as turtles also transmit the disease. *Salmonella* adhere to and invade enterocytes of both the small and large intestine, causing a profound inflammatory response. Within 10 to 48 hours after ingestion, nausea, vomiting, abdominal cramps, and diarrhea ensue. Diarrhea usually ends spontaneously within a week.

Treatment and Prevention

- **Treatment:** Fluid and electrolyte replacement are important if diarrhea is severe. Antibiotics are not normally used except in immunocompromised individuals to prevent systemic spread of the infection.
- **Prevention:** No vaccine or preventive drug is available. Prevention is accomplished by proper sewage disposal, correct handling of food, and good personal hygiene.

Laboratory Identification

- Organisms isolated from stool samples produce colorless colonies on MacConkey agar.

Gram (–) rods

Shigella species

Shigella sonnei
Shigella dysenteriae
Shigella flexneri
Shigella boydii

Common characteristics

- **Gram-negative rods**
- **Facultative anaerobes**
- **Most *Shigella* species are unable to ferment lactose, except *S. sonnei* does so weakly.**
- **Catalase-positive, oxidase negative**
- **Culture on Hektoen agar**

Pathogenesis/Clinical Significance

Shigella species *are* spread from person to person, with contaminated stools serving as a major source of organisms. Flies and contaminated food and water can also transmit the disease. The organism has a low infectious dose (less than 200 viable organisms are sufficient to cause disease). Therefore, secondary cases within a household are common, particularly under conditions of crowding and/or poor sanitation.

S. sonnei, which is a common cause of shigellosis in the United States, invades and destroys the mucosa of the large intestine but rarely penetrates to the deeper intestinal layers. *S. dysenteriae* also invades the colonic mucosa but, in addition, produces an exotoxin (**Shiga toxin**) with enterotoxic and cytotoxic properties.

- **Bacillary dysentery (shigellosis)**
  This disease is characterized by diarrhea with blood, mucus, and painful abdominal cramping. The disease is generally most severe in the young and in older adults, and among malnourished individuals, in whom shigellosis may lead to severe dehydration and even death.

Treatment and Prevention

- **Treatment:** Antibiotics such as ciprofloxacin or azithromycin can reduce the duration of illness and the period of shedding organisms, but usage should be guided by susceptibility tests.
- **Prevention:** Protection of the water and food supplies and personal hygiene are crucial for preventing *Shigella* infections. Vaccine development is currently experimental.

Laboratory Identification

- During acute illness, organisms can be cultured from stools using Hektoen agar or other media specific for intestinal pathogens.

Gram (+) cocci

Staphylococcus species

Staphylococcus aureus
Staphylococcus epidermidis
Staphylococcus saprophyticus

Common characteristics

- **Gram-positive, staining darkly**
- **Cocci tending to occur in bunches like grapes**
- **Facultative anaerobic organisms**
- **Cultured on enriched media containing broth and/or blood**

Staphylococcus aureus

Pathogenesis/Clinical Significance

S. aureus is part of the normal flora of certain mucous membranes (for example, the anterior nares, and vagina), and of the skin. It is also, however, the most virulent of the staphylococci.

Infection occurs during penetration of the skin (for example, due to a wound, or during surgery), typically resulting in an abscess. Subsequent disease can be caused by the actual infection, by toxins in the absence of infection (toxinosis), or by a combination of infection and intoxication. Important *S. aureus* virulence factors include: 1) cell wall virulence factors that can promote binding to mucosal cells and exert antiopsonic (and, therefore, antiphagocytic) effects; 2) cytolytic exotoxins (including hemolysins); and 3) superantigen exotoxins, including enterotoxins (which cause food poisoning), toxic shock syndrome toxin, and exfoliative toxin (which causes scalded skin syndrome in children, and also bullous impetigo). The most common diseases caused by *S. aureus* are the following.

- **Localized skin infections**

  These include 1) small, superficial abscesses involving sweat or sebaceous glands, or hair follicles (for example, the common **sty**); 2) subcutaneous abscesses (**furuncles** or **boils**) that form around foreign bodies such as splinters; and 3) larger, deeper infections (**carbuncles**) that can lead to bacteremia.

- **Diffuse skin infection—impetigo (pyoderma)**

  This is a superficial, spreading, crusty skin lesion generally seen in children.

- **Deep, localized infections**

  S. aureus is the most common cause of acute and chronic infection of the bone (**osteomyelitis**), and also the most common cause of arthritis resulting from acute infection of the joint space ("**septic joint**").

- **Other infections**

  S. aureus can cause **acute endocarditis**, **septicemia**, and severe, **necrotizing pneumonia**. [Note: *S. aureus* is one of the most common causes of hospital-acquired (nosocomial) infections. Progression to septicemia is often a terminal event.]

- **Toxinoses**

  Toxic shock syndrome is caused by strains of *S. aureus* that produce a specific, absorbable toxin. The syndrome results in high fever, rash, vomiting, diarrhea, hypotension, and multiorgan involvement (especially gastrointestinal, renal, and hepatic damage). Staphylococcal **gastroenteritis** is caused by ingestion of food contaminated with toxin produced by *S. aureus*. **Scalded skin syndrome** (mild cases are sometimes called **bullous impetigo**) involves the appearance of superficial bullae resulting from the action of an exfoliative toxin that attacks the intercellular adhesive of the stratum granulosum, causing marked epithelial desquamation.

[*STAPHYLOCOCCUS* SPECIES ARE CONTINUED ON THE NEXT PAGE.]

Treatment and Prevention

- **Treatment:** Serious *S. aureus* infections require aggressive treatment, including incision and drainage of localized lesions as well as systemic antibiotics. Acquired antibiotic resistance determinants are frequently present, complicating the choice of drug. For example, nearly all *S. aureus* isolates are resistant to penicillin G, and methicillin-resistant *S. aureus* (MRSA) is becoming prevalent. Nafcillin and oxacillin have replaced penicillin G because they are β-lactamase resistant. Vancomycin is also used to treat MRSA, but strains resistant to this drug have emerged.
- **Prevention:** No vaccine or preventive drug is available. Infection control procedures such as barrier precautions, washing of hands, and disinfection of fomites are important in the control of nosocomial *S. aureus* epidemics.

Laboratory Identification

- *S. aureus* stains strongly positive with Gram stain, and cells appear in grape-like clusters.
- *S. aureus* is catalase and coagulase positive.
- *S. aureus* forms deep yellow, hemolytic colonies on enriched media.

Staphylococcus epidermidis

Pathogenesis/Clinical Significance

S. epidermidis is part of the normal flora of the skin and anterior nares.

- **Important cause of infections from prosthetic implants**

  Surgical implants, such as heart valves and catheters, are easily infected by *S. epidermidis.* Cell envelope polysaccharides enable biofilm formation, which facilitates attachment to plastic surfaces. The ability to form a biofilm is an important virulence factor.

Treatment and Prevention

- **Treatment:** Acquired drug resistance by *S. epidermidis* is even more frequent than with *S. aureus.* Vancomycin sensitivity remains the rule, but vancomycin-resistant isolates have been reported.
- **Prevention:** No vaccine or preventive drug is available.

Laboratory Identification

- *S. epidermidis* stains strongly positive with Gram stain. The cocci appear in grape-like clusters.
- The organism produces white, nonhemolytic colonies on enriched agar. It is coagulase-negative, and novobiocin-sensitive.

Staphylococcus saprophyticus

Pathogenesis/Clinical Significance

S. saprophyticus is part of the normal vaginal flora.

- **Cystitis in women**

  S. saprophyticus is a frequent cause of cystitis in women. [Note: A urinary coagulase-negative staphylococcus is often presumed to be *S. saprophyticus,* and novobiocin resistance can be used for confirmation.]

Treatment and Prevention

- **Treatment:** *S. saprophyticus* tends to be sensitive to most antibiotics, even penicillin G.
- **Prevention:** No vaccine or preventive drug is available.

Laboratory Identification

- *S. saprophyticus* stains strongly positive with Gram stain. The cocci appear in grape-like clusters.
- The organism produces white, nonhemolytic colonies on enriched agar. It is coagulase negative and novobiocin resistant.

Gram (+) cocci ←

Streptococcus species

Streptococcus agalactiae
Streptococcus pneumoniae
Streptococcus pyogenes

Common characteristics

- **Gram-positive**
- **Ovoid to spherical in shape, occurring as pairs or chains**
- **Nonmotile, catalase negative**
- **Aerotolerant anaerobes**
- **Culture on blood agar**

Streptococcus agalactiae

Pathogenesis/Clinical Significance

S. agalactiae is a group B streptococcus. It is found normally in the genital tract of female carriers and the urethral mucous membranes of male carriers, as well as in the gastrointestinal tract (especially the rectum). Transmission occurs from an infected mother to her infant at birth, and via sexual transmission among adults.

S. agalactiae's polysaccharide capsule is antiphagocytic, which allows the bacterium to infect tissue and induce an inflammatory response.

- **Meningitis and septicemia in neonates**

  Infection occurs as the infant traverses the birth canal. *S. agalactiae* is a leading cause of these syndromes in neonates, with a high mortality rate.

- **Infections of adults**

  S. agalactiae is an occasional cause of endometritis in postpartum women and of septicemia or pneumonia in individuals with impaired immune systems.

Treatment and Prevention

- **Treatment:** All isolates remain sensitive to penicillin G and ampicillin, which are still the antibiotics of choice. In life-threatening infections, an aminoglycoside can be added to the regimen.
- **Prevention:** No vaccine or preventive drug is available.

Laboratory Identification

- Samples of blood, cervical swabs, sputum, or spinal fluid can be cultured on blood agar. Group B streptococci are β-hemolytic, with larger colonies and less hemolysis than group A streptococci.
- *S. agalactiae* can hydrolyze sodium hippurate, and is catalase-negative.

[*STREPTOCOCCUS* SPECIES ARE CONTINUED ON THE NEXT PAGE.]

Streptococcus pneumoniae

Pathogenesis/Clinical Significance

S. pneumoniae (formerly called *Diplococcus pneumoniae* and referred to as "pneumococcus") is the most common cause of pneumonia and otitis media, and an important cause of meningitis and bacteremia/sepsis. *S. pneumoniae* is carried in the nasopharynx of many healthy individuals. Infection can be either endogenous (in a carrier who develops impaired resistance to the organism) or exogenous (by droplets from the nose of a carrier).

Virulence factors include the polysaccharide capsule, which is antiphagocytic, and the cell-associated enzymes, pneumolysin and autolysin.

- **Acute bacterial pneumonia**
  Pneumonia, caused most frequently by *S. pneumoniae*, is a leading cause of death in older adults and those whose resistance is impaired. It is frequently preceded by an upper or middle respiratory viral infection, which predisposes to *S. pneumoniae* infection of pulmonary parenchyma. Mechanisms include increased volume and viscosity of secretions that are more difficult to clear and secondary inhibition of the action of bronchial cilia by viral infection.
- **Otitis media**
  Characterized by earache, this is the most common bacterial infection of children, and *S. pneumoniae* is its most common cause.
- **Meningitis**
  S. pneumoniae is a common cause of meningitis. This disease has a high mortality rate, even when treated appropriately.

Treatment and Prevention

- **Treatment:** Penicillin G has been the drug of choice, but resistant strains are regularly seen. Most resistant strains remain sensitive to vancomycin and ceftrixone, Therefore these antibiotics are the agents of choice for invasive infections by penicillin-resistant strains of *S. pneumoniae.*
- **Prevention:** An anti-pneumococcal capsular polysaccharide vaccine that immunizes against 23 serotypes of *S. pneumoniae* is indicated for the protection of high-risk individuals over age 2 years. A 13-valent vaccine has recently been approved for use in infants over the age of 6 weeks.

Laboratory Identification

- Under the light microscope, gram-positive *S. pneumoniae* appear as encapsulated, lancet-shaped organisms, occurring in pairs (hence the former name, "diplococcus").
- Samples obtained from a nasopharyngeal swab, blood, pus, sputum, or spinal fluid can be cultured on blood agar. The colonies are α-hemolytic.
- Capsular swelling (quellung reaction) is observed when the pneumococci are treated with type-specific antiserum.

Streptococcus pyogenes

Pathogenesis/Clinical Significance

Group A streptococcus that resides in infected patients and also healthy human carriers by adhering to skin and mucous membranes (especially the nasopharynx), as its habitat. Most common means of transmission are via aerosol from a carrier or someone who has streptococcal pharyngitis, or from direct contact with a skin carrier or a patient with impetigo.

S. pyogenes causes some of the most rapidly progressive infections known, including **cellulitis** (diffuse spreading inflammation) anywhere in the body. It also causes postinfectious sequelae, including rheumatic fever and acute glomerulonephritis. Like *Staphylococcus aureus, S. pyogenes* secretes a wide range of exotoxins.

- **Acute pharyngitis, or pharyngotonsillitis**
  S. pyogenes is the most common bacterial cause of sore throats, especially in patients ages 2 to 20 years, and pharyngitis (for example, **strep throat**) is the most common type of *S. pyogenes* infection. Toxigenic strains release a pyrogenic exotoxin which leads to an extensive rash, in the syndrome designated **scarlet fever**.
- **Acute rheumatic fever**
  This autoimmune disease can occur 2 to 3 weeks after initiation of pharyngitis. This disease is caused by cross-reactions between antigens of the heart and joint tissues, and streptococcal antigen.
- **Impetigo**
  This is a contagious, pus-forming infection of the skin, in which a thick, yellowish crust forms, usually on the face. It usually affects children, and can cause severe and extensive lesions on the face and limbs.

[*STREPTOCOCCUS PYOGENES* IS CONTINUED ON THE NEXT PAGE.]

Treatment and Prevention

- **Treatment:** Drainage and debridement are very important in treating necrotizing fasciitis/myositis. Antibiotics are used for all group A streptococcal infections. *S. pyogenes* has not acquired resistance to penicillin G, which remains the antibiotic of choice for acute streptococcal disease. For the penicillin-allergic patient, a macrolide, such as clarithromycin or azithromycin, is the preferred drug.
- **Prevention:** There is no vaccine against *S. pyogenes.* Rheumatic fever is prevented by rapid eradication of the organism by antibiotic treatment early in the infection.

Laboratory Identification

- Specimens obtained from throat swabs, pus and lesion samples, sputum, blood, or spinal fluid can be cultured on sheep blood agar. *S. pyogenes* forms characteristic small, opalescent colonies surrounded by a large zone of β-hemolysis.
- Serologic tests are used to detect a patient's antibody titer to streptolysin-O (ASO test).
- *S. pyogenes* is highly sensitive to bacitracin, and diagnostic disks with a very low concentration of the antibiotic inhibit growth in culture.

Streptococcus pyogenes (continued)

Pathogenesis/Clinical Significance

- **Erysipelas**

  Affecting all age groups, patients with erysipelas suffer from a fiery red, advancing erythema, especially on the face and lower limbs.

- **Puerperal sepsis**

  This infection is initiated during, or following soon after, the delivery of a newborn. A disease of the uterine endometrium, patients suffer from a purulent vaginal discharge, and are often very ill systemically, with high fever.

- **Invasive group A streptococcal (GAS) disease**

  Patients have a deep local invasion with or without necrosis. (The involvement of **necrotizing fasciitis/myositis** led to the term "**flesh-eating bacteria**.") GAS disease often spreads rapidly, even in otherwise healthy individuals, leading to bacteremia and sepsis.

Treatment and Prevention

Laboratory Identification

Spirochetes

Treponema species

Treponema pallidum

Common characteristics

- **Gram-negative but stain poorly and need to be visualized by other means**
- **Long, slender, flexible, spiral- or corkscrew-shaped rods**
- **Highly motile**
- **Does not grow in culture**

Pathogenesis/Clinical Significance

T. pallidum is a human parasite, transmitted primarily by sexual contact, where the infectious lesion is generally on the skin or mucous membranes of the genitalia.

T. pallidum secretes the enzyme hyaluronidase, which disrupts the ground substance, thereby facilitating the spread of infection. They have endoflagella (axial filaments) that lie beneath the outer sheath of the organism, providing motility.

- **Syphilis**

  T. pallidum multiplies at the site of initial infection, and spreads via the lymph to the blood. Within 2 to 10 weeks, a hard, painless ulcer (**chancre**) forms. Up to 10 weeks later, secondary lesions appear. These consist of a red **maculopapular rash**, seen primarily on the palms and soles, and pale, moist papules, seen primarily in the anogenital region (where they are called **condylomas**), the armpits, and the mouth. Both primary and secondary lesions are rich in *T. pallidum* organisms, and are extremely infectious, but both heal spontaneously. Secondary lesions may be accompanied by systemic involvement, such as **syphilitic hepatitis**, **meningitis**, **nephritis**, and **chorioretinitis**. In untreated individuals, the disease progresses to a tertiary stage, characterized by degenerative changes in the nervous system, cardiovascular lesions, and/or development of granulomatous lesions (**gummas**) in the liver, skin, and bones.

- **Congenital syphilis**

  A pregnant woman with syphilis can transmit *T. pallidum* through the placenta to her fetus after the first 10 to 15 weeks of pregnancy. Infection can cause death and spontaneous abortion of the fetus or cause it to be stillborn. Those infants that live develop the symptoms of congenital syphilis, including a variety of central nervous system and structural abnormalities.

Treatment and Prevention

- **Treatment:** Penicillin G is still the drug of choice. Erythromycin or tetracycline can be used for penicillin-allergic patients.
- **Prevention:** No vaccine or preventive drug is available, and protection from syphilis depends on safe sexual practice. Treatment of a woman with appropriate antibiotics during pregnancy prevents congenital syphilis.

Laboratory Identification

- *T. pallidum* cannot be seen in a Gram-stain. A darkfield examination of a clinical sample can show motile spirochetes.
- *T. pallidum* has not been cultured *in vitro.*
- Serologic tests include the nontreponemal antigen tests (BDRL, RPR, and Wasserman tests), and treponemal antibody tests (FTA-ABS, TPI, and TPHA tests).

Gram (–) rods

Vibrio species

Vibrio cholerae

Common characteristics

- **Gram-negative**
- **Short, curved rod**
- **Rapidly motile due to single polar flagellum**
- **Facultative anaerobes**
- **Growth of many *Vibrio* species requires or is stimulated by NaCl**
- **Culture on blood or MacConkey agar**

Pathogenesis/Clinical Significance

V. cholerae is transmitted by contaminated water and food. In the acquatic environment, a number of reservoirs have been identified, including crustaceans, phytoplankton and protozoa. Outbreaks of *V. cholerae* infection have been associated with raw or undercooked seafood harvested from contaminated waters.

Following ingestion, *V. cholerae* infects the small intestine. Adhesion factors are important for colonization and virulence. The organism is not invasive, and causes disease through the action of an enterotoxin (**cholera toxin**) that causes the activation of adenylyl cyclase by ADP-ribosylation. This initiates an outpouring of fluid into the intestine. Only *V. cholerae* strains that contain a lysogenic phage, which encodes cholera toxin, are pathogenic.

- **Cholera**

  Full-blown cholera is characterized by massive loss of fluid and electrolytes from the body. After an incubation period ranging from hours to a few days, profuse watery diarrhea (**rice-water stools**) begins. Untreated, the death from shock may occur in hours to days, with the death rate exceeding 50 percent.

Treatment and Prevention

- **Treatment:** Replacement of fluids and electrolytes is crucial in preventing shock, and does not require bacteriologic diagnosis. Antibiotics such as doxycycline can shorten the duration of diarrhea and excretion of the organism.
- **Prevention:** Public health measures that reduce fecal contamination of water supplies and food, and adequate cooking of foods, can minimize transmission.

Laboratory Identification

- *V. cholerae* from a stool sample grows on standard, nonselective media such as blood and MacConkey agars. Thiosulfate-citrate-bile salts-sucrose medium can enhance isolation.
- *V. cholerae* is oxidase-positive.

Gram (–) rods

Yersinia species

Yersinia pestis

Common characteristics

- **Gram-negative**
- **Small rod that stains bipolarly**
- **Nonmotile, encapsulated**
- **Culture on MacConkey or CIN (selective) agar**

Pathogenesis/Clinical Significance

Y. pestis is endemic in a variety of mammals, both urban and sylvatic, and is distributed worldwide. Infection is transmitted by fleas, which serve to maintain the infection within the animal reservoir. Humans are generally accidental and dead-end hosts. The organism can also be transmitted by ingestion of contaminated animal tissues and via the respiratory route.

Organisms are carried by the lymphatic system from the site of inoculation to regional lymph nodes, where they are ingested by phagocytes. *Y. pestis* multiplies in these cells. Hematogenous spread of bacteria to other organs and tissues may occur, resulting in hemorrhagic lesions at these sites.

- **Bubonic (septicemic) plague**

  The incubation period (from flea bite to development of symptoms) is generally 2 to 8 days. Onset of nonspecific symptoms, such as high fever, chills, headache, myalgia, and weakness that proceeds to prostration, is characteristically sudden. Within a short time, the characteristic, painful **buboes** develop, typically in the groin, but they may also occur in axillae or on the neck. Blood pressure drops, potentially leading to septic shock and death.

- **Pneumonic plague**

  If plague bacilli reach the lungs, they cause a purulent pneumonia that is highly contagious, and, if untreated, is rapidly fatal.

Treatment and Prevention

- **Treatment:** Streptomycin is the drug of choice, and gentamicin and tetracycline are acceptable alternatives. Because of the potential for overwhelming septicemia, rapid institution of antibiotic therapy is crucial. Supportive therapy is essential for patients with signs of shock.
- **Prevention:** A formalin-killed vaccine is available for those at high risk of acquiring plague. For individuals in enzootic areas, efforts to minimize exposure to rodents and fleas is important.

Laboratory Identification

- Laboratory identification can be made by a gram-stained smear, and culture of an aspirate from a bubo (or sputum in the case of pneumonic plague).
- The organism grows on both MacConkey and blood agars, although colonies grow somewhat more slowly than do those of other *Enterobacteriaceae*.

VIRUSES

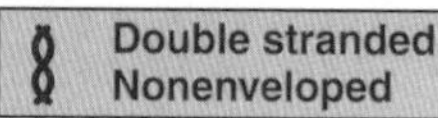

Adenoviridae

Adenoviruses

Common characteristics

- **Double-stranded, linear DNA**
- **Nonenveloped, icosahedral**
- **Replicates in nucleus, killing host cell**

Pathogenesis/Clinical Significance

The site of the clinical syndrome caused by adenovirus infection is generally related to the mode of virus transmission. Adenoviruses are primarily agents of respiratory disease, and are transmitted via the respiratory route. Those associated specifically with gastrointestinal disease are transmitted by the fecal–oral route, whereas ocular infections are transmitted by virus-contaminated hands, ophthalmologic instruments, or swimming pools.

- **Respiratory tract diseases**

  The most common manifestation of adenovirus infection of infants and young children is **acute febrile pharyngitis**, characterized by a cough, sore throat, nasal congestion, and fever. Acute respiratory disease occurs primarily in epidemics among new military recruits, and is facilitated by fatigue and crowded conditions. These syndromes may progress to true viral pneumonia, which, in infants, has a mortality rate of about 10 percent.

- **Ocular diseases**

  If both the respiratory tract and the eyes are involved, the syndrome is referred to as **pharyngoconjunctival fever**. A similar follicular conjunctivitis may occur as a separate, self-limiting disease. A more serious infection is **epidemic keratoconjunctivitis** in which the corneal epithelium is also involved and which may be followed by corneal opacity lasting several years. The epidemic nature of this disease arises in part from transmission by improperly sterilized ophthalmologic instruments.

- **Gastrointestinal diseases**

  Most of the human adenoviruses multiply in the GI tract and can be found in stools. However, these are generally asymptomatic infections. Two serotypes have been associated specifically with **infantile gastroenteritis**, and have been estimated to account for 5 to 15 percent of all viral diarrheal disease in children.

Treatment and Prevention

- **Treatment:** No antiviral agents are currently available for treating adenovirus infections.
- **Prevention:** A new vaccine was licensed for use among United States military personnel in 2011. This vaccine contains live, unattenuated adenovirus types 4 and 7, formulated for oral administration.

Laboratory Identification

- Isolation of virus for identification is not done on a routine basis but may be desirable in cases of epidemic disease or a nosocomial outbreak, especially in the nursery.
- Identification of the adenovirus serotype can be done by neutralization or hemagglutination inhibition using type-specific antisera.
- Enteric adenoviruses are detected by direct test of stool specimens by enzyme-linked immunosorbent assay (ELISA).

Single stranded
Positive strand
Icosadedral or helical
Enveloped

Flaviviridae

Hepatitis C viruses

Common characteristics

- **Positive-strand, single-stranded, nonsegmented RNA genome**
- **Enveloped, icosahedral nucleocapsid**
- **Genomic RNAs serve as messenger RNAs and are infectious**
- **Virions do not contain any enzymes**

Pathogenesis/Clinical Significance

Hepatitis C viruses (HCV) have, in the past, been the primary cause of non-A, non-B, transfusion-associated hepatitis. Tests to screen blood for HCV have been available for several years, so that HCV as a cause of transfusion-associated hepatitis is now unusual. This group of viruses is heterogeneous and can be divided into several types. Transmission is via blood (through transfusion, intravenous drug use, and renal dialysis treatment). In addition, there is evidence of sexual transmission, as well as vertical transmission.

- **Hepatitis C**

  HCV replication occurs in the hepatocyte, and probably also in mononuclear cells (lymphocytes and macrophages). Destruction of liver cells may result both from a direct effect of viral replication, and from the host immune response. The majority of infections with HCV are subclinical, but about 25 percent of infected individuals present with acute hepatitis including jaundice. More important, a significant proportion of infections progress to a chronic hepatitis and cirrhosis. Some of these individuals go on to develop hepatocellular carcinoma many years after the primary infection. Concomitant chronic infection with HBV results in more severe disease.

Treatment and Prevention

- **Treatment:** Treatment of patients with chronic hepatitis with α-interferon is sometimes of benefit but, in most cases, only for the period during which the patient is receiving the interferon. Chronic hepatitis caused by HCV that results in severe liver damage may be an indication for a liver transplant.
- **Prevention:** No vaccine or preventive drug is available at this time.

Laboratory Identification

- A specific diagnosis can be made by demonstration of antibodies that react with a combination of recombinant viral proteins.
- Sensitive tests are also now available for detection of viral RNA, for example, by polymerase chain reaction amplification of reverse-transcribed HCV RNA.

Double stranded
Enveloped

Hepadnaviridae

Hepatitis B virus

Common characteristics

- **Circular DNA, partly single-stranded, partly double-stranded, non–covalently closed genome, with four overlapping genes**
- **Enveloped, icosahedral nucleocapsid**
- **Multifunctional reverse transcriptase/DNA polymerase in virion**
- **Viral antigens: the capsid protein (hepatitis B capsid antigen, HBcAg), the envelope protein (hepatitis B surface antigen, HBsAg), and a second capsular antigen (HBeAg) that is secreted by infected cells**

Pathogenesis/Clinical Significance

Infectious hepatitis B virus (HBV) is present in all body fluids of an infected individual. Therefore, blood, semen, saliva, breast milk, etc. serve as sources of infection. In the United States, HBV is most frequently contracted by sexual intercourse and by intravenous drug use. In areas of high endemicity in developing countries, the majority of the population becomes infected at or shortly after birth from a chronically infected mother or from infected siblings.

The primary cause of hepatic cell destruction is the cell-mediated immune response by cytotoxic (CD8) T lymphocytes, which react specifically with fragments of the nucleocapsid proteins (HBcAg and HBeAg) expressed on the infected hepatocyte membrane.

[HEPATITIS B IS CONTINUED ON THE NEXT PAGE]

Treatment and Prevention

- **Treatment:** The drug of choice depends on multiple factors, including the antibody and antigen status of the patient. Interferon and pegylated interferon, lamivudine, adefovir, entecavir, telbivudine, and tenofovir are treatment options.

Laboratory Identification

- Hepatitis is established using liver function tests.
- Viral antigens and antiviral antibodies are detected using serologic techniques such as enzyme-linked immunosorbent assay and radioimmunoassay.
- Presence of IgM anti-HBc accompanied by HBsAg is a specific indicator of HBV infection.

Hepatitis B virus (continued)

Pathogenesis/Clinical Significance	Treatment and Prevention	Laboratory Identification
• **Acute hepatitis** In about two thirds of individuals infected with HBV, the primary infection is asymptomatic, even though such patients may later develop symptomatic chronic liver disease. In acute HBV infections, there is an incubation period of between 45 and 120 days, followed by a preicteric (prejaundice) period lasting several days to a week. This is characterized by mild fever, malaise, anorexia, myalgia, and nausea. The acute, icteric phase then follows, and lasts for 1 to 2 months. It is during this phase that dark urine, due to bilirubinuria and jaundice, are evident. There usually is also an enlarged and tender liver. During the acute phase, large quantities of viral antigens, nucleic acids, and antiviral antibodies appear in the blood. In 80 to 90 percent of adults, a convalescent period of several more months is followed by complete recovery. Following resolution of the acute disease (or asymptomatic infection), about 2 to 10 percent of adults, and over 80 percent of infants, remain chronically infected. • **Fulminant hepatitis** In 1 to 2 percent of acute symptomatic cases, much more extensive necrosis of the liver occurs during the initial acute illness. This is accompanied by high fever, abdominal pain, and eventual renal dysfunction, coma, seizures, and, in about 8 percent of cases, death. • **Primary hepatocellular carcinomas (HCC; hepatomas)** HCC is one of the major causes of death due to malignancy worldwide. Approximately 80 percent of HCCs occur in chronically HBV-infected individuals. However, the mechanisms relating HBV infection and HCC are not understood. Clinically, a patient with HCC exhibits weight loss, right-upper-quandrant pain, fever, and intestinal bleeding.	• **Prevention:** A vaccine is available that is composed of HBsAg. It is recommended as one of the routine infant immunization, and also for adults in health care professions, and those with life-styles that present a high risk of infection. Hepatitis B immunoglobulin is prepared from the blood of donors having a high titer of anti-HBs antibody. It provides passive immunization for individuals accidentally exposed to HBV and for infants born to women who are HBV-positive.	

Double stranded
Enveloped

Herpesviridae

Epstein-Barr virus
Herpes simplex virus, type 1
Herpes simplex virus, type 2
Human cytomegalovirus
Human herpesvirus, type 8
Varicella-zoster virus

Common characteristics

- **Linear, double-stranded DNA genome**
- **Replicate in the nucleus**
- **Envelope contains antigenic, species-specific glycoproteins**
- **In the tegument between the envelope and capsid are a number of virus-coded enzymes and transcription factors essential for initiation of the infectious cycle**
- **All herpesviruses can enter a latent state following primary infection, to be reactivated at a later time**

Epstein-Barr virus

Pathogenesis/Clinical Significance

Most transmission of Epstein-Barr virus (EBV) occurs by intimate contact with saliva that contains virus.

EBV replicates in mucosal epithelium. The virus then spreads to the lymph nodes, where it infects B cells. EBV next travels via the blood to other organs, particularly targeting liver and spleen. The B-cell infection leads to B-cell proliferation, accompanied by nonspecific increases in total IgM, IgG, and IgA.

- **Infectious mononucleosis (IM)**

  The "atypical lymphocytosis" characteristic of infectious mononucleosis is caused by the active cytotoxic T cell response to the EBV antigens expressed by infected B cells. The typical IM syndrome appears after an incubation period of 4 to 7 weeks, and includes pharyngitis, lymphadenopathy, and fever. Headache and malaise often precede and accompany the disease, which may last several weeks. Throughout life, healthy EBV carriers continue to have episodes of asymptomatic virus shedding.

- **Association with Burkitt lymphoma and other human neoplastic diseases**

  EBV infection has been found to be associated with Burkitt lymphoma, nasopharyngeal carcinoma, and Hodgkin disease. The exact role played by the EBV in these diseases is not clear.

Treatment and Prevention

- **Treatment:** Although acyclovir inhibits EBV replication, none of the antiherpes drugs have been effective in modifying the course or severity of IM due to EBV or in preventing development of EBV-related B-cell malignancies.
- **Prevention:** No vaccine or preventive drug is available.

Laboratory Identification

- The classic diagnostic test for EBV-associated mononucleosis is detection of heterophile antibodies that agglutinate sheep and horse red blood cells.
- Serologic tests, such as immunofluorescence reactions and enzyme-linked immunoaorbent assay (ELISA) to detect antibodies specific for viral proteins, are used to evaluate the stage of disease.

Herpes simplex virus, type 1

Pathogenesis/Clinical Significance

Herpes simplex virus type 1 (HSV-1) has a relatively rapid, cytocidal growth cycle. HSV-1 establishes latency in trigeminal ganglia after oropharyngeal infection. Transmission of HSV-1 is by direct contact with virus-containing secretions (usually saliva), or with lesions on mucosal surfaces.

- **Primary HSV-1 infections**

  The virus multiplies in the nuclei of epithelial cells on the mucosal surface onto which it has been inoculated, most frequently, that of the oropharyngeal region. Vesicles or shallow ulcers containing infectious HSV-1 are produced, primarily in the oropharynx. These cause sore throat, fever, gingivitis, and anorexia. The most common symptomatic HSV-1 infections of the upper body are **gingivostomatitis** in young children, and **tonsillitis** and **pharyngitis** in adults. Infection of the eye by HSV-1 can cause severe **keratoconjuctivitis**. [Note: HSV-1 infections of the eye are the second most common cause of corneal blindness in the United States (after trauma).] If HSV-1 infection spreads to the central nervous system, frequently fatal **encephalitis** can occur. In immunocompetent individuals, HSV-1 infection remains localized due to cytotoxic T cells that recognize HSV-specific antigens on the surface of infected cells, and kills them before progeny virus has been produced.

- **Latent HSV-1 infections**

  A life-long latent infection is usually established in the trigeminal ganglia as a result of entry of infectious virions into sensory neurons that end at the site of infection. Recurrent HSV-1 infections may be asymptomatic, but result in viral shedding in secretions. If symptoms occur, they usually include **herpes labialis** (formation of "**cold sores**" or "**fever blisters**") around the lips.

Treatment and Prevention

- **Treatment:** Herpesviruses encode considerably more enzymatic activities and regulatory functions than do viruses with smaller genomic size. A number of these activities duplicate the functions of host cell enzymes, but, because they are virus-specific, they provide excellent targets for anti-viral agents that are relatively non-toxic for the cell. Acycloguanosine (acyclovir) is selectively effective against HSV because it becomes an active inhibitor only after initially being phosphorylated by the HSV-coded thymidine kinase. The drug cannot cure a latent infection, but can minimize or prevent recurrences. Other inhibitors active against HSV DNA synthesis include famciclovir, foscarnet, and topically applied penciclovir.
- **Prevention:** No vaccine or preventive drug is available.

Laboratory Identification

- Cell tissue culture inoculated with a sample of vesicle scraping, fluid, or genital swab shows gross cytopathic changes in several days; individual infected cells can be detected within 24 hours by use of immunofluorescence or immunoperoxidase staining with antibodies against viral early proteins.
- Viral DNA (amplified by polymerase chain reaction) can be detected in clinical samples, including cerebrospinal fluid in patients with HSV encephalitis.

Herpes simplex virus, type 2

Pathogenesis/Clinical Significance

Herpes simplex virus, type 2 (HSV-2) has a relatively rapid, cytocidal growth cycle. HSV-2 establishes latency in sacral or lumbar ganglia. Transmission of HSV-2 generally occurs by sexual contact or by infection of a newborn during birth.

- **Primary HSV-2 infections**

  Primary genital tract lesions are similar to those of the oropharynx caused by HSV-1, but the majority of these infections are asymptomatic. When symptomatic, local symptoms such as pain and itching, and systemic symptoms of fever, malaise, and myalgias may be more severe than those that accompany primary oral cavity infections. Vesiculo-ulcerative lesions on the female's vulva, cervix, and vagina or the male's penis can be very painful. Neonatal herpes is contracted by the baby during birth. If untreated, a disseminated infection results, often involving the CNS, leading to a high mortality rate. [Note: Infection in utero appears to occur only rarely.]

- **Latent HSV-2 infections**

  HSV-2 remains latent in the sacral ganglia. Reactivation of HSV-2 genital infection occurs frequently, and may be asymptomatic. However, the infected individual sheds virus during the reactivation period regardless of symptoms, and can transmit the virus to a sexual partner during that period.

Treatment and Prevention

- **Treatment:** Same as for HSV-1.
- **Prevention:** No vaccine or preventive drug is available. Prevention of HSV transmission is enhanced by avoidance of contact with potential virus-shedding lesions and by safe sexual practices. Neonatal HSV can be prevented by delivery via cesarean section.

Laboratory Identification

- Same as for HSV-1.

Human cytomegalovirus

Pathogenesis/Clinical Significance

Human cytomegalovirus (HCMV) is transmitted by infected individuals through their tears, urine, saliva, semen or vaginal secretions, and breast milk. HCMV can also cross the placenta.

HCMV replicates initially in epithelial cells of the respiratory and GI tracts, followed by viremia and infection of all organs of the body. In symptomatic cases, kidney tubule epithelium, liver, and central nervous system, in addition to the respiratory and GI tracts, are most commonly affected. HCMV has a relatively slow replication cycle, with the formation of characteristic multinucleated giant cells, thus the name "cytomegalo-". Latency is established in nonneural tissues, primarily lymphoreticular cells, and glandular tissues.

- **HCMV infectious mononucleosis**

  Whereas most HCMV infections occur in childhood, primary infection as an adult may result in a mononucleosis syndrome that is clinically identical to that caused by Epstein-Barr virus (EBV). It is estimated that about 8 percent of infectious mononucleosis (IM) cases are due to HCMV. The major distinguishing feature of HCMV IM is the absence of the heterophile antibodies that characterize IM caused by EBV.

- **Cytomegalic inclusion disease**

  HCMV is the most common intrauterine virus infection. Of infants born to women experiencing their first HCMV infection during pregnancy, 35 to 50 percent will become infected, of which 10 percent will be symptomatic. The severity of the latter, referred to as cytomegalic inclusion disease, ranges from fetal death to various degrees of damage to liver, spleen, blood-forming organs, and components of the nervous system (a common cause of hearing loss and mental retardation).

- **HCMV infection of immunosuppressed transplant recipients**

  Such individuals are multiply at risk from 1) HCMV present in the tissue being transplanted, 2) virus carried in leukocytes in the associated blood transfusions, and 3) reactivation of endogenous latent virus. The resulting infection can cause destruction of GI tract tissues, hepatitis, and pneumonia, the latter being a major cause of death in bone marrow transplant recipients.

Treatment and Prevention

- **Treatment:** Treatment of HCMV infections is indicated primarily in immunocompromised patients. Acyclovir is ineffective because HCMV lacks a thymidine kinase. Ganciclovir is used for invasive infections of transplant recipients and acquired immune deficiency syndrome (AIDS) patients. Cidofovir is used for ganciclovir-resistant mutants. Foscarnet can be used in combination with ganciclovir or as an alternate treatment when resistant mutants appear.
- **Prevention:** No vaccine or preventive drug is available.

Laboratory Identification

- Serologic diagnosis using enzyme-linked immunosorbent assay techniques can distinguish primary from recurrent infection, by demonstrating either IgG seroconversion or the presence of HCMV-specific IgM.
- Determination of the presence and amount of viral DNA or proteins in white blood cells is used to evaluate invasive disease.
- Presence of extracellular virus in urine or saliva may simply be due to an asymptomatic recurrence.

[HUMAN CYTOMEGALOVIRUS CONTINUED ON THE NEXT PAGE.]

Human cytomegalovirus (continued)

Pathogenesis/Clinical Significance	Treatment and Prevention	Laboratory Identification

- **HCMV infection of AIDS patients**
  Invasive opportunistic HCMV infections are common in AIDS patients. These become increasingly important as CD4+ lymphocyte counts and immune competence decline. Any organ systems can be affected, but pneumonia, and blindness due to HCMV retinitis, are especially common. Encephalitis and dementia, esophagitis, enterocolitis, and gastritis are other significant problems.

Varicella-zoster virus

Pathogenesis/Clinical Significance

Varicella-zoster virus (VZV) has a relatively rapid, cytocidal growth cycle, and establishes latency in sensory nerve ganglia.

Transmission of VZV is usually via respiratory droplets, which results in initial infection of the respiratory mucosa, followed by spread to the regional lymph nodes. From there, progeny virus enters the bloodstream, undergoes a second round of multiplication in cells of the liver and spleen, and is disseminated throughout the body by infected mononuclear leukocytes.

- **Varicella ("chickenpox")**
  Following infection of a normal, healthy child, the first symptoms include fever, malaise, headache, and abdominal pain. Next is appearance of the virus-containing vesicles ("pox") characteristic of the disease. These begin on the scalp, face, or trunk about 10 to 23 days after exposure, causing severe itching, and then proceed to the extremities and mucous membranes, such as the oropharynx, conjunctiva, and vagina. The infected individual is contagious from 1 to 2 days before appearance of the vesicles. Varicella is more serious in adults and immunocompromised patients, potentially causing pneumonia, fulminant hepatic failure, and varicella encephalitis. Fetal infection during pregnancy is uncommon, but can result in multiple developmental anomalies.

- **Zoster ("shingles")**
  Due to the disseminated nature of the primary infection, latency is established in multiple sensory ganglia, the trigeminal and dorsal root ganglia being most common. On reactivation, there is substantial multiplication and horizontal spread of virus among the cells in the ganglion. Viral destruction of sensory ganglia leads to the pain associated with acute zoster. Debilitating postherpetic neuralgia and abnormal sensory phenomena may last as long as several months. The likelihood of reactivation increases with age and with depressed cellular immune competence.

Treatment and Prevention

- **Treatment for varicella:**
  Varicella in normal children does not require treatment. Treatment of primary varicella in immunocompromised patients, adults, and neonates is warranted by the severity of the disease. Acyclovir has been the drug of choice. Newer drugs, such asfamciclovir and valacyclovir, have greater activity against VZV.

- **Treatment for zoster:** Oral acyclovir reduces the time course and acute pain of zoster, but has little or no effect on the subsequent postherpetic neuralgia. Famciclovir, given early in the acute phase of zoster, decreases acute pain and the time to resolution of lesions, and also shortens the duration of postherpetic pain.

- **Prevention:** A live, attenuated vaccine is recommended as one of the routine childhood vaccines. It is also indicated for nonimmune adults who are at risk of contagion. Zostavax is a high-potency version of the chickenpox vaccine, which also contains live, attenuated virus. Zostavax has been approved for use in adults over age 50 years for prevention of zoster and, with it, the debilitating effects of postherpetic neuralgia.

Laboratory Identification

- Cell tissue culture inoculated with a sample of vesicle fluid shows gross cytopathic changes in several days, and individual infected cells can be detected within 24 hours by use of immunofluorescence or immunoperoxidase staining with antibodies against viral early proteins.

- More rapid diagnosis can be made by reacting epithelial cells scraped from the base of vesicles with the stains described above or doing *in situ* hybridization with VZV-specific DNA probes.

Single stranded
Negative strand
Helical
Enveloped

Orthomyxoviridae

Influenza virus

Common characteristics

- **Negative-strand RNA genome**
- **Spherical, enveloped, pleomorphic virus**
- **RNA is segmented into eight pieces**
- **Virion has two types of membrane protein spikes: H protein (hemagglutinin) and N protein (neuraminidase)**
- **Virion contains RNA polymerase**

Pathogenesis/Clinical Significance

Influenza is spread by respiratory droplets and is an infection solely of the respiratory tract. There is rarely a viremia or spread to other organ systems.

Influenza viruses are classified as types A, B, and C, depending on the antigenicity of their inner proteins (only A and B are of medical importance). Type A viruses are further broken down into subtypes based on antigens associated with the outer viral proteins, H and N. Influenza viruses have shown marked variation over the years in their antigenic properties, specifically of the H and N proteins. This variation is due primarily to antigenic shift.

- **Influenza (the "flu")**

  Following inhalation of influenza virus particles, respiratory epithelial cells are destroyed by the host immune response, specifically, cytotoxic T cells. Typically, influenza has an acute onset characterized by chills, followed by a high fever, muscle aches, and extreme drowsiness. The disease runs its course in 4 to 5 days, after which there is a gradual recovery. The most serious problems, such as pneumonia, occur in the very young, older adults, and people with chronic cardiac or pulmonary disease, or who are immunodeficient.

- **Reye syndrome**

  This is a rare and serious complication of viral infections in children, especially in those who have had chickenpox or influenza. Aspirin used to lower the virus-induced fever may contribute to the appearance of this syndrome. Therefore, acetaminophen is usually recommended for fevers of unknown origin in children.

Treatment and Prevention

- **Treatment:** Amantidine and rimantadine prevent the influenza virus from uncoating. They reduce both the duration and severity of flu symptoms in type A influenza infections, but only if given early in infection. Influenza viruses readily develop resistance to these compounds. Zanamivir and oseltamivir are newer drugs that inhibit viral neuraminidase, an enzyme required for release of virus from infected cells.
- **Prevention:** A vaccine consisting of formalin-inactivated influenza virus is available. It is of critical importance that the vaccine contain the specific subtypes of influenza virus present in the population that year. Given before the onset of symptoms, amantidine and rimantidine can also prevent disease, and are useful for treating high-risk groups. A live, attenuated influenza virus vaccine, administered intranasally, has also been approved.

Laboratory Identification

- Quantitation of antibodies that inhibit hemagglutination can be done for surveillance purposes.
- Demonstration of viral antigens in respiratory tract secretions is a more rapid method for diagnosis of influenza infection.
- Detection of viral RNA by reverse transcription polymerase chain reaction is sensitive and specific.

Double stranded
Nonenveloped

Papovaviridae

Papillomavirus

Common characteristics

- **Double-stranded, circular DNA**
- **Nonenveloped, icosahedral**
- **Over seventy types of human papillomaviruses currently recognized**

Pathogenesis/Clinical Significance

Transmission of human papillomavirus (HPV) infection requires direct contact with infected individuals or contaminated surfaces. All human papillomaviruses induce **hyperplastic epithelial lesions**, infecting either cutaneous (keratinizing) or mucosal (squamous) epithelium. The HPVs within each of these tissue-specific groups have varying potentials to cause malignancies. There are: 1) a small number of virus types that produce lesions having a high risk of progression to malignancy, such as in the case of **cervical carcinoma**; 2) other virus types produce mucosal lesions that progress to malignancy with lower frequency, causing, for example, **anogenital warts** (**condyloma acuminatum**, a common sexually transmitted disease) and **laryngeal papillomas** (the most common benign epithelial tumors of the larynx); 3) in those individuals with a genetic predisposition for the inability to control the spread of warts, some virus types cause multiple cutaneous warts that do not regress, but spread to many body sites (**epidermodysplasia verruciformis**) which give rise with high frequency to **squamous cell carcinomas** several years after initial appearance of the original warts; and 4) still other virus types that are associated only with benign lesions, for example, **common**, **flat**, and **plantar warts**.

Treatment and Prevention

- **Treatment:** Cutaneous warts generally require surgical removal or destruction of the wart tissue with liquid nitrogen, laser vaporization, or cytotoxic chemicals. Interferon, given orally, is effective in causing regression of laryngeal papillomas. When injected directly into genital warts, interferon is effective in about half of the patients. Cidofovir is also effective as a topical application.
- **Prevention:** Two vaccines are available to prevent infection with high-risk HPV types. One vaccine contains capsid proteins from HPV types 16 and 18 (high risk) and the other vaccine contains capsid proteins from HPV types 6, 11, 16, and 18. The vaccines are now recommended for both young females and males to prevent HPV-associated cancers.

Laboratory Identification

- Diagnosis of cutaneous warts generally involves no more than visual inspection.
- Typing of human papillomavirus is done either by immunoassays for viral antigens or polymerase chain reaction amplification.
- Human papillomavirus cannot be cultured in the laboratory.

Single stranded
Negative strand
Helical
Enveloped

Paramyxoviridae

Measles virus
Mumps virus
Parainfluenza virus
Respiratory syncytial virus

Common characteristics

- **Nonsegmented, negative-strand RNA**
- **Spherical, enveloped viruses**
- **Some contain RNA polymerase in their virions**
- **Envelope contains F (fusion) protein that allows virus to enter cells via a fusion process, rather than by receptor-mediated endocytosis**

Measles virus

Pathogenesis/Clinical Significance

Measles virus is transmitted by sneeze- or cough-produced respiratory droplets. The virus is extremely infectious, and almost all infected individuals develop a clinical illness.

- **Measles**

  Measles virus replicates initially in the respiratory epithelium, and then in various lymphoid organs. Classic measles begins with a prodromal period of fever, upper respiratory tract symptoms (cough and coryza), and conjunctivitis. Two to three days later, Koplik spots develop in the mouth and throat, and a generalized macular rash appears, beginning at the head and traveling slowly to the lower extremities. Soon after the rash appears, the patient is no longer infectious. A rare complication occurring within 2 weeks after the onset of the rash is **postinfectious encephalomyelitis,** an autoimmune disease. Children are particularly susceptible, especially those weakened by other diseases or hunger.

Treatment and Prevention

- **Treatment:** No antiviral drugs are available for measles.
- **Prevention:** A live, attenuated measles vaccine is available and is usually administered in the form of the measles-mumps-rubella (MMR) vaccine.

Laboratory Identification

- Demonstration of an increase in the titer of antiviral antibodies can be used in the diagnosis of measles.

Mumps virus

Pathogenesis/Clinical Significance

Mumps virus is spread by respiratory droplets.

- **Mumps**

  Although about one third of infections are subclinical, the classic clinical presentation and diagnosis center on infection and swelling of the salivary glands, primarily the parotid glands. However, mumps virus can enter the bloodstream, causing widespread infection. This may involve not only salivary glands, but also the pancreas, central nervous system, and testes. Male sterility occasionally occurs, due to bilateral infection of the testes (orchitis).

Treatment and Prevention

- **Treatment:** No antiviral drugs are available for mumps.
- **Prevention:** A live, attenuated vaccine is available and is usually administered in the form of the measles-mumps-rubella (MMR) vaccine.

Laboratory Identification

- Virus may be recoverable from saliva, blood, cerebrospinal fluid, or urine, and can be cultured.
- Serologic tests detect antiviral antibody in the blood.

Parainfluenza virus

Pathogenesis/Clinical Significance

There are four clinically important human parainfluenza viruses (hPIV), designated hPIV types 1 to 4. They are called "parainfluenza" because individuals may present with influenza-like symptoms, and, like influenza, the viruses have both hemagglutinating and neuraminidase activity. [Note:Unlike influenza, these activities are not subject to antigenic shift.]

Infection by these viruses is spread by respiratory droplets, and is confined to the respiratory tract.

- **Respiratory tract infections**

  Parainfluenza viruses cause **croup**, **pneumonia**, and **bronchiolitis**, mainly in infants and children. They are also a cause of the "**common cold**" in individuals of all ages.

Treatment and Prevention

- **Treatment:** No antiviral drugs are recommended for these infections. Symptoms can be treated as necessary.
- **Prevention:** No vaccine or preventive drug is available.

Laboratory Identification

- Serologic tests for antibody to the virus can aid in the diagnosis of parainfluenza virus infection.

Respiratory syncytial virus

Pathogenesis/Clinical Significance

Respiratory syncytial virus (RSV) is transmitted by respiratory droplets or by contaminated hands carrying the virus to the nose or mouth. Repeated infections are common.

- **Respiratory tract infections**

  RSV is the major viral respiratory tract pathogen in the pediatric population, and the most important cause of **bronchiolitis** in infants. It may also cause **pneumonia** in young children, an **influenza-like syndrome** in adults, and **severe bronchitis with pneumonia** in older adults. RSV does not spread systemically.

Treatment and Prevention

- **Treatment:** The only specific treatment for RSV infection is ribavirin, administered by aerosol, which is only of moderate benefit.
- **Prevention:** No vaccine or preventive drug is available. Spread of infection between people can be controlled by hand-washing and avoiding others with the infection.

Laboratory Identification

- Definitive diagnosis of RSV can be made by culture of virus from nasopharyngeal secretions, detection of viral RNA by reverse transcriptase polymerase chain reaction or detection of viral antigen by enzyme-linked immunosorbent assay techniques.

Single stranded
Positive strand
Icosadedral
Nonenveloped

Picornaviridae

Coxsackievirus
Hepatitis A virus
Poliovirus

Common characteristics

- **Positive-strand, single-stranded, nonsegmented RNA genome**
- **Non-enveloped, icosahedral**
- **Genomic RNAs serve as messenger RNAs and are infectious**
- **Virions do not contain any enzymes**

Coxsackievirus

Pathogenesis/Clinical Significance

Coxsackieviruses are members of the genus *Enterovirus*. Individuals are infected with coxsackieviruses by ingestion of contaminated food or water, or inhalation of aerosols containing the virus. These viruses are stable in the low pH of the stomach, replicate in the gastrointestinal tract, and are excreted in the stool (fecal–oral route). Coxsackieviruses also replicate in the oropharynx. They are carried by the blood to peripheral tissues, including the heart and central nervous system.

- **Coxsackievirus infections**

  These give rise to a large variety of clinical syndromes including upper respiratory infections, meningitis, gastroenteritis, herpangina (intense swelling of the throat), pleurisy, pericarditis, myocarditis, and myositis.

Treatment and Prevention

- **Treatment:** No antiviral agents or vaccines are currently available for treating coxsackievirus infections.

Laboratory Identification

- Viruses can be isolated and cultured from the stool or from various target organs.
- Evidence of infection can also be obtained by demonstration of a rise in antibody titer.

Hepatitis A virus

Pathogenesis/Clinical Significance

Hepatitis A virus (HAV) is a member of the genus *Hepatovirus*. It is the most common cause of viral hepatitis in the United States. Transmission is by the fecal–oral route, and the virus is shed in the feces. For example, a common mode of transmission of the virus is through eating uncooked shellfish harvested from sewage-contaminated water. Transmission via blood (similar to hepatitis B transmission) is rare.

- **Hepatitis A ("infectious hepatitis")**

  HAV infections are most commonly seen among children, especially those living in crowded accommodations such as summer camps. The main site of replication is the hepatocyte, where infection results in severe cytopathology, and liver function is severely impaired. The prognosis for patients with HAV is generally favorable, and development of persistent infection and chronic hepatitis is uncommon.

Treatment and Prevention

- **Treatment:** Immune globulin is used as postexposure prophylaxis. No antiviral agents are currently available for treating HAV infections.
- **Prevention:** Vaccines prepared from whole virus inactivated with formaldehyde are now available. Immune globulin has been used for many years, mainly as postexposure prophylaxis. Prevention of HAV infection requires taking measures to avoid fecal contamination of food and water.

Laboratory Identification

- HAV grows poorly in tissue culture.
- Evidence of infection can be gained by the demonstration of a rise in antibody titer.

Poliovirus

Pathogenesis/Clinical Significance

Poliovirus is a member of the genus *Enterovirus*. Individuals are infected with poliovirus by ingestion of contaminated food or water. Enteroviruses are stable in the low pH of the stomach, replicate in the GI tract, and are excreted in the stool (fecal–oral route). After replicating in the oropharynx and intestinal tract lymphoid tissue, poliovirus can enter the bloodstream and spread to the central nervous system.

- **Poliomyelitis**

  The great majority of poliovirus infections are asymptomatic. The classic presentation in those poliovirus-infected individuals who become ill is that of **flaccid paralysis**, most often affecting the lower limbs. This is due to viral replication in, and destruction of, the lower motor neurons in the anterior horn of the spinal cord. **Respiratory paralysis** may also occur, following infection of the brainstem.

Treatment and Prevention

- **Treatment:** No antiviral agents are currently available for treating poliovirus infections.
- **Prevention:** A killed poliovirus vaccine (Salk) that is injected, and a live, attenuated poliovirus vaccine (Sabin) that is given orally are available, and have led to the elimination of wild-type polio from Western Europe, Japan, and the Americas. The few cases that occur in the United States are either brought from other countries, or are caused by vaccine strains of virus that have reverted to a virulent form.

Laboratory Identification

- Poliovirus can be isolated and cultured from the stool or cerebrospinal fluid.
- Evidence of infection can also be obtained by demonstration of a rise in antibody titer.

Single stranded
Positive strand
Icosadedral or helical
Enveloped

Retroviridae

Human immunodeficiency virus

Common characteristics

- **Single-stranded, positive-sense, linear RNA; two copies per virion (diploid)**
- **Viral envelope contains glycoprotein that undergoes antigenic variation**
- **Virion contains reverse transcriptase**

Pathogenesis/Clinical Significance

Human immunodeficiency virus (HIV) is a nononcogenic retrovirus. Transmission occurs mainly by one of three routes: 1) sexually (it is present in both semen and vaginal secretions), 2) with blood or blood products (whole blood, plasma, clotting factors, and cellular fractions of blood by transfusion, or by inoculation with HIV-contaminated needles), and 3) perinatally (either transplacentally, during passage through the birth canal, or in breastfeeding).

The specific HIV cell surface receptor is the CD4+ molecule, located primarily on helper T cells. HIV enters the cell by fusion of the virus envelope with the plasma membrane. Reverse transcription takes place in the cytoplasm, with the viral RNA-dependent reverse transcriptase first synthesizing a DNA-RNA hybrid molecule, then degrading the parental RNA while replacing it with a second strand of DNA. The resulting linear molecule of double-stranded DNA is the provirus. It is transported to the nucleus and is randomly inserted into the host chromosome by viral enzymes. The integrated DNA is translated into viral mRNAs that code for viral proteins, and also will be packaged into progeny virus. Assembled virions bud through the plasma membrane. Production of virus is a continuous process, eventually killing the host cell.

- **HIV infection**

  Several weeks after the initial infection, one third to two thirds of individuals experience symptoms similar to those of infectious mononucleosis, during which there is a very high level of virus replication in CD4+ cells. Lymph nodes become infected, which are the sites of virus persistence during the asymptomatic period. The acute phase viremia resolves into a clinically asymptomatic or "latent" period lasting from months to many years. This period is characterized by persistent generalized lymphadenopathy, diarrhea, and weight loss.

- **Acquired immune deficiency syndrome (AIDS):**

  The progression from asymptomatic infection to AIDS occurs as a continuum of progressive clinical states. The number of infected CD4+ cells decreases, and T-cell precursors in the lymphoid organs are infected and killed, so the capacity to generate new CD4+ cells is gradually lost. Cells of the monocyte/macrophage lineage are also infected, and transport the virus into other organs, including the brain. When the CD4+ count falls below 200/µl, and increasingly frequent and serious opportunistic infections appear, the syndrome is defined as AIDS.

Treatment and Prevention

- **Treatment:** Inhibitors of viral reverse transcriptase include both nucleoside and non-nucleoside reverse transcriptase inhibitors. They prevent the establishment of HIV infection. Inhibitors of the viral protease delay the production of progeny virus. Because administering combinations of these drugs delays the appearance of resistant mutants, 3 or 4 drugs are given at the same time. This is referred to as "highly active anti-retroviral therapy" or HAART.
- **Prevention:** No vaccine is available. Perinatal transmission can be reduced with zidovudine (AZT) therapy of the pregnant woman, followed by several weeks of AZT to the newborn. Prevention can be achieved by screening blood and tissues prior to transfusion or transplant, using condoms during sexual intercourse, and strict adherence to universal precautions by health care workers.

Laboratory Identification

- Amplification of viral RNA or DNA proviruses by the polymerase chain reaction technique is the most sensitive method for detection of virus in blood or tissue specimens.
- For purposes of screening the blood supply, enzyme-linked immunosorbent assay (ELISA) testing for the p24 (CA) antigen in serum can detect infection about a week earlier than tests for antibody.
- For screening individuals, the ELISA procedure is also used to detect antibodies in serum. Any positive results must be confirmed using the Western blot technique.

Single stranded
Negative strand
Helical
Enveloped

Rhabdoviridae

Rabies virus

Common characteristics

- **Negative-strand, single-stranded, non-segmented RNA genome**
- **Enveloped, helical nucleocapsid**
- **Virus is bullet-shaped**
- **Virion contains RNA-dependent RNA polymerase**

Pathogenesis/Clinical Significance

Rabies virus is a member of the genus *Lyssavirus*. A wide variety of wildlife, such as raccoons, skunks, squirrels, foxes, and bats, provide a reservoir for the virus. In developing countries, domestic dogs and cats also constitute an important reservoir for rabies. Humans are usually infected by the bite of an animal, but, in some cases, infection is via an aerosol, for example, droppings from infected bats.

- **Rabies**

  Following inoculation, the virus may replicate locally, but then travels via retrograde transport within peripheral neurons to the brain, where it replicates primarily in the gray matter. From the brain, the rabies virus can travel along autonomic nerves, leading to infection of the lungs, kidney, adrenal medulla, and salivary glands. The incubation period is extremely variable, but generally lasts 1 to 8 weeks. Symptoms of the infection include hallucinations, seizures, weakness, mental dysfunction, paralysis, coma, and finally death from a fatal encephalitis with neuronal degeneration of the brain and spinal cord. Once symptoms begin, death is inevitable. Many, but not all, patients show the classic rabid sign of hydrophobia, a painful inability to swallow liquids, leading to avoidance.

Treatment and Prevention

- **Treatment:** Once an individual has clinical symptoms of rabies there is no effective treatment.
- **Prevention:** Preexposure prophylaxis, which is indicated for individuals at high risk (for example, veterinarians) consists of administration of a killed virus vaccine. In the United States, three vaccine formulations are Food and Drug Administration approved. All contain inactivated virus grown in cultured cells (chick embryo cells, human diploid cells [HDCV], or monkey lung cells) Postexposure prophylaxis is instituted after an animal bite or exposure to an animal suspected of being rabid. It consists of both passive immunization with antirabies immunoglobulin and active immunization with HDCV.

Laboratory Identification

- Diagnosis rests on a history of exposure and signs and symptoms characteristic of rabies. However, a reliable history of exposure is often not obtainable, and the initial clinical presentation may vary. Therefore, a clinical diagnosis may be difficult.
- Postmortem, characteristic cytoplasmic inclusions (Negri bodies) may be seen in regions of the brain such as the hippocampus.

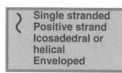

Single stranded
Positive strand
Icosadedral or helical
Enveloped

Togaviridae

Rubella virus

Common characteristics

- **Positive-strand, single-stranded, nonsegmented RNA genome**
- **Enveloped, icosahedral nucleocapsid**
- **Genomic RNAs serve as messenger RNAs and are infectious**
- **Virions do not contain any enzymes**

Pathogenesis/Clinical Significance

Rubella virus is a member of the genus *Rubivirus.* The virus is transmitted via respiratory secretions from an infected individual.

- **German measles**

  This is a mild clinical syndrome (not to be confused with rubeola, caused by the measles virus). The infection is characterized by a generalized maculopapular rash and occipital lymphadenopathy. In most cases, these symptoms may be hardly noticeable, and the infection remains subclinical.

- **Congenital rubella**

  The major clinical significance of rubella is that when a pregnant woman is infected with the virus, there can be significant damage to the developing fetus, especially in the first trimester. This damage can include congenital heart disease, cataracts, hepatitis, and abnormalities related to the tral nervous system, such as mental retardation, motor dysfunction, and deafness.

Treatment and Prevention

- **Treatment:** No antiviral drugs are currrently in use.
- **Prevention:** Fetal damage due to rubella infection is preventable by use of the live, attenuated rubella vaccine that is included with the routine childhood vaccinations. This vaccine is effective, has few complications, and ensures that when women reach childbearing age, they are immune to rubella infection. The vaccine should not be given to women who are already pregnant or to immunocompromised patients, including young babies.

Laboratory Identification

- A diagnosis of rubella infection can be made by measuring a rise in antibody titer.
- Pregnant women with anti-rubella IgM antibody are presumed to have been recently exposed to the virus.

Disease Summaries 33

I. OVERVIEW

The chapter describes diseases caused by organisms that have common features, including their modes of transmission or clinical syndrome associated with the disease. This summary is guided, in part, by the frequency of disease as reported to the Centers for Disease Control and Prevention (CDC) which monitors the incidence of more than fifty notifiable diseases, most of them organism-specific (Figure 33.1). [Note: A notifiable disease is one for which regular, frequent, and timely information regarding individual cases is considered necessary for prevention and control of the disease.] For example, data reported to the CDC show sexually transmitted diseases (diseases that have sexual contact as a common mode of transmission) are among the most common infectious diseases in the United States. However, some diseases included in this chapter are not reported by the CDC. These diseases are monitored by institutions, such as hospitals, where the reporting is as much clinical by syndrome as it is by organism. For example, a hospital keeps track of its nosocomial urinary tract infections or ventilator-associated pneumonias.

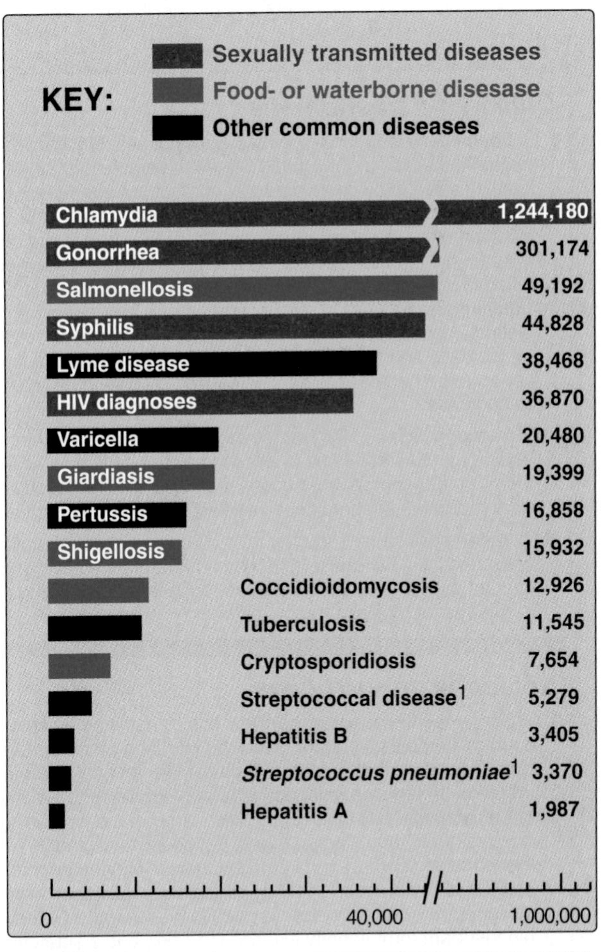

Figure 33.1
Reported cases of some notifiable diseases in the United States, 2009. [1]Invasive disease.

II. SEXUALLY TRANSMITTED DISEASES

Chlamydia remains the most commonly reported infectious disease in the United States, and its incidence is slowly increasing. Women, especially young women, are hit hardest by *Chlamydia*. Gonorrhea is the second most commonly reported infectious disease in the United States. Although the disease rate is falling to historic lows, the occurrence of drug resistance is on the rise. Other sexually transmitted agents are described in Figures 33.2.

SEXUALLY TRANSMITTED DISEASES

A Prevalence of common bacterial diseases

400
300
200
100
0
Approximate incidence (Cases per 100,000 population, United States)
Chlamydia
Gonorrhea
Syphilis
96 98 00 02 04 06 08 10
Year

Incidence of chlamydial infections and syphilis is increasing, whereas gonorrhea is decreasing.

B Classification of bacterial pathogens

Gram (–) rods

Neisseria gonorrhoeae
Haemophilus ducreyi

Spirochetes

Treponema pallidum

Mycoplasma

Ureaplasma urealyticum

Chlamydia

Chlamydia trachomatis

Chlamydia trachomatis

- *C. trachomatis* is the major causal agent of sexually transmitted bacterial disease in the United States. It affects both sexes. Transmission is by close personal contact (for example, during birth, or sexual contact). Men develop nongonococcal urethritis and possible other infections (for example, of the prostate or rectum). Women develop infection of the cervix, which may progress to pelvic inflammatory disease. Repeated or chronic exposures to *C. trachomatis* can lead to sterility and ectopic pregnancy. A clinically distinct infection causing lymphadenopathy, with destructive lesions on genitalia and adjacent tissue, is called lymphogranuloma venereum. This manifestation is caused by distinct serovars of *C. trachomatis*.
- *C. trachomatis* is an obligate intracellular parasite. The elementary body form uses adhesins to attach to susceptible host cell membrane receptors on mucous membranes. The reticulate body form replicates in phagocytic vesicles, eventually killing the host cell.
- *C. trachomatis* causes trachoma, a chronic keratoconjunctivitis that often results in blindness. Trachoma is transmitted by personal contact, by contaminated surfaces touched by hands and conveyed to the eye, or by flies.

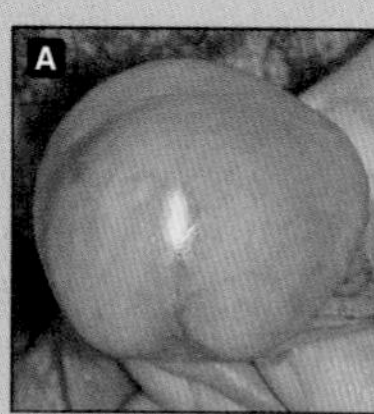

Urethritis

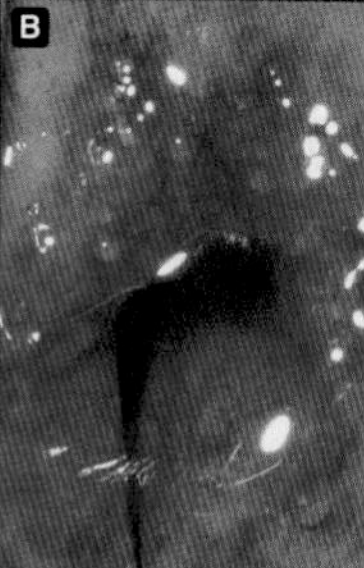

Chlamydial cervicitis

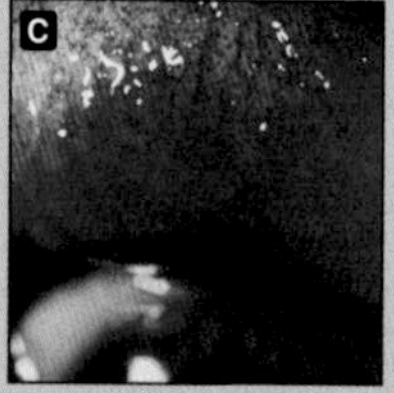

Chlamydial conjunctivitis

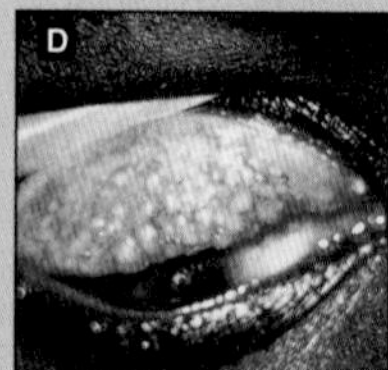

Trachoma

Neisseria gonorrhoeae

- *N. gonorrhoeae* causes gonorrhea. It is transmitted by sexual contact. In males, symptoms include infection of the urethra (gonococcal urethritis), purulent discharge, and pain during urination. In females, infection is usually localized to the endocervix, often causing a purulent vaginal discharge. If the woman's disease progresses to the fallopian tubes, gonococcal salpingitis (which may lead to tubal scarring and infertility), pelvic inflammatory disease, and fibrosis can occur. In many cases, the infection is asymptomatic in women. *N. gonorrhoeae* may cause disseminated infection via the bloodstream, prominently involving the skin and a small number of joints (arthritis-dermatitis syndrome).
- *N. gonorrhoeae* is highly sensitive to cool temperatures and dehydration. Bacterial proteins (pili and outer membrane proteins) enhance the attachment of the bacterium to host epithelial and mucosal cell surfaces, such as those of the urethra, rectum, cervix, pharynx, and conjunctiva, causing colonization and infections.

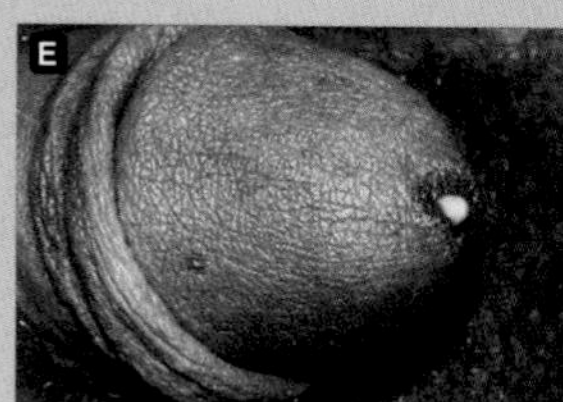

Gonococcal urethritis

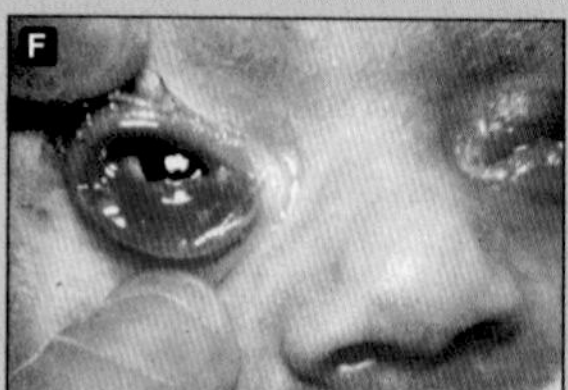

Gonococcal ophthalmia neonatorum

BACTERIA

Figure 33.2 (continued on the next page)
Characteristics of sexually transmitted diseases: bacterial pathogens.

SEXUALLY TRANSMITTED DISEASES

Treponema pallidum

- *T. pallidum* infection causes syphilis. It is transmitted primarily by sexual contact, in which the infectious lesion is generally on the skin or mucous membrane of the genitalia. Within 2 to 10 weeks after infection, a painless, hard ulcer (chancre) forms. Up to 10 weeks later, a secondary rash occurs that may be accompanied by systemic involvement, such as syphilitic hepatitis, meningitis, nephritis, or chorioretinitis. In untreated individuals, a tertiary stage occurs after a latent (asymptomatic) period. Tertiary syphilis is characterized by degenerative changes in the nervous system, cardiovascular lesions, and granulomatous lesions (gummas) in the liver, skin, and bones.
- *T. pallidum* can be transmitted across the placenta of an infected woman to her fetus, causing death and spontaneous abortion of the fetus, or causing it to be stillborn. Those infants that live have the symptoms of congenital syphilis, which include a variety of central nervous system (CNS) and structural abnormalities.

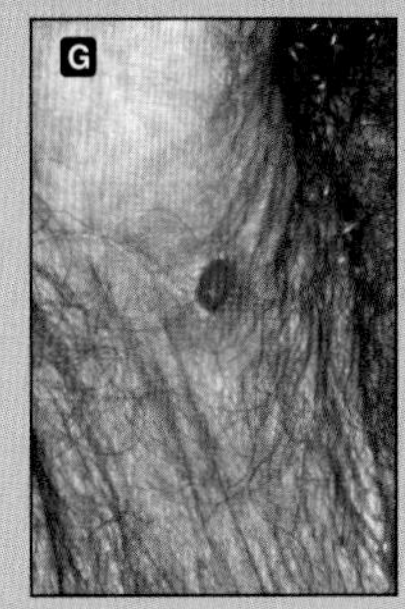

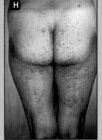

Primary syphilis chancres of the penis

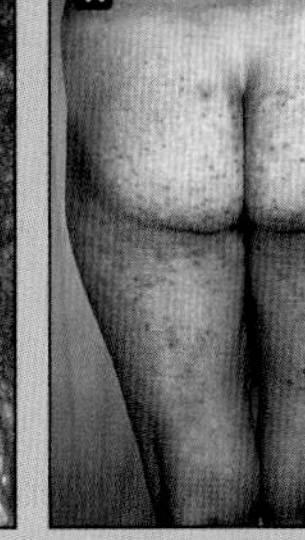

Secondary syphilis

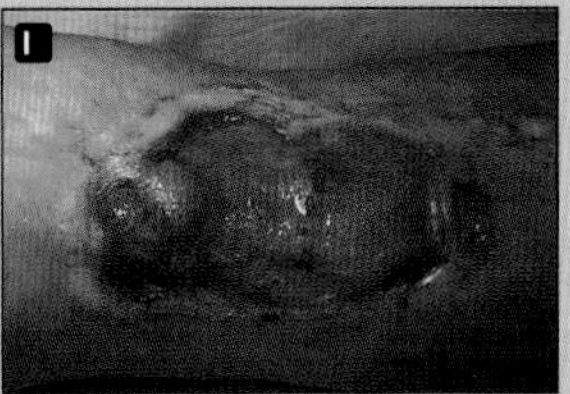

A gumma of tertiary syphilis

Ureaplasma urealyticum

- *U. urealyticum* causes nongonococcal urethritis, particularly in men. The organism has a high colonization rate among sexually active men and women.
- In women, *U. urealyticum* causes postpartum fever and chorioamnionitis. The organism has been isolated from cases of endometritis and from vaginal secretions of women who undergo premature labor or deliver low-birth-weight babies. These infants are often colonized, and *U. urealyticum* has been isolated from the infant's lower respiratory tract and the CNS, both with and without evidence of inflammatory response.

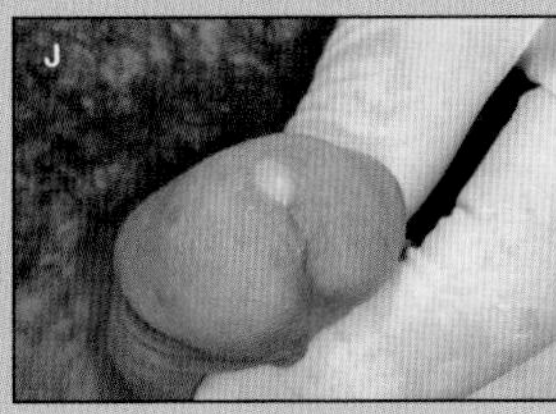

Non-gonococcal urethritis

Haemophilus ducreyi

- *H. ducreyi* causes chancroid (soft chancre), a sexually-transmitted, ulcerative disease. Chancroid is a major health problem in developing countries, although its incidence is low in the United States. *H. ducreyi* infection causes painful, ragged ulcers on the genitalia, and lymphadenopathy may occur. Untreated, this progresses to formation of a bubo (a swollen, painful lymph node), which then suppurates.
- Open genital sores facilitate the transmission of human immunodeficiency virus.

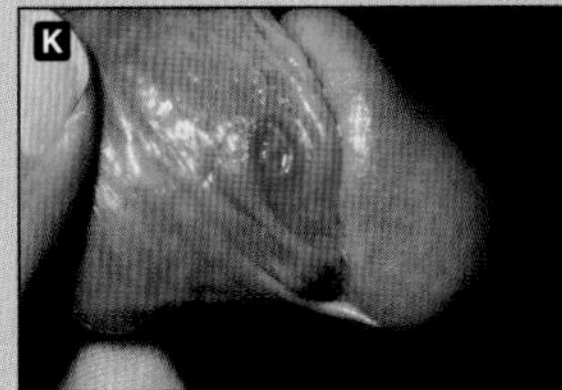

Chancroid

BACTERIA

Figure 33.2 (continued on the next page)
Characteristics of sexually transmitted diseases: bacterial pathogens.

SEXUALLY TRANSMITTED DISEASES

Candida albicans

- *C. albicans* is a yeast that is part of the normal body flora, which can be found in the skin, mouth, vagina, and intestines. It can also be introduced to the body, for example, during sexual contact. Overgrowth of candida (candidiasis) occurs when competing bacterial flora are eliminated, for example, by antibacterial antibiotics. Unlike *Trichomonas vaginalis*, which requires that the vagina have a pH of about 6.0 for growth, *C. albicans* grows at the normal vaginal pH of 4.0.
- **Vulvovaginal candidiasis** is a common clinical syndrome, often seen both in the physician's office and at sexually transmiteed disease clinics. This syndrome causes itching and burning pain of the vulva and vagina, accompanied by a white discharge that is usually thick and curd-like.

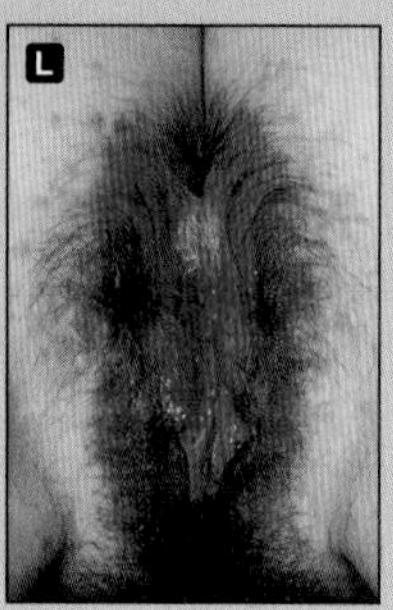

Vulvovaginal candidiasis

FUNGUS

Trichomonas vaginalis

- *T. vaginalis* causes trichomoniasis, the most common protozoal urogenital tract infection of humans. The disease is largely sexually transmitted. In females, it causes inflammation of the mucosal tissue of the vagina, vulva, and cervix, accompanied by a copious, yellowish discharge. Less commonly, it infects the male urethra, prostate, and seminal vesicles, producing a white discharge.
- The optimum pH for growth of *T. vaginalis* is about 6.0; therefore, the organism does not thrive in the normal, acidic vagina, which has a pH of about 4.0. Abnormal alkalinity of the vagina favors acquisition of the disease.

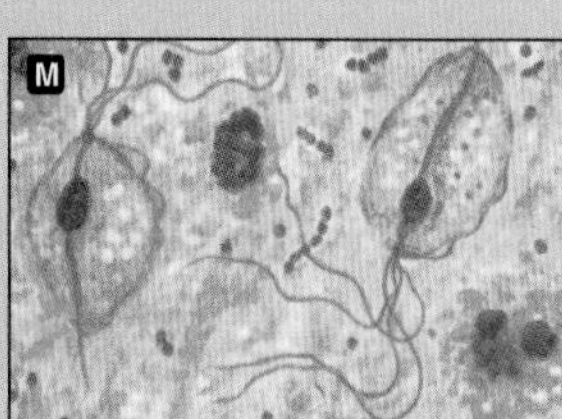

Trichomonas vaginalis

PROTOZOAN

A Prevalence of common viral diseases

Human papillomavirus

Herpes simplex virus

Human immunodeficiency virus

0 500,000 1,000,000

New cases per year in the United States

B Classification of viral pathogens

Double stranded Nonenveloped	Human papillomavirus
Double stranded Enveloped	Herpes simplex virus 2; Human cytomegalovirus
Single stranded Positive strand Icosadedral or helical Enveloped	Human immunodeficiency virus

Herpes simplex virus type 2 (HSV-2)

- HSV-2 transmission generally occurs by sexual contact or by infection during birth. The sexually transmitted infection causes genital tract lesions, most of which are asymptomatic. When symptomatic, local pain and itching and systemic symptoms of fever, malaise, and myalgias may occur. Vesiculoulcerative lesions on the vulva, cervix, and vagina, or the penis, can be painful. Neonatal herpes is contracted by a baby during birth. If untreated, a disseminated infection results, often involving the CNS, leading to a high mortality rate.
- HSV-2 has a relatively rapid, cytocidal growth cycle that establishes latency in nerve ganglia. Reactivation of HSV-2 genital infection occurs frequently and is often asymptomatic. The infected person sheds virus during the reactivation period regardless of symptoms and can transmit the virus to a sexual partner during that period.

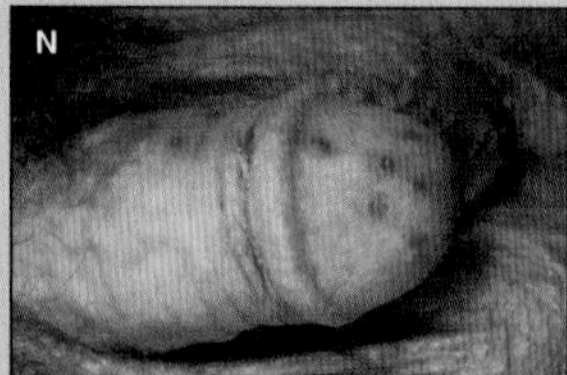

Herpes simplex lesions

VIRUSES

Figure 33.2 (continued on the next page)
Characteristics of sexually transmitted diseases: fungi, protozoa, and viruses.

SEXUALLY TRANSMITTED DISEASES

VIRUSES

Human papillomavirus (HPV)

- Infection by certain HPV causes anogenital warts (condylomata acuminata) verruca vulgaris. Transmission is through sexual contact or from mother to baby during birth.
- Lesions appear around the external genitalia, on the cervix, and/or inside the urethra or vagina, 4 to 6 weeks after infection. Some HPV infections are benign, but several types have been implicated as causes of different types of cancer, including cervical, rectal, penile, and oropharyngeal.

Condyloma acuminatum

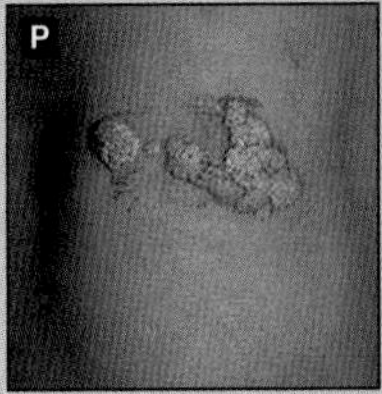

Verruca vulgaris (on a finger)

Human cytomegalovirus (HCMV)

- HCMV is the most common intrauterine viral infection. It is also the most common viral infection of neonates. HCMV is transmitted by infected individuals through tears, urine, saliva, semen or vaginal secretions, and breast milk. Of infants born to women experiencing their first HCMV infection during pregnancy, 35 percent to 50 percent will become infected, of which 10 percent will be symptomatic (cytomegalic inclusion disease). Manifestations of the latter can include various degrees of damage to liver, spleen, blood-forming organs, and components of the nervous system (a common cause of hearing loss and mental retardation) or fetal death. Invasive opportunistic HCMV infections are common in AIDS patients. Such infections are also a danger to transplant recipients and other immunocompromised individuals.
- HCMV replicates initially in epithelial cells, usually of the respiratory and gastrointestinal tracts. This is followed by viremia and infection of all organs of the body. Latency is established in non-neural tissues, primarily lymphoreticular cells and glandular tissues.

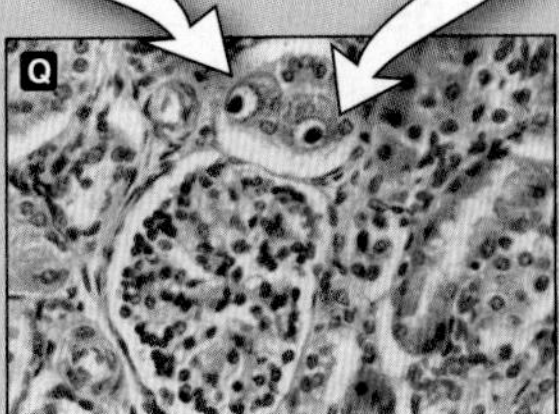

A single renal tube contains large intranuclear virus inclusion bodies that have a typical "owl-eye" appearance.

Cytomegalovirus infection. Section of kidney taken at autopsy from a 3-month-old boy.

Human immunodeficiency virus

- HIV infects CD4+ T-cells, T cell precursors, and cells of the monocyte/macrophage lineage, resulting in a state of immunodeficiency. Transmission of HIV occurs by three routes: 1) sexually (virus is present in both semen and vaginal secretions); 2) via blood or blood products; and 3) perinatally (vertically). Several weeks after the initial infection, some individuals experience symptoms similar to infectious mononucleosis. The acute-phase viremia resolves into a clinically asymptomatic latent period lasting from months to many years. The progression from asymptomatic infection to acquired immune deficiency syndrome occurs as a continuum of progressive clinical states. Infected cells of the monocyte/macrophage system transport the virus into other organs including the brain. Death usually occurs from opportunistic infections, such as those shown at right.
- HIV is a nononcogenic retrovirus. It binds to a surface CD4 molecule, located primarily on helper T cells. HIV enters the cell by fusion of the virus envelope with the plasma membrane, followed by reverse transcription. This results in formation of a molecule of double-stranded DNA that is integrated into a host cell chromosome. Progeny virus are produced continuously, and the process eventually kills the host cell.

Opportunistic Infections of AIDS

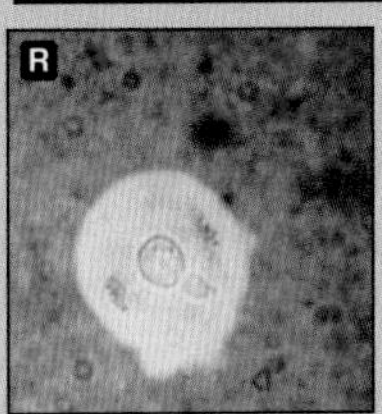

Cryptococcus present in the cerebrospinal fluid.

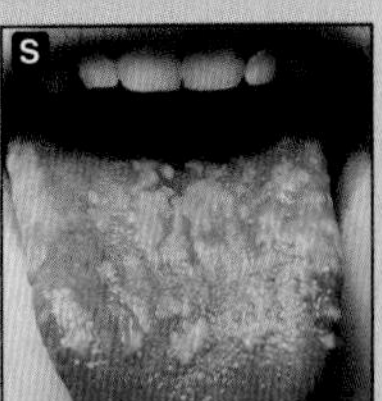

Oral thrush, or candidiasis

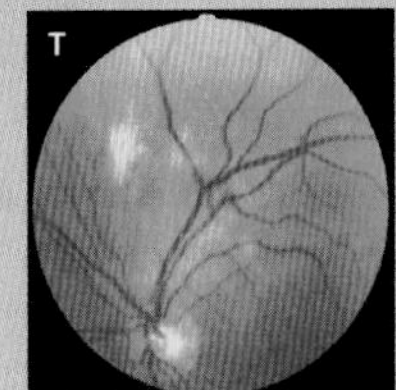

Cytomegalovirus retinitis

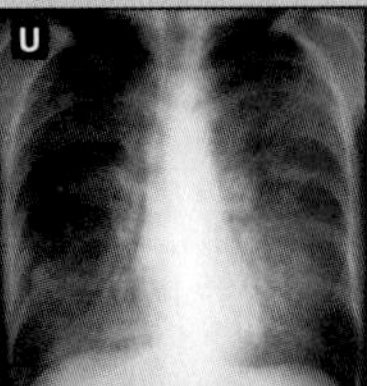

Pneumocystis pneumonia

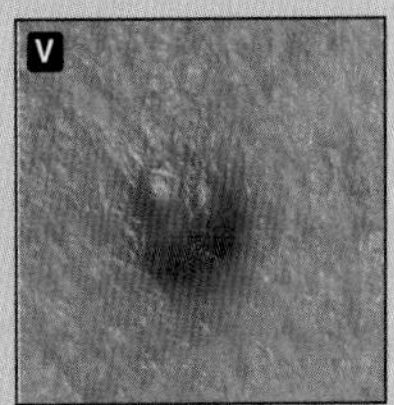

Kaposi sarcoma

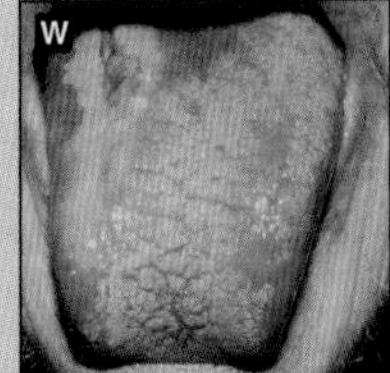

Hairy leukoplakia

Figure 33.2 (continued)
Characteristics of sexually transmitted diseases: viruses.

FOODBORNE ILLNESS (bacterial)

A Common causes of foodborne illness

Organism	Estimated number of illnesses (millions)
Salmonella species	
Clostridium perfringens	
Campylobacter species	
Staphylococcus aureus	

0 0.25 0.5 0.75 1.0
Millions
Estimated number of illnesses in the United States (2011)

B Classification of pathogens

Gram (+) cocci
- *Staphylococcus aureus*

Gram (–) rods
- *Escherichia coli*
- *Campylobacter jejuni*
- *Salmonella* species
- *Shigella* species
- *Vibrio cholerae*

Anaerobic organisms
- *Clostridium botulinum*
- *Clostridium perfringens*

C Common complaints[1]

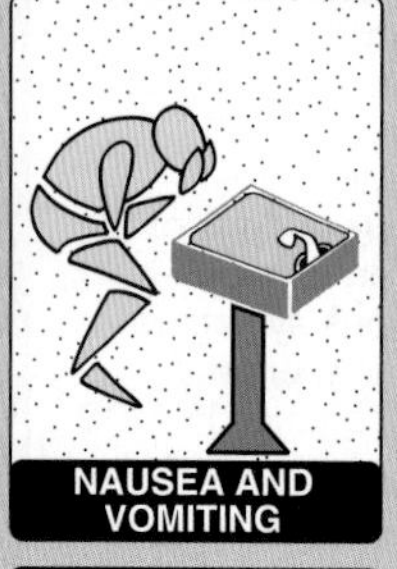

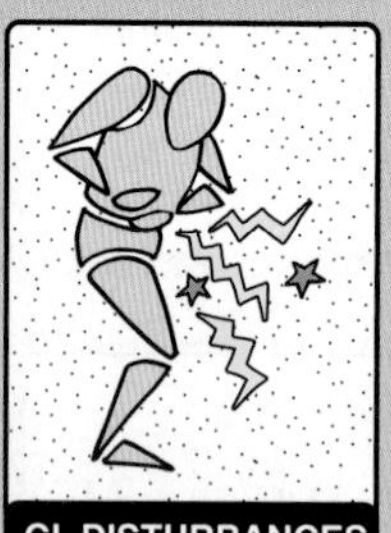

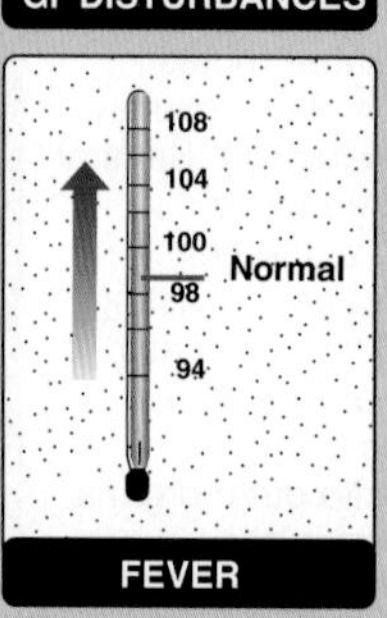

Salmonella species

- Nontyphoidal *Salmonella* serovars, particularly Typhimurium and Enteritidis, cause a localized gastroenteritis in which the symptoms result from causative bacteria proliferating in the intestine of affected individuals. Transmission is usually via food, especially chickens, eggs, and egg products.
- These organisms all invade host cells by injection of effector proteins directly into the host cytoplasm. Widespread antibiotic resistance among these organisms requires sensitivity testing to determine the appropriate antibiotic treatment, if any is given.

Clostridium species

- *Clostridium perfringens* is a major cause of food poisoning in the United States. The occurrence of clinical symptoms requires a large inoculum of 10^8 organisms or greater. Therefore, a typical episode of clostridial food poisoning involves cooking that fails to inactivate spores, followed by holding the food for several hours under conditions that allow bacterial germination and several cycles of growth.
- *Clostridium perfringens* secretes various exotoxins, enterotoxins, and hydrolytic enzymes that facilitate the disease process. Symptoms involved in clostridial food poisoning typically include nausea, abdominal cramps, and diarrhea, occurring 8 to 18 hours after eating contaminated food. Fever is absent and vomiting rare. The attack is usually self-limited, with recovery within 1 to 2 days.
- *Clostridium botulinum* causes botulism. A neurotoxin produced by the bacteria results in flaccid paralysis. Contact with the organism itself is not required, and hence, the disease is a pure intoxication.

Campylobacter jejuni

- *C. jejuni* is the leading cause of foodborne disease in the United States. It also causes traveler's diarrhea and pseudoappendicitis. *C. jejuni* is transmitted to humans primarily via the fecal–oral route—through direct contact, exposure to contaminated meat (especially poultry), or contaminated water supplies.
- *C. jejuni* infects the intestine, and it can cause ulcerative, inflammatory lesions in the jejunum, ileum, or colon. In otherwise healthy individuals, it typically causes an acute enteritis following a one- to seven-day incubation. The disease lasts days to several weeks, and generally is self-limiting. Symptoms may be both systemic (fever, headache, myalgia) and intestinal (abdominal cramping and diarrhea, which may or may not be bloody). Bacteremia may occur, most often in infants and older adults.

Staphylococcus aureus

- *S. aureus* gastroenteritis is caused by ingestion of food containing the bacterial enterotoxin. Often contaminated by a food-handler, these foods tend to be protein-rich and/or salty (for example, egg salad, cream pastry, or ham) and improperly refrigerated.
- The toxin stimulates the vomiting center in the brain by binding to neural receptors in the upper gastrointestinal tract. Symptoms such as nausea, vomiting, and diarrhea are acute following a short incubation period (less than 6 hours). The attack is usually self-limiting.

Figure 33.3 (continued on the next page)
Disease summary of some major organisms causing bacterial food poisoning.
[1]Other complaints may include headache and myalgias.

FOODBORNE ILLNESS (bacterial)

Shigella species

- *Shigella* species cause shigellosis (bacillary dysentery)—a human intestinal disease that occurs commonly among young children. Shigellae are typically spread from person to person, with food or water contaminated with fecal material serving as a major source of organisms.
- Shigellae invade and destroy the mucosa of the large intestine. The resulting bacillary dysentery is characterized by diarrhea with blood, mucus, and painful abdominal cramping. The disease is generally most severe in the very young and elderly, and among malnourished individuals, in whom shigellosis may lead to severe dehydration, and sometimes death.

Vibrio species

- *Vibrio cholerae* secretes a toxin which causes cholera, an infection in the small intestine. The cholera toxin causes an outflowing of ions and water to the lumen of the intestine. After an incubation period ranging from hours to a few days, profuse watery diarrhea ("rice-water" stools) begins. Untreated, death from severe dehydration causing hypovolemic shock may occur in hours to days, and the death rate may exceed 50 percent. Appropriate treatment reduces the death rate to less than 1 percent.
- Transmission occurs primarily by drinking water or eating food that has been contaminated by the feces of an infected person, including one with no apparent symptoms.
- Worldwide, cholera affects 3–5 million people and causes 100,000–130,000 deaths a year as of 2010. This occurs mainly in the developing world.

Escherichia coli

- *E. coli* is part of the normal flora of the colon, but pathogenic virotypes have acquired new virulence factors allowing them to be more pathogenic both inside and outside of the GI tract. Transmission of intestinal disease is commonly by the fecal-oral route, with contaminated food (such as beef and unpasteurized milk) and water serving as the vehicles.
- Several types of intestinal infections with *E. coli* have been identified. These differ in their pathogenic mechanisms. Among the most important are: 1) enterotoxigenic *E. coli* (ETEC)—a common cause of traveler's diarrhea in developing countries. ETEC colonizes the small intestine and produces enterotoxins. These cause prolonged hypersecretion of chloride ions and water by the intestinal mucosal cells while inhibiting the reabsorption of sodium, resulting in significant watery diarrhea over a period of several days. 2) Enterohemorrhagic *E. coli* (EHEC) binds to cells in the large intestine, where it produces an exotoxin (Shiga-like toxin) that destroys microvilli, causing a severe form of copious, bloody diarrhea (hemorrhagic colitis) in the absence of mucosal invasion or inflammation. Serotype O157:H7 is the most common strain of *E. coli* that produces Shiga-like toxin.

Figure 33.3 (continued)
Disease summary of major organisms causing bacterial food poisoning. [Note: Adequate fluid and electrolyte replacement and maintenance are key to managing diarrheal illnesses.]

III. FOODBORNE ILLNESS (bacterial)

Foodborne illness results from eating food contaminated with organisms or toxins (Figure 33.3). Foodborne illness tends to occur at picnics, school cafeterias, and large social functions. These are commonly situations in which food may be left unrefrigerated or food preparation techniques are insufficiently safe. Foodborne illness often occurs from undercooked meats or dairy products that have remained at room temperature for extended periods. In patients with foodborne illness, fluid consumption is important to avoid dehydration. Children with diarrhea may be given an over-the-counter electrolyte product. Solid foods should not be eaten until the diarrhea has passed, and dairy should be avoided, as it can worsen diarrhea temporarily.

Intravenous fluid may be indicated in patients with severe diarrhea who are unable to drink fluids (for example, caused by nausea or vomiting)

Most patients spontaneously recover from the most common types of foodborne illnesswithin a couple of days. Antibiotic therapy is usually not indicated, except in cases of severe illness. Infants and elderly people have the greatest risk for oodborne illness. It is estimated that foodborne gastroenteritis causes 48 million illnesses, 127,000 hospitalizations, and 3,000 deaths in the United States annually.

URINARY TRACT INFECTIONS

A Common causes of urinary tract infection (UTI)[1]

Escherichia coli

Staphylococcus saprophyticus

Klebsiella

Proteus

Pseudomonas aeruginosa

0 10 20 30 40 50 60 70 80 90

Approximate prevalence (%)

B Classification of pathogens

Gram (+) cocci

Staphylococcus saprophyticus

Gram (–) rods

Escherichia coli
Klebsiella species
Proteus species
Pseudomonas aeruginosa

Escherichia coli

- *E. coli* is the most common cause of UTI, including cystitis and pyelonephritis. Women are particularly at risk for infection. Acquisition is frequently from the patient's flora.
- Uncomplicated cystitis (the most commonly encountered UTI) is caused by uropathogenic strains of *E. coli*, characterized by P fimbriae (an adherence factor). Complicated UTI (pyelonephritis) often occurs in settings of obstructed urinary flow, and may be caused by nonuropathogenic strains of *E. coli*. UTI requires treatment with antibiotics.

Staphylococcus saprophyticus

- *S. saprophyticus* is a frequent cause of cystitis in women, probably related to its occurrence as part of normal vaginal flora. It is also an important agent of hospital-acquired infections associated with the use of catheters.
- *S. saprophyticus* is a coagulase-negative staphylococcal species. It tends to be sensitive to most antibiotics, even penicillin G. It can be distinguished from most other coagulase-negative staphylococci by its natural resistance to novobiocin.

C Common complaints

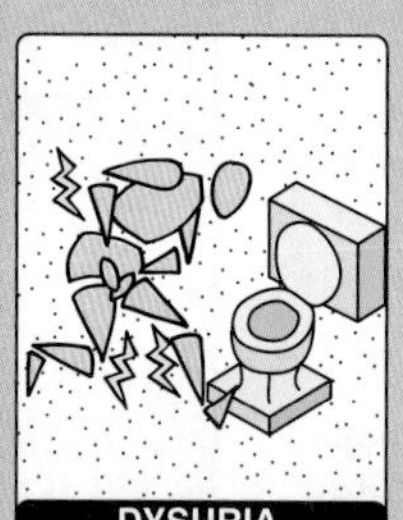

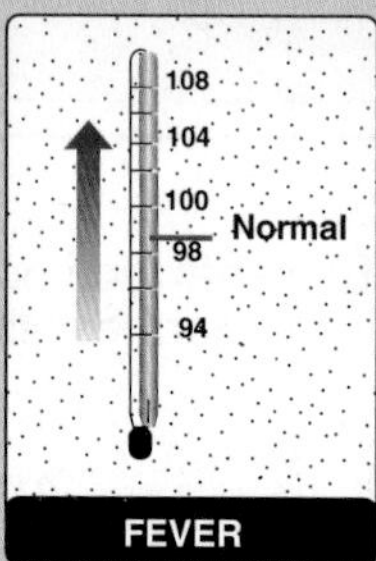

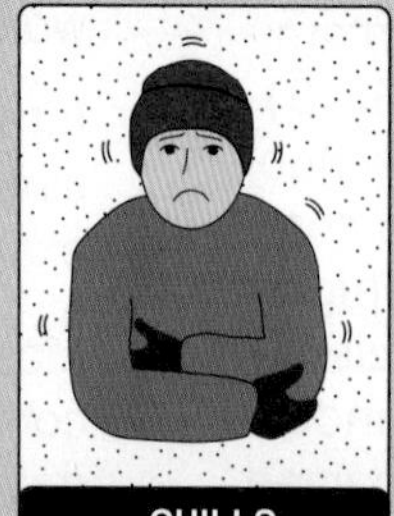

Other enterobacteria

- Other genera of *Enterobacteriaceae*, such as *Klebsiella*, *Enterobacter*, *Proteus*, and *Serratia*, which can be found as normal inhabitants of the large intestine, include organisms that are primarily opportunistic and often nosocomial pathogens. They all frequently colonize hospitalized patients, especially in association with antibiotic treatment, indwelling catheters, or invasive procedures, causing extra-intestinal infections such as those of the urinary tract.
- Wide-spread antibiotic resistance among these organisms necessitates sensitivity testing to determine the appropriate antibiotic treatment.

Pseudomonas aeruginosa

- *P. aeruginosa* is a significant opportunistic pathogen and a major cause of hospital-acquired (nosocomial) infections such as UTI, particularly in patients who have been subjected to catheterization, instrumentation, surgery, or renal transplantation, or prior antibiotic therapy.
- *P. aeruginosa* disease begins with attachment and colonization of host tissue. Pili on the bacteria mediate adherence, and an alginate capsule reduces the effectiveness of normal clearance mechanisms. Host tissue damage facilitates adherence and colonization. Because *Pseudomonas* infections typically occur in patients with impaired defenses, aggressive antimicrobial therapy is generally required.

Figure 33.4
Disease summary of urinary tract infections. [1]Uncomplicated cystitis.

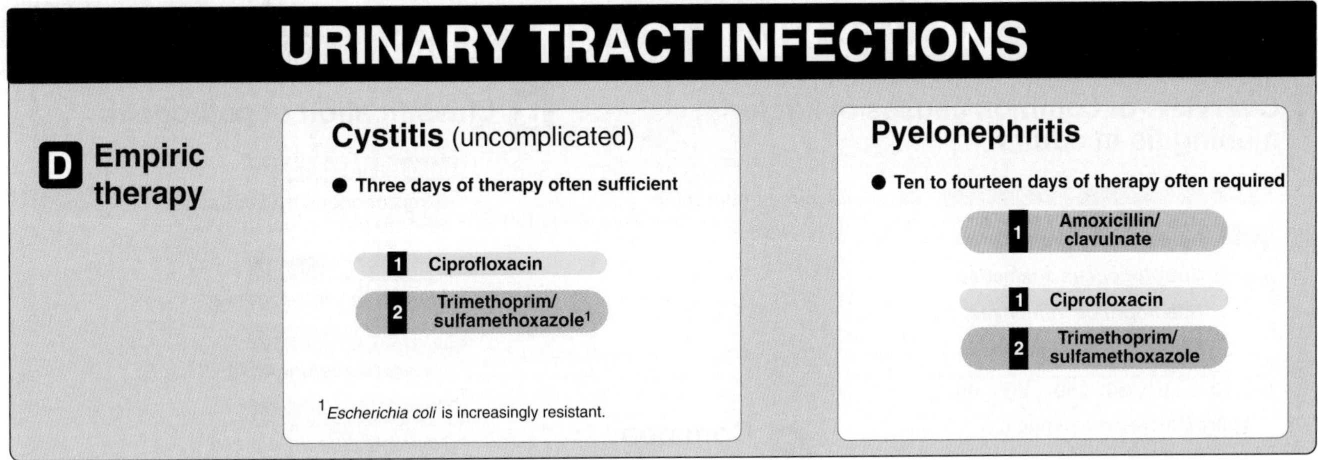

URINARY TRACT INFECTIONS
D Empiric therapy
Cystitis (uncomplicated)
Three days of therapy often sufficient
1 Ciprofloxacin
2 Trimethoprim/ sulfamethoxazole[1]
[1] Escherichia coli is increasingly resistant.
Pyelonephritis
Ten to fourteen days of therapy often required
1 Amoxicillin/ clavulnate
1 Ciprofloxacin
2 Trimethoprim/ sulfamethoxazole

Figure 33.4 (continued)
Disease summary of urinary tract infections. 1 Indicates first-line drugs; 2 indicates alternative drugs.

IV. URINARY TRACT INFECTIONS

Urinary tract infections (UTIs) most commonly affect either the lower urinary tract (infection of the urethra or bladder) or, less frequently, the upper urinary tract (acute pyleonephritis, or infection of the kidney). UTIs are termed "uncomplicated" when there is no underlying condition that increases the risk of infection, such as obstruction or urologic dysfunction. Most patients with UTI have uncomplicated cystitis, which is one of the most common infections in the United States, especially in sexually active women.

Escherichia coli is the most common cause of uncomplicated cystitis and pyelonephritis (70 to 95 percent of infections, Figure 33.4). Fecal contamination can lead to entry of an organism such as *E. coli* (one of the most common facultative organisms found in stool) into the urethra. These bacteria then move up into the bladder (and sometimes ascend into the kidney), producing infection. UTIs occur much more frequently in women as a result of the proximity of the urethral opening to the anus and the shorter length of the urethra before it opens into the bladder in women.

Staphylococcus saprophyticus as a causative agent is a distant second to *E. coli*, causing 5 to 20 percent of infections. *S. saprophyticus*, although less common than *E. coli*, often presents as a more aggressive disease with approximately one half of the patients showing involvement in the upper urinary tract. These patients are also more likely to have recurrent infection.

Patients with uncomplicated UTI usually present with dysuria, urinary frequency, urinary urgency, and/or suprapubic pains. Pyuria (the production of urine that contains white blood cells) is commonly found in UTIs. Fever or flank tenderness could indicate pyelonephritis. If the features suggestive of vaginitis or urethritis described above are present, a pelvic examination and appropriate cultures should be performed.

The risk of UTI, both cystitis and pyelonephritis, can be increased by several factors, especially sexual intercourse, particularly with a new sexual partner. The use of spermicides, particularly in combination with a diaphragm, also increases the risk of a woman developing a UTI.

BACTERIAL MENINGITIS

A Overview of common causes of bacterial meningitis in adults[1]

Organism	Approximate prevalence (%) (2003–2007)
Streptococcus pneumoniae	~60
Neisseria meningitidis	~10
Streptococcus agalactiae	~7
Haemophilus influenzae	~5
Listeria monocytogenes	~4

B Classification of pathogens

Gram (+) cocci

Streptococcus agalactiae
Streptococcus pneumoniae

Gram (+) rods

Listeria monocytogenes

Gram (–) cocci

Neisseria meningitidis

Gram (–) rods

Haemophilus influenzae

C Common complaints[2]

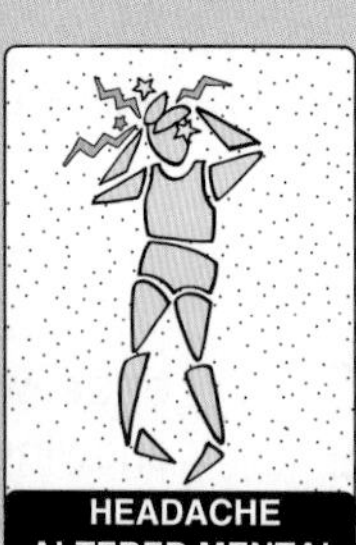

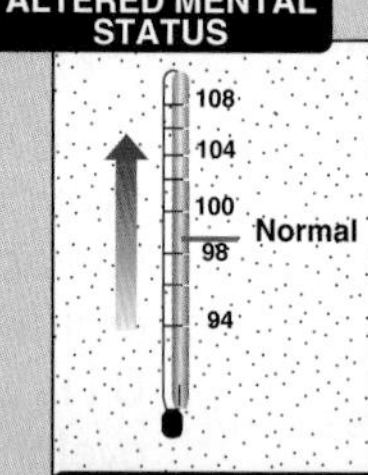

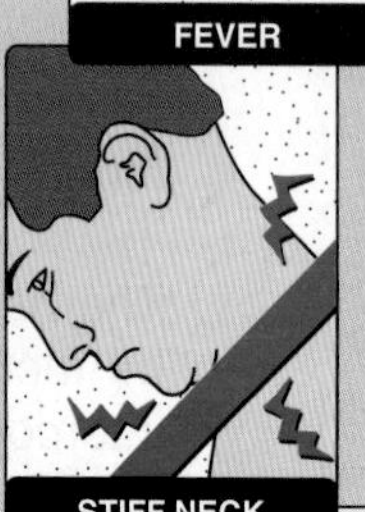

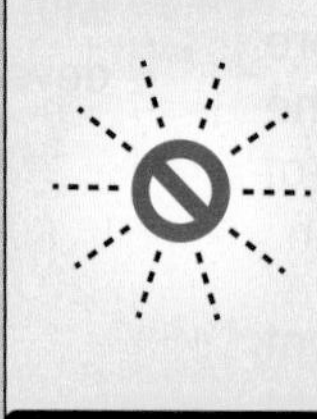

Streptococcus pneumoniae

- *S. pneumoniae* is an important cause of meningitis and pneumonia. It is carried in the nasopharynx of many healthy individuals. Infection can be either endogenous (in a carrier who develops impaired resistance to the organism) or exogenous (by droplets from the airway of a carrier).
- *S. pneumoniae* infections can result in a bacteremia leading to infection of several sites in the human body, including the central nervous system (CNS). This meningitis has a high mortality rate, even when treated appropriately. *S. pneumoniae* is the most common cause of bacterial meningitis in adults.

Neisseria meningitidis

- *N. meningitidis* is a common cause of meningitis. Transmission is via respiratory droplets. Pili allow the attachment of *N. meningitidis* to the nasopharyngeal mucosa.
- If meningococci penetrate the epithelial lining of the nasopharynx and enter the bloodstream, they rapidly multiply, causing meningococcemia. If *N. meningitidis* crosses the blood–brain barrier, it can infect the meninges, causing an acute inflammatory response that results in a purulent meningitis. The initial fever and malaise can rapidly evolve into severe headache, rigid neck, vomiting, and sensitivity to bright light. Coma can occur within a few hours. *N. meningitidis* is the most common cause of bacterial meningitis between the ages of 2 and 18 years.

Haemophilus influenzae

- *H. influenzae* is a normal resident of the human upper respiratory tract. Transmission is by respiratory droplets.
- After attaching to and colonizing the respiratory mucosa, the infection can become systemic, with bacteria spreading via the blood to the CNS. *H. influenzae* was a leading cause of bacterial meningitis, especially in infants and young children. A conjugated vaccine against *H. influenzae* capsular polysaccharide type b is now administered to infants and has dramatically lowered the number of meningitis cases attributable to this organism.

Streptococcus agalactiae

- *S. agalactiae* causes meningitis and septicemia in neonates. It is found normally in the genital tract of female carriers and the urethral mucous membranes of male carriers, as well as in the gastrointestinal (GI) tract (especially the rectum). Transmission occurs during birth and is sexually transmitted among adults.
- Infection of an infant occurs as it traverses the birth canal. *S. agalactiae* infection is a leading cause of neonatal meningitis, and it has a high mortality rate.

Listeria monocytogenes

- *L. monocytogenes* infections are most common among older adults, pregnant women, fetuses or newborns, and immunocompromised individuals. Meningitis is a common presentation. Listeria infections, which may occur as sporadic cases or in small epidemics, are usually foodborne, with the organism entering the body via the GI tract.

Figure 33.5 (continued on next page)
Characteristics of organisms causing bacterial meningitis.

[1] *Escherichia coli* is a major cause of meningitis in the newborn. Viral meningitis is more common than the bacterial form and generally (but not always) less serious. Viral meningitis is often caused by enteroviruses and sometimes herpes simplex virus.
[2] Other complaints include chills and cardiac arrhythmias.

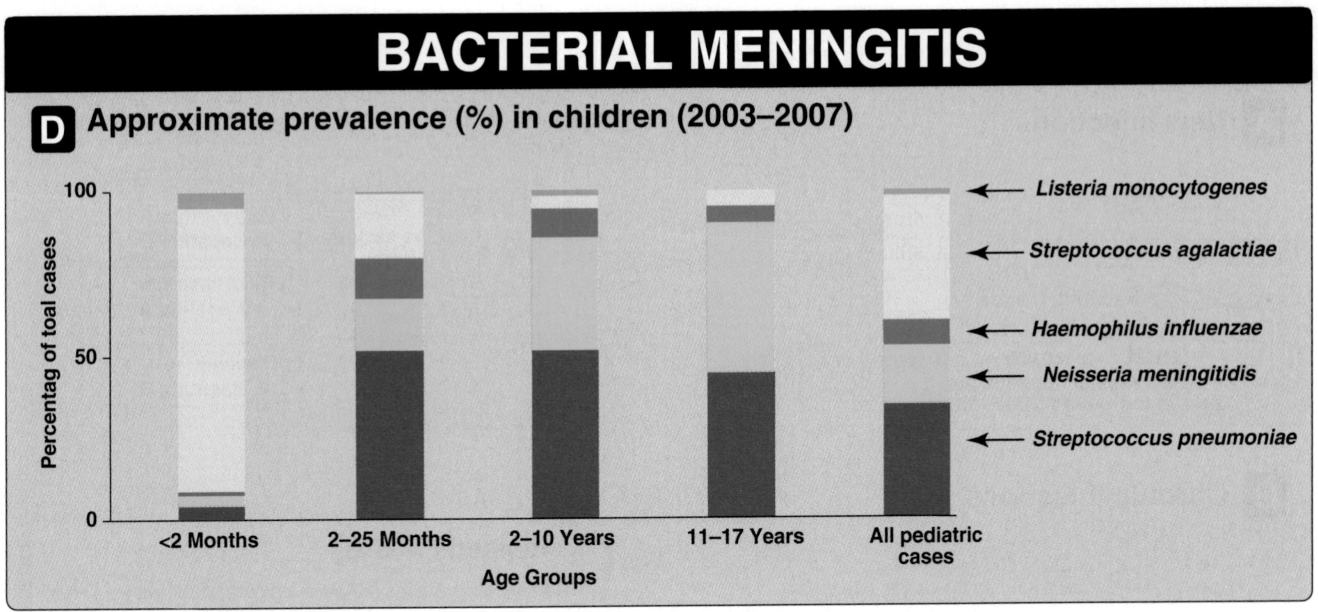

Figure 33.5 (continued)
Characteristics of organisms causing bacterial meningitis.

V. MENINGITIS

Bacterial meningitis is a medical emergency that requires immediate diagnosis and treatment. Untreated disease is virtually 100% lethal and, even with optimal therapy, there is a high mortality rate.

Virtually all patients with community-acquired bacterial meningitis show at least one of the classic triad of symptoms, which includes fever, neck stiffness, and altered mental status (Figure 33.5). These symptoms can develop over several hours, or they may take 1 to 2 days. Other symptoms may include nausea, vomiting, discomfort with bright lights, confusion, and sleepiness. *Streptococcus pneumoniae* and *Neisseria meningitidis* are responsible for 80% of all cases of bacterial meningitis.

Initial blood cultures are positive in 50 to 75 percent of adults with bacterial meningitis. A specimen of cerebrospinal fluid (CSF) should be obtained for cell count and differential, glucose and protein concentration, Gram stain, and culture. Characteristic findings in bacterial meningitis include decreased glucose concentration, elevated protein and white blood cell count in the CSF. Some patients may require computed tomography (CT) scan as a precaution before lumbar puncture.

Therapy for bacterial meningitis requires bactericidal antimicrobial agents that can cross the blood–brain barrier into the CSF. Oral antibiotics should not be used because the dose and tissue levels tend to be considerably lower than with parenteral agents. Antibiotic therapy should be initiated immediately after lumbar puncture. If imaging is performed before lumbar puncture, therapy should be initiated before the patient is sent for neuroimaging. Delay in the initiation of antimicrobial therapy increases the risk of death or brain damage.

Most authorities recommend that an intravenous glucocorticoid such as dexamethasone be given immediately prior to or together with the first dose of antibiotic because of damage to the central nervous system caused by the inflammatory response to the infecting organism.

Initial therapy may be empiric with cefotaxime or ceftriaxone. However, the availability of Gram stain of organisms in the CSF should guide the selection of intravenous antibiotics. Antibiotic therapy should also be reviewed once the CSF culture and *in vitro* susceptibility studies are available.

HEPATITIS

A New infections

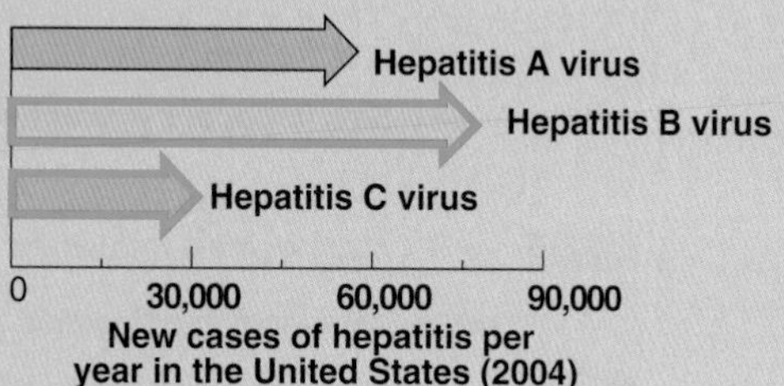

Double stranded Enveloped	Hepadnaviridae • Hepatitis B
Single stranded Positive strand Icosadedral Nonenveloped	Caliciviridae • Hepatitis E
	Picornaviridae • Hepatitis A
Single stranded Positive strand Icosadedral or helical Enveloped	Flaviviridae • Hepatitis C

B Chronic infections

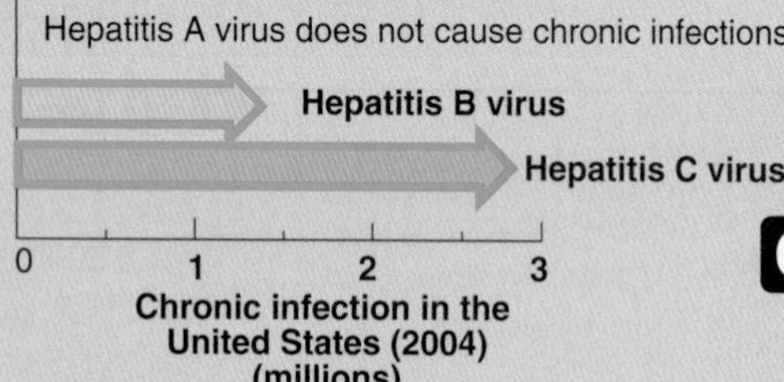

Hepatitis A virus

- Hepatitis A virus (HAV) is a picornavirus, with a linear, single-stranded, positive-sense RNA genome. The virus is nonenveloped.
- Transmission is by the fecal–oral route. The main site of replication is the hepatocyte, where infection results in severe cytopathology, and liver function is severely impaired. The prognosis for patients with HAV is generally favorable, and development of persistent infection and chronic hepatitis is uncommon.
- Prevention of infection requires taking sanitary measures. Immune globulin has been used for many years, mainly as postexposure prophylaxis. A formalin-inactivated whole virus vaccine is available.

C Common complaints

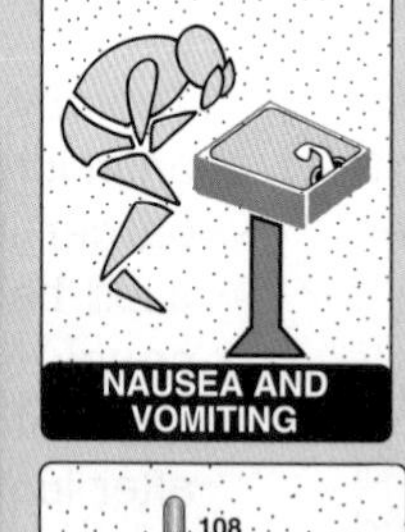

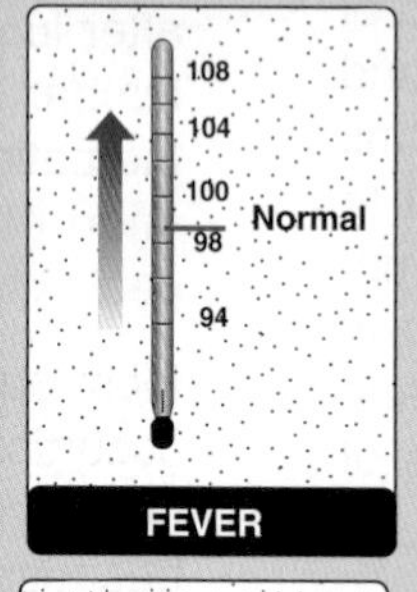

ALT
BILIRUBIN

ELEVATED LIVER ENZYMES; JAUNDICE

Hepatitis B virus

- Hepatitis B virus (HBV) is a hepadnavirus and the only human hepatitis virus that has a DNA genome. A unique feature of HBV is that the viral DNA replicates via an RNA intermediate. HBV is enveloped.
- Infectious HBV is present in all body fluids of an infected individual, including blood, semen, saliva, and breast milk. In the United States, HBV is most frequently contracted by adults through sexual intercourse or by intravenous (IV) drug use. In developing countries, it is transmitted primarily from mother to infant.
- The primary cause of hepatic cell destruction by HBV is the specific reaction of cytotoxic T lymphocytes with viral HBc and HBe antigens expressed on the infected cell's membrane. HBV infections can be acute (accompanied by mild fever, malaise, and myalgia, followed by jaundice and bilirubinuria, with an enlarged and tender liver) or chronic. Chronic carriers may be asymptomatic, but have a higher risk of developing severe chronic hepatitis, leading to progressive liver damage that may result in cirrhosis and/or hepatocellular carcinoma.
- A highly effective vaccine produced in genetically engineered cells is now available. It is included among routine childhood immunizations.

Hepatitis C virus

- Hepatitis C virus (HCV) is a member of the Flaviviridae. It has a linear, single-stranded, positive-sense RNA genome. HCV is enveloped.
- HCV was a major cause of post-transfusion hepatitis ("non-A, non-B"). IV drug users and patients on hemodialysis are also at high risk for infection with HCV. The virus can be transmitted sexually and from mother to infant.
- HCV replication occurs in hepatocytes and mononuclear cells. Both viral replication and the host immune response contribute to destruction of liver cells. Most infections are subclinical, but about 25 percent of infected individuals present with acute hepatitis, including jaundice. A significant proportion of infections progress to a chronic hepatitis and cirrhosis, and some of these individuals develop hepatocellular carcinoma. Coinfection with HBV is often present in those manifesting these more serious consequences. Combination treatment with ribavirin plus interferon provides a higher rate of success in eradicating viral infection in adults than does interferon alone.

Figure 33.6 (continued on the next page)
Characteristics of hepatitis. [ALT = alanine aminotransferase.]

HEPATITIS

Hepatitis D virus

- Hepatitis D virus (HDV, or delta agent) is found in nature only as a result of coinfection with HBV, and it requires HBV to serve as a helper virus for infectious HDV production. HDV has a circular, single-stranded negative-sense RNA genome and an envelope with a protein that is provided by HBV.
- HDV can be transmitted by the same routes as HBV. Pathologically, liver damage is essentially the same as in other viral hepatitides, but the presence of HDV usually results in more extensive and severe damage. No specific treatment for HDV infection is available.

Hepatitis E virus[1]

- Hepatitis E virus (HEV) is a calicivirus, with a linear, single-stranded, positive-sense RNA genome. HEV is non-enveloped.
- HEV is a major cause of enterically transmitted, waterborne hepatitis in developing countries.[1] The peak incidence is in young adults, and the disease is especially severe in pregnant women, in whom death can result from HEV infection.
- No antiviral treatment or vaccine is currently available.

	Drug	Vaccine
Hepatitis A	None	This inactivated virus vaccine offers 99 percent effective immunization against hepatitis A virus infection. Neutralizing antibodies persist for more than 3 years.
Hepatitis B	Lamivudine α-Interferon Adefovir Entecavir	Recombinant hepatitis B vaccine is a noninfectious subunit viral vaccine. The vaccine is derived from hepatitis B surface antigen (HBsAg) produced through recombinant DNA techniques. Following a three-dose series, immunity lasts approximately 5 to 7 years.
Hepatitis C	α-Interferon Ribavirin	None

Figure 33.6 (continued)
Characteristics of hepatitis.
[1]No cases of hepatitis E have been reported in the United States

VI. HEPATITIS

Hepatitis is inflammation of the liver. The disease can be caused by infections from parasites, bacteria, or viruses (such as hepatitis A, B, or C, as shown in Figure 33.6). Liver damage can also result from alcohol, drugs, or poisonous mushrooms. Hepatitis A, B, and C are clinically the most important forms of viral liver disease. Hepatitis A does not lead to chronic infection. Infection provides life-long immunity

Persons at risk of hepatitis B infection include 1) individuals with multiple sex partners; 2) men who have sex with men; 3) sex contacts of infected persons; 4) injection drug users; and 4) household contacts of chronically infected persons. Death from chronic hepatitis B occurs in 15 to 25 percent of chronically infected persons.

Most hepatitis C infections result from illegal injection drug use. Transfusion-associated cases occurred prior to blood donor screening, but now the incidence is less than 1 per 2 million transfused units of blood. Fifty percent of those with hepatitis C go on to have chronic liver disease and, possibly, liver failure (cirrhosis) or liver cancer. Hepatitis C is the number one reason for receiving a liver transplant in the United States.

COMMUNITY-ACQUIRED PNEUMONIA[1]

A Common pathogens[2]

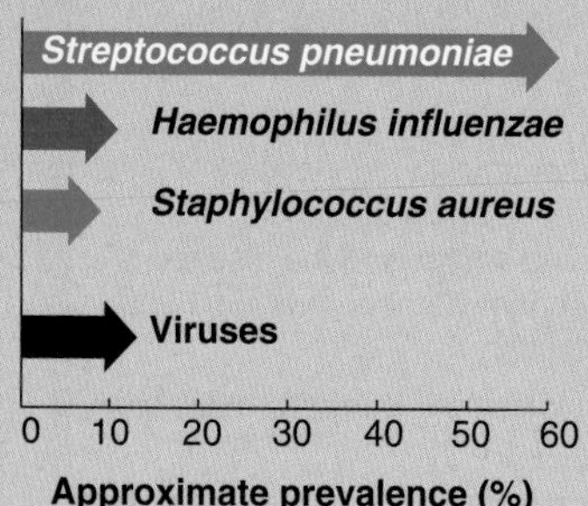

B Classification of pathogens

Gram (+) cocci

Staphylococcus aureus
Streptococcus pneumoniae

Gram (–) rods

Haemophilus influenzae

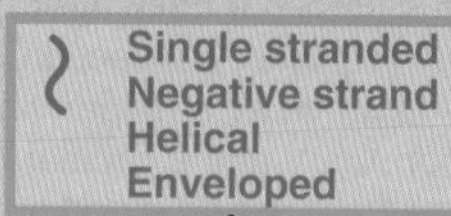

Paramyxoviridae
- Influenza virus types A and B
- Respiratory syncytial virus

Streptococcus pneumoniae

- *S. pneumoniae* is the most common cause of pneumonia. It is the leading cause of death in the older adults and those with impaired resistance.
- Because it is carried in the nasopharynx of many healthy individuals, infection may be endogenous or exogenous (by droplets from the nose of a carrier).
- A prior virus infection (for example, with influenza virus) that causes increased volume and viscosity of bronchial secretions and inhibition of the action of the bronchial cilia predisposes the patient to secondary infection by *S. pneumoniae*.

Haemophilus influenzae

- Transmission is by respiratory droplets.
- *H. influenzae* causes pneumonia, especially in older adults and immunocompromised individuals.
- After attaching to and colonizing the respiratory mucosa, the infection can become systemic, with bacteria spreading via the blood to the central nervous system.

Staphylococcus aureus

- *S. aureus* infections are most common in IV drug users, older adults, in people with a recent influenza virus infection, and in individuals with cystic fibrosis.
- *S. aureus* is transmitted via direct contact. If it infects the lungs, it causes severe, necrotizing pneumonia. Cell wall virulence factors promote binding to mucosal cells.

C Common complaints

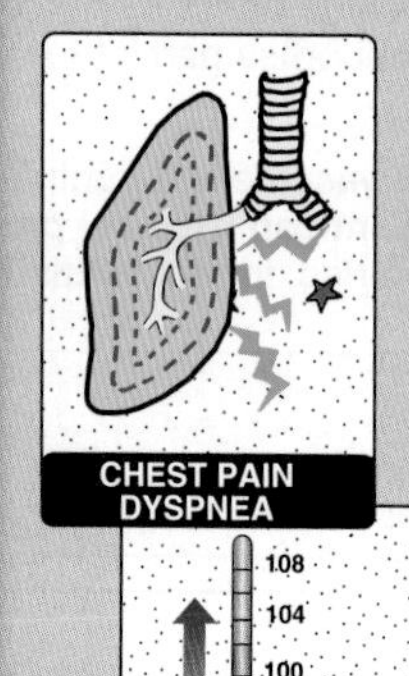

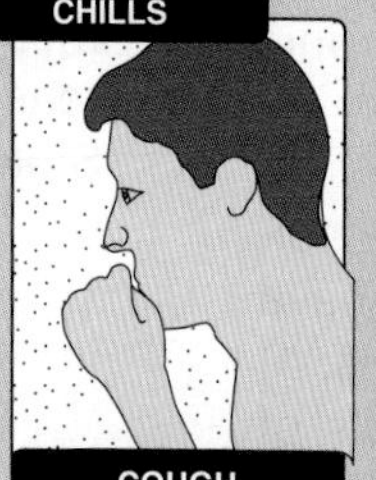

Influenza virus types A and B

- Influenza, spread by respiratory droplets, is an infection solely of the respiratory tract.
- Following inhalation of influenza virus particles, infected respiratory epithelial cells are destroyed by cytotoxic T cells.
- Pneumonia following a bout of influenza occurs in the young, older adults, in people with chronic cardiac or pulmonary disease, or those who are immunodeficient. Pneumonia can be caused by influenza virus or by secondary infection with bacteria such as *S. pneumoniae*.

Parainfluenza viruses

- Human parainfluenza viruses Types 1–4 cause influenza-like symptoms.
- Infection by these viruses is spread by respiratory droplets and is confined to the respiratory tract.
- Human parainfluenza viruses cause pneumonia, as well as croup and bronchiolitis, mainly in infants and children.

Respiratory syncytial virus

- Transmission is by respiratory droplets or by contaminated hands carrying the virus to the nose or mouth.
- RSV is the major viral respiratory tract pathogen in the pediatric population. It can cause pneumonia in young children and severe bronchitis with pneumonia in the elderly.

Figure 33.7
Characteristics of community-acquired pneumonia.

[1]Disease may be "typical" or "atypical." "Typical" pneumonia is characterized by shaking chills, purulent sputum, and x-ray abnormalities that are proportional to the physical signs. "Atypical" pneumonia is characterized by insidious onset, scant sputum and x-ray abnormalities greater than predicted by physical signs.
[2]Additional causes of community-acquired pneumonia are described in Figure 33.8.

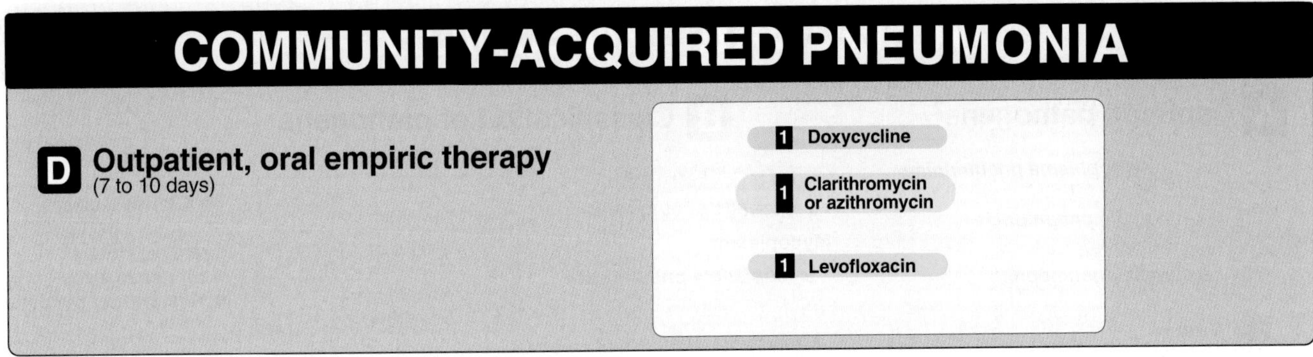

Figure 33.7 (continued)
Characteristics of community-acquired pneumonia. 1 Indicates first-line drugs.

VII. COMMUNITY-ACQUIRED PNEUMONIA

The term "community-acquired pneumonia" refers to a pneumonia in a previously healthy person who acquired the infection outside a hospital (or a long-term care facility).

Typical pneumonia usually is caused by bacteria (left-hand column of Figure 37.7) and tends to be the most serious and, in adults, the most common cause of pneumonia. Atypical pneumonia usually is caused by the influenza virus, *Mycoplasma*, *Chlamydia*, *Legionella*, adenovirus, or other unidentified microorganisms. *Streptococcus pneumoniae* is the most common cause of community-acquired bacterial pneumonia.

Respiratory viruses are the most common causes of pneumonia in young children, peaking between ages 2 and 3 years. By school age, *Mycoplasma pneumoniae* becomes more common.

Tests for a microbial diagnosis are usually not done in outpatients because most patients with community-acquired pneumonia are treated empirically, based on the most common pathogens associated with the condition. Drugs of choice include doxycycline, azithromycin or levofloxacin.

Choosing between outpatient and inpatient treatment is a crucial decision because of the possible risk of death. Many infected individuals can be treated as outpatients with oral antibiotics. In the presence of an underlying chronic disease or severe symptoms, the patient will likely require hospitalization for intravenous antibiotics and oxygen therapy. Infants and the older adults are more commonly admitted for treatment of pneumonia. With treatment, most patients will improve within several days to 2 weeks. Elderly or debilitated patients who fail to respond to treatment may die from respiratory failure.

The pneumococcal vaccine prevents *S. pneumoniae* pneumonia caused by those serotypes included in the vaccine. Flu vaccine prevents pneumonia and other infections caused by influenza viruses. It must be given yearly to protect against new viral strains. Hib vaccine prevents pneumonia in children from *Haemophilus influenzae* type b.

"ATYPICAL" PNEUMONIA[1]

A Common pathogens[2]

Pathogen	Approximate prevalence (%)
Mycoplasma pneumoniae	~20
Chlamydia pneumoniae	~10
Legionella pneumophila	~7
Viruses	~7

Approximate prevalence (%): 0 10 20 30 40 50 60

B Classification of pathogens

Gram (–) rods
Legionella pneumophila

Mycoplasma
Mycoplasma pneumoniae

Chlamydia
Chlamydia pneumoniae

Double stranded, Nonenveloped — • Adenoviruses

Single stranded, Negative strand, Helical, Enveloped — Paramyxoviridae
- Influenza virus
- Respiratory syncytial virus

Mycoplasma pneumoniae

- *M. pneummoniae* is the most common cause of primary atypical pneumonia (also called "walking pneumonia" because the patient usually remains ambulatory throughout the illness). The highest incidence of disease occurs in older children and young adults (ages 6 to 20 years). *M. pneumoniae* infection of the lower respiratory tract is transmitted by respiratory droplets.
- P1 protein (a cytoadhesin) allows *M. pneumoniae* to adhere tightly to the cell surface of host ciliated bronchial epithelial cells, inhibiting ciliary action. Patches of affected mucosa desquamate, causing an inflammatory response in bronchial tissues.

Chlamydia pneumoniae

- *C. pneumoniae* is a major cause world wide of atypical pneumonia as well as community-acquired respiratory infections such, as pharyngitis, laryngitis, and bronchitis. Transmission from human to human occurs primarily by the aerosol route.
- *C. pneumoniae* is an obligate intracellular parasite. It uses adhesins to attach to susceptible host cell membrane receptors, usually in columnar or transitional epithelia. They replicate in phagocytic vesicles, eventually killing the host cell.

Legionella pneumophila

- *L. pneumophila* causes Legionnaires disease, an atypical pneumonia with multisystem symptoms. Infections generally result from inhalation of contaminated aerosol from commercial water handling systems, such as air conditioners. Human-to-human transmission does not occur.
- *L. pneumophila* replicates in cells of the monocyte–macrophage system in the alveoli, causing a necrotizing, multifocal pneumonia. In the environment, *L. pneumophila* replicates in amebas.

C Common complaints[2]

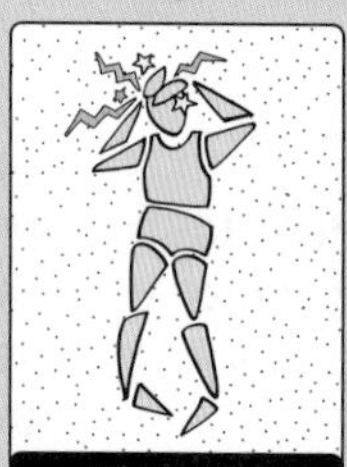

FEVER

108
104
100
98
94
Normal

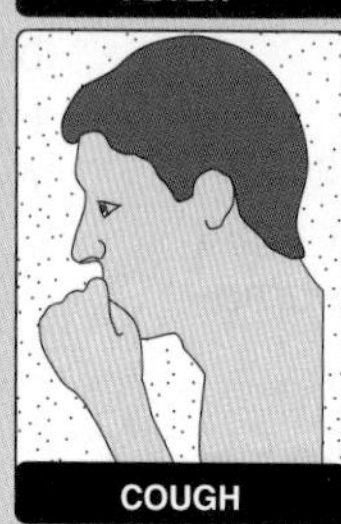

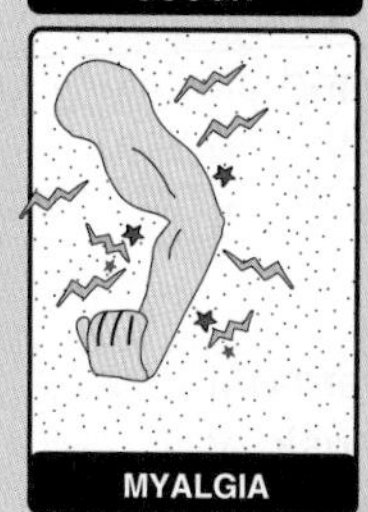

Influenza viruses

- Influenza epidemics regularly occur worldwide. Influenza infections are the most significant causes of viral pneumonia in adults. Influenza, spread by respiratory droplets, is an infection solely of the respiratory tract. There is rarely a viremia or spread to other organ systems.
- Following inhalation of influenza virus particles, infected ciliary respiratory epithelial cells desquamate and lose their ability to mechanically clear the respiratory tract. This may result in secondary bacterial pneumonia.

Respiratory syncytial virus (RSV)

- RSV is the major viral respiratory tract pathogen in the pediatric population and the most important cause of bronchiolitis and pneumonia in infants under age 1 year. It also causes atypical pneumonia in young children, an influenza-like syndrome in adults, and severe bronchitis with pneumonia in the older adults. RSV is transmitted by respiratory droplets or by contaminated hands carrying the virus to the nose or mouth. Repeated infections are common.
- Infection by RSV causes necrosis of epithelial cells in the alveoli, bronchioles, and bronchi. Mucus, dead cells, and fibrin clog the airways.

Adenovirus

- Adenoviruses cause outbreaks of lower respiratory tract infections, especially in crowded environments such as military bases. Adenoviruses are generally spread by respiratory droplets. Infected infants most commonly suffer from febrile pharyngitis, Acute respiratory disease occurs primarily in epidemics among new military recruits. These respiratory syndromes can progress to true pneumonia.
- Adenoviruses replicate well in epithelial cells, the replicative infection resulting in cell death. Systemic infections are rare.

Figure 33.8
Characteristics of atypical pneumonia.

[1]"Atypical" pneumonia is characterized by insidious onset, scant sputum and x-ray abnormalities greater than predicted by physical signs.

[2]Other pathogens include *Chlamydia psittaci*, *Pneumocystis jiroveci*, varicella-zoster virus, and parainfluenza viruses.

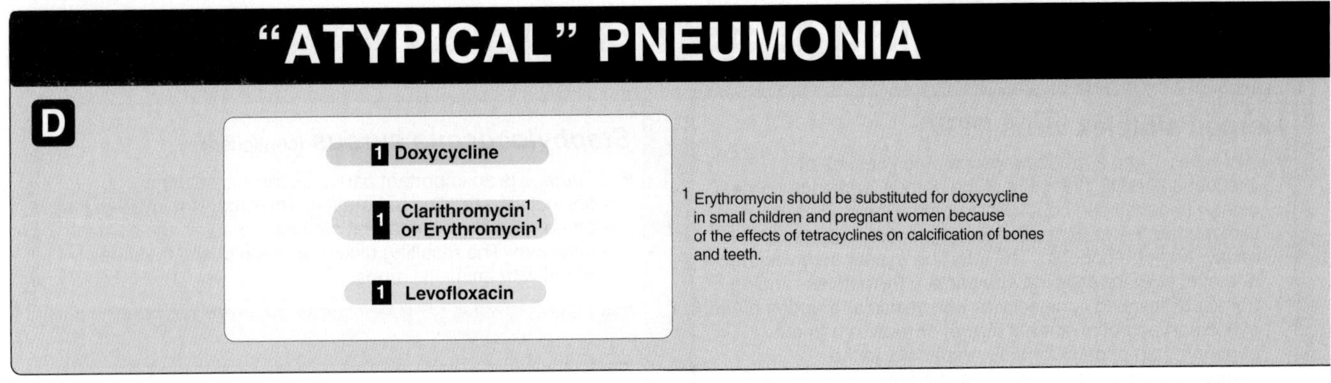

"ATYPICAL" PNEUMONIA
D
1 Doxycycline
1 Clarithromycin[1] or Erythromycin[1]
1 Levofloxacin
[1] Erythromycin should be substituted for doxycycline in small children and pregnant women because of the effects of tetracyclines on calcification of bones and teeth.

Figure 33.8 (continued)
Characteristics of atypical pneumonia (continued). 1 Indicates first-line drugs.

VIII. ATYPICAL PNEUMONIA

Pneumonia is often divided into "typical" pneumonia caused by pyogenic bacteria such as *Streptococcus. pneumoniae* or *Haemophilus influenzae*, and "atypical" pneumonia caused by organisms such as *Mycoplasma pneumoniae*, *Chlamydia pneumoniae,* and *Legionella pneumophilia* (Figure 33.8).

Atypical pneumonia caused by *M. pneumoniae* and *C. pneumoniae* usually cause milder forms of pneumonia. It is characterized by a more drawn-out course of symptoms unlike other forms of pneumonia that can come on more quickly with more severe early symptoms. In contrast, pneumonia caused by *Legionella pneumophilia* occurs particularly among older adults and those with chronic diseases and weakened immune systems. It is associated with a higher mortality rate. Atypical pneumonias: 1) exhibit a nonlobar, patchy, ill-defined infiltrate on chest radiography; and 2) failure to show a causative organism on Gram stain or culture of sputum as routinely performed.

Despite the identification of multiple causative organisms, *M. pneumoniae* is responsible for more cases of this syndrome than any other single organism.

Mycoplasma pneumonia often affects younger people and may be associated with anemia, rashes, and neurologic syndromes.

Chlamydial pneumonia is usually mild with a low mortality rate. In contrast, atypical pneumonia caused by *Legionella* accounts for 2–6 percent of pneumonias and has a higher mortality rate.

Elderly individuals, smokers, and people with chronic illnesses and weakened immune systems are at higher risk for atypical pneumonia. Contact with contaminated aerosol systems (like infected air conditioning systems) has also been associated with pneumonia caused by *Legionella.*

Patients with atypical pneumonia can generally be treated with empirical antibiotic therapy as outpatients. The drugs of choice are doxycycline and erythromycin (or azithromycin). Severe cases of atypical pneumonia, especially common with pneumonia caused by *Legionella*, may require intravenous antibiotics and oxygen supplementation. Empiric treatment of community-acquired pneumonia should always include treatment for atypical organisms.

There are no proven methods for preventing atypical pneumonia. A vaccine is administered to members of the military to prevent adenovirus infections.

DISEASES OF THE EYE

Herpes simplex virus (HSV)

- HSV types 1 and 2 are the most common causes of infectious keratitis (infection of the cornea leading to corneal ulcers) in developed countries. Symptoms include a red eye with moderately severe pain, tearing, decreased visual acuity, and photophobia. The infection usually involves only one eye. HSV keratitis may be primary (symptoms ranging from subclinical to conjunctivitis with vesicular eruption of the eyelid and potential corneal ulcers) or recurrent (more common than primary keratitis, especially in the immunocompromised, in whom symptoms generally include mild irritation and photophobia). [Note: The conjunctiva is a thin, translucent, mucous membrane that lines the eyelid and covers the white portion of the eyeball. Viral conjunctivitis is more common than bacterial conjunctivitis in developed countries.] Treatment involves application of topical antiherpes agents, such as trifluridine.
- Other herpesviruses also cause eye infections. For example, cytomegalovirus infection is particularly dangerous in acquired immune deficiency syndrome (AIDS) patients, in whom it causes a variety of diseases. One of these syndromes can cause blindness if untreated (for example, with ganciclovir or foscarnet). Varicella-zoster virus (VZV) is also dangerous for AIDS patients, causing acute retinal necrosis that is treated with acyclovir. VZV reactivation can cause zoster, which can involve the eyelid or cornea.

Adenovirus

- Adenovirus infection is a common cause of acute conjunctivitis, especially in children. This infection may occur while the child is experiencing acute febrile pharyngitis, in which case the syndrome is referred to as pharyngoconjunctival fever. Adenoviruses may be transmitted via the hands, contaminated eyedrops, or insufficiently chlorinated swimming pools. Adenoviral conjunctivitis usually resolves after seven to ten days without therapy.
- A more serious infection is epidemic keratoconjunctivitis, which involves formation of a painful ulcer of the corneal epithelium. The ulcer may result in corneal opacity lasting several years. The epidemic nature of this disease arises in part from transmission by improperly sterilized ophthalmologic instruments. No antiviral agents are currently available for adenovirus infections.

Staphylococcus aureus

- *S. aureus*, a member of the normal flora of the body, is a major cause of infections of the eyelid and cornea. For example, *S. aureus* can infect the glands of the eyelid, resulting in the production of a sty (a painful red swelling on the margin of the eyelid). Treatment consists of warm compresses applied regularly and topical antibiotic ointment (for example, bacitracin ointment).

Staphylococcus aureus (continued)

- *S. aureus* is an important cause of chronic bacterial conjunctivitis, leading to keratitis. The organism invades the cornea following trauma that causes a break in the corneal epithelium. The resulting ulcers are painful and must be treated with antibiotic drops.

Neisseria gonorrhoeae

- *N. gonorrhoeae* is the most common cause of hyperacute bacterial conjunctivitis, the most severe form of conjunctivitis. Untreated, it can lead to keratitis and corneal perforation. Ceftriaxone can be used to treat gonococcal conjunctivitis.
- Ophthalmia neonatorum (ON) refers to any conjunctival inflammation of the newborn. It is acquired by the infant during its passage through the birth canal of a mother infected with the gonococcus. [Note: Gonococci are the most serious infectious cause of ON, although *Chlamydia* are the most common cause.] If untreated, acute conjunctivitis may lead to blindness or rupture of the eye. Treatment is with IV or IM ceftriaxone.

Chlamydia trachomatis

- *C. trachomatis*, serotypes A, B, Ba, and C cause chronic keratoconjunctivitis (trachoma) that often results in blindness. Trachoma is a leading cause of blindness in endemic areas of northern India, the Middle East, and North Africa. Trachoma is transmitted by personal contact, for example, by eye-to-eye via droplets, by contaminated surfaces touched by hands and conveyed to the eye, or by flies. Because of persistent or repeated infection over several years, the inflammatory response with attendant scarring leads to permanent opacities of the cornea and distortion of eyelids.
- Over 50 percent of infants born to women infected with *C. trachomatis* serotypes D–K will contract ophthalmia neonatorum (see *N. gonorrhoeae*, above) on passage through the birth canal. The most common presentation is inclusion conjunctivitis of the newborn. This acute, purulent conjunctivitis (named for the inclusion bodies seen in infected conjunctival epithelial cells) usually heals without permanent damage to the infant's eye. Treatment is with oral erythromycin. Individuals of any age may develop a transient purulent inclusion conjunctivitis due to *C. trachomatis* serotypes D–K. Such individuals are often found to be genitally infected as well. Treatment includes any of a number of broad-spectrum antibacterial agents, such as azithromycin, erythromycin, or tetracycline (in patients older than age 8 years).

Figure 33.9

Examples of bacteria and viruses that cause diseases of the eye.
Other viruses causing eye diseases include influenza virus and rubella virus. Other bacteria causing eye diseases include *Staphylococcus pneumoniae*, *Streptococcus pyogenes*, *Haemophilus* species, *Pseudomonas aeruginosa*, *Treponema pallidum*, and *Mycobacterium tuberculosis*.

IX. DISEASES OF THE EYE

Trachoma is the most prevalent eye infection in the world (Figure 33.9). However, physicians in developed countries are more likely to encounter patients with: 1) conjunctivitis (or pink eye), marked by pus or watery discharge and crust on the eyelashes; 2) styes, an abscess in the follicle of an eyelash; and 3) blepharitis, inflammation of the eyelids. Conjunctivitis is a condition which is often treated with antibiotics even though a minority of cases are caused by bacterial infection. Although it has characteristic signs, herpes simplex keratitis can be misdiagnosed as conjunctivitis.

Gonococcal eye infections are never treated topically and are always treated parenterally. Whether used for prophylaxis in an infant whose mother is known to have gonococcal cervicitis or for treatment of established gonococcal ophthalmia neonatorum, the CDC's recommendations are limited to IV or IM ceftriaxone. This is separate from the prophylactic use of erythromycin in the eyes of newborns regardless of the status of the mother, which is widely recommended and in many jurisdictions required by law.

X. OPPORTUNISTIC INFECTIONS OF HIV

Individuals with advanced human immunodeficiency virus (HIV) infection are vulnerable to infections and malignancies called "opportunistic infections" because they take advantage of the opportunity offered by a weakened immune system (Figure 33.10). The clinical symptoms of HIV infection are mainly caused by the emergence of opportunistic infections and cancers that the immune system would normally prevent. Infections that are rarely seen in those with normal immune systems are deadly to those with HIV.

Different opportunistic infections typically occur at different stages of HIV infection. Patients with early HIV disease can develop tuberculosis, malaria, bacterial pneumonia, herpes zoster, staphylococcal skin infections, and septicemia. These are diseases that can affect individuals with normal immune systems, but occur at a much higher rate, and with greater severity, in HIV patients.

When the immune system is very weak due to advanced HIV disease, opportunistic infections such as *Pneumocystis jiroveci*, toxoplasmosis, and cryptococcosis develop. Many of the opportunistic infections that occur at this late stage can be fatal.

The development of highly active antiretroviral therapies (HAART, p. 303) has greatly decreased the morbidity and mortality from HIV. HAART is effective in preventing opportunistic infections and should be considered for all HIV-infected persons.

However, certain patients are unable to take HAART, and others have not responded to HAART regimens. Such patients will benefit from prophylaxis against opportunistic infections. In addition, prophylaxis against specific opportunistic infections continues to provide survival benefits even among persons who are receiving HAART. With HAART, antimicrobial prophylaxis for opportunistic infections may not need to be lifelong.

Antiretroviral therapy can restore immune function. The period of susceptibility to opportunistic processes continues to be accurately indicated by $CD4^+$ T-lymphocyte counts for patients receiving HAART. Stopping prophylactic regimens can simplify treatment, reduce toxicity and drug interactions, lower cost of care, and potentially facilitate adherence to antiretroviral regimens.

OPPORTUNISTIC INFECTIONS OF HIV

A Bacteria

Mycobacterium avium complex

- *Mycobacterium avium-intracellulare complex* (MAC) is a complex of acid-fast bacilli, serotypes of which infect birds and various mammals. MAC is ubiquitous, and individuals can easily acquire a MAC infection.
- In the United States, disseminated (miliary) disease caused by MAC is the most common systemic bacterial infection in aquired human immune deficiency syndrome (AIDS) patients and is responsible for significant morbidity. Serious pulmonary diseases include chronic bronchitis and pneumonia. Cervical lymphadenitis, chronic osteomyelitis, and renal or skin infections can occur. Clinical presentation usually includes fevers, night sweats, chills, and weight loss. In AIDS patients undergoing HAART treatment, cases of MAC-caused disease have sharply declined.
- Diseases caused by MAC are particularly refractory to chemotherapy. Because of the large number of resistant variants, treatment of disease and prevention of reinfections requires two to four drugs given simultaneously. Relapses are common.

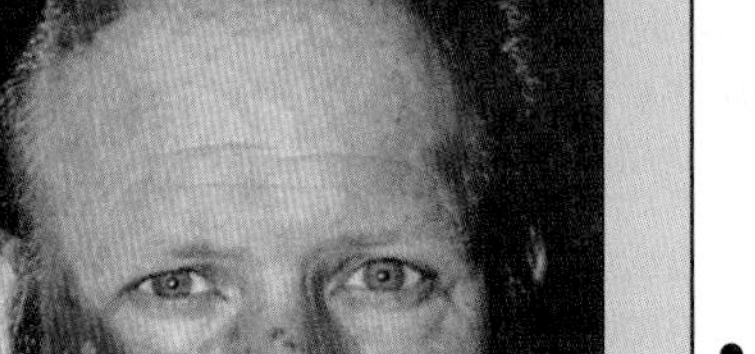

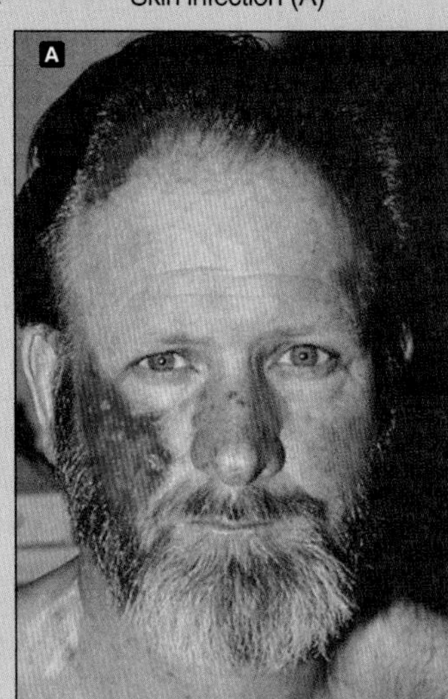

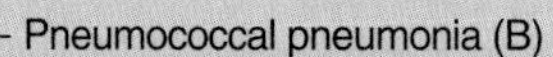

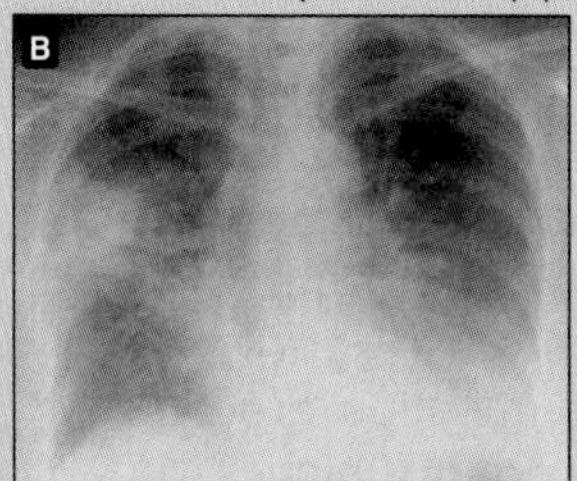

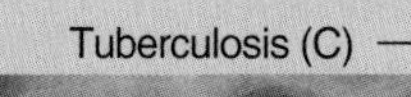

Streptococcus pneumoniae

- *S. pneumoniae* (pneumococci) are gram-positive, nonmotile, encapsulated cocci that tend to occur in pairs (diplococci). They can be found in the nasopharynx of many healthy individuals. *S. pneumoniae* can be spread endogenously (if the carrier develops impaired resistance to the organism) or exogenously (by droplets from the nose of a carrier).
- *S. pneumoniae* is the most common bacterial respiratory pathogen in HIV-positive patients. The *S. pneumoniae* cell-associated virulence factors autolysin and pneumolysin contribute to its pathogenicity. The organism causes acute bacterial pneumonia and is a leading cause of death. *S. pneumoniae* also causes bacteremia/sepsis and meningitis.
- Those *S. pneumoniae* strains that are resistant to penicillin G remain sensitive to third-generation cephalosporins and vancomycin.

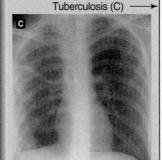

Mycobacterium tuberculosis

- Once a disease mainly of older adults, clinical tuberculosis has become more prevalent among younger individuals (ages 25 to 44 years) and among children. In the United States, the increase is attributed to the high prevalence of mycobacterial disease in AIDS patients (for whom it is a major health threat) and the increase in immigrants, particularly from southeast Asia.
- Transmission occurs when patients with active pulmonary tuberculosis shed large numbers of organisms by coughing. The organisms are resistant to desiccation and can remain viable in the surroundings for a long time. Individuals with a depressed immune system, especially those who are HIV positive, are particularly susceptible to infection.
- In the primary disease, *M. tuberculosis* survives and grows within host cells such as macrophages, which can carry the organisms to additional sites. Productive (granulomatous) lesions known as tubercles can develop at those sites. In AIDS patients, as their immunity wanes, the primary infection is generally progressive, and one or more of the tubercles may expand, leading to destruction of tissue and clinical illness, for example, chronic pneumonitis, tuberculous osteomyelitis, or tuberculous meningitis. If active tubercles develop throughout the body, the condition is known as miliary (disseminated) tuberculosis. Reactivation of preexisting tubercles is caused by an impairment in immune status, such as that seen in AIDS.
- Because of the large number of drug-resistant strains of *M. tuberculosis*, treatment includes two or more drugs to prevent outgrowth of resistant strains. Principal drugs used include isoniazid, ethambutol, pyrazinamide and rifampin. The bacille Calmette-Guerin antituberculosis vaccine should not be given to AIDS or other immunosuppressed individuals because it contains live organisms, and has occasionally become virulent.

Figure 33.10 (continued on next page)
Organisms frequently causing infections in patients infected with human immunodeficiency virus (HIV). [Note: Other important bacterial species causing infection in HIV patients include *Haemophilus influenzae* (pneumonia), *Campylobacter* species (diarrhea), *Shigella* species (diarrhea and bacteremia).]
HAART = highly active antiviral therapy.

OPPORTUNISTIC INFECTIONS OF HIV

A Bacteria (continued)

Salmonella species

- *Salmonella* are flagellated, motile, gram-negative bacilli, routinely found in the GI tract of humans and other animals. *Salmonella* are transmitted most frequently by the fecal–oral route (often with food as an intermediary) but can also be transmitted to humans by pets such as turtles. Serovar Typhimurium is of particular concern because it is increasingly drug-resistant.
- *Salmonella* invade epithelial cells of the small intestine. In immunocompromised hosts, the infection can become systemic with disseminated foci. In HIV-infected individuals, a high-grade bacteremia can occur, in which *Salmonella* seed distant organs, and in older patients, tends to seed pre-existing atherosclerotic plaque. Fever can last indefinitely in untreated focal *Salmonella* infection. *Salmonella* infections also cause severe gastroenteritis, characterized by nausea, vomiting, and diarrhea.
- The treatment for *Salmonella* infections in an immunocompromised host is typically ciprofloxacin. Alternative treatments (depending on drug resistance) include ampicillin or trimethoprim-sulfamethoxazole. In patients with AIDS, relapse is a major problem. Therefore, months of therapy are required.

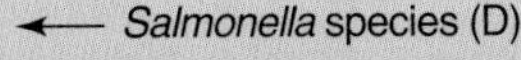

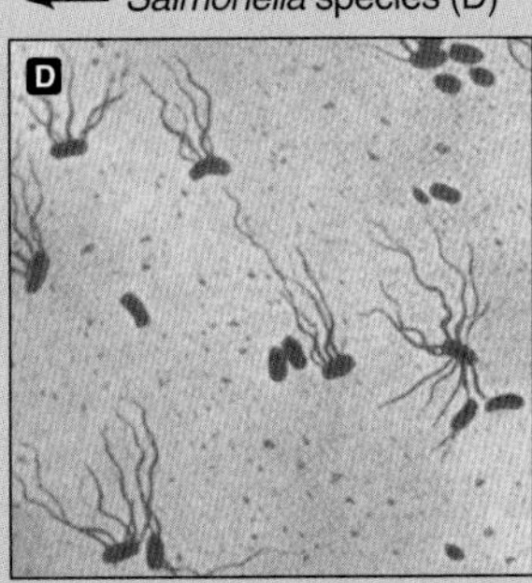

Pulmonary histoplasmosis (E)→

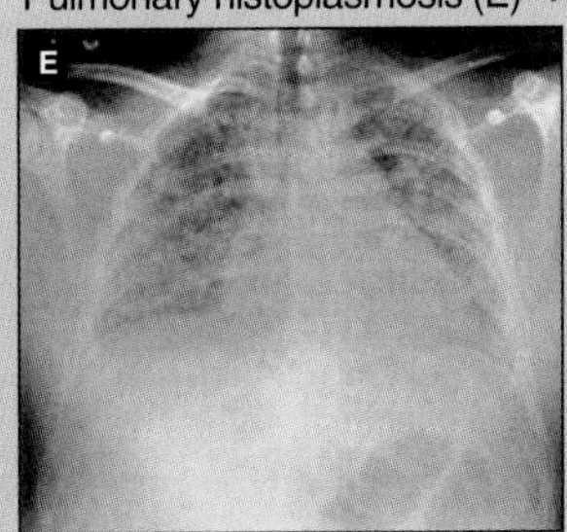

Histoplasma capsulatum

- *H. capsulatum* is a soil fungus that is found worldwide but is most prevalent in central North America. The organism produces spores that, when airborne, enter the lungs and germinate into yeast-like cells. These yeast cells are engulfed by macrophages in which they multiply.
- In healthy individuals, pulmonary infections with *H. capsulatum* may be acute but self-limiting. In HIV-infected persons, nearly all cases are disseminated at the time of diagnosis. Dissemination results from invasion of cells of the reticuloendothelial system, which distinguishes this organism as the only fungus to exhibit intracellular parasitism. Disseminated histoplasmosis causes fever, weight loss, hypertension, and pulmonary distress. If untreated, it can lead to respiratory and liver failure.
- *H. capsulatum* infection is treated with itraconazole, with amphotericin B as an alternative. Life-long maintenance therapy may be required to prevent reoccurrence of the disease in HIV-positive patients.

B Fungi

Candida species

- *Candida albicans* and other *Candida* species are part of the normal body flora. They are found in the skin, mouth, vagina, and intestines. Candidiasis is the most common fungal infection of HIV-positive individuals. The presence of esophageal candidiasis is a hallmark of the progression from HIV infection to AIDS.
- Candidiasis is generally limited to oral, esophageal, or vaginal mucosa. Oral candidiasis (thrush) presents as raised, white plaques on the oral mucosa, tongue, or gums. The plaques can become confluent and ulcerated and can spread to the esophagus (an indicator of full-blown AIDS). Vaginal candidiasis presents as itching and burning pain of the vulva and vagina, accompanied by a thick or thin white discharge. Vaginal candidiasis frequently recurs. Systemic candidiasis is rare.
- Candidiasis is treated with fluconazole or itraconazole. However, azole-resistant strains of *Candida* require alternative treatment, for example, with amphotericin B.

← Oral candidiasis (F)

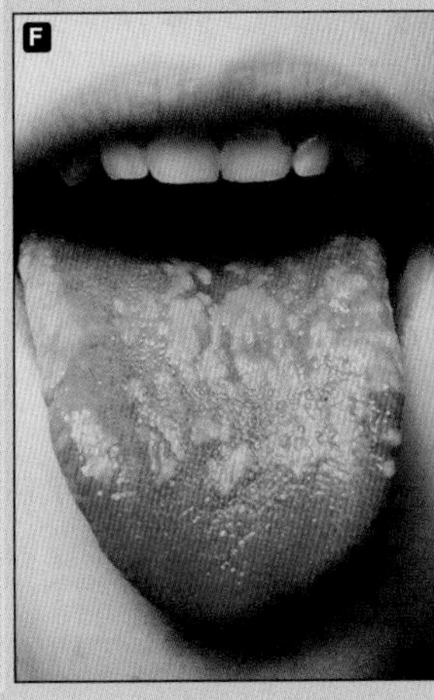

Cryptococcus neoformans

- *C. neoformans* is a yeast that is found world wide. It is especially abundant in soil containing bird droppings. Its spores are inhaled.
- In healthy persons, cryptococcosis is generally a mild, subclinical lung infection. In AIDS patients, cryptococcosis is the second most common fungal infection and potentially the most serious. In these individuals, the infection often disseminates to the brain and meninges, causing meningitis, frequently with fatal consequences. Presenting symptoms include fever, headache, and malaise. Patients are often forgetful and lethargic.
- Cryptococcal meningitis is treated with fluconazole, with amphotericin B as an alternative. This therapy should be continued lifelong to prevent reoccurrence of the infection.

Cutaneous cryptococcosis (G)

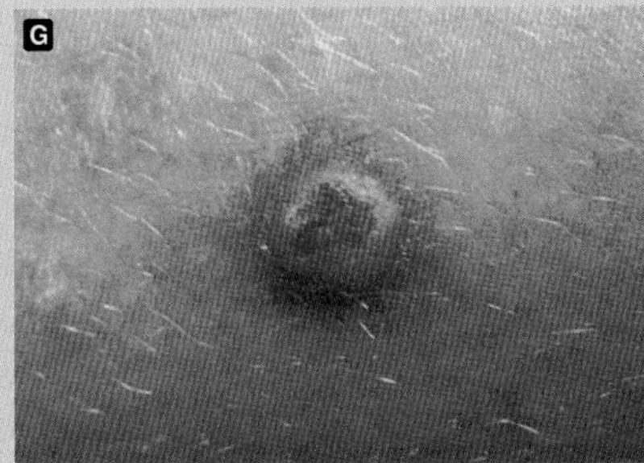

Figure 33.10 (continued on next page)
Organisms causing opportunistic infections in patients infected with human immunodeficiency virus (HIV). [Note: Other opportunistic fungal infections include aspergillosis and coccidioidomycosis.]

OPPORTUNISTIC INFECTIONS OF HIV

C Other

Pneumocystis jiroveci

- *P. jiroveci* is a unicellular eukaryote. It is the most common opportunistic pathogen in AIDS patients.
- *P. jiroveci* causes frequently fatal *P. jiroveci* pneumonia (PJP). Before the use of immunosuppressive drugs and the AIDS epidemic, PJP was a rare disease. It is almost 100 percent fatal if untreated.
- Prophylaxis with trimethoprim-sulfamethoxazole is recommended for HIV-infected patients with fewer than 200 CD4+ cells/µl. However, individuals infected with HIV who are undergoing treatment with HAART have shown a significant decrease in incidence of PJP.

Cryptosporidium species

- *Cryptosporidium* is an intracellular parasite that inhabits the epithelial cells of the villi of the lower small intestine. The source of infection is often the feces of domestic animals and farm run-off has been implicated as a source of cryptosporidium contamination of drinking water.
- Infection of healthy individuals may be asymptomatic or may cause mild cases of diarrhea, which are generally self-limiting. However, in AIDS patients, the infection may be severe and intractable. Cryptosporidiosis causes diarrhea that varies from mild to a fulminant, persistent cholera-like illness. Patients experience nausea, vomiting, abdominal pain, and weight loss.
- In AIDS patients, no treatment for cryptosporidiosis has proven completely effective, although paromomycin has provided some improvement.

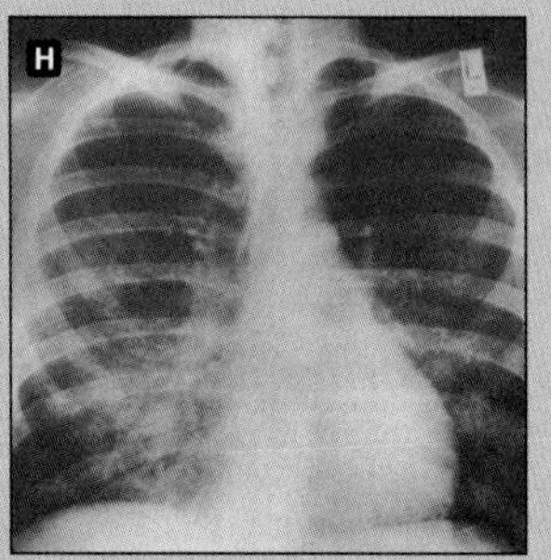

Pneumocystis pneumonia

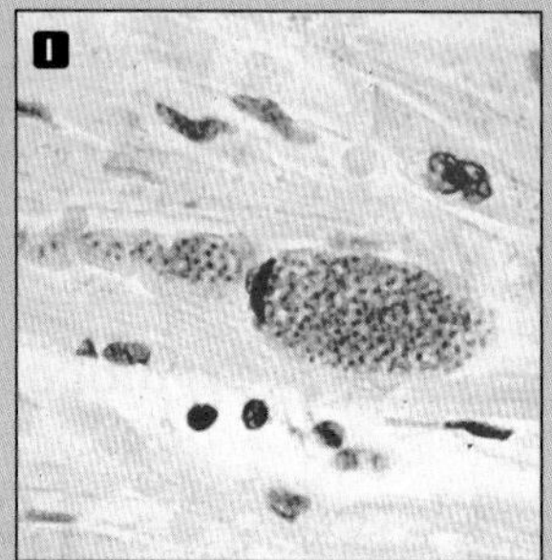

Toxopolasma gondii

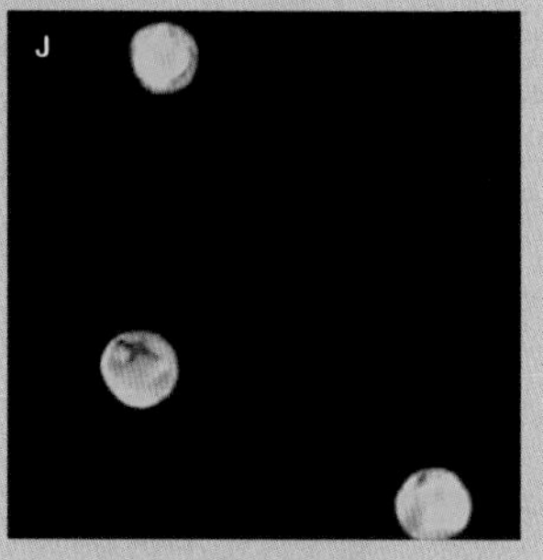

Cryptosporidium species

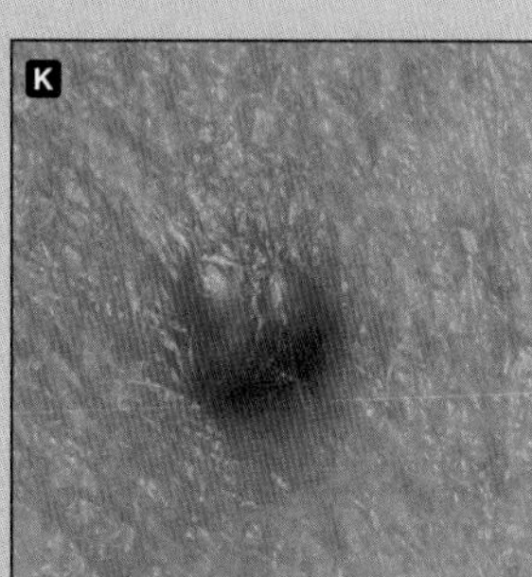

Kaposi sarcoma

D Parasites

Toxoplasma gondii

- *T. gondii* is a sporozoan, distributed worldwide, which infects all vertebrate species, although the definitive host is the cat. Transmission is by accidental ingestion of oocysts present in cat feces, eating raw or undercooked meat, congenitally from an infected mother, or from a blood transfusion. Rapidly growing *T. gondii* trophozoites establish early, acute infections. Slowly growing trophozoites encyst in muscle and brain tissue and in the eye.
- *T. gondii* infections of healthy humans are asymptomatic and common, but they are the most common cause of focal encephalitis in AIDS patients. Toxoplasmosis in this population is usually due to reemergence of encysted organisms, rather than from new, exogenous infection. Clinical presentation of encephalitis can include weakness, confusion, seizures, or coma. Disseminated toxoplasmosis can involve the heart, skeletal muscle, lung, colon, and other organs.
- *T. gondii* infection is treated with a combination of sulfadiazine and pyrimethamine. Lifelong secondary prophylaxis involves sulfadiazine plus pyrimethamine.

E Viruses

Human herpesvirus type 8 (HHV-8)

- HHV-8 (also known as Kaposi sarcoma-associated herpesvirus) is a member of the Herpesviridae family. It is enveloped, with a double-stranded DNA genome.
- In the United States, antibodies to HHV-8 antigens are found primarily in the same populations at risk for HIV infection, leading to the conclusion that the primary mode of transmission is sexual. The frequency of perinatal transmission of HHV-8 appears low.
- HHV-8 has been detected in over 90 percent of patients with Kaposi sarcoma (KS), but in less than 1 percent of non-KS tissues. KS was the most common neoplasm in AIDS patients but has essentially disappeared from those HIV-infected individuals with access to HAART treatment. There is no established independent drug treatment for HHV-8 infected individuals.

Figure 33.10 (continued on the next page)
Organisms causing opportunistic infections in patients infected with human immunodeficiency virus (HIV).

OPPORTUNISTIC INFECTIONS OF HIV

E Viruses (continued)

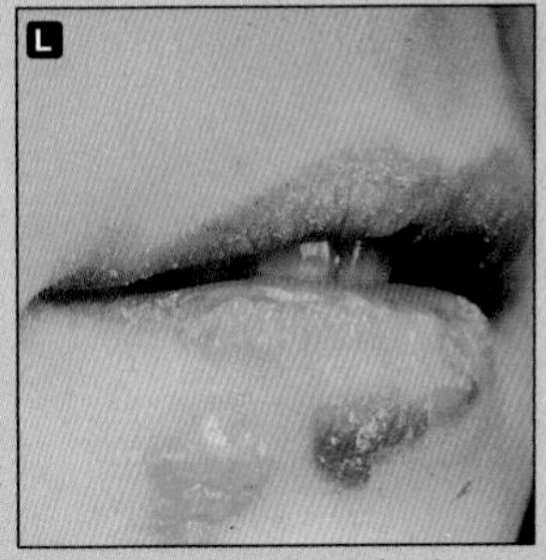

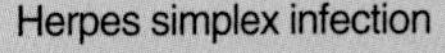
Herpes simplex infection

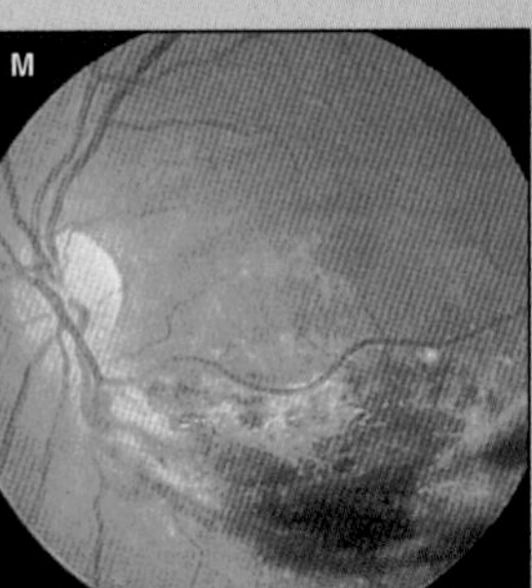

Cytomegalovirus retinitis

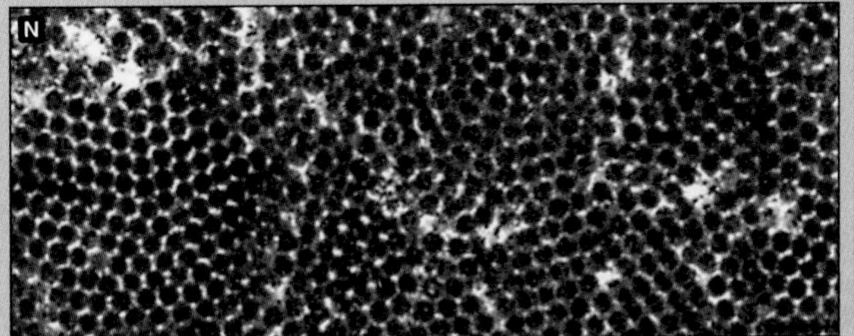

JC virus particles from an infected oligodendrocyte nucleus

Herpes simplex virus (HSV)

- HSV types 1 and 2 are members of the *Herpesviridae* family. They are enveloped, with a double-stranded DNA genome. Initial infection with HSV is by direct contact with virus-containing secretion, or with lesions on mucosal surfaces. HSV can also be transmitted during birth. HSV coinfection of patients with HIV infection occurs frequently, probably because of their similar modes of transmission.
- Initial replication of the virus is in epithelial cells of the mucosal surface onto which they have been inoculated. In individuals with depressed immune systems, the virus reproduces and can be transported to various sites in the body. It also establishes lifelong latent infections in the regional ganglia.
- Reactivation of latent virus leading to invasive HSV infections in AIDS patients becomes increasingly important as CD4+ lymphocyte counts decline. Herpetic ulcers occur on the face, hand, or genitals, and oral ulcers occur. Recurrence of genital herpes can be more frequent and severe in HIV-infected persons.
- If primary or recurrent herpes episodes are particularly frequent and/or severe, acyclovir or, alternatively, famciclovir can be administered.

JC virus (JCV)

- JCV is a member of the *Papovaviridae* family, *Polyomaviridae* subfamily. It is a nonenveloped virus containing supercoiled, double-stranded, circular DNA.
- As HIV-infected individuals become increasingly immunocompromised, approximately 5 percent of them will develop progressive multifocal leukoencephalopathy (PML), so called because the lesions are restricted to the white matter of the brain. In PML, reactivated JCV carries out a cytocidal infection of the brain's oligodendrocytes. This leads to demyelination caused by loss of capacity of myelinated cells to maintain their sheaths. Early development of impaired speech and mental capacity is rather rapidly followed by paralysis and sensory abnormalities, with death commonly occurring within 3 to 6 months of the initial symptoms.
- JCV is transmitted by droplets from the upper respiratory tract of infected persons and possibly through contact with their urine. The virus spreads from the upper respiratory tract to the kidneys, where it may persist in an inactive state in the tubular epithelium of healthy individuals.
- A regimen of HAART plus cidofovir is currently showing some promise in patients experiencing PML. Because infection with JCV is nearly universal and asymptomatic, and PML represents reactivation of latent virus in the immunocompromised host, there are no viable preventive measures at present.

Human cytomegalovirus (HCMV)

- HCMV is a member of the *Herpesviridae* family. It is enveloped, with a double-stranded DNA genome. Initial infection with HCMV commonly occurs during childhood. Transmission is via body fluids such as tears, urine, saliva, milk, semen, and vaginal secretion or organ transplants, or by blood transfusions. HCMV can also be transmitted transplacentally. HCMV coinfection of patients with HIV infection occurs frequently, probably because of their similar modes of transmission.
- Initial replication of the virus in epithelial cells of the respiratory and GI tracts is followed by viremia and infection of all organs of the body, including the kidney tubule epithelium, liver, CNS, and respiratory and GI tracts. The virus establishes latency, predominantly in the monocytes and macrophages, among other cells.
- Reactivation of latent virus leading to invasive HCMV infections in AIDS patients becomes increasingly frequent as CD4+ lymphocyte counts decline. Any organ system can be affected, but blindness due to HCMV chorioretinitis is especially common, developing in more than 20 percent of AIDS patients whose CD4+ count is less than 50/µl. Encephalitis, dementia, esophagitis, enterocolitis, and gastritis are other significant problems caused by HCMV. In addition, coinfection with HCMV may accelerate the progression of AIDS. At autopsy, 90 percent of AIDS patients are shown to be infected with HCMV. However, the incidence of HCMV chorioretinitis has been significantly decreased in HIV-infected individuals being treated with HAART.
- The drug regimen for both primary prophylaxis (when recommended) and prevention of recurrence of HCMV infections in AIDS patients includes ganciclovir, cidofovir, and/or foscarnet. Oral valganciclovir is also licensed for the treatment of HCMV chorioretinitis.

Figure 33.10 (continued)
Organisms causing opportunistic infections in patients infected with human immunodeficiency virus (HIV). [Note: Other opportunistic viral infections include shingles and oral hairy leukoplakia.]

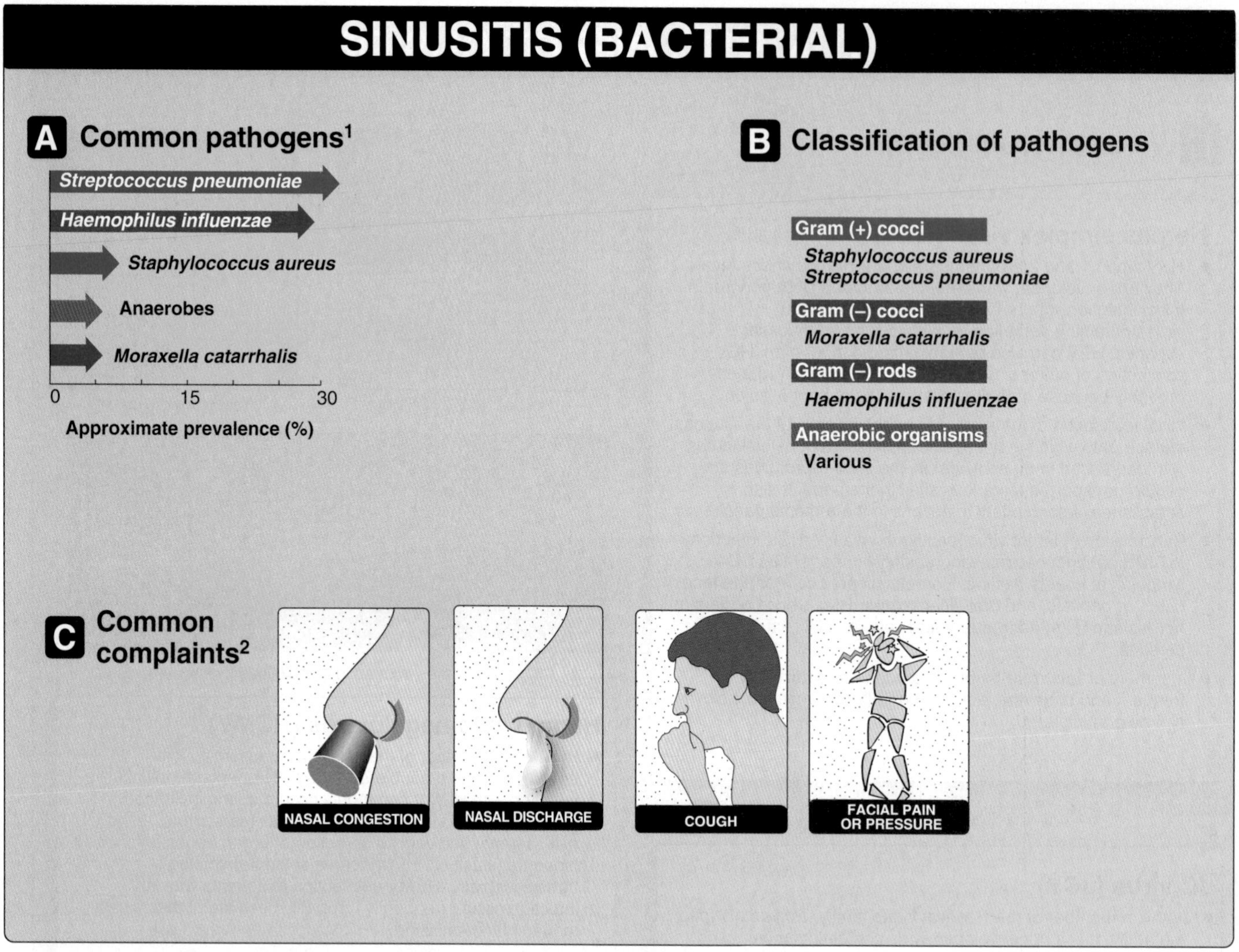

SINUSITIS (BACTERIAL)

A Common pathogens[1]

Streptococcus pneumoniae
Haemophilus influenzae
Staphylococcus aureus
Anaerobes
Moraxella catarrhalis
0 15 30
Approximate prevalence (%)

B Classification of pathogens

Gram (+) cocci
Staphylococcus aureus
Streptococcus pneumoniae
Gram (–) cocci
Moraxella catarrhalis
Gram (–) rods
Haemophilus influenzae
Anaerobic organisms
Various

C Common complaints[2]

NASAL CONGESTION
NASAL DISCHARGE
COUGH
FACIAL PAIN OR PRESSURE

Figure 33.11
Characteristics of bacterial sinusitis.
[1]Experts vary widely in their recommendations for antibiotics. [2]Other symptoms include maxillary tooth discomfort, hyposmia (diminished sense of smell), headache, fever (nonacute), halitosis, fatigue, ear pain, and ear fullness.

XI. BACTERIAL SINUSITIS

Acute sinusitis is an infection of one or more of the paranasal (alongside the nose) sinuses. A viral infection accompanying the common cold is the most frequent cause of acute sinusitis. Viral infection is also the most common predisposing condition associated with acute bacterial sinusitis. However, only approximately 2 percent of viral sinusitis is complicated by acute bacterial sinusitis. There appear to be no signs and symptoms of acute respiratory illness that are both sensitive and specific in making the distinction between bacterial and viral infection. Bacterial sinusitis is usually a self-limited disease, with 75 percent of cases resolving without treatment in one month. However, individuals with untreated acute bacterial sinusitis are at risk of developing intracranial and orbital complications as well as chronic sinus disease.

Viral sinusitis is associated with the presence of rhinovirus, parainfluenza, and influenza viruses in sinus aspirates. Other viruses which cause acute respiratory disease can also presumably produce viral sinusitis.

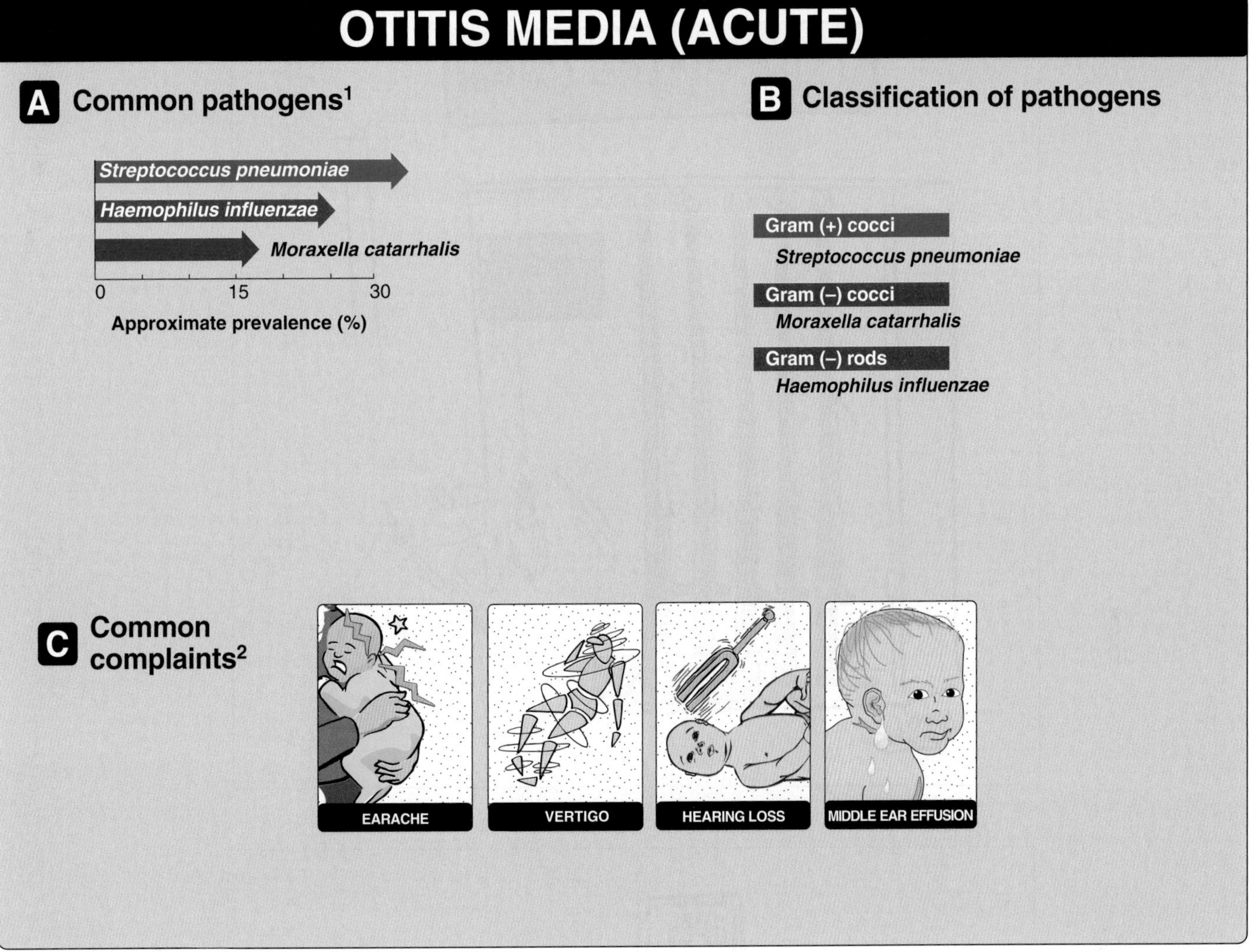

Figure 33.12
Some characteristics of acute bacterial otitis media.
[1]Other pathogens include *Staphylococcus aureus*, group A Streptococcus, and *Pseudomonas aeruginosa*.
[2]Nonspecific symptoms and signs include fever, irritability, headache, apathy, anorexia, vomiting, and diarrhea.

XII. OTITIS MEDIA

Otitis media is one of the most frequent diagnoses in sick children visiting physicians' offices and accounts for almost one third of all antibiotic prescriptions for children in the United States.

Acute otitis media is characterized by the presence of fluid in the middle ear accompanied by acute signs of illness, and usually occurs in young children. Fluid may persist for weeks to months after the onset of signs of acute otitis media, despite appropriate therapy. Whenever fluid fills the middle ear space, there is some loss of hearing, which may lead to problems of development of speech, language, and cognitive abilities in the child.

Otitis media often follows a upper respiratory tract viral infection or allergy that results in congestion of the respiratory mucosa of the nose, nasopharynx, and eustachian tube. Congestion of the mucosa in the eustachian tube causes an obstruction which can lead to accumulation of secretions produced by the mucosa of the middle ear. These secretions have no way to exit and accumulate in the middle ear space. Viruses and bacteria that colonize the upper respiratory tract can reach the middle ear and may result in suppuration (formation of pus) with clinical signs of acute otitis media.

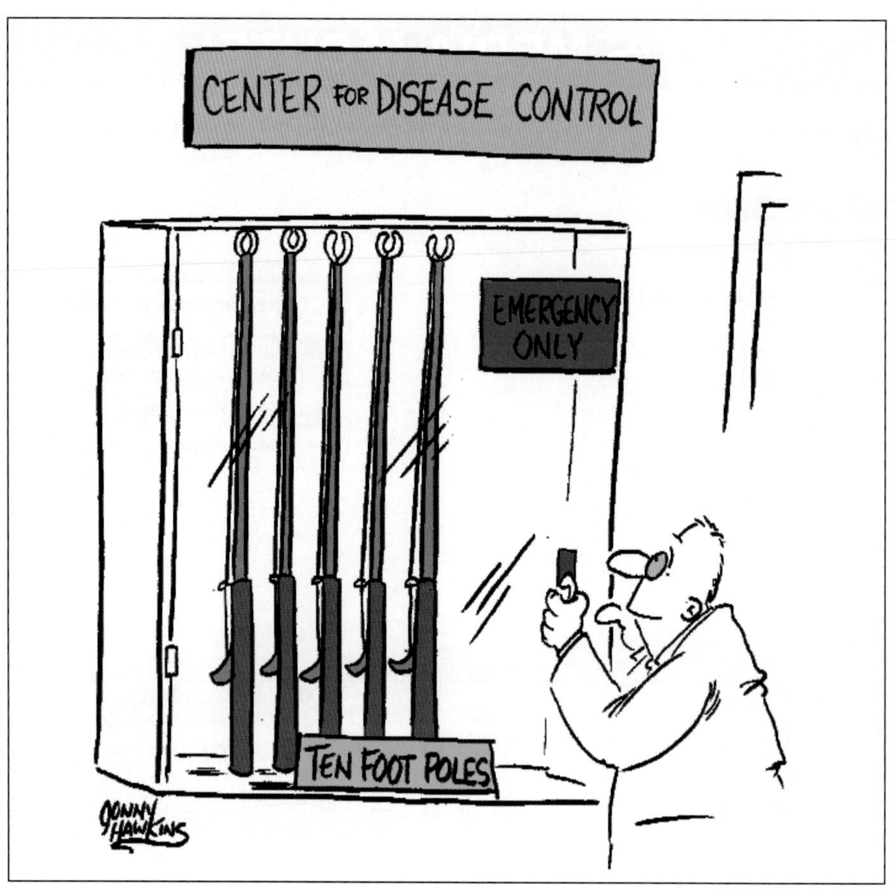

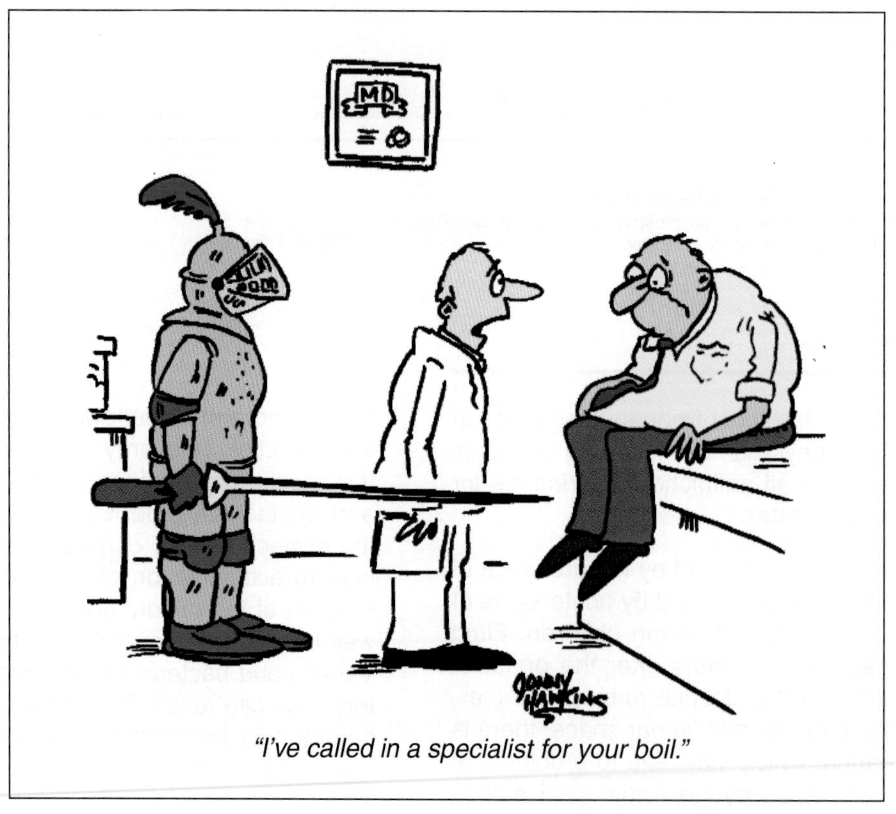

"I've called in a specialist for your boil."

Illustrated Case Studies

34

I. OVERVIEW

These extended case studies complement the basic information presented in Chapters 1 through 31. They reinforce basic principles of clinical microbiology, such as the role of a Gram stain, and the patient's history in instituting effective antimicrobial therapy—concepts useful in answering examination questions, and in the clinics. Most of the cases provide clinical information obtained from a single patient, although a few cases describe a composite of typical features derived from several patients.

Case 1: Man with necrosis of the great toe

This 63-year-old man with a long history of diabetes mellitus was seen in consultation because of an abrupt deterioration in his clinical status. He was admitted to the hospital for treatment of an ulcer, which had been present on his left great toe for several months. Figure 34.1 shows a typical example of lower extremity ulcer in a diabetic man.

Because of the inability of medical therapy (multiple courses of oral antibiotics) to resolve the ulcer, he underwent amputation of his left leg below the knee. On the first postoperative day he developed a temperature of 101°F, and on the second postoperative day he became disoriented and his temperature reached 105.2°F. His amputation stump was mottled with many areas of purplish discoloration, and the most distal areas were quite obviously necrotic (dead). Crepitus (the sensation of displacing gas when an area is pressed with the fingers) was palpable up to his patella. An X-ray of the left lower extremity showed gas in the soft tissues, extending beyond the knee to the area of the distal femur. A Gram stain of a swab from the necrotic tissue is shown in Figure 34.2.

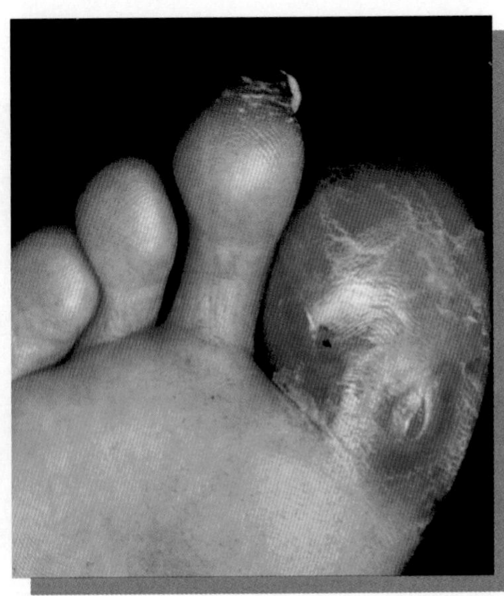

Figure 34.1
Perforating ulcer of the great toe.

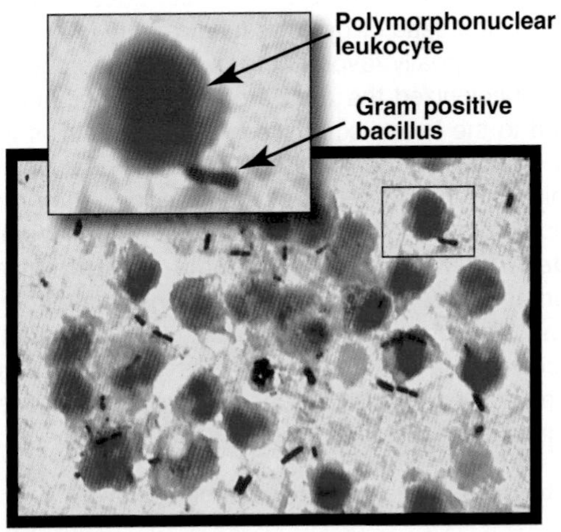

Figure 34.2
Gram stain of material swabbed from deep within a crepitant area. There are numerous polymorphonuclear leukocytes and many large gram-positive bacilli, as well as a few gram-negative bacilli and cocci.

34.1 Based on the morphology of the gram-positive organisms, their most likely identification is:

A. *Streptococcus pyogenes.*
B. *Escherichia coli.*
C. *Actinomyces israelii.*
D. *Clostridium perfringens.*
E. *Staphylococcus aureus.*

The correct answer is **D** (*Clostridium perfringens*), which is a rather large, gram-positive bacillus. **A** (*Streptococcus pyogenes*) cannot be correct because it is a gram-positive coccus, not a bacillus. **B** (*Escherichia coli*) is incorrect because it is a gram-negative rod, not a gram-positive organism. **C** (*Actinomyces israelii*) is, in fact a gram-positive bacillus, but it is thin to the point of being described as filamentous and characteristically branched and, therefore, is essentially impossible to mistake for a *Clostridium*. **E** (*Staphylococcus aureus*) is a gram-positive coccus, not a bacillus.

The patient was treated with massive intravenous doses of aqueous penicillin G, together with intravenous gentamicin. He underwent an above-knee amputation of his leg and, after a very stormy period of hectic fever and hypotension, he began to improve. Cultures from deep within his necrotic amputation stump grew *Clostridium perfringens* and *Pseudomonas aeruginosa*. Throughout his course his hemoglobin, which was tested repeatedly while he was very ill, remained stable.

Discussion: This patient had *Clostridium perfringens* gas gangrene, one of the dreaded complications that may follow lower extremity amputation in diabetics. Diabetics sometimes require amputation of part or all of a lower extremity because the blood supply to these limbs is reduced by accelerated atherosclerosis, which occludes blood vessels. The resulting dead or dying tissue has very low oxygen tension, which greatly favors the growth of anaerobes. *C. perfringens* colonized the area around the anus, and may be spread to the lower extremities. If the amputation is insufficient, it may leave behind tissue whose blood supply is compromised to the point that oxygen tension in the remaining stump favors the growth of anaerobes. The elaboration, by *C. perfringens*, of large amounts of gas that are not absorbed by the tissues allows the clostridial organisms to spread along fascial planes, which are separated by the pressure of the gas as the clostridia grows. Thus gas production acts as a "virulence factor," which makes this organism quite ferocious.

Why be concerned about the hemoglobin level?

The reason that the physicians were worried about the stability of the patient's hemoglobin is that another virulence factor of *C. perfringens* is an exotoxin (the α-toxin) with lecithinase activity. Because red blood cell membranes are rich in lecithin, this toxin, which is secreted by the bacteria directly into the bloodstream, destroys red blood cell membranes, causing cells to lyse. Patients who die of overwhelming *C. perfringens* infection may have their red blood cells destroyed so rapidly that the resulting anemia is itself fatal.

How do you explain the presence of *Pseudomonas* in the wound?

Pseudomonas was probably selected for by the antibiotics that the patient received prior to his surgery, during the attempts to treat his ulcer as an out-patient. Antibiotics exert great pressure on the microbial flora of the skin and bowel. Less resistant organisms on his skin and in his bowel were replaced by those that could withstand many antibiotics such as *Pseudomonas aeruginosa*. Anaerobic infections tend to be mixed with facultative anaerobic and aerobic bacteria, as this one was.

Case 2: Adult conjunctivitis

This 15-year-old boy was admitted because of pain and redness of his left eye, which had lasted for 4 days. He had previously been well. Four days prior to medical evaluation he awoke with pain in his left eye, accompanied by a thick, yellow discharge from the conjunctiva. He saw an ophthalmologist, who obtained a culture of the yellow discharge, and prescribed tobramycin ophthalmic antibiotic drops, which the patient began to use the same day.

The patient's eye remained severely inflamed after 4 days of treatment with eye drops (Figure 34.3). The conjunctiva was very swollen and injected (the blood vessels were very dilated, or "bloodshot"). At a follow-up visit on the fourth day of treatment, the patient reported minimal improvement in his symptoms. The culture taken at the first visit had grown a gram-negative diplococcus that utilized only glucose.

A swab of the yellow discharge from this patient's eye

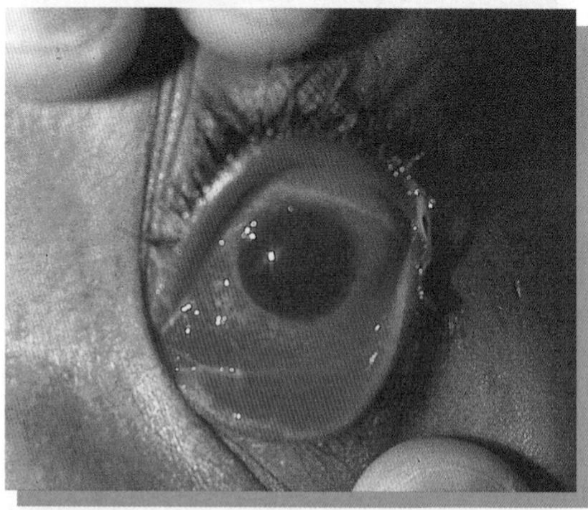

Figure 34.3
Inflamed eye of patient.

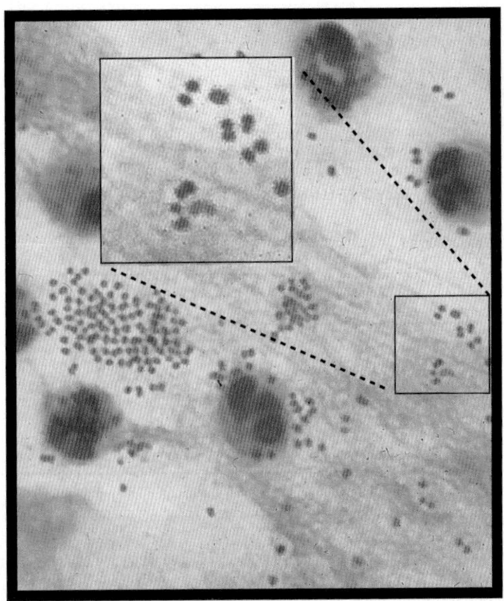

Figure 34.4
Gram stain of discharge from eye.

would have the appearance of Figure 34.4 on Gram stain, with numerous polymorphonuclear leukocytes, several containing kidney bean–shaped, gram-negative diplococci.

34.2 Based on the morphology and carbon source utilization profile of the organism that grew in the culture, the most likely etiology of this eye infection is:

A. *Escherichia coli.*
B. *Neisseria gonorrhoeae* (gonococcus).
C. *Neisseria meningitidis* (meningococcus).
D. *Streptococcus pneumoniae* (pneumococcus).
E. *Staphylococcus aureus.*

The correct answer is **B** (*Neisseria gonorrhoeae*). It is a gram-negative diplococcus that utilizes glucose, not maltose or lactose, and it is known to cause serious ocular infections when it is inoculated directly in the eye (see below). **A** (*Escherichia coli*) is incorrect because *E. coli* is a gram-negative bacillus, not a coccus. **C** (*Neisseria meningitidis*) is not acceptable because, although it is a gram-negative diplococcus, it utilizes both maltose *and* glucose, eliminating it from consideration based on the information available. **D** (*Streptococcus pneumoniae*) is incorrect because it is a gram-*positive* diplococcus, not a gram-*negative* one. **E** (*Staphylococcus aureus*) is incorrect because it is a gram-*positive* coccus and is characteristically arranged in clusters, not in pairs.

The patient was treated with ceftriaxone, and his eye cleared dramatically. At the time of his second visit to the ophthalmologist, he was asked whether he had had any genital symptoms. He related that he had had a purulent (full of pus) discharge from his penis for several days before the onset of his ocular symptoms. He was not sure whether his current female sexual partner had been having any vaginal discharge.

34.3 The most likely source from which this organism entered the patient's eye is:

A. his unwashed hands after touching a toilet seat.
B. his unwashed hands after touching his penis.
C. kissing his girlfriend's cheek.
D. a public swimming pool.
E. a dry cotton towel that he used to dry his face.

The correct answer is **B** (his unwashed hands after touching his penis). *Neisseria gonorrhoeae* most commonly causes urethritis (inflamed urethra) in males, and it is most probable that this patient inadvertently rubbed his eyes with his hands after contaminating them with material from his penis. **A** (his unwashed hands after touching a toilet seat) is unlikely because gonococci do not survive on inanimate objects **(fomites)** and, although many an unfaithful husband or boyfriend would like his partner to believe that toilet seats are good sources of acquiring gonorrhea, it just doesn't happen that way. **C** (his girlfriend's cheek) is very unlikely because facial skin is seldom involved with gonorrhea, and he would have had to rub his eye directly on an infectious lesion to get *N. gonorrhoeae* into it. **D** (a public swimming pool) is very unlikely because of the dilution effect of the water in a pool and the probable inhibition of the growth of gonococci, which are very fastidious, by chlorine or other antibacterial substances in a public swimming pool. **E** (a dry cotton towel that he used to dry his face) is incorrect because *N. gonorrhoeae* is very susceptible to drying and because cotton contains fatty acids that actually inhibit this organism. In fact, it is recommended that swabs, which are used to obtain material for gonococcal cultures, **not** be made of cotton. In addition, the environmental fragility of the gonococcus is such that it is important that specimens for gonococcal culture be transferred promptly from the patient either to the definitive culture plate or to a reliable transfer medium until they can be inoculated onto culture plates. This is especially true for a specimen taken from an eye, because other fastidious organisms, such as *Haemophilus* species, may cause conjunctivitis that is clinically indistinguishable from that caused by *N. gonorrhoeae.*

Discussion: This patient had adult gonococcal conjunctivitis. In this syndrome, the gonococcus is carried from a genital discharge to the patient's own eye by his or her hands. In newborns who acquire gonococcal eye infections by passing through the uterine cervix and vagina of mothers with active gonorrhea, the syndrome is called "ophthalmia neonatorum."

Is adult gonococcal conjunctivitis really so serious? What was incorrect with just using antibiotic eye drops to treat it?

Because of antibiotic resistance and the potential of *N. gonorrheae* to penetrate deep into the eyeball, topical therapy with antibiotic drops is inadequate to treat gonococcal conjunctivitis. It is an infection that requires therapy with a

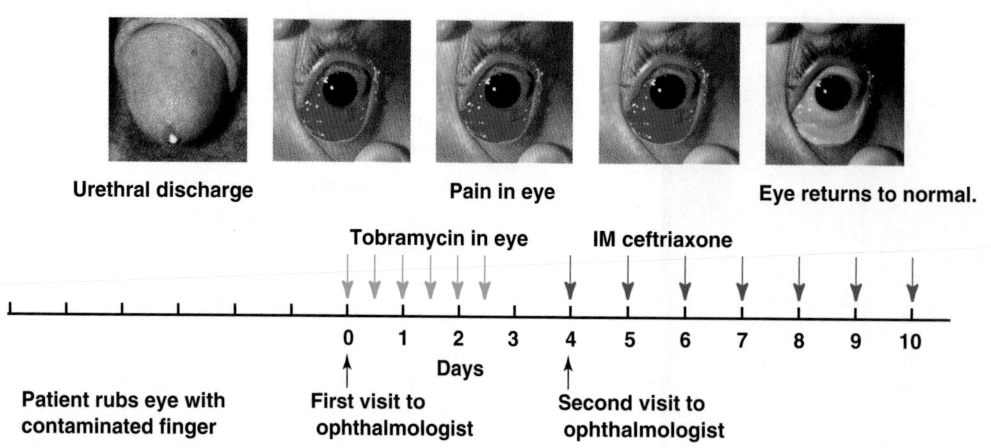

Figure 34.5
Summary of case. IM = intramuscular.

systemically administered (for example, intravenous or intramuscular) antibiotic. If proper treatment is not given, the organism may invade more deeply into the eye, causing it to rupture.

Are there ways that this eye infection could have been prevented?

If this patient's urethritis had been treated earlier, his ocular infection might have been prevented because the spread of the contagion to his hands might not have occurred. Although it is not always a "sure thing," diligent attention to handwashing after handling the genitalia would also have reduced the likelihood of contamination of the hands. We all frequently put our hands on our eyes, so anything that would improve hand hygiene helps to prevent the spread of infection from hands to eyes. Finally, the "usual" measures that prevent the spread of sexually transmitted infections (barriers such as condoms, limiting the number of sexual contacts, to name two) may have effectively kept this young man from acquiring this potentially serious eye infection. Figure 34.5 summarizes the chronology of the case.

Case 3: Gas within a bulla

This 60-year-old woman was seen in consultation because of a skin lesion and fever that had been present for 24 hours. She had been in failing health for many years because of chronic active hepatitis. Recently, because of progressive liver disease, oral prednisone at a dose of 60 mg daily was begun. The day prior to admission to the hospital she developed fever and chills, and she was admitted for intravenous antibiotics. When she arrived at the hospital, she complained of pain in her right knee and thigh.

Physical examination revealed a stuporous woman (unresponsive to verbal stimuli, barely responsive to painful stimuli). Her temperature was 100°F. Remarkable findings, in addition to her mental status, included edema of the right thigh and leg and areas of erythema (redness due to tiny dilated blood vessels in the skin) of both thighs and legs. On the medial aspect of the right lower extremity, proximal and distal to the knee, there was an area of purpura (hemorrhage into the skin) as shown in Figure 34.6. Within this area, there were bullae (large blisters), one of which was filled with red fluid. At the top of the fluid in this bulla there floated many tiny bubbles (Figure 34.7). There was marked asterixis of the hands (a flapping tremor indicative of metabolic encephalopathy that, in a stuporous patient, can be elicited by holding the wrists in slight extension).

Because of the presence of a cellulitis with purpura and a bulla with cherry-red fluid and gas, a presumptive diagnosis of *Clostridium perfringens* sepsis was made, with the plan being to treat the patient with very high doses of penicillin G. However, Gram stain of the fluid aspirated from the bulla revealed the appearance seen in Figure 34.8.

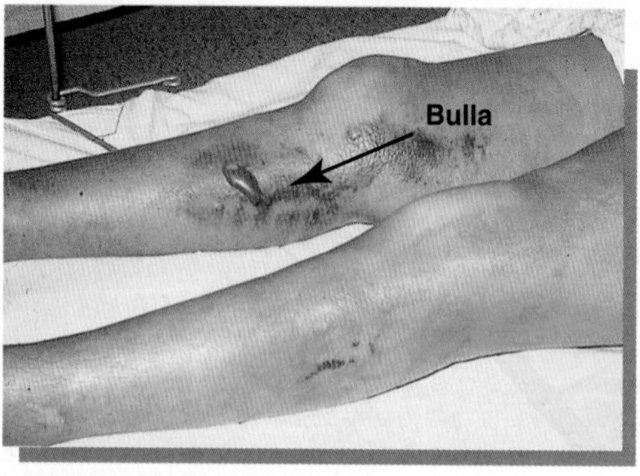

Figure 34.6
Erythema of the thighs and legs and a patch of purpura, proximal and distal to the right knee. Within the more distal purpuric area is a bulla.

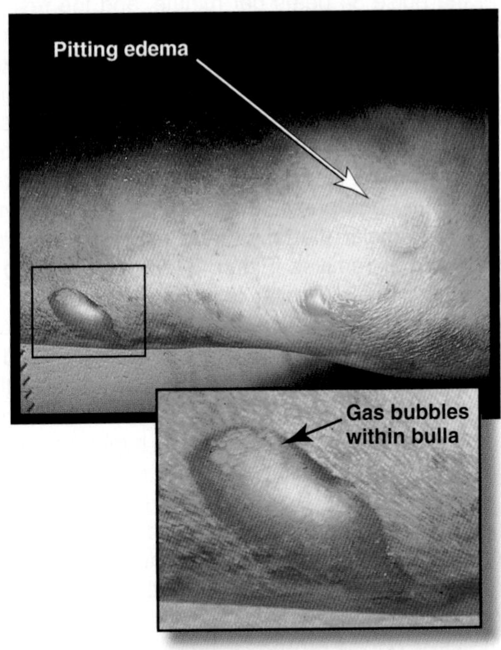

Figure 34.7
Close-up of the area in Figure 34.6, showing the bulla with bubbles. To the right is a depression caused by thumb pressure, illustrating pitting edema.

34.4 The organism seen in this Gram stain is most likely to be:

A. *Clostridium perfringens.*
B. *Streptococcus pyogenes.*
C. *Escherichia coli.*
D. *Neisseria meningitidis.*
E. *Lactobacillus casei.*

The correct answer is **C** (*Escherichia coli*), which is the only gram-negative rod on the list. **A** (*Clostridium perfringens*) is associated with gas-forming infections and bullae filled with red fluid, but it is a gram-positive rod. Skin infections due to **B** (*Streptococcus pyogenes*) may also form bullae, some even with reddish fluid. However, *Streptococcus pyogenes* is a gram-positive coccus, not a gram-negative rod. **D** (*Neisseria meningitidis*) is a gram-negative organism associated with purpuric skin lesions, but it is a coccus (usually seen in pairs) and not a rod. **E** (*Lactobacillus casei*) is a gram-positive rod that is seldom involved in invasive disease.

To the surprise of the consultant, this patient did not have a clostridial infection. *E. coli* alone grew from blood cultures and from the bulla fluid. It turned out to be susceptible to all the antibiotics against which it was tested, including ampicillin and gentamicin, but this information was not available for 48 hours. The patient was empirically treated with ampicillin, clindamycin, and gentamicin, beginning as soon as the results of the Gram stain were available. However, the morning after the initial consultation visit, in spite of treatment with two drugs effective against her *E. coli*, she died in hepatic failure.

Discussion: This patient illustrates many important clinicomicrobiologic points. First, many organisms may cause similar-appearing clinical lesions, so that as much hard microbiological data as possible must be collected prior to treatment. Pretreatment cultures, for example, are extremely important. Determining the exact identity of an organism and its susceptibility to antibiotics permits prediction of efficacy of the chosen antibiotic regimen and the selection of alternatives if, for some reason (such as an allergic reaction), treatment needs to be changed before the total course of therapy is completed.

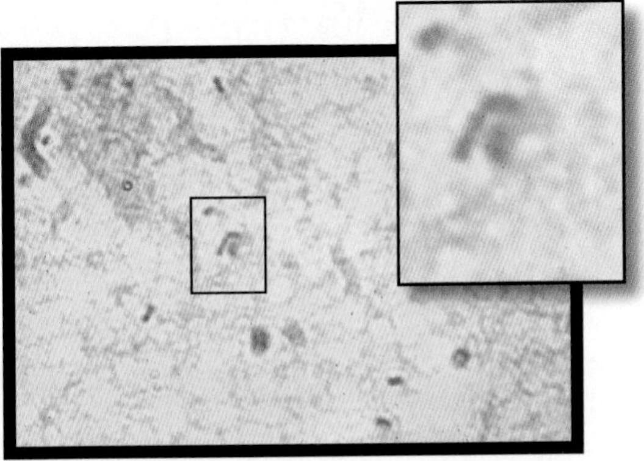

Figure 34.8
Gram stain of the bulla fluid shows gram-negative organisms, probably rods. The shorter forms probably represent rods seen at an angle, from their ends.

Why is the Gram stain important in general but especially for the management of this specific patient?

The Gram stain was the initial tip that, despite the clinical appearance of the lesion, this was not a gram-positive anaerobic process but a gram-negative process, allowing optimal antibiotic selection within minutes of assessment of the patient. Second, this patient reminds us that not all gas-forming infections are due to the notorious clostridial genus. Gas is produced by the metabolism of a wide variety of microorganisms of quite varied morphologies. With *E. coli*, gas does not accumulate as it does with clostridial species because the gas produced by *E. coli* is mainly carbon dioxide, which is absorbed by the tissues almost as fast as it is produced by the microorganism. Culture is necessary for speciation and to allow antibiotic susceptibility testing. Finally, the patient died even though she was treated quite promptly with the right drugs. It was reassuring to have cultures that proved the *in vitro* efficacy of her antibiotic regimen. It is probable that her underlying liver disease was so advanced that this episode of sepsis caused her to go into irreversible hepatic coma. In addition, the steroid therapy may have interfered with her ability to fight off any infection. Although her physicians were dismayed at her death, they could feel confident that she did not die because of inadequate antibiotic therapy or incorrect antibiotic choices. The appropriateness of the initial antibiotic regimen resulted from the clinical-microbiologic correlation of the lesion and the Gram stain. However, note the rapidity with which gram-negative organisms can result in death due to endotoxemia.

Case 4: Man with a rash

This 25-year-old man was admitted to the hospital for shortness of breath, which had been present for 1 day. He had been well until 3 days before admission, in mid-June, when he developed sneezing and a runny and stuffy nose. The next day he noted a nonproductive cough. Red blotches were observed on his face the following day, at which time the patient began to complain of retro-orbital headache and feverishness. One day later there was more rash on his face, and it had spread to his arms and trunk. Progressive malaise and shortness of breath prompted hospital admission.

There had been no known tick exposure. At age 3 months the patient's mother was told that an illness with rash, which the patient had, was measles. He had never received a dose of measles vaccine.

34.5 The illness in the differential diagnosis that prompted the question about tick exposure is:

A. dengue fever.
B. measles (rubeola).
C. German measles (rubella).
D. meningococcemia.
E. Rocky Mountain spotted fever.

The correct answer is **E** (Rocky Mountain spotted fever), which is the only tick-borne disease on this list. This patient's rash made the physician of record think of Rocky Mountain spotted fever, especially because it occurred in June, when ticks are quite active in many areas of the United States. (See below for further elaboration on this point.) **A** (dengue fever) is, in fact, a disease carried by an arthropod vector, but the vector of dengue fever is a mosquito and not a tick. **B** (measles), **C** (German measles), and **D** (meningococcemia) are not vector borne but are transmitted by inhalation of contagious material that may be breathed out by an infected individual into ambient air, a simpler and more direct mode of transmission.

On physical examination, the patient's temperature was 100°F, the pulse 84 beats per minute, and the respirations mildly labored at a rate of 22 per minute. [Note: Normal respiratory rate is somewhere between 14 and 18. It takes real work to breathe at 22 per minute, and this is often quite obvious when you look at a patient, for which reason the respirations are described as "labored."] The skin was warm and dry. The face was completely erythematous (red, but blanching upon pressure) and there was an erythematous maculopapular (flat spots and raised bumps) rash on the trunk and extremities (Figure 34.9), with large confluent areas on the back. Similar lesions were present on the palms. There were shotty anterior cervical and supraclavicular lymph nodes. [Note: The term shotty is used in describing the feel of lymph nodes when they are palpated through the skin. Shotty lymph nodes are hard and round like shotgun pellets.] The conjunctivae were hyperemic (too red, from dilated blood vessels) along the outer margins of the lids. The throat was extremely hyperemic. The buccal mucosa contained several raised white spots, each the size of a grain of salt, opposite the lower molars. The chest was resonant and clear. The remainder of the physical examination was unremarkable.

The white blood cell count was 3,100/μl (lower than the lower limit of normal, which in many laboratories is 4,000/μl), with a differential of 70 percent polymorphonuclear leukocytes, 22 percent band forms, 7 percent lymphocytes, 1 percent monocytes. [Note: These results are very suggestive of a viral infection.] The partial pressure of oxygen in arterial blood, with the patient breathing air enriched to make its oxygen content 24 percent, was 110 mm Hg

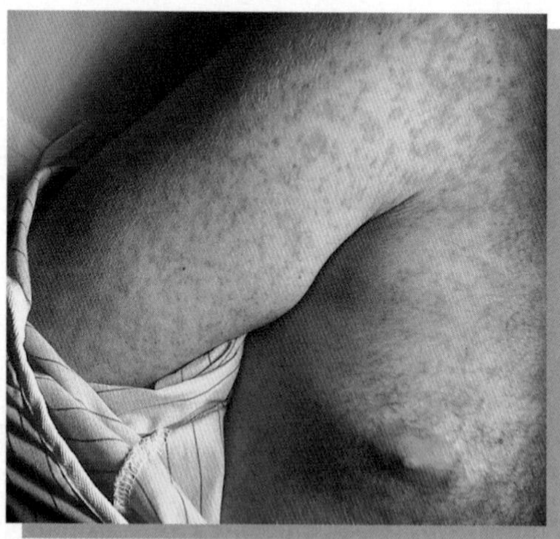

Figure 34.9
Extensive erythematous maculopapular rash covering the trunk and extremities. Not shown are the patient's face, on which the lesions were so confluent that his entire face was erythematous, and back, which had many large confluent areas of erythema.

(abnormally low, for such a high percentage of oxygen in inspired air at sea level). The chest film revealed interstitial infiltrates (not involving the actual alveolar spaces but mainly the interalveolar septa) in both lower lobes.

Because of clinical suspicions raised by the history and physical examination, antibodies against rubeola virus were measured, with the following results:

Complement fixation	Hemagglutination inhibition
Hospital day 3	
<1: 8	1:20
10 days later	
1:64	1:80

Using acute and convalescent phase sera for a retrospective immunologic diagnosis, the presence of at least a fourfold rise in these antibodies is considered conclusive proof that the illness, which is clinically compatible with measles, was, in fact, measles, and not one of its late spring/early summer mimics, such as Rocky Mountain spotted fever, an enterovirus infection, or early meningococcemia.

34.6 The clinical clues that would make the consultant consider measles prominently in the differential diagnosis included all of the following EXCEPT the:

A. pattern of spread of the rash.
B. white spots on the buccal mucosa.
C. appearance of the illness in June.
D. interstitial pneumonia.
E. relatively low total white blood cell count.

The correct answer is **C** (appearance of the illness in June). Unlike many vector-borne illnesses, measles in the United States is a disease of cooler weather, quite typically the winter. Although it is not impossible to see measles in June (after all, this patient got it in June), it is not among the data that would heighten suspicion that an illness is measles. The other answers are incorrect because they are data that do heighten the suspicion of measles: **A** (pattern of spread of the rash) is very typical of the way in which measles evolves on the skin, that is, from the face to the trunk and extremities, in contrast to Rocky Mountain spotted fever, which classically begins at the periphery (wrists and ankles) and spreads centripetally; **B** (white spots on the buccal mucosa) were Koplik spots, an enanthem (mucosal rash) that is felt to be pathognomonic (distinctly characteristic) of measles; **D** (interstitial pneumonia), while nonspecific, is quite compatible with an illness such as measles, which characteristically causes an interstitial "giant cell" pneumonia, interfering with the transport of oxygen across the alveolar septa into the pulmonary capillaries; **E** (relatively low white blood cell count) is also what is expected in many viral illnesses, including measles.

Discussion: This patient had serologically proven measles at age 25 years. He somehow had escaped laws requiring measles immunization for entry into school, perhaps because he was thought to have had actual measles in infancy. Whether he actually had measles at age 3 months will never be known with certainty, but it is unlikely. Because of the very high degree of immunity to measles in adults of his mother's age, the presence of specific maternal antimeasles antibody crossing the placenta into his circulation, should have protected him from measles for many months after his birth. On the other hand, if he did actually have measles at age 3 months, it is unlikely that he would have acquired durable immunity to this virus, owing to the immaturity of the immune system in so young an infant.

However, this patient had Koplik spots (Figure 34.10). In the setting of a compatible febrile illness with rash, Koplik spots are very good evidence of measles. Serologic evidence was obtained because, at the time of his illness, in his state of residence, the measles situation was unstable, and the State Health Department was very interested in unassailable proof that a suspicious illness was, in fact, measles. Whereas viral cultures could have been obtained, serologic evidence was used to prove the etiology of this patient's illness, for reasons of convenience and cost. This is a common practice for documenting the viral etiology of diseases in the clinical setting.

This lucky patient gradually improved and was discharged from the hospital. Many individuals with measles, especially adults and very young children, suffer severe illness with measles, often with serious immediate complications (such as bacterial pneumonia) and long-term sequelae that involve the central nervous system.

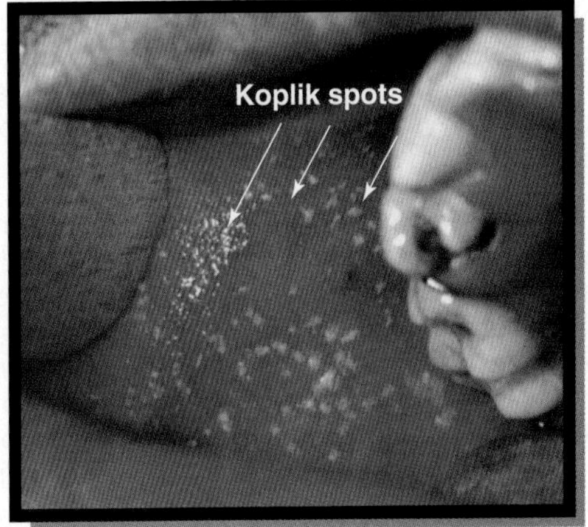

Figure 34.10
Koplik spots.

Why should a physician in the United States be concerned about a disease that is nearly extinct here?

Although immunization is among the most successful of all public health interventions in the history of U.S. medicine, there are still outbreaks of vaccine-preventable disease such as measles. In recent years, in addition to outbreaks of measles in the United States, there have been serious increases in the incidence of mumps (that have involved a broad age spectrum that included fully immunized individuals) and whooping cough (pertussis). Sometimes the index case (first patient) is someone who has traveled abroad, sometimes it is an international adoptee, and sometimes it is associated with immigration from a country in which the illness is still prevalent. Sometimes the source is very difficult to identify. All of the vaccine-preventable diseases can have serious consequences, and it is important to be able to recognize them so that their spread into susceptible populations can be prevented or, at least, contained. Moreover, such outbreaks sometimes teach us that the conventional wisdom about what constitutes an adequate course of immunization (number of doses of vaccine) is incorrect. This was true for measles, mumps, rubella, chickenpox, and pertussis.

Case 5: Woman with cough

This 39-year-old woman was admitted with fever and cough, which had been present for several days. She had daily cough productive of green sputum (indicating the presence of inflammatory cells, most probably polymorphonuclear leukocytes) and was treated with inhaled bronchodilators for what was believed to be asthma. The patient had a long history of productive cough (cough yielding sputum), and, in 1976, invasive studies documented bronchiectasis (a condition in which inflammation has caused permanent dilation of the walls of bronchi). She was treated with antibiotics and had no further physician contact until 1982, when she developed pneumonia. This resolved with antibiotics.

In 1991 (2 years prior to the current admission) she again developed pneumonia. Noninvasive studies, including computerized tomographic (CT) scan of the chest, confirmed bronchiectasis of the left lower lobe including the lingula. The patient's physicians believed that there was also bronchiectasis elsewhere in the lungs. With antibiotics, this pneumonia resolved, and for several months prior to this admission she took cefaclor, an oral second-generation cephalosporin, 1 out of every 4 weeks. This was changed to azithromycin (a macrolide with antimicrobial spectrum broader than that of erythromycin). Shortly before admission, because of increasing fever and productive cough, the antimicrobial regimen was again changed, this time to trimethoprim-sulfamethoxazole. Her symptoms became worse, and she agreed to be admitted to the hospital. There was no exposure to dusts, fumes, danders, or toxins. A parrot was the only house pet.

34.7 Pets are sometimes important sources of infection to their owners. The organism that is most closely associated with parrots is:

A. *Pasteurella multocida.*

B. *Mycobacterium marinum.*

C. *Francisella tularensis.*

D. *Chlamydia psittaci.*

E. *Coxiella burnetii.*

The correct answer is **D** (*Chlamydia psittaci*). This organism, which does not grow in culture media, is closely associated with many types of birds, not only the "psittacine" birds (parrots, parakeets) from which it gets its specific name. The birds need not appear ill to be capable of transmitting *C. psittaci* to humans. The other choices are all associated with animals or their environments, but not birds. **A** (*Pasteurella multocida*) is found in the mouths of animals, especially cats and dogs, and is a gram-negative rod. **B** (*Mycobacterium marinum*) is an acid-fast bacillus that infects traumatic wounds that are sustained in salt or brackish water. **C** (*Francisella tularensis*) is classically associated with handling freshly killed rabbits, although it has also been acquired from other mammals. **E** (*Coxiella burnetii*) is categorized with the rickettsiae and causes Q fever, an infection that may occur after exposure to livestock (for example, parturient sheep).

The patient's temperature was 103°F. She was alert and in no distress. Examination of the chest revealed it to be normally resonant throughout, with diffuse coarse wheezes (musical sounds indicating constriction of bronchi and consistent with, but not diagnostic of, asthma). There was mild clubbing of the fingers and toes (bulbous swellings of the distal digits seen in patients with a variety of chronic illnesses, especially those involving the lungs).

The chest film revealed right lower lobe pneumonia. Gram stain of expectorated sputum revealed many filamentous, branched gram-positive rods (Figure 34.11). These failed to grow in cultures but had grown, aerobically, from sputum cultured.

34.8 From this Gram stain, the possible genera into which the organism fits include:

A. *Candida.*

B. *Nocardia.*

C. *Clostridium.*

D. *Actinomyces.*

E. *Pseudomonas.*

Both **B** (*Nocardia*) and **D** (*Actinomyces*) are correct answers, as both are gram-positive filamentous rods with prominent branching. Their fine, threadlike (filamentous) diameter distinguishes them immediately from the much larger fungal genera such as **A** (*Candida*). Multiple overlapping pseudohyphae of *Candida* species may appear to be branches, but their much larger size makes their identity as fungi, and not bacteria, quite evi-

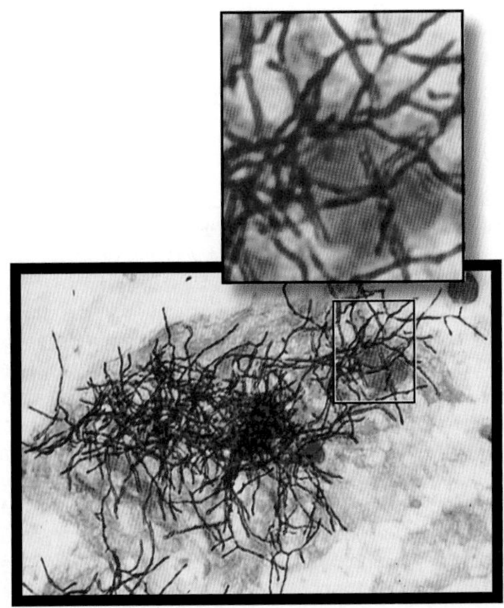

Figure 34.11
Gram stain of sputum shows many filamentous, branched, gram-positive rods. The fine caliber and the prominent presence of branching are important distinguishing morphologic characteristics.

dent. **C** (*Clostridium*) is, indeed, a gram-positive rod, but it is not branched, and its width is much greater than that of *Nocardia* or *Actinomyces*. **E** (*Pseudomonas*) cannot be correct for many reasons, the most important of which is that it is a gram-negative rod.

The patient was treated with high doses of trimethoprim-sulfamethoxazole, intravenously at first. It was then given orally, because of the decrease in her temperature and marked improvement in her cough. Subsequent Gram stains of her sputum showed near disappearance of the filamentous gram-positive rods (that had been identified as *Nocardia asteroides* in 1991).

Discussion: The *Nocardia* had probably never been eradicated from her lungs in 1991 and had most likely smoldered there until it finally reached a quantity adequate to cause symptoms and radiographic changes of pneumonia. The absence of treatment effective against *Nocardia*, after resolution of the 1991 pneumonia, made this very likely to occur. Bronchiectasis made this patient's mucociliary clearance mechanisms ineffective, allowing persistence of bacteria in areas that are normally sterile. *Nocardia* may be quite tenacious under these circumstances, making it necessary to maintain this patient, probably for years, on a regimen that will at least suppress the organism to levels that do not make her ill.

Is sputum handled differently from other specimens in the microbiology laboratory?

Expectorated sputum is not usually cultured for anaerobes, because there would be contamination of the sputum with mouth flora, heavy in anaerobes, on its way from lungs to collection container. Documentation of an anaerobe, such as *Actinomyces*, as the cause of a lung lesion requires that the specimen be obtained without passing through the mouth. One way to do this is to pass a needle through the chest wall, under CT scan guidance, directly into the lesion. This was never done to this patient, whose filamentous, branched gram-positive rods did not grow in sputum obtained during this episode of pneumonia. It was, after all, not cultured anaerobically, so that *Actinomyces*, if present, would not have grown. But her physicians felt confident that *Nocardia* was the culprit for two reasons: 1) *Nocardia* was what had been in her sputum previously, and 2) there was a clear response to trimethoprim-sulfamethoxazole, which would not be expected to have a significant effect on *Actinomyces*. Unfortunately, not every organism that causes disease, including *Nocardia*, will be successfully grown in cultures every time. That (and the rapid availability of the presumptive answer) is why Gram stain is such an important tool in the clinical application of microbiology.

Case 6: Woman with swollen wrist

This 25-year-old woman was admitted because of swelling and pain of her left wrist of ten days' duration. She had previously been well. Twelve days before admission she was bitten on the left hand by her pet cat. Two days later she developed pain, redness, and swelling of her hand, and her physician treated her with oral cloxacillin (a penicillin derivative, active against *Staphylococcus aureus* and *Streptococcus pyogenes*, with the ability to withstand staphylococcal β-lactamase). After transient improvement in her symptoms and signs of inflammation, she became worse, so that by the time of admission, she was unable to close her fingers or move her wrist. In addition, she noted evening fevers as high as 100.2°F.

On physical examination, her temperature was 99.7°F. The left wrist and thenar eminence were erythematous (red, but with blanching of the redness on pressure, indicating dilation of cutaneous blood vessels—the "rubor" of the classic signs of inflammation). There was markedly reduced range of motion, both extension and flexion, of the fingers. Extension and flexion of the wrist were limited to just a few degrees. The patient's wrist and hand are shown in Figure 34.12.

The white blood cell count was 13,000/μL, with a marked increase in the percentage of immature granulocytes (the "left shift" of an acute inflammatory process). Gram stain of the wrist fluid, which was cloudy when aspirated, revealed sheets of polymorphonuclear leukocytes and many gram-negative rods (Figure 34.13).

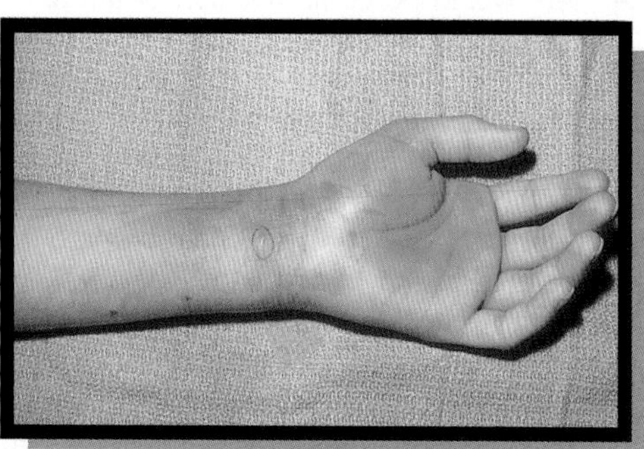

Figure 34.12
The thenar eminence is swollen, and the patient is only able to flex and extend her wrist and fingers minimally, due to pain. This photo was taken just prior to removal of wrist joint fluid from a point within the circle on the volar aspect of the wrist.

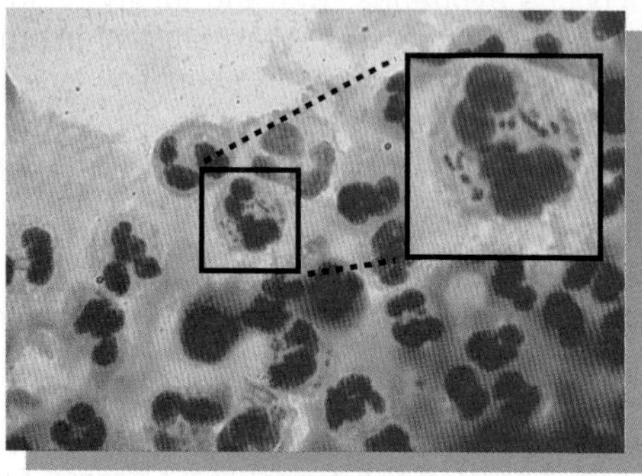

Figure 34.13
Gram stain of wrist fluid. There are innumerable (sheets) polymorphonuclear leukocytes and many gram-negative rods.

34.9 From among the following, the gram-negative rod that is most commonly associated with cat bites is:

A. *Pasteurella multocida.*

B. *Bartonella henselae.*

C. *Streptobacillus moniliformis.*

D. *Streptococcus pyogenes.*

E. *Lactobacillus casei.*

The correct answer is **A** (*Pasteurella multocida*), a gram-negative rod that frequents the mouths of some animals, particularly cats, but also dogs. The extreme sharpness of feline teeth causes enormous pressure at the site of the puncture during a bite, allowing inoculation of the organism deep into tissues. **B** (*Bartonella henselae*) is incorrect, although it is a gram-negative rod associated with exposure to cats. In immunocompetent hosts, the principal condition caused by this organism, which is carried mainly on the paws of cats, is cat scratch disease, whose name implies transmission by cat scratches not cat bites. **C** (*Streptobacillus moniliformis*) is also a gram-negative rod, pleomorphic, which is most commonly acquired by the bite or scratch of rats or mice. Although it may be carried—and transmitted—by carnivores that prey on these rodents, it is less characteristically associated with cat-induced injuries than with rat or mouse exposure. The simplest reason that **D** (*Streptococcus pyogenes*) is incorrect is that it is a gram-positive coccus, not a gram-negative rod. Likewise, **E** (*Lactobacillus casei*) cannot be a correct answer because it is a gram-positive rod, not a gram-negative one.

Culture of the wrist joint fluid yielded *P. multocida* and *P. aeruginosa*. The patient underwent open debridement of her wrist, which showed extensive damage of the joint space and tendons in the vicinity of the joint space. With intravenous penicillin G (aimed at the *P. multocida*) and gentamicin (aimed at the *P. aeruginosa*), together with intensive physical therapy, she had complete recovery of flexion and extension of her wrist and fingers.

Discussion: *P. multocida* is a notorious cause of infection induced by animal bites, especially those of cats. It has a propensity to invade osteoarticular tissues, which are often very near to the point at which the animal bites. Serious illness has occurred in newborns who have been licked by the family cat, presumably due to inoculation of *P. multocida* onto the infant, and invasion of the bloodstream because of the immaturity of the neonatal immune system.

What is the single most important part of this patient's history that helps to suspect the correct microorganism?

The single most important part of this patient's history is the fact that her infection was preceded by the bite of a cat. The primary care physician treated the patient as if she had an uncomplicated break in the skin with ingress of bacteria that ordinary live on skin surfaces (*Staphylococcus aureus* and *S. pyogenes*). It is important to think of the clinical association of animals and *P. multocida*, because this organism is resistant to a number of antibiotics, yet sensitive to penicillin G, which ordinarily would not be used to treat infection due to most gram-negative rods and much skin flora.

Case 7: Man with endophthalmitis

This 66-year-old man with non–insulin-dependent diabetes mellitus had been feeling well until 1 week earlier. At that time he noted the sudden onset of shaking chills lasting about 20 minutes, associated with low back pain that radiated into the medial aspect of both thighs. These episodes occurred several times over the next few days. About 2 days after the onset of these chills, he developed pain, swelling, and erythema (redness that blanches with pressure, due to dilation of superficial blood vessels as part of the inflammatory response—"rubor") of his left hand. The next day he noted a "black spot" obscuring his vision on his right eye, progressing over the next day to complete loss of vision in his right eye. His ophthalmologist found a hypopyon (collection of pus in the anterior chamber) and treated him with a subconjunctival injection of gentamicin (an aminoglycoside antibiotic) 80 mg, methylprednisolone (a glucocorticoid anti-inflammatory agent) 40 mg, topical gentamicin, and atropine (an anticholinergic to keep the pupil dilated) eye drops. The patient's diabetes had been well controlled with chlorpropamide (a sulfonylurea oral hypoglycemic agent) and diet. There was no history of trauma to the eye.

The pain in his back and his left hand became worse the next day, and the following day, because the hypopyon was much worse, the ophthalmologist admitted the patient to the hospital. The anterior chamber was opaque (Figure 34.14) and the intraocular pressure was increased.

Physical examination revealed the temperature to be 97.8°F, the pulse regular at 90 beats per minute, and the blood pressure 160/90 mm Hg. The cornea of the right eye was opaque, with a dense hypopyon along its lower half.

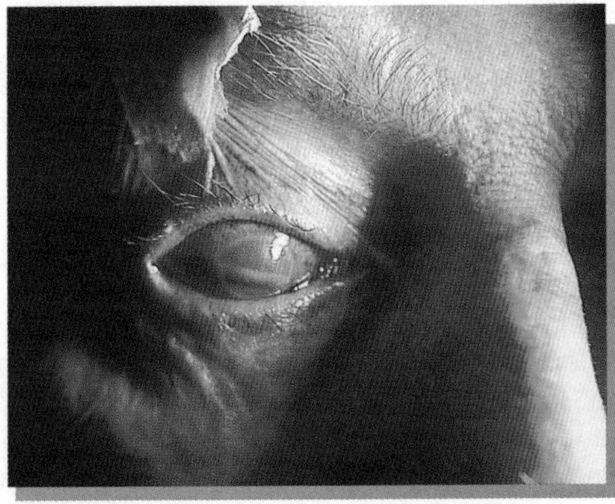

Figure 34.14
The patient's right eye at the time of admission to the hospital. The cornea is cloudy and there is a collection of white blood cells (hypopyon) behind it in the anterior chamber.

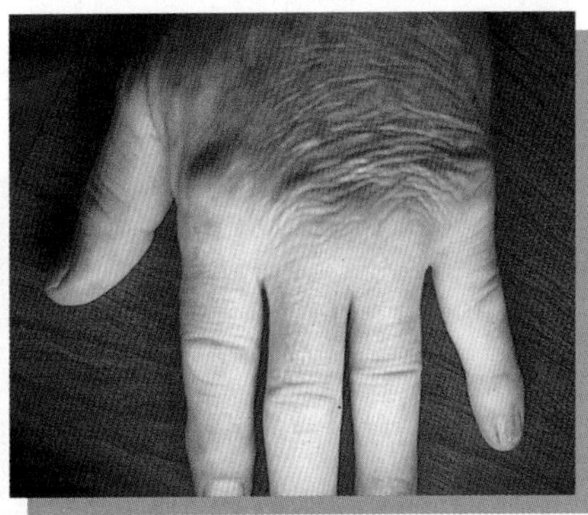

Figure 34.15
The patient's left hand at the time of admission to the hospital. The lateral three MCP joints are swollen, with erythema especially visible over the fourth MCP joint. MCP = metacarpophalangeal.

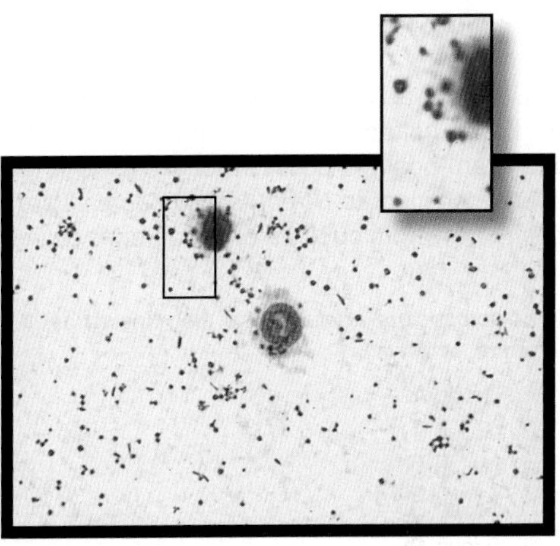

Figure 34.16
Gram stain of the anterior chamber fluid taken at the time of admission to the hospital. There are polymorphonuclear leukocytes and many gram-positive cocci, some distorted to an elongated shape.

The retina could not be visualized behind this hypopyon. The left hand revealed erythema, swelling, warmth, tenderness, and very decreased range of motion of the third, fourth, and fifth metacarpophalangeal (MCP) joints (Figure 34.15). There was a small, healing laceration of the left shin.

The white blood cell (WBC) count was 16,500/μl (normal 5,000 to 10,000), with 78 percent polymorphonuclear leukocytes, 20 percent band forms, and 2 percent lymphocytes (a "left shift" toward immature granulocytes, consistent with an acute inflammatory process). Gram stain of fluid aspirated from the anterior chamber of the right eye (Figure 34.16) revealed many polymorphonuclear leukocytes and large numbers of gram-positive cocci, some irregular in shape (a reflection of partial efficacy of the injected gen-

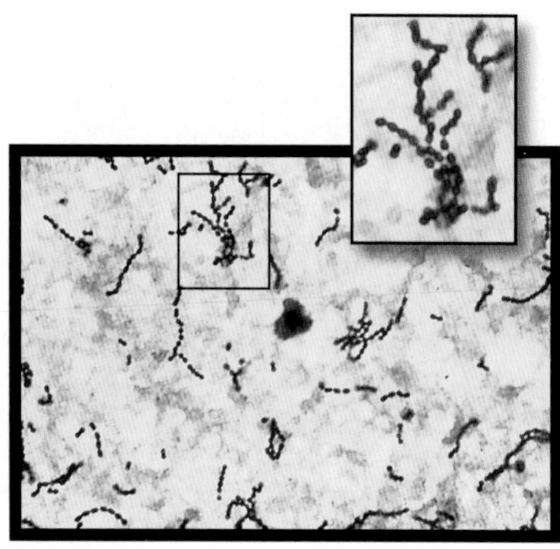

Figure 34.17
Gram stain of organisms grown from blood cultures. These are gram-positive cocci in chains, consistent with *Streptococcus* species.

tamicin, which was inhibiting these organisms without killing them). Blood cultures taken at the time of hospitalization yielded gram-positive cocci in long chains (Figure 34.17) that were identified as *Streptococcus agalactiae*. The same organism grew from cultures of the anterior chamber fluid.

34.10 *Streptococcus agalactiae* is also known by its Lancefield group, which is:

A. Group A
B. Group B
C. Group C
D. Group D
E. Group G

The correct answer is **B** (Group B). Because *Streptococcus agalactiae* is in Group B, all of the other choices are incorrect.

This patient went on to have a stormy course, with intense pain in his eye, where the inflammation increased for several days before it started to improve (Figure 34.18).

He was found on further study to have infective endocarditis (an infection of a heart valve, with growths of bacteria, called "vegetations," which may break off into the arterial circulation). He thus had "showers" of bacteria-laden material in his arterial tree, explaining his low back pain, the acute arthritis of his left hand, and the very active infection of his eye. The "portal of entry" of this bacterial infection was most probably the laceration of his shin.

What are the clues that suggest *S. agalactiae* as the culprit in this man's infection?

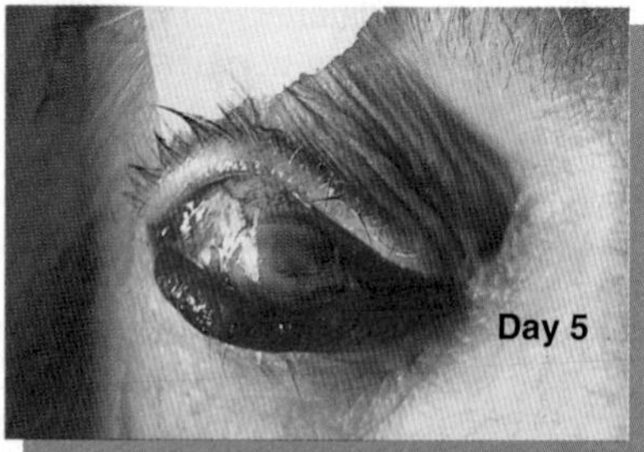

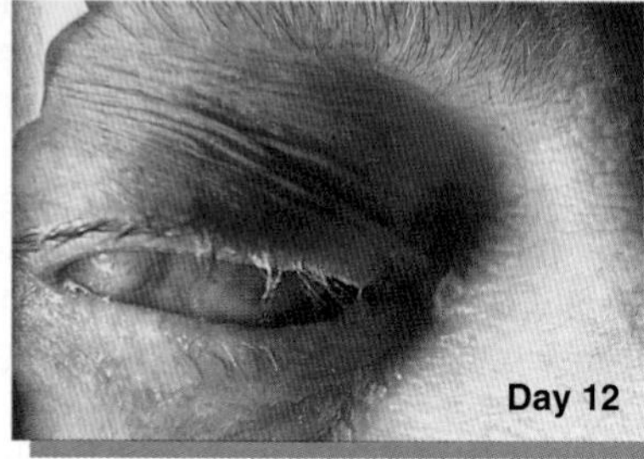

Figure 34.18
Top: The patient's right eye after 5 days of intravenous penicillin G, showing persistence of the hypopyon and intense chemosis (edema of the conjunctiva, which has swelled to the point that it is hanging over the lower eyelid). Bottom: The patient's right eye after 10 days of intravenous penicillin G, with resolution of the chemosis but persistence of corneal opacification.

The first clue, as is so often the case, came from the Gram stain. There were Gram-positive cocci in the anterior chamber, and these formed very long chains in the blood culture medium. Unlike healthy people, diabetics are more likely to harbor *S. agalactiae* on their skin, especially on the lower extremities. Because his diabetes impaired his ability to contain a localized infection, he was more prone to having the bacteria that contaminated the laceration invade his bloodstream, from which some of them colonized a heart valve and, from there, further seeded tissues with end-artery circulation (eye, hand, vertebral column). He was treated for a total of 6 weeks with intravenous aqueous penicillin G, 4 million units every 4 hours, and he eventually got better, but the vision in his right eye was permanently lost.

Case 8: Man with fever and paraplegia

This 32-year-old man complained of fever and myalgias (muscle pain) for 1 week. He had always been in good health. In late July he visited a grassy area of rural New Jersey. Two days later he developed diarrhea, fever, malaise (a general feeling of not being well), and a rash. He saw a physician 3 days after the onset of these symptoms and, because of elevated serum transaminase levels, was told he had hepatitis. The diarrhea had stopped, and he now complained of headache, primarily frontal and retro-orbital (over and behind the eyes).

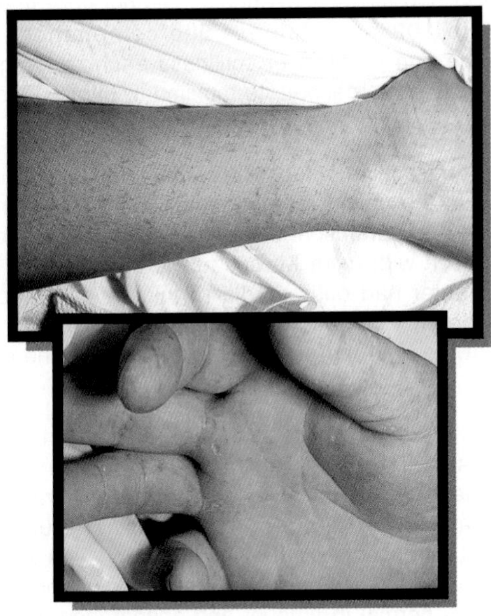

Figure 34.19
Top: The patient's ankle, showing numerous, tiny, cutaneous hemorrhages (petechiae). Bottom: The patient's right hand showing edema to the extent that he cannot flex his fingers further than shown in this photo.

There was no travel outside New Jersey, and there was no history of injecting drug use, multiple sexual partners, or homosexual contact.

On examination he was well developed, well nourished, and comfortable. His temperature was 103.5°F, and his pulse 120 beats per minute (a rapid heart rate consistent with his fever). The conjunctivae were injected (bloodshot), and the pharynx slightly more red than normal. A diffuse, confluent, erythematous macular rash covered the back and chest (red, but blanching when pressed, or "erythematous," and not raised above the level of surrounding skin—"macular"). The liver was slightly enlarged, with a total span measuring 13 cm. Its edge was tender (painful to the touch of the examiner). The muscles of the patient's arms and legs were also tender. Numerous petechiae were present on the extremities, as shown in Figure 34.19. His hands were edematous, preventing him from closing them into a fist (see Figure 34.19).

The hemoglobin was 13.4 g/dl (slightly less than the lower limit of normal of 14), the white blood cell (WBC) count 13,500/μl (normal 5,000 to 10,000), with 68 percent polymorphonuclear leukocytes, 20 percent band forms, 7 percent lymphocytes, and 5 percent monocytes. [Note: A high total WBC with increased percentage of immature granulocytes indicates an acute inflammatory process.] The platelet count was 91,000/μl (normal 140,000 to 400,000). Serum aspartate aminotransferase (AST) was 273 (normal up to 40), and serum alanine aminotransferase (ALT) was 198 (normal up to 45). [Note: The abnormal transaminases are consistent with an inflammatory process of the liver.] The chest film was normal. Blood cultures drawn at the time of admission to the hospital did not result in any bacterial growth.

Because of the season during which this illness occurred, and because of its involvement of several systems (skin, muscles, liver, alimentary canal), the physicians caring for this man suspected Rocky Mountain spotted fever and began therapy with doxycycline (a long-acting tetracycline). One day after institution of this treatment, he became paraplegic and stuporous, recovering, with physical therapy, over the next several weeks. The doxycycline was continued for a total of 10 days.

34.11 The diagnosis of Rocky Mountain spotted fever is ordinarily confirmed by which of the following tests?

A. Blood cultures
B. Weil-Felix ("febrile") agglutinins
C. Antibodies against *Rickettsia rickettsii*
D. Antibodies against *Rickettsia prowazekii*
E. Antibodies against *Salmonella typhi*

The correct answer is **C** (antibodies against *Rickettsia rickettsii*). *R. rickettsii* is the microbial etiology of Rocky Mountain spotted fever. **A** (blood cultures) is incorrect. In clinical practice, because rickettsiae are obligate intracellular pathogens, ordinary liquid blood culture media, which are cell free, cannot support their growth. In addition, laboratory accidents that have resulted in aerosolization of rickettsial cultures have caused fatalities, and most clinical laboratories are unwilling to work with these organisms in culture. **B** (Weil-Felix "febrile" agglutinins), which are antibodies directed against Proteus OX-19 and OX-2 antigens, are not specific enough, cross-reacting with antigens of other rickettsial species. Thus, B is incorrect. **D** (antibodies against *Rickettsia prowazekii*) is not correct because *R. prowazekii* is the etiology of epidemic typhus, not Rocky Mountain spotted fever. **E** (antibodies against *Salmonella typhi*) is incorrect because *S. typhi* is one of the etiologies of enteric fever, not Rocky Mountain spotted fever. The name "typhoid" fever may make one think about a possible relationship to a rickettsial species that causes "typhus," but the two should never be confused.

Complement-fixing antibody titers against *R. rickettsii* were positive at a dilution of 1:32 on day 10 of illness and 1:128 3 weeks later. This fourfold rise in specific antibody confirms that the illness that this young man suffered was Rocky Mountain spotted fever.

Discussion: There is much about this patient's story that is very typical of Rocky Mountain spotted fever and is, therefore, very instructive. He became ill at the height of the summer, when ticks are most active. He spent time in a grassy area of a state that is well within the range of *Dermacentor variabilis*, the dog tick, which is a competent vector of *R. rickettsii*. The cell that *R. rickettsii* infects is the vascular endothelial lining cell. Thus, it makes sense that Rocky Mountain spotted fever involves many different organ systems (which all have a blood supply), and causes the kind of leakiness of blood vessels that leads to edema and petechial hemorrhages. The vascular injury, together with certain immune-mediated events, may result in disseminated intravascular coagulation, consuming platelets and leading to the low platelet count that was seen in this patient. Any tissue can be involved, but the skin and central nervous system seem to be preferred targets of *R. rickettsii*, explaining the extent of his rash and the complication of paraplegia.

If this patient received appropriate antibiotic therapy, why did he become paraplegic after treatment was begun?

The onset of paraplegia after appropriate therapy was begun warrants special comment. In addition to causing blood vessels to leak, vasculitis may also result in occlusion of blood vessels. It is probable that, prior to the administration of the doxycycline, infection of this patient's spinal cord vessels had progressed to the point that spinal cord ischemia (impaired blood supply) was inevitable, causing injury and even death of enough motor neurons to lead to paraplegia. One of the reasons that Rocky Mountain spotted fever is such a frightening disease is its potential to cause infarction of tissue.

Early treatment, based on clinical suspicion before definitive proof is available, is very important with Rocky Mountain spotted fever. In one series of observations that included fatal cases, it was noted that fatalities only occurred when treatment was begun at least 5 days after the onset of symptoms. Although individual symptoms are nonspecific, clues—such as multisystem illness with fever occurring at a time of year when ticks are active in a region in which Rocky Mountain spotted fever occurs—should raise the level of suspicion of Rocky Mountain spotted fever enough to warrant treatment directed at this disease.

Case 9: Woman with fever

This 28-year-old woman developed fever the day after the birth of her second child. She had always been well and had emigrated to the United States from India 7 years earlier. Her first pregnancy, 4 years later, resulted in a healthy baby girl, who was well at home throughout the patient's second pregnancy. The patient was admitted to the hospital in active labor at term (that is, after the full 9 months) of her second pregnancy. Vaginal examination revealed amniotic fluid stained with meconium, and so the patient was taken to the operating room for emergency cesarean section. [Note: Meconium is fetal feces, and when it is present in the amniotic fluid prior to birth, it indicates that the baby is in enough distress to warrant quick delivery.] Prior to the administration of anesthesia, labor had progressed to the point that a healthy, full-term female infant was delivered vaginally.

The mother developed a temperature of 102°F on the first postpartum (after delivery) day. She was treated with oral ampicillin 500 mg every 6 hours. Temperature maxima of 101°F to 102°F continued. She complained of mild headache and a sense of chilliness each evening, when her temperature reached its maximum. [Note: This is not unusual in patients with fever.]

Further questioning at the time of the consultant's visit indicated that the patient is a vegetarian and had, during the week prior to parturition, consumed several meals consisting of pizza with extra Mexican-style cheese. Her 3-year-old daughter had otitis media (a middle ear infection) 2 weeks before the patient went into labor but was well at home at the time the patient was admitted to the obstetric unit.

Physical examination done in the early afternoon of the third postpartum day revealed an alert woman in no distress. Her temperature was 99°F. The general physical examination was within normal limits. The uterus was enlarged as expected following a delivery. The lochia (the normal bloody vaginal discharge that follows the birth of a baby) was normal in amount and appearance and did not have a foul smell.

The blood count was within normal limits, as was the chest film. Blood cultures, taken at the onset of fever, yielded a gram-positive bacillus, morphologically identical to that shown in Figure 34.20. Aerobic subculture on blood agar yielded colonies that were β-hemolytic. Further subculture revealed the organism to be motile. The same organism grew in cultures of the lochia.

34.12 The most likely etiology of this patient's bacteremia is:

A. *Streptococcus pyogenes.*
B. *Escherichia coli.*
C. *Propionibacterium acnes.*
D. *Clostridium perfringens.*
E. *Listeria monocytogenes.*

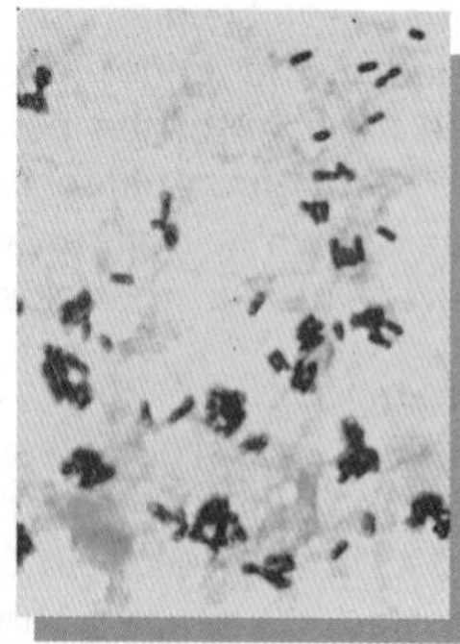

Figure 34.20
Gram stain of blood culture shows gram-positive diphtheroid-like rods, many of which are at angles to one another. The material in the background is debris from the red cells in the blood inoculated into the liquid blood culture medium.

The correct answer is **E** (*Listeria monocytogenes*). It is a gram-positive rod that may easily be mistaken for a diphtheroid. However, its β-hemolysis and motility distinguish it from diphtheroids, which are much less likely to be hemolytic, and are nonmotile. Although **A** (*Streptococcus pyogenes*) and **B** (*Escherichia coli*) may cause postpartum bacteremia, both are incorrect answers to the question, because *S. pyogenes* is a gram-positive not a bacillus, and *E. coli* is a gram-negative bacillus. Although **D** (*Clostridium perfringens*) is a gram-positive bacillus, it is an incorrect answer because it is anaerobic and would be most unlikely to grow in aerobic subculture. The absence of a foul smell from the lochia, although not entirely ruling out anaerobic infection, lessens the probability that anaerobes are present.

The organism that grew from the cultures was *L. monocytogenes.* Ampicillin was continued, but the route was changed from oral to intravenous, and the dose raised to 3 g every 6 hours. [Note: The reason is that high blood levels of ampicillin are required to eradicate a bacteremia due to an organism susceptible to this drug. Such high blood levels could not be achieved with oral administration of ampicillin.] Fever resolved rapidly, and the remainder of the postpartum course was uneventful for the patient. However, her baby became quite ill on its second day of life, and had to be transferred to a neonatal intensive care unit, requiring assisted ventilation for several days. Blood cultures from the baby grew out the same gram-positive bacillus. After much intensive care and many days of antibiotics, the baby also recovered.

Discussion: This patient had perinatal listeriosis. *L. monocytogenes* is an especially important pathogen among immunocompromised individuals, pregnant women, and newborns. The portal by which *L. monocytogenes* entered the mother's bloodstream was shown by cultures of her lochia to be her genital tract. It is probably from there that it entered the baby as well.

Is there a clue in the history about the source of *L. monocytogenes* from which this patient acquired it?

L. monocytogenes is now known to be a foodborne pathogen. The most likely source from which she acquired *L. monocytogenes* was the cheese on her pizza. Although *L. monocytogenes* is present in a number of different foods, dairy products are among the most important sources of foodborne listeriosis. Unlike many other microorganisms, Listeria has the ability to grow at refrigerator temperatures, making it possible to reach high concentrations in contaminated foods even with refrigeration. Cured meats and certain noncooked vegetable products, such as coleslaw, may harbor this organism, and refrigeration is not enough to prevent these foods from causing trouble once they are contaminated with it. The association with certain dairy products is so strong that pregnant women, especially in the third trimester, and immunocompromised individuals are advised not to eat soft cheeses. Because of its superficial resemblance to commensal diphtheroids, it is easy to miss *L. monocytogenes* in cultures. The combination of β-hemolysis and the motility it exhibits in special agar tubes when cultured at 20°C to 25°C serve to distinguish this important pathogen from nonpathogenic lookalikes, allowing appropriate treatment of patients and rewarding vigilance in the clinical laboratory.

Case 10: Man in coma

This 52-year-old man was found unresponsive at home on the day of admission. He had a long history of alcoholism, complicated by a seizure disorder. For several days prior to admission he had been drinking heavily. He was found by relatives at home, unresponsive, with continuous epileptiform movements (he did not regain consciousness between seizures). In the Emergency Room, his temperature was 105°F, and his neck was stiff. Chest examination suggested pneumonia involving the upper and middle lobes of the right lung. A chest X-ray was taken (Figure 34.21). There was no response to verbal stimuli, and he was in a coma.

Because of the fever and unconsciousness, lumbar puncture was done promptly to examine the cerebrospinal fluid (CSF). The CSF was very cloudy. There were 561 WBC/μl (98 percent polymorphonuclear leukocytes). The protein concentration was 380 mg/dl, the glucose concentration 5 mg/dl. [Note: These findings are typical for acute bacterial meningitis.]

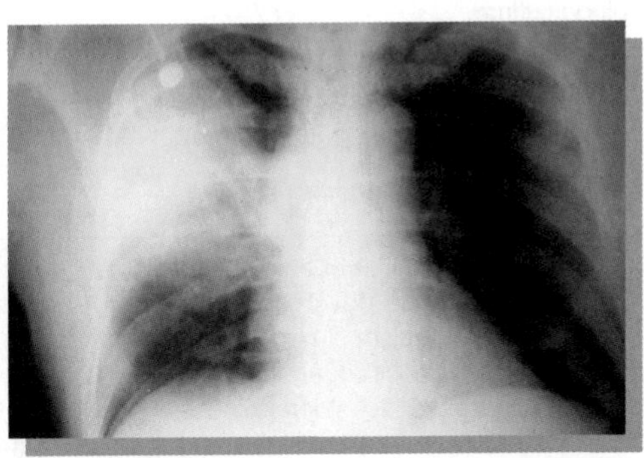

Figure 34.21
Chest film. The white areas are "liquid density," and the black areas are "air density." The central shadow represents the patient's heart. The wedge-shaped white areas on the left are the radiographic appearance of pneumonia involving the middle and upper lobes of the right lung.

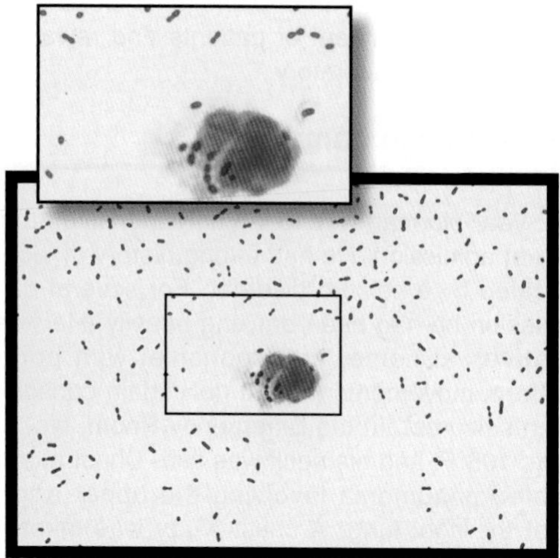

Figure 34.22
Gram stain of the sediment of cerebrospinal fluid, showing a single polymorphonuclear leukocyte and large numbers of gram-positive cocci in pairs.

34.13 The test that will yield the most rapidly available information about the presumptive bacterial cause of this patient's infection is:

A. blood culture.
B. cerebrospinal fluid culture.
C. cerebrospinal fluid Gram stain.
D. urine culture.
E. sputum Gram stain.

The correct answer is **C** (cerebrospinal fluid Gram stain). Although the Gram stain does not tell the exact genus and species of an organism, it narrows down the choices so that an intelligent guess regarding the probable microbial etiology is possible, considering the morphology and the overall clinical situation. Because the Gram stain takes only minutes to perform, precious time is saved in initiating therapy that is as specific as possible. **A** (blood culture) and **B** (cerebrospinal fluid culture) are both incorrect answers because of the time required for visible growth to appear in cultures and the additional time required to identify organisms that do grow. Also, sometimes organisms may be so fastidious that they do not grow easily, further increasing the time it takes to identify them. **D** (urine culture) is incorrect because the site of the clinically evident infection is not the urinary tract. **E** (sputum Gram stain) is incorrect primarily because it may be difficult to obtain reliable sputum from an unconscious patient, resulting in unnecessary delays. Also, in patients whose infection involves the meninges, regardless of the source, defining the central nervous system process takes priority over most other diagnostic considerations and is most likely to lead to the most specific possibility because of the absence of "normal" resident flora in the cerebrospinal fluid (CSF).

Gram stain of the CSF showed scant polymorphonuclear leukocytes (PMNs) and very large numbers of gram-positive cocci in pairs (Figure 34.22). The chest film confirmed pneumonia of the right upper and middle lobes. The peripheral white blood cell (WBC) count was 4,700/ml (73 percent PMNs, 19 percent bands). (For a patient with this degree of illness due to infection, this WBC count is unusually low and reflects his inability to mount appropriate defenses against his infection.)

34.14 In this patient with lobar pneumonia and cerebrospinal fluid that has a heavy concentration of gram-positive cocci in pairs (diplococci), the most likely microbial etiology of his infections is:

A. *Neisseria meningitidis.*
B. *Staphylococcus haemolyticus.*
C. *Streptococcus pneumoniae.*
D. *Listeria monocytogenes.*
E. *Cryptococcus neoformans.*

The correct answer is **C** (*Streptococcus pneumoniae*), which is a gram-positive coccus that often occurs in pairs and is a notorious cause of community-acquired pneumonia, especially in heavy alcohol users. It has a propensity to invade the central nervous system (CNS), causing meningitis. **A** (*Neisseria meningitidis*) is incorrect because it is a gram-negative diplococcus, albeit an important cause of meningitis in adults. **B** (*Staphylococcus haemolyticus*) is incorrect because this organism, indeed a gram-positive coccus, is not likely to be arrayed in pairs, but rather in clusters. Moreover, it is not often associated with lung infections, or with meningitis unless there is an antecedent break in the meninges, as with surgery or trauma. **D** (*Listeria monocytogenes*) is incorrect because the organism is a gram-positive bacillus and not a coccus, although it is a well-known cause of meningitis, especially in heavy alcohol users. **E** (*Cryptococcus neoformans*) is incorrect because, in spite of its name, it is not a coccus but a yeast, which is considerably larger than a coccus. [Note: Although cryptococcus appears to be a gram-positive organism in Gram stains and can cause both pneumonia and meningitis, one would never mistake it for a bacterium, both because of its size and because it has the morphologic property of budding.]

Penicillin (which, when this patient was treated, was the drug of choice for *S. pneumoniae* infections) in very high doses was given within minutes of the lumbar puncture. The patient never regained consciousness, continuing to have seizures almost constantly for the next 2 days, despite aggressive anticonvulsant treatment. His heart rate slowed, and his blood pressure became immeasurably low. Resuscitation attempts failed, and he was pronounced dead on his third hospital day.

An α-hemolytic, gram-positive coccus, morphologically identical to the organism that was seen in the cerebrospinal fluid (CSF) Gram stain, grew from cultures of blood and CSF. It was identified as *S. pneumoniae.*

Discussion: *S. pneumoniae*, commonly known as the pneumococcus, is the most frequent cause of meningitis in adults and usually enters the bloodstream (and from there the CNS) via the lungs. Occasionally, even with the most intensive supportive care and the earliest possible specific antimicrobial treatment, patients with pneumococcal infections die.

Was there something about this patient that put him at a disadvantage in his battle with *S. pneumoniae*?

This patient was at a particular disadvantage because his heavy alcohol use diminished his ability to fight many types of infection by reducing the capacity of his bone marrow to mount a response of the types of cells, polymorphonuclear leukocytes (PMNs), needed to engulf pneumococci and destroy them. The relatively small number of PMNs in his CSF were unable to keep up with the rapid proliferation of pneumococci in his subarachnoid space (where the CSF is located). Ordinarily, when CSF is cloudy in meningitis, it is because of a large number of PMNs in it. This patient's CSF was cloudy more from the massive numbers of pneumococci it contained. [Note: When this patient was seen, penicillin-resistant pneumococci were very rare. Nowadays, empiric therapy would be vancomycin.]

Case 11: Man with recurrent fever

This 21-year-old male university student had fever intermittently for several weeks. The patient had previously been well and was a varsity football player at an East Coast university. Shortly after the end of the school year, he spent 6 weeks in North Carolina at an encampment on a military base. During this time, he recalled multiple tick bites. He personally removed a number of ticks that had been embedded in his skin. He spent the remainder of the summer at his family's home in eastern Washington and at their summer cabin in Idaho. After several weeks in the West, he developed fever as high as 105°F, accompanied by headache, myalgias (muscle pains), arthralgias (joint pains), nausea, and occasional vomiting. After 5 days, his symptoms abated, and he felt well. Ten days after the resolution of these symptoms he had them again, but they were less severe and only lasted about 2 days. Ten days after the second febrile illness he had a third, similar episode that also resolved after about 2 days.

He returned to his university at the end of the summer, and, about 2 weeks after his last febrile episode, he again developed fever, this time mild, and accompanied by generalized malaise. When he was examined, his temperature was 98°F, and his pulse 72 beats per minute. His physical examination was completely within normal limits except that his spleen tip was palpable about 4 cm below his left costal margin with deep inspiration. His hemoglobin concentration was 12.6 g/dl (lower limit of normal is 14), his white blood cell count was normal at 4,500/μl, his platelet count was 135,000/μl (lower limit of normal is 140,000). An incidental observation was made by the laboratory technician who examined the patient's peripheral blood smear for the blood count. What was seen is shown in Figure 34.23.

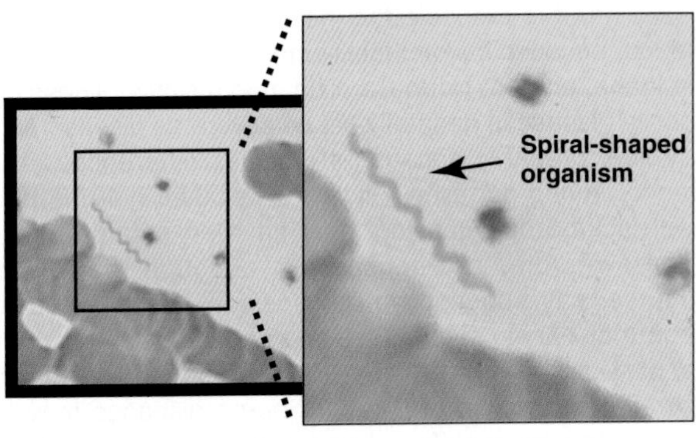

Figure 34.23
Wright stain of this patient's peripheral blood smear, revealing a spiral-shaped organism among (but not within) the circulating blood cells.

34.15 Which of the following tick-borne infections is compatible with the microbial morphology shown in Figure 34.23?

A. Rocky Mountain spotted fever (*Rickettsia rickettsii*)
B. Colorado tick fever (Coltivirus)
C. Ehrlichiosis (*Ehrlichia* species)
D. Relapsing fever (*Borrelia* species)
E. Babesiosis (*Babesia microti*)

The correct answer is **D** (relapsing fever), which is caused by a spirochetal organism of the genus *Borrelia*. Spirochetes do not appear on Gram stain, but those that cause relapsing fever may be seen in Wright stain smears of peripheral blood. **A** (Rocky Mountain spotted fever) is incorrect because rickettsiae are not visible with ordinary stains, and they do not have the spiral morphology seen in Figure 34.23. **B** (Colorado tick fever) is an incorrect answer because viruses are generally too small to be seen with light microscopy. Pathologic changes that some viruses cause (for example, inclusion bodies) are visible with light microscopy, but the virus itself is not. **C** (ehrlichiosis) is not caused by a spirochete. The abnormality that it creates is seen in circulating leukocytes and, because of its fancied resemblance to a mulberry, is called a morula. **E** (babesiosis) also is not caused by a spirochete. The etiologic agent, a protozoan that resembles malarial forms, may, however, be seen in Wright stain preparations of peripheral blood.

The patient was treated with doxycycline 200 mg per day for 10 days. Shortly after his first dose of doxycycline, he had severe fever and chills. He subsequently felt better and recovered completely. Of note is the fact that six of his family members, who also spent time at the home in Idaho, also had an illness characterized by recurrent episodes of fever and other constitutional symptoms.

Discussion: This young man had a very typical case of relapsing fever, an illness that is transmitted by lice or ticks. Ticks are responsible for endemic disease. Those ticks that transmit *Borrelia* species that cause relapsing fever prefer humid environments and altitudes of 1,500 to 6,000 feet. Although this patient remembered tick bites in North

Carolina, it is probable that he acquired relapsing fever in Idaho, because several family members who were with him in Idaho, and not North Carolina, had a similar illness. Tick-borne disease is generally not as severe as disease spread by lice, probably because of species differences in virulence among borreliae. Slightly fewer than half the people with tick-borne relapsing fever have an enlarged spleen. The symptoms are nonspecific, although the relapsing course may suggest the diagnosis. However, other tick-borne diseases, such as malaria and babesiosis, may present with similarly nonspecific symptomatology that may occur in episodes. Several tick-borne diseases may have characteristic manifestations visible in peripheral blood smears. The need to pay attention to findings seen in peripheral blood is well illustrated by this patient.

Why did this patient, who seemed to be getting better before he was treated, get worse after treatment with doxycycline was begun?

His apparent exacerbation of symptoms with the initial treatment is typical of relapsing fever (and a few other spirochetal diseases, including syphilis and Lyme disease). Rapid lysis of spirochetes causes production of several cytokines and the attendant symptoms, which may be severe, including fever, chills, hypotension, and leukopenia. With illness due to the *Borrelia* species that are the agents of louse-borne relapsing fever, this "Jarisch-Herxheimer" reaction may be fatal and should be anticipated so that patients can be observed for a time after the first dose of antibiotic. The reaction is clinically similar to an exaggeration of the febrile episodes observed with untreated relapsing fever.

Case 12: Woman from Ecuador with cough

This 23-year-old woman had been having pain in her left anterior and posterior chest for 1 month. A native of Ecuador, the patient had been in the United States for 4 years and had previously been well. Two months prior to the current visit, she developed cough productive of whitish sputum, worse in the early morning. There was no attendant shortness of breath, and she had not noted any particular odor of the sputum. She had not had hemoptysis (the coughing up of blood). About 1 month after the onset of the cough, she began to have intermittent pleuritic (worse with coughing or deep breathing) left chest pain. In the 1 1/2 months leading up to the current visit, she had noted increasing fatigue and weight loss of 10 pounds but no loss of appetite. There was no history of fever or night sweats.

The patient had never injected drugs. She had a total of two sexual partners, her last sexual contact having occurred 2 years earlier.

The physical examination revealed a well-developed, well-nourished young woman in no distress, with a temperature of 98°F, a pulse of 98 beats per minute, respiratory rate of 18 per minute, and blood pressure 102/60. There was no significant lymphadenopathy (swollen lymph nodes). The chest revealed fine crackles in the suprascapular areas bilaterally, greater on the left than on the right. [Note: There was probably fluid in the alveoli of the upper lobes.] The left upper lobe area was dull to percussion. [Note: There was probably enough fluid in at least most of the alveoli in this area to cause the lungs to seem solidified ("consolidated") on the physical examination.] The remainder of the physical examination was unremarkable. The patient's chest film (Figure 34.24) shows infiltrates of both upper lobes, with at least two cavities in the left upper lobe and a probable cavity of the right lung (arrows).

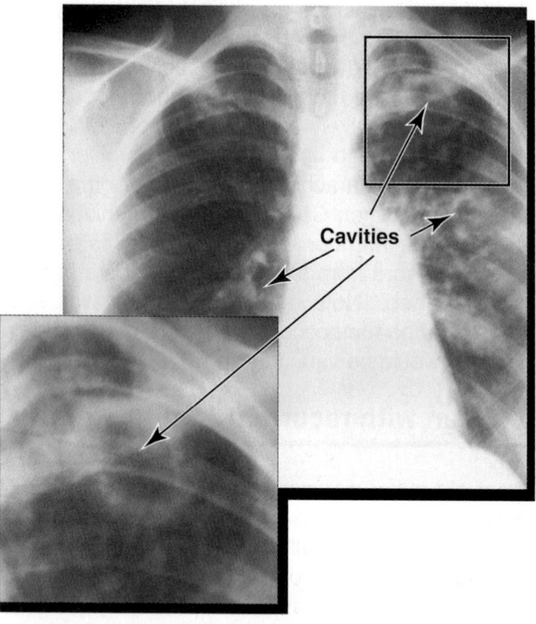

Figure 34.24
Chest radiograph reveals infiltrates in both lungs, with two cavities in the left upper lobe and probably another in the right lung.

34.16 Because of the history of productive cough and weight loss in a woman from South America, with cavitary pulmonary infiltrates seen on the chest film, the physicians caring for this patient suspected tuberculosis. Which of the following studies will give the most rapid presumptive support to the diagnosis of active pulmonary tuberculosis?

A. Tuberculin skin test
B. Sputum culture for acid-fast bacilli
C. Sputum Gram stain
D. Sputum acid-fast stain
E. Sputum assay for *Mycobacterium tuberculosis* by polymerase chain reaction

The correct answer is **D** (sputum acid-fast stain), which takes just minutes to perform and, when positive in a compatible clinical setting (which this patient certainly provides), is very strong presumptive evidence of active tuberculosis. **A** (tuberculin skin test) is not correct because a positive tuberculin reaction indicates infection with tuberculosis but not necessarily active disease. **B** (sputum culture for acid-fast bacilli [AFB]) is incorrect because cultures may take up to 6–8 weeks to yield growth of organisms. Cultures are important to confirm the diagnosis of tuberculosis and to provide an isolate whose susceptibility to antituberculous drugs can be tested, but sputum cultures do not contribute to rapid presumptive diagnosis. **C** (sputum Gram stain) is incorrect because tubercle bacilli (and other AFB) are not visualized with Gram stain. **E** (sputum assay for *Mycobacterium tuberculosis* by polymerase chain reaction) takes several hours and is not usually available in ordinary community-based clinical laboratories. When it is positive (see below) it is very helpful.

The physicians caring for this patient obtained sputum for AFB stain and culture. The AFB stain (Figure 34.25) showed large numbers of AFB, some of which had the typical beaded appearance of *M. tuberculosis*.

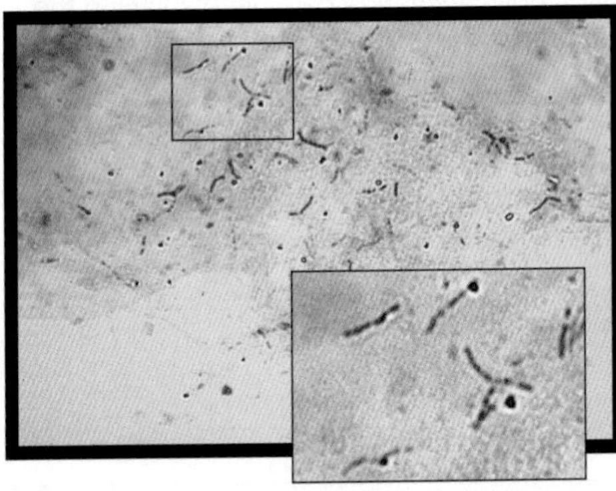

Figure 34.25
Acid-fast stain of sputum, showing many acid-fast bacilli. Beaded appearance of several of the AFB (inset) is characteristic, although not definitively diagnostic, of *Mycobacterium tuberculosis*.

34.17 The "classic" solid medium that is used to cultivate *Mycobacterium* species is:

A. Sabouraud agar.
B. Lowenstein-Jensen medium.
C. MacConkey agar.
D. Thayer-Martin medium.
E. sheep blood agar.

The correct answer is **B** (Lowenstein-Jensen medium), an egg-based solid medium that supports the growth of *Mycobacterium* species, including *Mycobacterium tuberculosis*. **A** (Sabouraud agar) is used to cultivate fungi, not acid-fast bacilli (AFB). **C** (MacConkey agar) is a medium that is selective for gram-negative bacilli, not AFB. **D** (Thayer-Martin medium) is chocolate agar to which certain antibiotics have been added and is a medium selective for *Neisseria gonorrhoeae* in specimens taken from nonsterile sites such as genital secretions. **E** (sheep blood agar) is a general-purpose medium for bacteria that does not support the growth of mycobacteria.

This patient's sputum was cultured in a liquid medium that produced fluorescence in the presence of actively respiring *Mycobacterium*, allowing growth to be detected in 9 days. The presence of *M. tuberculosis* in this culture was confirmed by DNA probe. The organism was later found to be susceptible to all antituberculous medications tested. On the basis of the positive AFB stain of her sputum, the patient was treated with isoniazide, rifampin, pyrazinamide, and ethambutol. She gained weight and stopped coughing shortly after the onset of treatment. She continued to respond very well to her treatment. Laboratory studies later confirmed that she was not co-infected with human immunodeficiency virus (HIV).

Discussion: One could hardly ask for a more classical presentation of pulmonary tuberculosis (TB). The patient comes from an area of high endemicity for TB, and the constellation of weight loss, productive cough, and cavitary pulmonary infiltrates is extremely characteristic of TB. [Note: If she had fever and night sweats, her presentation would have been "classic."]

Where and when did this person acquire her infection with *M. tuberculosis*?

Although it is possible that she acquired TB after coming to the United States, it is likely that her active disease represents recrudescence (reactivation) of an infection that she acquired many years earlier. The total number of patients with active TB identified per year and the incidence of new cases of active disease in the United States are at an all-time low. But, since 2001, more than half of the patients with active TB in the United States are emigrants from abroad. Her geographic origin made TB the most likely cause of her rather lengthy cough illness.

Is there an association between active TB and immunosuppression?

Sound cell-mediated immunity (CMI) has been found to be of great importance in containing tuberculous infection. It is not surprising, therefore, that TB is one of the infections that is especially severe in patients whose CMI is impaired by HIV infection. The association between active TB and HIV disease is so strong that the presence of active TB is felt to be a reason to look for concomitant HIV infection. That is why this patient was tested for HIV.

Case 13: Woman with headache

This 68-year-old, right-handed woman was admitted to the hospital because of headaches that began about 1 month earlier.

She was in good general health. About 1 month prior to admission, she developed progressively severe headaches and vertigo (a sensation that her environment was spinning around her). Shortly after the onset of these complaints, she noted photophobia (discomfort from light, to the extent that room lighting caused her eyes to hurt). The photophobia increased to the point that she had to wear sunglasses to cope with Christmas tree lights indoors. She was observed by her family to become increasingly lethargic (drowsy) and forgetful, prompting her hospitalization.

Physical examination revealed a lethargic woman who was oriented to person and place but not to time. She knew her name and where she was, but not the month or the year or that Christmas and New Year's Day had just passed. The temperature was 98.9°F. There was moderate resistance to anterior flexion of her neck beyond 60°. The lungs had crackles at both bases (consistent, in this instance, with findings described below in the chest X-ray). Neurologic examination revealed pain when her straightened legs were raised beyond 45° (evidence, with the resistance to neck flexion, that there was at least moderate inflammation of the meninges). In addition, when reaching for objects with her hands, she consistently overreached and missed them ("past-pointing," indicative of cerebellar dysfunction). This latter finding was worse on the left than on the right.

Computerized tomography of the head revealed only mild cerebral atrophy (shrinkage—probably age related). Because of the signs of meningeal irritation, a lumbar puncture was performed shortly after admission to the hospital.

The peripheral white blood cell (WBC) count was 11,800/µl (normal between 5,000 and 10,000), with 83 percent polymorphonuclear leukocytes, 9 percent band forms, 4 percent lymphocytes, and 4 percent monocytes (a slight increase in immature granulocytes, suggesting an acute inflammatory process somewhere within the patient). The chest X-ray revealed diffuse interstitial infiltrates of both lower lobes (that is, increased fluid in the septa separating very minute air spaces).

The cerebrospinal fluid (CSF) obtained during the lumbar puncture was clear and colorless, with a total white blood cell count of 18/µl (normal up to 4), with 75 percent polymorphonuclear leukocytes and 25 percent lymphocytes. [Note: Polymorphonuclear leukocytes are never normally present in CSF.] The CSF glucose was 28 mg/dl with simultaneous blood glucose of 119 mg/dl. [Note: The blood glucose was within normal limits, but CSF glucose considerably less than 50 percent of blood glucose suggests that a viable microorganism is present in the subarachnoid space.] The CSF protein concentration was 58 mg/dl (very slightly above the upper limit of normal for this patient's age).

While performing the WBC count on the CSF, an alert laboratory technician observed structures that did not resemble WBCs. A sample of CSF was centrifuged, and the sediment resuspended in India ink. Under the microscope, in dramatic relief among the India ink particles, were the organisms shown in Figure 34.26.

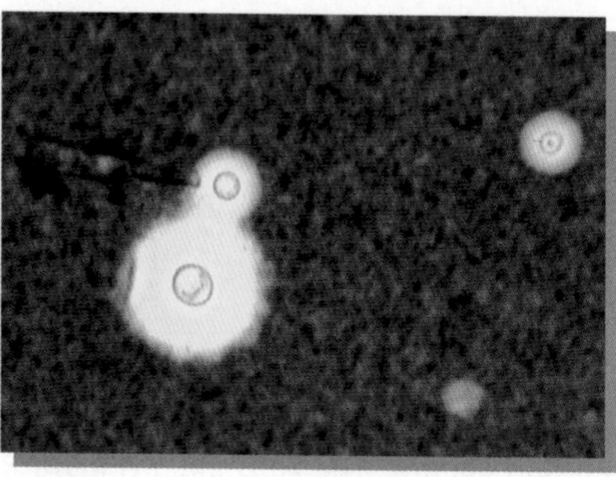

Figure 34.26
India ink preparation of cerebrospinal fluid. A cell and its clear zone appears to be separating from a larger, similar cell. This process, called "budding," is characteristic of yeast cells. The clear zone surrounding the cells is actually a polysaccharide capsule displacing the India ink particles.

34.18 The most likely etiology of this patient's meningitis is:

A. *Streptococcus pneumoniae.*
B. *Candida albicans.*
C. *Histoplasma capsulatum.*
D. *Clostridium perfringens*
E. *Cryptococcus neoformans.*

The correct answer is **E** (*Cryptococcus neoformans*). It is a yeast that reproduces by budding and is characterized by a polysaccharide capsule. The presence of the polysaccharide capsule is very helpful for rapid diagnosis in microscopic examination of clinical specimens such as cerebrospinal fluid (CSF). The capsule may appear Gram negative, and the yeast cell itself gram-positive, in Gram stains. But India ink very dramatically brings the capsule into view under the microscope. **A** (*Streptococcus pneumoniae*) is incorrect because, being a bacterium, it is much smaller than yeast and it does not manifest budding. *S. pneumoniae* progeny are the same size as its parent cell. It also does not display its polysaccharide capsule in ordinary preparations. **B** (*Candida albicans*) is a yeast that manifests budding, but it is not encapsulated. Therefore, this cannot be a correct answer. **C** (*Histoplasma capsulatum*) is incorrect for the same reason—it does not display a polysaccharide capsule in clinical specimens. **D** (*Clostridium perfringens*) is incorrect because, although larger in size than many bacteria, it is still much smaller than a yeast cell. Also, clostridia are not encapsulated and are not round, as are yeast cells.

The organism that grew from cultures of CSF and blood was *C. neoformans*. Despite very aggressive therapy with amphotericin B, both intravenously and instilled directly into a lateral cerebral ventricle, the patient followed a relentless downhill course and died on the eighth day of treatment. Autopsy confirmed severe meningitis due to *C. neoformans*.

What does the presence of infection due to *C. neoformans* suggest about the status of the patient's adaptive immune system?

Discussion: Invasive disease due to this organism is strongly suggestive of a defect in cell-mediated immunity (CMI), and its presence in this patient caused the clinicians caring for her to suspect that she had a malignant lymphoma. [Note: This patient was treated in the early 1980s, prior to the emergence of human immunodeficiency virus (HIV) as a significant cause of severely impaired CMI. Moreover, she had none of the known risk factors that might lead to HIV infection.] In addition to the cryptococcal disease itself, autopsy revealed a clinically inapparent malignant lymphoma that was limited to the patient's urinary bladder and fallopian tubes.

The lymphoma did not cause this patient's death the way many cancerous tumors do, that is, by causing failure of a vital organ. Instead, the profound defect in CMI that accompanies lymphomas (as well as a number of other clinical entities) created in this patient a predisposition to infection with an organism whose progression she could not resist. As *C. neoformans* often does, it attacked her central nervous system preferentially. By the time this infection created clinical symptoms of headache, photophobia, and vertigo, it had passed the point of reversibility and caused her death.

What is the connection between lymphoma and infection?

It is characteristic of malignancies that are accompanied by an immune defect that death is the result of an overwhelming infection. By correlating the immune defect with the underlying disease, one may often anticipate the complicating infection, and intervene in time to effect a favorable clinical outcome. Or, as with this patient, the presence of an opportunistic infection (one that takes particular advantage of individuals with an immune compromise) may herald the clinical onset of an immune-compromising disease. It is, therefore, quite important to be able to match an organism with the list of illnesses associated with the corresponding immune defect.

Case 14: Hematuria in an Egyptian-born man

This 34-year-old man had always enjoyed good health. Several months before the current office visit he began to notice gross hematuria (blood in his urine). The hematuria was unaccompanied by fever, pain, or burning on urination or by any increased sense of urgency to void. He had not had unexplained weight loss.

Born in Cairo, Egypt, he spent his childhood summers on his grandparents' farm in the Nile Delta. He recalled swimming in the Nile twice, the last time when he was in his early 20s. He finished college in Egypt and was well enough to complete military service there. His only infirmity was loss of vision in his right eye since childhood, for reasons unknown to the patient. He had not been back to Egypt since entering the United States 10 years before the onset of the hematuria. He was working as a computer technician. There was no history of exposure to toxins either at work or during recreational activities.

The physical examination was completely within normal limits, except for a red opacity of the lens of the right eye, which was blind. His hemoglobin, 13.5 g/dl, was just below the lower limit of normal of 14. The rest of the laboratory studies were all normal.

Because of concern that the hematuria might herald a malignancy, the patient underwent fiberoptic cystoscopy (an examination that directly visualizes the inside of the urinary bladder). A mass was noted in the fundus of the bladder, biopsy of which is shown in Figure 34.27.

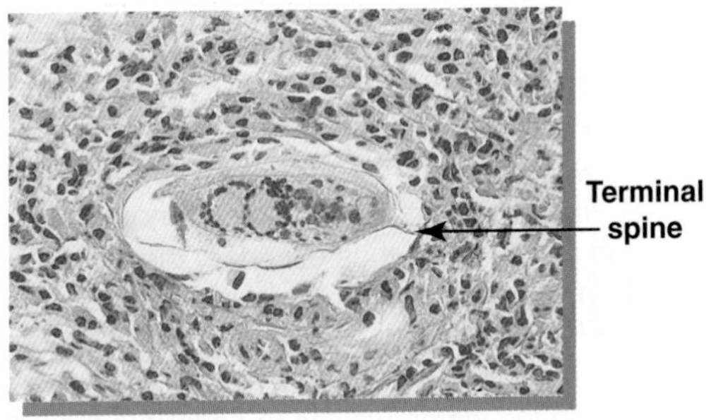

Figure 34.27
Biopsy of the urinary bladder shows areas of inflammation, some containing an ovum with a terminal spine. The presence of this spine at the end of the ovum identifies *Schistosoma haematobium*.

34.19 The part of the history that is most specifically connected with the diagnosis of infection with *Schistosoma haematobium* is which of the following?

A. Gross hematuria
B. The patient's origin in Egypt
C. Swimming in the Nile
D. Concurrent blindness
E. Mild anemia (hemoglobin 13.5 g/dl)

The correct answer is **C** (swimming in the Nile). *Schistosoma haematobium* is a fluke that requires a very specific snail to complete its life cycle. This snail is found only in certain bodies of water in Africa, most notably the Nile River. **A** (gross hematuria) is a symptom that results from the propensity of *S. haematobium* to invade bladder veins, where adult flukes lay their eggs. However, gross hematuria may occur with many conditions and, thus, is not as specifically connected with *S. haematobium* infection as is exposure to the snail vector caused by swimming in the Nile. **B** (the patient's origin in Egypt) is of itself not enough to suspect schistosomiasis, because Egyptians who have not swum in water that is infested with the specific snail vector are not at risk of acquiring this parasite. **D** (concurrent blindness) is part of another parasitic infection associated with fresh water: onchocerciasis ("river blindness"). The roundworm *Onchocerca volvulus* is transmitted to humans by the bite of the black fly, which frequents the fresh water rapids of certain rivers, including some in Africa. **E** (mild anemia) is part of many disease processes and so is not necessarily a hint to the diagnosis of *S. haematobium* infection.

A person from the Nile Valley who has gross hematuria should be suspected of having infection with *S. haematobium* regardless of what other diagnoses may need to be entertained by the rest of the history. The fluke's life cycle illustrates why this is true. Infected humans inevitably excrete *S. haematobium* eggs in their urine, which finds its way into the water. Once thus excreted, these eggs develop into a very motile form called a miracidium that "homes in" on the intermediate host, which is a snail. In the snail, the fluke metamorphoses into a form called a cercaria, which swims freely in the water, waiting to penetrate the intact skin of a person who may be swimming or wading in this water. Once in the human, *S. haematobium* develops into adults, which migrate to the veins of the vesical plexus around the bladder. The female lays eggs, which create an inflammatory response that leads to bleeding, which is perceived by the infected individual as gross hematuria. The passage of these eggs, in urine, into water inhabited by the correct species of snail, completes the life cycle.

This patient was treated with praziquantel, a potent drug that is effective against a number of helminths, including *Schistosoma* species. His hematuria resolved, and repeat cystoscopy revealed resolution of the infective process. He was warned not to swim in the Nile if he should return to Egypt.

Would it be possible to eradicate the snail from its habitat so that people who are exposed to these waters will not be at risk of infection?

The snails are so numerous and so widespread, and so very difficult to kill, that eradicating them would probably have a devastating effect on the overall ecology of the endemic region and the potability of the water. Sometimes it is necessary to avoid risk-associated behaviors. The difficulty is in promoting this behavioral change in populations at risk.

Case 15: Multisystem illness with skin changes

This 35-year-old man was well prior to admission, when he underwent a right inguinal hernia repair. His subsequent course was uneventful until the fifth postoperative day. On that day he developed fever, chills, and diarrhea consisting of five to six watery stools per day. The diarrhea was accompanied by nausea and vomiting. There was no abdominal pain. These gastrointestinal symptoms lasted for 4 days and were accompanied by what the patient described as total anuria (the complete suppression of urinary secretion by the kidneys). He also reported what he perceived to be delusions, especially when trying to fall asleep at night. At about the same time, he developed generalized erythroderma (redness of the skin that blanches when the red areas are pressed), which lasted a few days. His wife, a nurse, observed petechiae (pinpoint intracutaneous hemorrhages) on his lower legs. With all of these symptoms, he refused to consider visiting a physician.

One week after the onset of the fever, his herniorrhaphy wound opened and serosanguineous (mixed blood and serum) fluid began to ooze from it. He continued to feel malaise. The day prior to admission, he was seen by his surgeon, who began treatment with oral tetracycline (because of a history of serious allergy to β-lactam drugs, having manifested as urticaria). However, because of the severity of his symptoms and because of abnormal blood tests, he was admitted to the hospital the next day.

The temperature was 100.8°F, the pulse regular at 90 per minute, and the blood pressure 130/75. The herniorrhaphy wound was open, with tender, indurated (hardened), erythematous (red, with blanching on pressure) margins. Serosanguineous material was oozing from it.

After debridement of his wound and 1 day of treatment with clindamycin and tobramycin, he noted distinct improvement in his sense of well-being. His temperature fell to normal. Intravenous clindamycin was continued for a total of 7 days, followed by another 3 days orally. On about the fifth hospital day, 16 days after the onset of his fever, he noted peeling of the skin of the palmar surfaces of his thumbs. This was followed, over the next 3 days, by generalized desquamation of the skin of his hands and knees and, to a lesser extent, his feet (Figure 34.28).

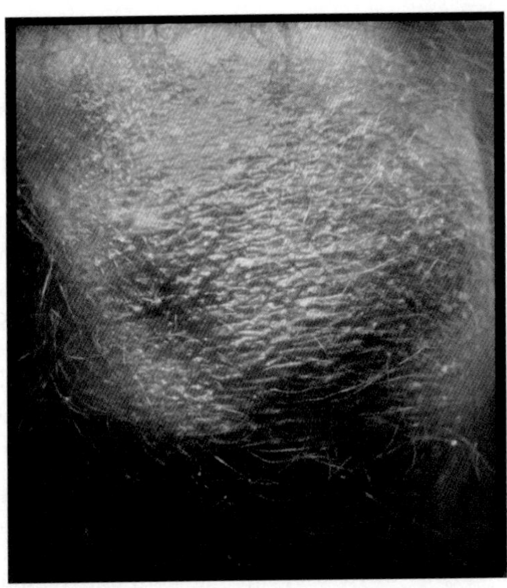

Figure 34.28
Desquamation of skin (knee).

34.20 An organism grew from the serosanguineous wound drainage but not from the blood cultures. From the list below, the most likely organism to cause this constellation of clinical and laboratory findings is:

A. *Escherichia coli.*
B. *Neisseria gonorrheae.*
C. *Pseudomonas aeruginosa.*
D. *Staphylococcus aureus.*
E. *Clostridium perfringens.*

The correct answer is **D** (*Staphylococcus aureus*). This patient has a classical presentation of the staphylococcal toxic shock syndrome (see below). There is nothing specific about this patient to suggest that **A** (*Escherichia coli*) has caused his illness, and that organism would be somewhat unusual as a cause of a cutaneous wound infection in an otherwise healthy person. The skin lesions of **B** (*Neisseria gonorrheae*) are isolated pustules, not desquamation, and these are associated with infection that is disseminated through the bloodstream, which is often accompanied by positive blood cultures. **C** (*Pseudomonas aeruginosa*) is incorrect also because this organism is not associated with desquamation. The skin lesion that may suggest P. aeruginosa is a necrotic area called ecthyma gangrenosum. Although **E** (*Clostridium perfringens*) is associated with a skin manifestation, this is gas gangrene, and involves both muscle and skin.

How does *S. aureus* cause such multisystem disease?

Discussion: *S. aureus* can elaborate a number of pyrogenic exotoxins called superantigens. These include toxic shock syndrome toxin-1 (TSST-1) and staphylococcal entertoxins. These superantigens bypass the usual activation of the immune system, with activation of a very large percentage of T cells, with massive release of cytokines. This results in a shock state similar to that from endotoxin. This patient had fever, diffuse erythroderma, and involvement of his liver (elevated transaminase and alkaline phosphatase), blood (anemia and very high white blood cell count that was out of proportion to the inflammation of his wound—which did not have purulent drainage), kidneys (elevated creatinine that was not corrected with hydration), diarrhea, and abnormal mental status. His platelet count was probably low at the time that he was noted to have petechiae, further evidence of a transient blood dyscrasia. Additionally, his wound grew out *S. aureus*, which was later shown to produce staphylococcal enterotoxin B.

Staphylococcal TSS gained notoriety in the early 1980's, with its association with the use of super-absorbency tampons. However, the syndrome was first described in children with staphylococcal osteomyelitis, and, with the withdrawal of super-absorbency tampons from the commercial market, nonmenstrual staphylococcal TSS is much more common than that associated with menstrual products. The reduced inflammation of the wound is probably from the TSST-1 itself, which interferes with migration of phagocytic cells into the wound. Desquamation of skin during convalescence is also a characteristic of staphylococcal TSS and helped to confirm the diagnosis of staphylococcal TSS. Further confirmation was obtained by proving that his specific strain of *S. aureus* produced the appropriate toxins.

Case 16: Diarrhea acquired in South America

This 18-year-old woman was admitted to the hospital 7 days after the onset of severe diarrhea. Always in good health, the patient had emigrated to the United States from Ecuador several years earlier. She returned to her native country to enter a university in the capital. About 8 days prior to admission, she ate in a restaurant. All who were with her ate fish, as she did, but she was the only one who ate fresh vegetables.

Two days later she developed severe watery diarrhea, passing voluminous amounts of stool several times per day. Two days after that, she began to vomit. These symptoms persisted until her departure for the United States a few days later. She described her stools as "rice water." At no time did she experience fever or chills.

When she was examined, her temperature was 98.4°F, her blood pressure low at 88/50, and her pulse was 72 per minute. Her skin was dry, with decreased turgor. Her eyes appeared to be sunken into their orbits, and her oral mucosal surfaces were dry. The remainder of the physical examination was within normal limits.

The hemoglobin was 15.8 g/dL (normal 12–18 g/dL), the white blood cell count 16,300/mL (normal to 10,000). A specimen of arterial blood revealed the pH to be 7.32 (normal 7.40), the PO_2 103 torr (normal), and the PCO_2 25.4

torr (abnormally low). The blood urea nitrogen was 36 mg/dL, and the serum creatinine was 3.1 mg/dL (normal about 1.0). The concentration of bicarbonate in venous blood was 14 mEq/L (normal 22–28). Wright stain of stool revealed no leukocytes. The stool was negative for occult blood.

34.21 Culture of stool yielded an organism. The most likely organism to cause this illness, taking into consideration all of the clinical and laboratory data, is:

A. *Escherichia coli* O157:H7.
B. *Salmonella typhi.*
C. *Clostridium difficile.*
D. *Shigella sonnei.*
E. *Vibrio cholerae.*

The correct answer is **E** (*Vibrio cholerae*). It causes disease by elaborating a toxin that greatly increases the influx of ions and water into the lumen of the intestine. As a secretory, noninflammatory diarrhea, it is not characterized by fecal leukocytes or blood. **A** (*Escherichia coli* O157:H7) causes hemorrhagic colitis, with copious stool as this patient had, but patients with this infection usually have very bloody stools. The reservoir is cattle, not fish or vegetables. **B** (*Salmonella typhi*) causes enteric fever (this patient was never febrile) and, when there is diarrhea, it is often preceded by constipation. It is an inflammatory process, so that there are fecal leukocytes. **C** (*Clostridium difficile*) usually, but not always, causes disease in relation to health care, especially during or after administration of antibiotics. The associated diarrhea is intensely inflammatory with very numerous fecal leukocytes. **D** (*Shigella sonnei*) is also a cause of extremely inflammatory diarrhea, with so many fecal leukocytes that pus may be visible in stool without magnification.

Discussion: This patient had moderately severe cholera. It had been absent from the Western Hemisphere for some 70 years, until the early 1990's, when it entered Peru in shipments of fish from Asia. Once introduced to an area in which safe drinking water was not widely available, it spread over the next few years throughout South and Central America.

Did this patient make a mistake that caused her to become infected with *V. cholerae*?

This patient violated a cardinal rule of food safety in the developing world by eating uncooked vegetables. [Note: *V. cholerae* persists in nature in aquatic environments, and, when contaminated, uncooked water is consumed, infection is transmitted. It is almost impossible to avoid infection when fresh vegetables that have been either irrigated or rinsed with contaminated water are consumed.] Because cholera is a toxin-mediated noninflammatory process, constitutional symptoms, such as fever, are uncommon. Stool volume may be so great that it may be difficult to keep up with fluid losses. For this patient, dehydration was so severe that she had mild renal failure, with a creatinine of 3.1 mg/dL.

This patient had a metabolic acidosis. How did that happen?

Her acid–base balance was affected by her diarrheal illness, perhaps in part by the renal failure, which causes metabolic acidosis. However, it is more likely that her metabolic acidosis was caused not by accumulation of hydrogen ions, but rather by extreme bicarbonate losses. Stool is alkaline, and when there is massive, prolonged diarrhea such as that experienced by this patient, the result can be metabolic acidosis, just as this patient had. The buffering function of bicarbonate is reduced when there are such huge losses of this cation in stool.

Why bother with so simple a test as microscopic examination of stool for leukocytes?

Among the various ways to categorize diarrhea, one that is useful clinically is inflammatory versus noninflammatory. A simple, inexpensive screening test is the microscopic examination of stool for leukocytes. When they are present, diarrhea is described as "inflammatory," and when they are absent, it is "noninflammatory." Four of the five proposed answers in this case discussion are causes of inflammatory diarrhea. The absence of fecal leukocytes virtually ruled them out. The epidemiologic setting and the large volumes of watery stool further supported the diagnosis of a noninflammatory diarrhea such as cholera. The links to South America and to fresh vegetables added credence to this diagnosis. This patient illustrates the importance of the history and simple laboratory test in making a clinical-microbiological correlation.

She was treated with doxycycline and intravenous hydration. She rapidly recovered and returned to university in Ecuador—after reinforcement of her understanding of safe food practices there.

Figure 34.29 shows a child with cholera.

Case 17: Painful Rash

This 39-year-old man had previously been well. In early March, 7 days prior to this visit, he developed burning pain and paraesthesias (tingling and numbness) of his left scalp and forehead. About 2 days later, he noted several papules (raised bumps) on his scalp (Figure 34.30), followed the next day by several more on his forehead over the left eyebrow and on his left upper eyelid. These evolved into small blisters on which crusts (scabs) formed. As the older lesions became crusted, new papules appeared in the same general area. A physician told him it was poison ivy and advised that he use a topical glucocorticoid cream. Two days later (the fifth day after the onset of the rash), he had not improved and sought consultation with an infectious diseases physician.

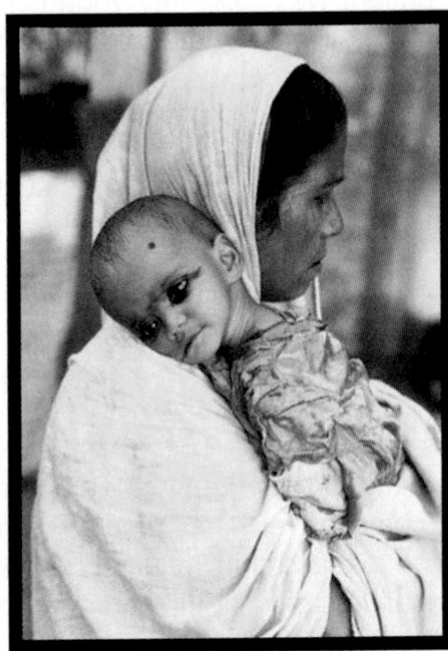

Figure 34.29
Child showing severe dehydration charactistic of cholera.

There had been no contact with plant matter in the several days prior to the onset of the rash.

On physical examination, his temperature was 98°F, and the pulse 88 beats per minute and regular. There were several erythematous (red, but blanching with pressure) papules, groups of clear-fluid–filled vesicles with erythematous bases, and crusted papules in an area that included the left anterior scalp, forehead, and upper eyelid. Several of the vesicles had tiny indentations in their centers ("umbilications"). The tip of the nose was spared.

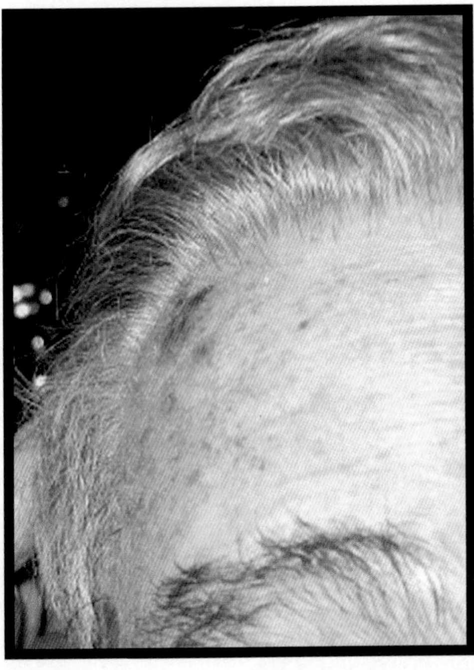

Figure 34.30
39-Year-old man several papules (raised bumps) on his scalp.

There were three healthy children at home, ranging in age from 12 months to 5 years. His wife, age 36 years, and the three children had all been well for the several weeks before this patient developed this rash. For about 2 weeks after all of the lesions healed, the patient complained of burning pain in the area where the rash had been.

34.22 The most likely microbial etiology for this patient's illness is:

A. rubeola virus.
B. varicella-zoster virus.
C. *Clostridium perfringens.*
D. *Streptococcus pyogenes.*
E. *Rickettsia rickettsii.*

The correct answer is **B** (varicella-zoster virus). The key is the evolution, appearance, and distribution of the rash. **A** (rubeola virus) definitely causes a rash (that is, measles), but it is not vesicular (blister causing), and it is more generalized than this patient's rash. Measles is also characterized by an enanthem, lesions inside the mouth. **C** (*Clostridium perfringens*) can cause blisters, but they usually are large and filled with bloody fluid. In addition, patients with systemic disease due to *C. perfringens* are usually very ill, rapidly deteriorating if intervention is not early and aggressive. **D** (*Streptococcus pyogenes*) can cause skin lesions, including vesicles. These may be filled with clear fluid and may crust, but they do not usually come in "crops" (see below). **E** (*Rickettsia rickettsii*) characteristically causes skin lesions, and these may go from papule to vesicle. They usually spread from the periphery toward the center of the body (centripetally) and often evolve into gangrenous lesions because the organism infects blood vessel walls, causing interruption of blood supply to organs, leading to necrosis.

Discussion: Although one could do laboratory tests to "confirm" the diagnosis, such as a microscopic examination of material scraped from the base of a newly unroofed vesicle (Tzanck preparation), or even viral cultures, this patient's illness is classical for zoster. Zoster results from the "reawakening" of varicella virus that remains dormant in sensory ganglion cells in the brainstem and spinal cord.

How does the distribution of the rash help to support the clinical diagnosis of zoster?

The rash is distributed in the territory of the nerve whose root is the site of the newly activated viral particles, following the pattern called a "dermatome." In the case of this patient, the dermatome is that of the first division of the fifth (trigeminal) cranial nerve. Every feature of this patient's rash was classical for zoster. Varicella virus causes lesions that evolve from papules to vesicles filled with clear fluid. The roof of the vesicle often is umbilicated, a characteristic that is common to certain members of the herpesvirus family, including varicella-zoster and herpes simplex. The fluid becomes cloudy, and, eventually, the roof of the vesicle breaks down, leaving a crusty scab in its place. Extremely characteristic of zoster is the appearance of pain and/or paraesthesias in the area that will eventually have the rash, usually a day or two before the rash is evident. [Note: If the clinician takes a careful history, and if the pain or paraesthesias follow a dermatome, he or she can look really smart if he or she (correctly) tells the patient to expect a rash in that area in a day or two.] None of the features of this patient's rash would be expected if it were due to poison ivy.

What is the patient's prognosis with regard to the symptoms he experienced?

One of the worst features of zoster is the pain that may linger for weeks after the rash has healed. This is called "postherpetic neuralgia" and may be extremely severe, especially in older adults. A vaccine has been developed for individuals age 60 years and older that can prevent or lessen the severity of the rash and the postherpetic neuralgia. At present, a single dose of this vaccine is all that is recommended, once in the patient's lifetime. The virus is the same as that in the varicella (chickenpox) vaccine but 15 times more concentrated than the varicella vaccine.

Because this patient was relatively young when he developed zoster, the likelihood of prolonged postherpetic neuralgia is very small. In fact, he experienced it for only 2 weeks.

Systemically administered antiviral drugs such as acyclovir or valacyclovir may promote more rapid healing of the rash and may reduce the severity of postherpetic neuralgia. To be effective, they must be given within 72 hours of the onset of the rash. This patient's diagnosis was correctly made too late for him to benefit from antiviral therapy.

When patients have severe or extensive zoster lesions, which have live virus in them, they may spread the virus to individuals who have never been infected with the varicella-zoster virus. The disease that results is chickenpox, which is the clinical manifestation of infection due to this virus in individuals who have never had it before. Zoster only occurs in individuals who have had chickenpox in the past. The patient's 12-month-old son had not yet received varicella vaccine and was, thus, susceptible to it. However, he remained well and received his first dose of varicella vaccine several months after his father recovered, according to the schedule recommended by the Centers for Disease Control and Prevention and the National Institutes of Health.

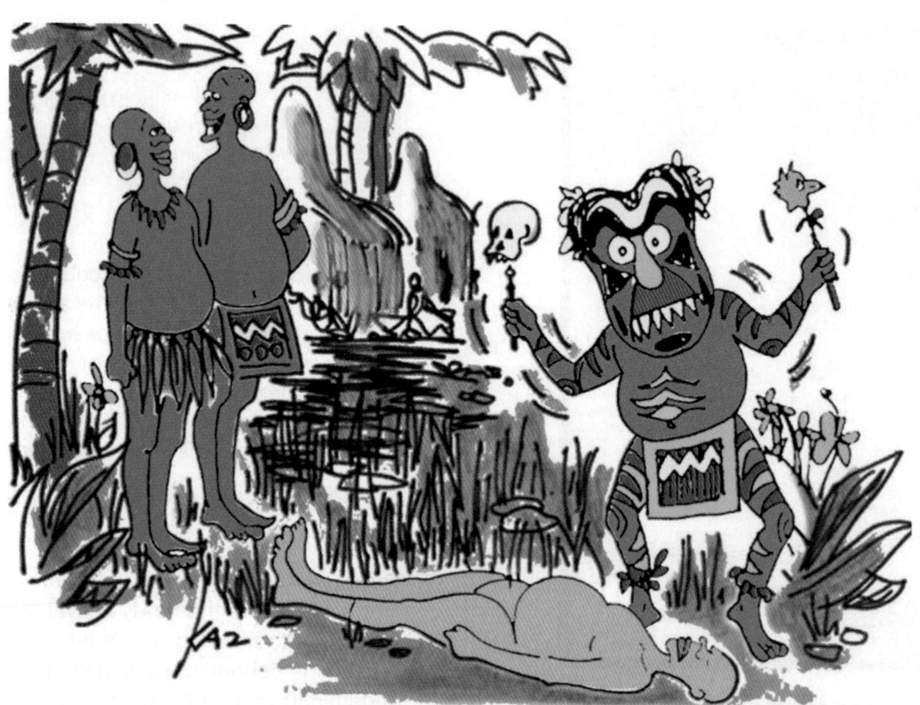

"It's a very effective dance when followed by a shot of penicillin."

Information contained in this Index

Page numbers in **boldface** indicate the most extensive discussion of the topic. Entries in ALL CAPITAL letters indicate diseases and syndromes. *See* cross-references direct the reader to the synonymous term. *See also* cross-references direct the reader to related topics. [Note: Positional and configurational designations in chemical names (for example, α-, β-, and *N*-) are ignored for alphabetizing.

A

B

D

F

G

H

I

N

Q

R

S

T

U

V

W

Y

Z

Figure Sources

Fig. 2.1: Courtesy of Bernard A. Cohen, MD, Christoph U. Lehmann, MD, DermAtlas, Johns Hopkins University.

Fig. 4.1 Meridian Diagnostics, Inc, Cincinnati, Ohio.

Fig. 4.1: Forbes, B. A., Sahm, D. I. F., and Weissfeld, A. S. *Baily & Scott's Diagnostic Microbiology.* Mosby, Inc. 1988. Fig. 14-11, p. 200.

Fig. 4.4: Wistreich, G. *Microbiology Perspectives: A Photographic Survey of the Microbial World.* Prentice-Hall, Inc. 1999. Fig. 193, p. 86.

Fig. 4.6: Bottone, E. J., Girolami, R., and Stamm, J. M., *Schneierson's Atlas of Diagnostic Microbiology,* Ninth Edition, Abbott Laboratories, 1984, p. 49.

Fig. 4.7: Becton-Dickinson Microbiology Systems.

Fig. 4.8: Mahon, C. R. and Manuselis, G., *Textbook of Diagnostic Microbiology,* W. B. Saunders Company, 1995. Fig. 9-2A, p. 310.

Fig. 4.9: Alexander, S. K. and Strete, D. *Microbiology: A Photographic Atlas for the Laboratory.* Benjamin Cummings, 2001. Fig. 5.6, p. 71.

Fig. 4.9: Cappuccino, J. G. and Sherman, N., *Microbiology: A Laboratory Manual,* Fourth Edition, Benjamin/Cummings Publishing Company, Inc, 1996. Color plate 28.

Fig. 4.9: de la Maza, L. M., Pezzlo, M. T. and Baron, E. J., *Color Atlas of Diagnostic Microbiology,* Mosby, *1997.* Fig. 8-16, p. 61.

Fig. 4.9: Forbes, B. A., Sahm, D. I. F., and Weissfeld, A. S. *Baily & Scott's Diagnostic Microbiology.* Mosby, Inc. 1988. Fig. 13.8, p. 173.

Fig. 4.9: Gillies, R.R. and Dodds, T.C., *Bacteriology Illustrated,* Third Edition, Williams and Wilkins Company, 1973, p. 41.

Fig. 4.13: Forbes, B. A., Sahm, D. I. F., and Weissfeld, A. S. *Baily & Scott's Diagnostic Microbiology.* Mosby, Inc. 1988. Fig. 15-6, p. 212.

Fig. 6.10: Lim, D. *Microbiology,* Second Edition. MCB/McGraw-Hill, 1998. Fig. 3.13, p. 55.

Fig. 8.6: Visuals Unlimited.

Fig. 8.7: Couresty of Dr. Gary E. Kaiser.

Fig. 8.11: Peters, G., Gray, E. D., and Johnson, G. M. in Bisno, A. L. and Waldvogel, F. A. *Infections Associated with Indwelling Medical Devices.* American Society for Microbiology, 1989. Fig. 1, p. 62.

Fig. 8.12 (middle row, left): Courtesy of The Canadian Infectious Diseases Society

Fig. 8.12 (middle row, center): Courtesy of Dr. John Bezzant.

Fig. 8.12 (middle row, right): Courtesy of Dr. John Bezzant.

Fig. 8.12 (bottom row, left): Costerton, J. W. and Lappin-Scott, H. M. ASM News 55 (12):653,

Fig. 8.12 (bottom row, center): Schenfeld, L. A. *N Engl J Med.* 342:1177 (2000).

Fig. 8.12 (bottom row, right): Courtesy of Dr. John Bezzant.

Fig. 9.5: Meltzer,D. L. and Kabongo, M. *American Family Physician,* July, 1997; pp. 145, 147.

Fig. 9.10: MacFaddin, J. F. *Biochemical Tests for Identification of Medical Bacteria.* Lippincott Williams & Wilkins, 2000. Fig. 3.1, p. 806.

Fig. 9.10 Gillies, R.R. and Dodds, T.C., *Bacteriology Illustrated,* Third Edition, Williams and Wilkins Company, 1973, p. 58.

Fig. 9.10: Hart, T. and Shears, P., *Color Atlas of Medical Microbiology,* Mosby-Wolfe. 1996. Fig. 123, p. 97.

Fig. 9.14: Courtesy Dr. David Rayner, University of Alberta Lab Med & Pathology.

Fig. 9.15 (top row, left): Courtesy of Dr. Donna Duckworth.

Fig. 9.15 (top row, right): Courtesy of Dr. Donna Duckworth.

Fig. 9.15 (bottom row, left): Bisno, A. L. and Stevens, D. L., *N Engl J Med.* 334: (#4), 241 (1996).

Fig. 9.15 (bottom row, middle): Peterson, P. K. and Dahl, M. V., *Dermatologic Manifestations of Infectious Diseases.* The Upjohn Company, 1982. Fig. 48-1, p. 105.

Fig. 9.15 (bottom row, right): Mir, M. A., *Atlas of Clinical Diagnosis,* W. J. B. Saunders Company Ltd., 1995. Fig. 2.103; p. 86.

Fig. 10.3: 2000 Red Book: Report of the Committee on Infectious Diseases, American Academy of Pediatrics.

Fig. 10.4: Public Health Image Library, Centers for Disease Control and Prevention.

Fig. 10.5 (left): Alexander, S. K. and Strete, D. Microbiology: *A Photographic Atlas for the Laboratory.* Benjamin Cummings, 2001. Fig. 2.7, p. 13.

Fig. 10.5 (right): Courtesy Harriet CW Thompson, M.S., Department of Microbiology, Immunology &, Parasitology, Louisiana State University Health Sciences Center, New Orleans,

Fig. 10.5 (bottom): Farrar, W. E., Wood, M. J., Innes, J. A., Tubbs, H., *Infectious Diseases.* Second Edition, Gower Medical Publishing, 1992. Fig. 1.35. p. 1.11.

Fig. 10.7 (upper left): Bottone, E. J., Girolami, R., and Stamm, J. M., *Schneierson's Atlas of Diagnostic Microbiology,* Ninth Edition, Abbott Laboratories, 1984. p. 5.

Fig. 10.7 (upper right): Bottone, E. J., Girolami, R., and Stamm, J. M., *Schneierson's Atlas of Diagnostic Microbiology,* Ninth Edition, Abbott Laboratories, 1984. p. 5.

Fig. 10.7 (bottom): Public Health Image Library, Centers for Disease Control and Prevention.

Fig. 11.2: Bottone, E. J., Girolami, R., and Stamm, J. M., *Schneierson's Atlas of Diagnostic Microbiology,* Ninth Edition, Abbott Laboratories, 1984. p. 37.

Fig. 11.2: Sherris, J. C., Editor. *Medical Microbiology,* Second Edition, Appelton & Lange, 1990. Fig. 19.3, p. 349.

Fig. 11.4: Schaechter, M., Engleberg, N. C., Eisenstein, B. I., and Medoff, G. *Mechanism of Microbial Disease,* Third Edition. Williams and Wilkins, 1998. Fig. 14.6, p. 166.

Fig. 11.5: Hoeprich, P. D., Jordan, M. C. and Ronald, A. R., *Infectious Diseases, a Treatise of Infectious Processes,* Fifth Edition, J.B. Lippincott Company, Philadelphia, 1994. Fig. 70-6, p. 681.

Fig. 11.7: Bottone, E. J., Girolami, R., and Stamm, J. M., *Schneierson's Atlas of Diagnostic Microbiology,* Ninth Edition, Abbott Laboratories, 1984. p. 37.

Fig. 11.8: Images in Clinical Medicine. *N Engl J Med,* 336:707 (1997).

Fig. 11.11: Beeching, N.J. and Nye, F.J., *Diagnostic Picture Tests in Clinical Infectious Disease,* Mosby- Wolfe, 1996. Fig. 61, p. 33.

Fig. 11.14 (left): Bottone, E. J., Girolami, R., and Stamm, J. M., *Schneierson's Atlas of Diagnostic Microbiology,* Ninth Edition, Abbott Laboratories, 1984. p 37.

Fig. 11.140 (right): Bottone, E. J., Girolami, R., and Stamm, J. M., *Schneierson's Atlas of Diagnostic Microbiology,* Ninth Edition, Abbott Laboratories, 1984. p. 37.

Fig. 11.14 (left, center row) : McMilan, A. and Scott, G. R. *Sexually Transmitted Diseases.* Churchill Livingstone, 1991. Fig. 17, p. 12.

Fig. 11.14 (right, center row): Brown, T. J., Yen-Moore, A., and Tyring, S. K. *Journal of the American Academy of Dermatology.* Volume 41, Number 4. October 1999. Fig. 10.

Fig. 12..5 (top, left): Atlas, R. M. *Microorganisms in our World.* Mosby, 1995, p. 41.

Fig. 12.7: Wistreich, G. *Microbiology Perspectives: A Photographic Survey of the Microbial World.* Prentice-Hall, Inc. 1999. Fig. 131, p. 59.

Fig. 12.8: Koneman, E. W., Allen, S. D., Janda, W. M., Schreckenberger, P. C. and Winn, W. C., *Color Atlas and Textbook of Diagnostic Microbiology,* Fifth Edition, J. B. Lippincott Company, 1997. Plate 6-1A.

Fig. 12.10 (left): Koneman, E. W., Allen, S. D., Janda, W. M., Schreckenberger, P. C. and Winn, W. C., *Color Atlas and Textbook of Diagnostic Microbiology,* Fourth Edition, J. B. Lippincott Company, 1992. Plate 5-1A.

Fig. 12.10 (right): Varnam, A. H. and Evans, M. G. *Foodborne Pathogens.* Mosby-Yearbook, Inc. 1991. Fig. 170, p. 228.

Fig. 12..12 (right): Leboffe, M. J. and Pierce, B. E. *A Photographic Atlas for the Microbiology Laboratory.* Morton Publishing Company. 1999. Fig. 11-35, p.137.

Fig. 12.14: Copyright Dennis Kunkel

Microscopy, Inc.

Fig. 12.15: Public Health Image Library, Centers for Disease Control and Prevention.

Fig. 12.17 (top, left): Leboffe, M.J. and Pierce, B. E. *A Photographic Atlas for the Microbiology Laboratory.* Morton Publishing Company. 1999. Fig. 11-21, p. 131.

Fig. 12.17 (top, right): Xia, H.X., Kean, C.T., and O'Morain. *European J. Clin. Microbiol. & Inf. Dis.* 13: 406 (1994).

Fig. 12..17 (bottom): Genta, R. M., and Graham, D. Y. *N Engl J Med.* 335:250 (Number 4) 1996.

Fig. 13.2: Musher, D. *J. Infectious Diseases,* 149:4, 4/84.

Fig. 13.5 (left): Quintiliani, R. and Bartlett, R. C., *Examination of the Gram-Stained Smear.* Hoffman-La Roche Inc., 1994. Fig. 7.

Fig. 13.5 (bottom): Farrar, W. E., Wood, M. J., Innes, J. A., Tubbs, H., *Infectious Diseases.* Second Edition, Gower Medical Publishing, 1992. Fig. 3.3, p. 3.4.

Fig. 13.9 (upper left): Alexander, S. K. and Strete, D. *Microbiology: A Photographic Atlas for the Laboratory.* Benjamin Cummings, 2001. Fig. 9.2, p. 123.

Fig. 13.9 (upper right): Koneman, E. W., Allen, S. D., Janda, W. M., Schreckenberger, p. C. and Winn, W. C., *Color Atlas and Textbook of Diagnostic Microbiology,* Fourth Edition, J. B. Lippincott Company, Philadelphia, 1992. Plate 7-2 E.

Fig. 13.9 (bottom): NIBSC/Science Photo Library/Photo Researcher, Inc.

Fig. 13.11 (left): Leboffe, M. J. and Pierce, B. E. *A Photographic Atlas for the Microbiology Laboratory.* Morton Publishing Company. 1999. Fig. 11-23, p. 132.

Fig. 13.11 (right): Koneman, E. W., Allen, S. D., Janda, W. M., Schreckenberger, P. C. and Winn, W. C., *Color Atlas and Textbook of Diagnostic Microbiology,* Fourth Edition, J. B. Lippincott Company, 1992. Plate 8-1 E.

Fig. 13.11 (bottom): Farrar, W. E., Wood, M. J., Innes, J. A., Tubbs, H., *Infectious Diseases.* Second Edition, Gower Medical Publishing, 1992. Fig. 2.29, p. 2.11

Fig. 13.12: Kassirer, J. P., *Images in Clinical Medicine,* Massachusetts Medical Society, 1997. p. 203.

Fig. 13.15 (left): Leboffe, M.J. and Pierce, B. E. *A Photographic Atlas for the Microbiology Laboratory.* Morton Publishing Company. 1999. Fig. 11-7, p. 124.

Fig. 13.15 (right): de la Maza, L. M., Pezzlo, M. T. and Baron, E. J., *Color Atlas of Diagnostic Microbiology, Mosby, 1997.* Fig. 9-18, p. 77.

Fig. 13.16: Volk, W. A., Gebhardt, B. M., Hammarskjold, M. and Kadner, R. J., *Essentials of Microbiology,* Fifth Edition, Lippincott-Raven, Philadelphia, 1996. Fig. 27-5, p 393.

Fig. 13.17: Courtesty of Dr. Sellers, Emory Uuniversity, Public Health Image Library, Centers for Disease Control and Prevention.

Fig. 13.18 (top, left): Koneman, E. W., Allen, S. D., Janda, W. M., Schreckenberger, P. C. and Winn, W. C., *Color Atlas and Textbook of Diagnostic Microbiology,* Fifth Edition, J. B. Lippincott Company, 1997. Plate 8-3H.

Fig. 13.18 (top, right): Koneman, E. W., Allen, S. D., Janda, W. M., Schreckenberger, P. C. and Winn, W. C., *Color Atlas and Textbook of Diagnostic Microbiology,* Fourth Edition, J. B. Lippincott Company, 1992. Plate 7-2J.

Fig. 13.18 (bottom): Center for Disease Control, Atlanta.

Fig. 13.20: Wistreich, G. *Microbiology Perspectives: A Photographic Survey of the Microbial World.* Prentice-Hall, Inc. 1999. Fig. 140, p. 63.

Fig. 13.21: Leboffe, M. J. and Pierce, B. E. *A Photographic Atlas for the Microbiology Laboratory.* Morton Publishing Company. 1999. Fig. 11-44; p. 142.

Fig. 13.23: Hart, T. and Shears, P., *Color Atlas of Medical Microbiology,* Mosby-Wolfe. 1996. Fig. 221, p. 150.

Fig. 13.23: Krammer, T. T. *Comparative Pathogenic Bacteriology* (Filmstrip). W. B. Saunders Company 1972. Slide: 34.

Fig. 14.4 Stephens, M. B. *Postgraduate Medicine,* Vol 99, No. 4, April 1996. p. 218.

Fig. 14.5: Bottone, E. J., Girolami, R., and Stamm, J. M., *Schneierson's Atlas of Diagnostic Microbiology,* Ninth Edition, Abbott Laboratories, 1984. p. 9.

Fig. 14.8: Courtesy of Dr. Gary E. Kaiser, The Community College of Baltimore County.

Fig. 14.9 (top, right): Finegold, S. M. and Sutter, V. L., *Anaerobic infections.* The Upjohn Company, 1986. Fig. 60, p. 51.

Fig. 14.9 (bottom, left): Finegold, S. M., Baron, E. J. and Wexler, H. M. *A Clinical Guide to Anaerobic Infections.* Star Publishing Company, 1992. Fig. 70, p. 69.

Fig. 14.9 (bottom, center): Finegold, S. M., Baron, E. J. and Wexler, H. M. *A Clinical Guide to Anaerobic Infections.* Star Publishing Company, 1992. Fig. 86, p. 82.

Fig. 14.9 (bottom, right): Kelly, C. P., Pothoulakis, C., and LaMont, J. T. *N Engl J Med.* 330:257-262 (1994).

Fig. 15.3: McMilan, A. and Scott, G. R. *Sexually Transmitted Diseases.* Churchill Livingstone., 1991 Fig. 63, p. 42.

Fig. 15.4: Brown, T. J., Yen-Moore, A. and Tyring, S. K. *Journal of the American Academy of Dermatology.* Volume 41, Number 4. October 1999. Fig. 1.

Fig. 15.4: Brown, T. J., Yen-Moore, A. and Tyring, S. K. *Journal of the American Academy of Dermatology.* Volume 41, Number 4. October 1999. Fig. 4.

Fig. 15.4: McMilan, A. and Scott, G. R. *Sexually Transmitted Diseases.* Churchill Livingstone, 1991 Fig. 63, p. 42.

Fig. 15.4: Brown, T. J., Yen-Moore, A. and Tyring, S. K. *Journal of the American Academy of Dermatology.* Volume 41, Number 4. October 1999. Fig. 8,

Fig. 15.5: McMilan, A. and Scott, G. R. *Sexually Transmitted Diseases.* Churchill Livingstone., 1991. Fig. 136, p. 92.

Fig. 15.7 (left): McMillan, A. and Scott, G. R. *Sexually Transmitted Diseases.* Churchill Livingstone, 1991. Fig. 64, p. 42.

Fig. 15.7 (right): Brown, T. J., Yen-Moore, A. and Tyring, S. K. *Journal of the American Academy of Dermatology.* Volume 41, Number 4. October 1999. Fig. 1.

Fig. 15.9: Verdon, M. E., Sigal, Leonard H., *American Family Physician.* August 1997. p. 429,

Fig. 15.9: Department of Dermatology, Uniformed Services University, Bethesda, Maryland.

Fig. 15.12 (next to bottom): American Society Microbiology (Microbelibrary.org). Jeffrey Nelson, Rush University.

Fig. 15.12 (bottom): Ledbetter, L. S., Hsu, S., and Less, J. B., *Po*

Fig. 15.14: Wistreich, G. *Microbiology Perspectives: A Photographic Survey of the Microbial World.* Prentice-Hall, Inc. 1999. Fig. 72, p. 39.

Fig. 15.14 (bottom): Farrar, W. E., Wood, M. J., Innes, J. A., Tubbs, H., *Infectious Diseases.* Second Edition, Gower Medical Publishing, 1992. Fig. 13.40., p. 13.15

Fig. 16.5 (top, right): Michael Gabridge/Visuals Unlimited.

Fig. 16.5 (top, left): Kassirer, J. P., *Images in Clinical Medicine,* Massachusetts Medical Society, 1997, p. 38.

Fig. 16.5 (bottom): Farrar, W. E., Wood, M. J., Innes, J. A., Tubbs, H., *Infectious Diseases.* Second Edition, Gower Medical Publishing, 1992. Fig. 2.25, p. 2.8.

Fig. 17.2: Cutlip, R. C., National Animal Disease Center. United States Department of Agriculture. Agricultural Research Service.

Fig. 17.5: Courtesy of Dr. Umberto Benelli, Online Atlas of Ophthalmology

Fig. 17.8 (top center): Wistreich, G. *Microbiology Perspectives: A Photographic Survey of the Microbial World.* Prentice-Hall, Inc. 1999. Fig. 158-B, p. 71.

Fig. 17.8 (middle row, center): Courtesy of Dr. Umberto Benelli, Online Atlas of Ophthalmology.

Fig. 17.8 (middle row, right): Courtesy of Vanderbilt University Medical Center, Department of Emergency Medicine.

Fig. 17.8 (bottom row, left): McMillan, A. and Scott, G. R. *Sexually Transmitted Diseases.* Churchill Livingstone, 1991. Fig. 25, p. 16.

Fig. 17.8 (bottom row, middle): Courtesy of Dr. Umberto Benelli, Online Atlas of Ophthalmology.

Fig. 17.8 (bottom row, right): McMillan, A. and Scott, G. R. *Sexually Transmitted Diseases.* Churchill Livingstone, 1991. Fig. 24, p. 18.

Fig. 18.2: Courtesy Dr. George P. Kubica, Public Health Image Library, Centers for Disease Control and Prevention.

Fig. 18.2: Alexander, S. K. and Strete, D. *Microbiology: A Photographic Atlas for the Laboratory.* Benjamin Cummings. Fig. 2.17, p. 15.

Fig. 18.3: Center for Disease Control, Atlanta, 1999.

Fig. 18.4: Tortora G. J., Funke, B. R. and Case C. E. *Microbiology, An Introduction.* Addison Wesley Longman, Inc. 1998. Fig. 24.10, p. 639.

Fig. 18.5: Iseman, Michael D., S/M Infectious Diseases Division. National Jewish Medical Research Center.

Fig. 18.7: Talaro, K. P. and Talaro, A. *Foundations in Microbiology, 3rd Edition.* WCB/McGraw-Hill, 1999. Fig. 19.19, p. 612.

Fig. 18.9: Courtesy Dr. George P. Kubica, Public Health Image Library, Centers for Disease Control and Prevention.

Fig. 18.13: Binford, C.H and Connor D.H. *Pathology of Tropical and Extraordinary Diseases: An Atlas*, Washington, D.D. 1976, Armed Forces Institute of Pathology.

Fig. 18.14 (top, left): Wistreich, G. *Microbiology Perspectives: A Photographic Survey of the Microbial World.* Prentice-Hall, Inc. 1999. Fig. 193, p. 86.

Fig. 18.14 (top, right): Center for Disease Control, Atlanta.

Fig. 18.14 (bottom, left): WebPath, courtesy of Edward C. Klatt MD, Florida State University College of Medicine.

Fig. 18.14 (bottom, right): Hogeweg, M. *Tropical Doctor* Suppl. 1, p. 15-21, 1992.

Fig. 18.15: Public Health Image Library, Centers for Disease Control and Prevention.

Fig. 19.2: Volk, W. A., Gebhardt, B. M., Hammarskjold, M. and Kadner, R. J., *Essentials of Microbiology*, Fifth Edition, Lippincott-Raven, Philadelphia, 1996. Fig. 34-1, p. 459.

Fig. 19.3: Public Health Image Library, Centers for Disease Control and Prevention.

Fig. 19.5: Greer, Ken/Visuals Unlimited.

Fig. 20.2(A): Larone, D. H. *Medically Important Fungi. A Guide to Identification.* Third Edition. American Society for Microbiology, 1995. p. 71.

Fig. 20.2(B): Schaf, David /Peter Arnold, Inc.

Fig. 20.3(A): Champe, S. P. and Simon, L. D. Cellular Differentiation and Tissue Formation in the Fungus Aspergillus nidulan, in *Morphogenesis.* Edited by Rossomando, E. F. and Alexander, S. Marcel Dekker, Inc. 1992. Fig. 2.

Fig. 20.3(B): Champe, S. P. and Simon, L. D. Cellular Differentiation and Tissue Formation in the Fungus Aspergillus nidulan, in *Morphogenesis.* Edited by Rossomando, E. F. and Alexander, S. Marcel Dekker, Inc. 1992. Fig. 3.

Fig. 20.4: Volk, W. A., Gebhardt, B. M., Hammarskjold, M. and Kadner, R. J., *Essentials of Microbiology*, Fifth Edition, Lippincott-Raven, Philadelphia, 1996. Fig. 35-3, p.477.

Fig. 20.5(A): Habif, Thomas p. *Clinical Dermatology, A Color Guide to Diagnosis and Therapy.* Mosby. 1996. Fig. 13-7, p. 367.

Fig. 20.5(B): Habif, Thomas p. *Clinical Dermatology, A Color Guide to Diagnosis and Therapy.* Mosby. 1996. Fig. 13-21, p. 374.

Fig. 20.5(C): Habif, Thomas p. *Clinical Dermatology, A Color Guide to Diagnosis and Therapy.* Mosby. 1996. Fig. 13-38, p. 383.

Fig. 20.5(D): Habif, T. P. *Clinical Dermatology, A Color Guide to Diagnosis and Therapy.* Mosby. 1996. Fig. 13-16, p. 371.

Fig. 20.5 (E): Mir, M. A., *Atlas of Clinical Diagnosis*, W. J. B. Saunders Company Ltd., 1995. Fig. 10.21; p. 203.

Fig. 20.6(A): Dr. Lucille K. Georg, Public Health Image Library, Centers for Disease Control and Prevention..

Fig. 20.6(C): Courtesy of Prince Leopold Institute of Tropical Medicine.

Fig. 20.7: Rubin, E. and Farber, J. L. *Pathology*, Second Edition. J. B. Lippincott Company, 1994. Fig. 9-60, p. 419.

Fig. 20.8 (A): Rubin, E. and Farber, J. L. *Pathology*, Second Edition. J. B. Lippincott Company, 1994. Fig. 9-57, p. 416.

Fig. 20.8 (B): Rubin, E. and Farber, J. L. *Pathology*, Second Edition. J. B. Lippincott Company, 1994. Fig. 9-58.

Fig. 20.8(C): Dr. Libero Ajello, Public Health Image Library, Centers for Disease Control and Prevention.

Fig. 20.8(D): Koneman and Roberts, *Practical Laboratory Mycology.* Williams and Wilkins.

Fig. 20.9: Center for Disease Control, Atlanta.

Fig. 20.10: Murray, p. R., Kobayashi, G. S., Pfaller, M. A. and Rosenthal, K. S., *Medical Microbiology, Second Edition*, Mosby, 1994. Fig. 44-3, p. 418.

Fig. 20.10: Murray, P. R., Kobayashi, G. S., Pfaller, M. A. and Rosenthal, K. S., *Medical Microbiology, Second Edition*, Mosby, St. Louis, 1994. Fig. 44-3, p. 418.

Fig. 20.11: Goldman, M., Johnson, p. C. and Sarosi, G. A.. *Clinics in Chest Medicine.* W. B. Saunders Company, 1999. Fig. 3. Volume 20, Number 3, September 1999.

Fig. 20.13: Kassirer, J. P., *Images in Clinical Medicine*, Massachusetts Medical Society, 1997. p. 44.

Fig. 20.14: Rubin, E. and Farber, J. L. *Pathology*, Second Edition. J. B. Lippincott Company, 1994. Fig. 9-51, p. 409.

Fig. 20.15: Rubin, E. and Farber, J. L. *Pathology*, Second Edition. J. B. Lippincott Company, 1994. Fig. 9-55, p. 414.

Fig. 20.16: McGee, J., Isaacson, P. G., and Wright, N. A. *Oxford Textbook of Pathology.* Oxford Press, 1992. Fig. 6.30.

Fig. 20.18: Volk, W. A., Gebhardt, B. M., Hammarskjold, M. and Kadner, R. J., *Essentials of Microbiology*, Fifth Edition, Lippincott-Raven, 1996. Fig. 35-18, p. 492.

Fig. 20.19: CDC/ Dr. Edwin P. Edwin, Jr. 1984.

Fig. 20.20: Emond, R. T. D., Rowland, H.A.K. and Welsby, P. D., *Color Atlas of Infectious Diseases*, Third Edition, Mosby-Wolfe. 1995. Fig. 339. p. 283.

Fig. 21.3: Gillies, R. R. and Dodds, T. C., *Bacteriology Illustrated*, Third Edition, Williams and Wilkins Company, 1973. p. 194.

Fig. 21.4 CDC – DPDx – Laboratory Identification of Parasites of Public Health Concern.

Fig. 21.5: Public Health Image Library, Centers for Disease Control and Prevention.

Fig. 21.7: Gillies, R. R. and Dodds, T. C., *Bacteriology Illustrated*, Third Edition, Williams and Wilkins Company, 1973. p. 198.

Fig. 21.12: Sun, T. *Parasitic Disorders. Pathology, Diagnosis and Management,* Second Edition. Williams and Wilkins, 1999. Fig. 5.7, p. 23.

Fig. 21.14: Public Health Image Library, Centers for Disease Control and Prevention.

Fig. 21.15: Sethi, S., Alcid, D., Kesarwala, H. and Tolan, R.W. Emerging Infectious Disease Journal, Volume 15, Number 5—May 2009, Centers for Disease Control and Prevention.

Fig. 22.2: de la Maza, L. M., Pezzlo, M. T. and Baron, E. J., *Color Atlas of Diagnostic Microbiology, Mosby, 1997.* Fig. 15-104, p. 170.

Fig. 22.4: H. Zaiman. *A Pictorial Presentation of Parasites.* Slide 16.

Fig. 22.6: Kassirer, J. P., *Images in Clinical Medicine*, Massachusetts Medical Society, 1997. p. 295.

Fig. 22.9: Kassirer, J. P., *Images in Clinical Medicine*, Massachusetts Medical Society, 1997. p. 306.

Fig. 24.4(B): Ordoukhanian, E. and Lane, Alfred T., *Postgraduate Medicine*, 101, February, pp. 223-232, 1997.

Fig. 24.4(C): Ordoukhanian, E. and Lane, Alfred T., *Postgraduate Medicine*, 101, February, pp. 223-232, 1997.

Fig. 24.7: Arthur, R. R, Shah, K.V. *Papovaviridae* In: The Polyomavirues. In Lennette E.H., Halonen P., Murphy, F. A., eds. *Laboratory Diagnosis of Infectious Diseases: Principles and Practices*, vol. II, Springer-Verlag 1988: 317-332.

Fig. 24.8(B): Ginsberg, H. S. *The Adenoviruses*, Plenum Publishers,1984.

Fig. 24.8(C): Volk, W. A., Benjamin, D. C., Kadner, R. J. and Parsons, J. T., *Essentials of Microbiology*, Fourth Edition, J. B.Lippincott Company,1991. Fig. 41.4, p. 563,

Fig. 24.11: Kassirer, J. P., *Images in Clinical Medicine*, Massachusetts Medical Society, 1997, p. 19.

Fig. 25.2: Volk, W. A., Gebhardt, B. M., Hammarskjold, M. and Kadner, R. J., *Essentials of Microbiology*, Fifth Edition, Lippincott-Raven, Philadelphia, 1996. Fig. 38-4A, p. 522. lippincott book.

Fig. 25.4: Courtesy of Bernard A. Cohen, MD, Christoph U. Lehmann, MD, DermAtlas, Johns Hopkins University.

Fig. 25.5 (top): Public Health Image Library,

Centers for Disease Control and Prevention.

Fig. 25.5(bottom): Public Health Image Library, Centers for Disease Control and Prevention.

Fig. 25.11: Habif, T. P. *Clinical Dermatology, A Color Guide to Diagnosis and Therapy*. Mosby. 1996. Fig. 12-34, p. 345.

Fig. 25.12: Stephen K., *Hospital Practice.* July 15, 1996. Fig. 2, p. 139.

Fig. 25.14: Courtesy of Joan Barenfanger, Laboratory Medicine, Memorial Medical Center, Springfield, IL

Fig. 25.15: Ball, A. P. and Gray, J. A., *Colour Guide Infectious Diseases*, Churchill Livingstone, Edinburgh, 1992. Fig. 56, p. 40.

Fig. 25.18: Custom Medical Stock Photo.

Fig. 25.19: Hall, C.B., Long, C.E., Schnabel, K.C., et al. *N Engl J Med.* 331:432-438 (1994).

Fig. 25.23: Public Health Image Library, Centers for Disease Control and Prevention.

Fig. 25.24: WebPath, courtesy of Edward C. Klatt MD, Florida State University College of Medicine.

Fig. 25.26: Henderson, D. A., et al. *Journal American Medical Association* 281:2130, 1999.

Fig. 26.3: Volk, W. A., Benjamin, D. C., Kadner, R. J. and Parsons, J. T., *Essentials of Microbiology*, Fourth Edition, J. B.Lippincott Company,1991. Fig. 45-1, p. 601.

Fig. 26. 7: Murray, P. R., Kobayashi, G. S., Pfaller, M. A. and Rosenthal, K. S., *Medical Microbiology, Second Edition*, Mosby, St. Louis, 1994. Fig. 68-12, p 714.

Fig. 27.2: Volk, W. A., Benjamin, D. C., Kadner, R. J. and Parsons, J. T., *Essentials of Microbiology*, Fourth Edition, J. B. Lippincott Company,1991. Fig. 46-1, p. 608.

Fig. 27.7: Moyer, L., Warwick, M., and Mahoney, F. J. *American Family Physician.* Fig. 2, 54: (Number 1) p. 112 (1996).

Fig. 28.5: Cotras, *Robbins Pathologic Basis of Disease*, Sixth Edition, W. B. Saunders Company, 1996. Fig. 7-38.

Fig. 28.6: Talaro, K. P. and Talaro, A. *Foundations in Microbiology, 3rd Edition.* WCB/McGraw-Hill, 1999. Fig. 25.12, p.801.

Fig. 28.15: Antman, K. and Change, Y. *N Engl J Med.* 342 (number 14) 1027 (2000).

Fig. 28.19: Armstrong, D. and Cohen, J., *Infectious Diseases.* Mosby 1999. Fig. 10.5, p. 8.10.4.

Fig. 28.20: Beilke, M.A. and Murphy, E.L., The human T-lymphotropic leukemia viruses 1 and 2. In: Volberding, P.A. and Palefsky, J., eds. Viral and Immunological Malignancies. Hamilton, Ontario: BC Decker; 2006:332.

Fig. 29.2(A): Fields, B. N., Knipe, D. M. and Howley, P. M.. *Virology, Third Edition*, Lippincott Williams and Wilkins, 1996. Fig. 1, p. 1140.

Fig. 29.2(B): Fields, B. N., Knipe, D. M. and Howley, P. M.. *Virology, Third Edition*, Lippincott Williams and Wilkins, 1996.

Fig. 29.4: http://www.pathguy.com/lectures/rabies.jpg

Fig. 29.6: Center for Disease Control, Atlanta.

Fig. 29.7: Courtesty Dr. Heinz F. Eichenwald, Public Health Image Library, Centers for Disease Control and Prevention.

Fig. 29.8: Mir, M. A., *Atlas of Clinical Diagnosis*, W. J. B. Saunders Company Ltd., 1995. Fig. 1.211, p. 42.

Fig. 29.10(A): Fields, B. N., Knipe, D. M. and Howley, P. M.. *Virology, Third Edition*, Lippincott Williams and Wilkins, 1996. Fig. 2, p. 1401.

Fig. 29.12: Fields, B. N., Knipe, D. M. and Howley, P. M. *Virology, Third Edition*, Lippincott Williams and Wilkins, 1996. Fig. 2, p. 1357. Photo courtesy of George Leser, Northwestern University, Evanston, Il.

Fig. 29.15: Jensen, M. M., Wright, D. N., and Robison, R. A. *Microbiology for the Health Sciences.* Prentice Hall, 1995. Fig. 33-2, p. 420.

Fig. 29.16: Treanor, J., et al., *Journal American Medical Association*, 283:1016-1024 (2000). Fig. 2, p. 1020.

Fig. 29.17: Courtesy Cynthia Goldsmith,Public Health Image Library, Centers for Disease Control and Prevention.

Fig. 30.2: Kapikian, A. Z., Kim, H. W., and Wyatt, R. G. Science 185:1049-1053, 1974.

Fig. 31.2: Hart, T. and Shears, P., *Color Atlas of Medical Microbiology*, Mosby-Wolfe. 1996. Fig. 16, p. 16.°

Fig. 33.2 (B): Connie Celum, Walter Stamm, Seattle STD/HIV Prevention Training Center.

Fig. 33.2 (C): Courtesty Diane P. Yolton, Pacific University.

Fig. 33.2 (D): Beeching, N.J. and Nye, F.J., *Diagnostic Picture Tests in Clinical Infectious Disease*, Mosby- Wolfe, London, 1996.Fig. 83, p. 46.

Fig. 33.2 (E): Courtesty Diane P. Yolton, Pacific University.

Fig. 33.2 F: Armstrong, Donald, and Cohen, Jonathan. *Infectious Diseases.* Mosby 1999. Fig. 25.9, p. 8.25.6.

Fig. 33.2 (G): CDC – National Center for HIV, STD and TB Prevention Division of Sexually Transmitted Diseases – STD Prevention – Syphilis Fact.

Fig. 33.2 (H): CDC – National Center for HIV, STD and TB Prevention Division of Sexually Transmitted Diseases – STD Prevention – Syphilis Fact.

Fig. 33.2 (I): MacMilan, A., Scott, G. R. *Sexually Transmitted Diseases*, Churchill Livingstone. 1991. Fig. 52, p. 34.

Fig. 33.2 (K): Salkind, M. R. *A Slide Atlas of Common Diseases*, Parthenon Publishing Group, 1994. Fig. 175.

Fig. 33.2 (L): Salkind, M. R. *A Slide Atlas of Common Diseases*, Parthenon Publishing Group, 1994. Fig. 183.

Fig. 33.2 (M): Gillies, R. R. and Dodds, T.C., *Bacteriology Illustrated*, Third Edition, Williams and Wilkins Company, Baltimore, 1973. p.198. 59.

Fig. 33.2 (N): Salkind, M. R. *A Slide Atlas of Common Diseases*, Parthenon Publishing Group, 1994. Fig. 172.

Fig. 33.2 (O): Brown, T. J., Yen-Moore, A. and Tyring, S. K. *Journal of the American Academy of Dermatology.* Volume 41, Number 5. November 1999. Fig. 1.

Fig. 33.2 (Q): Kassirer, J. P., *Images in Clinical Medicine*, Massachusetts Medical Society, 1997. p. 28.

Fig. 33.2 (R): Stone, D. R. and Gorbach, S. L. *Atlas of Infectious Diseases.* W. B. Saunders Company, 2000. Fig. 6-26, p. 103.

Fig. 33.2 (S): Salkind, M. R. *A Slide Atlas of Common Diseases*, Parthenon Publishing Group, 1994. Fig. 59.

Fig. 33.2 (T): Courtesy of Dr. Umberto Benelli, Online Atlas of Ophthalmology

Fig. 33.2 (U): Copyrighted image used with permission of the authors, Virtual Hospital (TM), www.vh.org

Fig. 33.2 (V): Salkind, M. R. *A Slide Atlas of Common Diseases*, Parthenon Publishing Group, 1994. Fig. 25.

Fig. 33.2 (W): Salkind, M. R. *A Slide Atlas of Common Diseases*, Parthenon Publishing Group, 1994. Fig. 60.

Fig. 33.10 (A): Wistreich, George. *Microbiology Perspectives: A Photographic Survey of the Microbial World.* Prentice-Hall, Inc. 1999. Fig. 199, p. 87.

Fig. 33.10 (B): Katz, D. S. and Leung, A. N. Radiology of Pneumonia. *Clinics in Chest Medicine.* Fig. 2. Volume 20. Number 3, September 1999. W. B. Saunders Company.

Fig. 33.10 (C): Katz, D. S. and Leung, A. N. Radiology of Pneumonia. *Clinics in Chest Medicine.* Fig. 4. Volume 20. Number 3, September 1999. W. B. Saunders Company.

Fig. 33.10 (D): Public Health Image Library, Centers for Disease Control and Prevention.

Fig. 33.10 (E): Goldman, M., Johnson, P. C. and Sarosi, G. A. Pneumonia: Fungal Pneumonias. *Clinics in Chest Medicine.* Volume 20, Number 3, September 1999. W. B. Saunders Company. Fig. 1.

Fig. 33.10 (F): Salkind, M. R. *A Slide Atlas of Common Diseases*, Parthenon Publishing Group, 1994. Fig. 59.

Fig. 33.10 (G): Courtesty Dr. David Ellis, University of Adelaide.

Fig. 33.10 (H): Emond, R. T. D., Rowland, H. A. K. and Welsby, P. D., *Color Atlas of Infectious Diseases*, Third Edition, Mosby-Wolfe. 1995. Fig. 339. p. 283.

Fig. 33.10 (J): Center for Disease Control, Atlanta.

Fig. 33.10 6(K): Salkind, M. R. *A Slide Atlas of Common Diseases*, Parthenon Publishing Group, 1994. Fig. 25.

Fig. 33.10 (L): Salkind, M. R. *A Slide Atlas of Common Diseases*, Parthenon Publishing Group, 1994. Fig. 9.

Fig. 33.10 (N): Arthur, R. R, Shah, K.V. *Papovaviridae* In: The Polyomavirues. In Lennette E.H., Halonen P., Murphy, F. A., eds. *Laboratory Diagnosis of Infectious Diseases: Principles and Practices*, Vol. II, Springer-Verlag 1988: 317-332.